PEDIATRIC EMERGENCY MEDICINE
Self-Assessment and Review

PEDIATRIC EMERGENCY MEDICINE
Self-Assessment and Review

Referenced to Pediatric Emergency Medicine: Concepts and Clinical Practice,
edited by Roger M. Barkin et al, ed 2, St. Louis, 1997, Mosby

Editors

DAVID H. RUBIN, MD, FAAP
Director, Department of Pediatric Emergency Medicine,
New York Flushing Hospital, Flushing, New York;
Clinical Associate Professor of Pediatrics,
Cornell University Medical College,
New York, New York

STUART M. CAPLEN, MD, FACEP
Chief, Department of Emergency Medicine,
Englewood Hospital Medical Center,
Englewood, New Jersey

EDWARD E. CONWAY, Jr., MS, MD, FCCM
Chief, Division of Pediatric Critical Care,
Beth Israel Medical Center;
Associate Professor of Pediatrics and Critical Care Medicine,
Albert Einstein College of Medicine,
Bronx, New York

ROGER M. BARKIN, MD, MPH, FAAP, FACEP
Vice President for Pediatric and Newborn Programs,
Columbia Health-ONE;
Professor of Surgery, Division of Emergency Medicine,
University of Colorado Health Sciences Center,
Denver, Colorado

SECOND EDITION

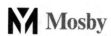

St. Louis Baltimore Boston Carlsbad Chicago Minneapolis New York Philadelphia Portland
London Milan Sydney Tokyo Toronto

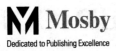
Mosby
Dedicated to Publishing Excellence

A Times Mirror
Company

Publisher: Laura DeYoung
Managing Editor: Kathryn Falk
Project Manager: Patricia Tannian
Production Editor: Gail Stobaugh
Design Manager: Gail Morey Hudson
Manufacturing Manager: Linda Ierardi
Cover Design: Teresa Breckwoldt

SECOND EDITION

Composition by Graphic World, Inc.
Printing/binding by Plus Communications

Mosby–Year Book, Inc.
11830 Westline Industrial Drive
St. Louis, Missouri 63146

International Standard Book Number 1-55664-453-1

98 99 00 01 02 / 9 8 7 6 5 4 3 2

Contributors

Editors:

David H. Rubin, MD, FAAP
Director, Department of Pediatric Emergency Medicine,
New York Flushing Hospital, Flushing, New York;
Clinical Associate Professor of Pediatrics,
Cornell University Medical College, New York, New York

Stuart M. Caplen, MD, FACEP
Chief, Department of Emergency Medicine,
Englewood Hospital Medical Center, Englewood, New Jersey

Edward E. Conway, Jr., MS, MD, FCCM
Chief, Division of Pediatric Critical Care,
Beth Israel Medical Center, New York, New York;
Associate Professor of Pediatrics and Critical Care Medicine,
Albert Einstein College of Medicine, Bronx, New York

Roger M. Barkin, MD, MPH, FAAP, FACEP
Vice President for Pediatric and Newborn Programs,
Columbia Health-ONE;
Professor of Surgery, Division of Emergency Medicine,
University of Colorado Health Sciences Center, Denver,
    Colorado

Contributors:

Won Baik-Han, MD, FAAP, FAAAI
Director, Pediatric Allergy/Immunology,
Attending Physician, Department of Pediatric Emergency
    Medicine and Pediatrics,
New York Flushing Hospital, Flushing, New York

Karen Balzanto, MD, FAAP
Assistant Professor of Pediatrics, Section of Pediatric
    Emergency Medicine,
University of Chicago Children's Hospital, Chicago, Illinois

David E. Bank, MD, FAAP
Director, Pediatric Emergency Services,
New York Hospital—Cornell Medical Center;
Assistant Clinical Professor of Pediatrics,
Cornell University Medical College, New York, New York

Holly M. Bannister, MD, FAAP
Clinical Instructor in Pediatrics,
New York University School of Medicine;
Attending Physician, Pediatric Emergency Services,
Bellevue Hospital Center, New York University Medical
    Center, New York, New York

Theodore M. Barnett, MD, FAAP
Attending Physician, Pediatric Emergency Medicine;
Assistant Professor of Pediatrics, Section of Emergency
    Medical Services,
The Children's Mercy Hospital, Kansas City, Missouri

Anne F. Brayer, MD, FAAP
Senior Instructor in Pediatrics and Emergency Medicine,
University of Rochester Medical Center;
Attending Physician,
Strong Memorial Hospital, Rochester, New York

Stuart M. Caplen, MD, FACEP
Chief, Department of Emergency Medicine,
Englewood Hospital Medical Center, Englewood, New Jersey

Laura C. Carlson, MD
Assistant Professor of Emergency Medicine, Department of
    Emergency Medicine,
Medical College of Georgia, Augusta, Georgia

Anthony J. Ciorciari, MD, FACEP
Attending Physician, Emergency Department,
Jacobi Medical Center;
Assistant Clinical Instructor in Emergency Medicine,
Albert Einstein College of Medicine, Bronx, New York

Edward E. Conway, Jr., MS, MD, FCCM
Chief, Division of Pediatric Critical Care,
Beth Israel Medical Center, New York, New York;
Associate Professor of Pediatrics and Critical Care Medicine,
Albert Einstein College of Medicine, Bronx, New York

Robert Crupi, MD
Associate Director and Attending Physician, Department of
    Emergency Medicine
New York Flushing Hospital, Flushing, New York

Sandra Cunningham, MD
Assistant Director and Attending Physician, Pediatric
    Emergency Services,
Jacobi Medical Center;
Assistant Professor of Pediatrics,
Albert Einstein College of Medicine, Bronx, New York

Peter S. Dayan, MD, FAAP
Instructor in Clinical Pediatrics,
Columbia-Presbyterian Medical Center and Babies Hospital,
    New York, New York

Jeffrey S. Fine, MD, FAAP
Clinical Instructor in Pediatrics,
New York University School of Medicine;
Attending Physician, Pediatric Emergency Medicine,
Bellevue Hospital Center, New York, New York

George L. Foltin, MD, FAAP, FACEP
Director, Pediatric Emergency Medicine,
Bellevue Hospital Center, New York University Medical
    Center;
Assistant Professor of Clinical Medicine,
New York University School of Medicine, New York,
    New York

Jessica C. Foltin, MD, FAAP
Director, Pediatric Emergency Medicine,
Beth Israel Medical Center, New York, New York;
Assistant Professor of Pediatrics and Emergency Medicine,
Albert Einstein College of Medicine, Bronx, New York

Jill C. Glick, MD, FAAP
Medical Director, Child Protective Services;
Associate Director, Pediatric Emergency Medicine,
University of Chicago Children's Hospital;
Assistant Professor of Pediatrics, University of Chicago,
    Chicago, Illinois

Steve Gottesfeld, DO
Attending Physician, Department of Emergency Medicine,
New York Hospital Medical Center of Queens, Flushing,
    New York;
Clinical Instructor of Medicine,
Cornell University Medical College, New York, New York

Adolfo Grieg, DO
Director, Division of Neonatology, Department of Pediatrics,
New York Flushing Hospital, Flushing, New York

Jackie Grupp-Phelan, MD
Senior AHCPR Fellow, Attending Physician, Pediatric
    Emergency Medicine,
Children's Hospital Medical Center, Seattle, Washington

Waseem Hafeez, MD, FAAP
Attending Physician, Pediatric Emergency Medical Services,
Montefiore-North Central Bronx Hospitals;
Assistant Professor of Pediatrics,
Albert Einstein College of Medicine, Bronx, New York

Martin G. Hellman, MD, FAAP, FACEP
Assistant Clinical Professor of Medicine,
Case Western Reserve University;
Attending Physician, Emergency Medicine,
Mt. Sinai Hospital of Cleveland, Cleveland, Ohio

Dennis Heon, MD, FAAP
Assistant Professor of Clinical Pediatrics,
New York University School of Medicine;
Attending Physician, Pediatric Emergency Medicine,
Bellevue Hospital Center, New York, New York

Arthur Klein, MD, FAAP, FACC
Executive Vice-Chairman, Department of Pediatrics,
New York Hospital–Cornell Medical Center;
Professor of Clinical Pediatrics, Department of Pediatrics,
Cornell University Medical College, New York, New York

Tom Kwiatkowski, MD, FACEP
Chairman, Department of Emergency Medicine,
Long Island Jewish Medical Center;
Associate Professor of Emergency Medicine,
Albert Einstein College of Medicine, Bronx, New York

Peter H. Lee, MD
Fellow, Division of Pediatric Emergency Services,
New York Hospital—Cornell Medical Center, New York,
    New York

Steven Lelyveld, MD
Associate Professor and Section Chief, Pediatric Emergency
    Medicine,
University of Chicago Children's Hospital, Chicago, Illinois

Robert Lembo, MD, FAAP
Associate Clinical Professor of Pediatrics,
New York University School of Medicine, New York,
    New York

Deborah A. Levine, MD
Senior Fellow, Pediatric Emergency Medicine,
New York University School of Medicine, Bellevue Hospital
    Center, New York, New York

Deborah M. Lopez, MD
Senior Fellow, Pediatric Critical Care,
Montefiore Medical Center, Albert Einstein College of
    Medicine, Bronx, New York

Adriana Manikian, MD
Fellow, Pediatric Emergency Medicine,
New York University School of Medicine, Bellevue Hospital
    Center, New York, New York

Francisco A. Medina, MD, FAAP
Medical Director, Department of Pediatric Emergency
    Medicine,
Baptist Hospital of Miami, Miami, Florida

Larry B. Mellick, MS, MD, FAAP, FACEP
Professor and Chairman, Department of Emergency Medicine,
    Director of Pediatric Emergency Medicine,
Medical College of Georgia, Augusta, Georgia

Michael A. Mojica, MD, FAAP
Clinical Instructor in Pediatrics,
New York University School of Medicine;
Attending Physician, Pediatric Emergency Medicine,
Bellevue Hospital Center, New York, New York

Ndidi Nwokorie, MD
Director, Pediatric Emergency Medicine,
Sinai Hospital of Baltimore, Baltimore, Maryland

Shari L. Platt, MD, FAAP
Clinical Instructor in Pediatrics,
New York University School of Medicine;
Assistant Director, Pediatric Emergency Medicine Fellowship,
Attending Physician, Pediatric Emergency Medicine,
New York University School of Medicine, Bellevue Hospital
  Center, New York, New York

Susana Rapaport, MD
Associate Chairperson, Department of Pediatrics,
New York Flushing Hospital, Flushing, New York

Ruby F. Rivera, MD
Attending Physician, Division of Pediatric Emergency
  Medicine,
Montefiore Medical Center;
Assistant Professor of Pediatrics,
Albert Einstein College of Medicine, Bronx, New York

David H. Rubin, MD, FAAP
Director, Department of Pediatric Emergency Medicine,
New York Flushing Hospital, Flushing, New York;
Clinical Associate Professor of Pediatrics,
Cornell University Medical College, New York, New York

Morton Salomon, MD, FAAP, FACEP
Vice-Chairman, Emergency Medicine,
Albert Einstein College of Medicine;
Director of Emergency Services,
Montefiore-North Central Bronx Hospitals;
Associate Professor of Pediatrics and Emergency Medicine,
Albert Einstein College of Medicine, Bronx, New York

Javier Sanchez, MD, FAAP
Attending Physician, Pediatric Critical Care,
Albany Medical College;
Assistant Professor of Pediatrics,
Albany Medical College, Albany, New York

Lucia J. Santiago, MD
Senior Fellow, Pediatric Emergency Medicine,
New York University School of Medicine, Bellevue Hospital
  Center, New York, New York

Jeffrey Schor, MD, MPH
Director, Pediatric Emergency Medicine
New York Hospital Medical Center of Queens, Flushing,
  New York
Clinical Assistant Professor of Pediatrics,
Cornell University Medical College, New York, New York

Cathy Schwartz, MD
Attending Physician, Emergency Department,
New York Downtown Hospital, New York, New York

Christopher Shields, MD, FACEP
Associate Chairman, Department of Emergency Medicine,
New York Hospital Medical Center of Queens, Flushing,
  New York;
Clinical Assistant Professor of Medicine,
Cornell University Medical College, New York, New York

Lewis P. Singer, MD, FAAP
Director, Pediatric Critical Care and Pulmonary Medicine,
Associate Professor of Pediatrics,
Albert Einstein College of Medicine-Montefiore Medical
  Center, Bronx, New York

Diane M. Sixsmith, MD
Chairman, Department of Emergency Medicine,
New York Hospital Medical Center of Queens, Flushing,
  New York;
Clinical Assistant Professor of Medicine,
Cornell University Medical College, New York, New York

F. Meridith Sonnett, MD
Associate Director, Division of Pediatric Emergency Medicine,
Babies and Children's Hospital, Columbia-Presbyterian
  Medical Center;
Assistant Professor of Clinical Pediatrics,
Columbia University College of Physicians and Surgeons, New
  York, New York

Arabella C. Stock, MD
Fellow, Division of Pediatric Critical Care and Pulmonary
  Medicine,
Albert Einstein College of Medicine-Montefiore Medical
  Center, Bronx, New York

J.S. Supure, MD, FAAP, FACEP
Clinical Professor of Pediatrics,
University of Nevada School of Medicine, Las Vegas, Nevada

Anju Tejani, MD
Fellow, Pediatric Emergency Medicine,
New York University School of Medicine, Bellevue Hospital
  Center, New York, New York

Alexandra E. Trinkoff, JD
Formerly Chief Legal Counsel,
George Washington University Hospitals, Washington, DC

Dawn E. Williamson, MD
Assistant Director, Department of Emergency Medicine,
New York Flushing Hospital, Flushing, New York;
Associate Physician, Department of Medicine,
Mt. Sinai School of Medicine, New York, New York

Gary B. Zuckerman, MD, FAAP
Associate Director, Division of Pediatric Critical Care
  Medicine,
Assistant Professor of Clinical Pediatrics, Department of
  Pediatrics,
Robert Wood Johnson Medical School, New Brunswick,
  New Jersey

Preface

Pediatric emergency medicine continues to evolve into one of the most exciting and newly recognized specialties in pediatrics. This second edition of *Pediatric Emergency Medicine: Self-Assessment and Review* contains more than 1200 multiple choice type of questions designed to teach and review core material in this important specialty. This textbook may be used as a study guide and self-assessment instrument by medical students, pediatric and adult emergency medicine residents, attending physicians, nurses and nurse practitioners, and pediatricians.

The structure of *Pediatric Emergency Medicine: Self-Assessment and Review* is designed to force the reader to consider each question and correct response in relation to the specific topic being studied. Each correct answer, with discussion, is noted in the "answer" section at the end of each chapter and refers to the newly published second edition of Dr. Roger M. Barkin's comprehensive text *Pediatric Emergency Medicine: Concepts and Clinical Practice* (St. Louis, Mosby, 1997). The reader is strongly encouraged to consult the appropriate page(s) for a broader understanding and description of the material presented in each question.

The questions presented in *Pediatric Emergency Medicine: Self-Assessment and Review* are designed and chosen to encompass a broad basic core of material that the contributors and editors believe is essential in under-standing the pathophysiology and management of sick infants and children. Even though many certifying examinations are eliminating "except" type questions ("all of the following are true *except*"), we have included this type of question to allow the reader to consider each possible response.

We are indebted to all of the contributors and to Kathy Falk, Robin Sutter, and Laurel Craven of Mosby for their enthusiastic effort and support of this project. We also would like to extend our appreciation to each individual author of Dr. Barkin's textbook *Pediatric Emergency Medicine: Concepts and Clinical Practice,* who provided the material on which the text is based.

Finally, we hope that you find this textbook challenging and educational and a source for increasing your knowledge of this subject. We have made every effort to ensure that the information is current and accurate. However, we cannot be responsible for the continued currency of the information or for any efforts or omissions in this book or any other consequences arising therefrom.

David H. Rubin, MD
Stuart M. Caplen, MD
Edward E. Conway, Jr., MD, MS
Roger M. Barkin, MD, MPH

Contents

PEDIATRIC EMERGENCY MEDICINE
Self-Assessment and Review

1

Approach to the Pediatric Patient in the Emergency Department

Susana Rapaport • Arabella C. Stock

See Barkin et al: Chapter 1.

For questions 1 to 10, match the age noted with the suggested age-appropriate emergency department [ED] interventions. Each answer may be used once, more than once, or not at all.

A. Newborn.
B. 1 month.
C. 4 months.
D. 6 months.
E. 9 months.
F. 1 year.
G. 2 years.
H. 3 years.
I. 6 years.
J. 8 years.

1. _____ Uses three simple words other than "mama."
2. _____ Has a visual preference for the human face.
3. _____ Smiles responsively.
4. _____ Climbs on furniture.
5. _____ Balances on one foot.
6. _____ Rolls from front to back.
7. _____ Sits unsupported.
8. _____ Bears weight.
9. _____ Visually follows a moving object.
10. _____ Stands momentarily on one foot.

11. A 6-month-old boy is seen in the ED because the mother is concerned that her son is not a good eater and is not gaining weight as fast as his older sibling did. The infant's birth weight was 2.8 kg (5th percentile) and height was 46 cm (5th percentile). At present his weight is 6.2 kg (5th percentile) and height is 64 cm (5th percentile). Your next step should be:
    A. Admit the child to the hospital for a 24-hour calorie count.
    B. Initiate a full workup for failure to thrive.
    C. Reassure the mother that her child is normal for his age.
    D. Recommend outpatient dietary consult.
    E. Schedule an upper gastrointestinal series to exclude gastrointestinal reflux.

12. You are evaluating a child who was brought to the ED after he was found abandoned in a supermarket. He is alert, active, and playful. He bears weight on his feet, does not walk, and imitates the sounds of your speech. You show him the otoscope, and then hide it, and he attempts to find it. His earliest approximate age is:
    A. 12 months.
    B. 9 months.
    C. 6 months.
    D. 15 months.
    E. None of the above.

13. A 2-month-old girl is evaluated because the mother is concerned with the rapid growth of her child's head. Her head circumference at birth was 35 cm. At present her head circumference should be:
    A. 37 cm.
    B. 35 cm.
    C. 39 cm.
    D. 41 cm.
    E. None of the above.

For questions 14 to 17, match the age with the developmental milestones and the physical findings at the age of earliest occurrence. Each answer may be used once, more than once, or not at all.

A. 12 months.
B. Adolescence.
C. 2 years.
D. 18 months.

14. _____ Traumatic injuries become a major cause of ED visits.
15. _____ Decrease in appetite compared with infancy.
16. _____ High systolic blood pressure and low pulse rate.
17. _____ Birth weight triples.

ANSWERS   [See Barkin et al: Chapter 1.]

For questions 1 to 10, questions and answers are taken from Table 1-2, Screening Developmental Milestones, page 4 in Barkin et al.

1. **F**
2. **A**
3. **B**
4. **G**
5. **I**
6. **C**
7. **D**
8. **E**
9. **B**
10. **H**
11. The answer is **C,** page 4.
    The weight of most infants doubles within 5 months and triples within a year.
    The length increases by 30 cm within the first year.
12. The answer is **B,** page 4.
    A 9-month-old bears weight, cruises, plays pat a cake, imitates speech, and tries to find a hidden object.
13. The answer is **C,** page 4.
    The head circumference of an infant increases by 2 cm a month for the first 3 months and by 1 cm a month for months 3 to 6; thereafter it increases by 0.5 cm a month.

For questions 14 to 17, questions and answers are taken from pages 4 to 7.

14. **C**
15. **D**
16. **B**
17. **C**

Pediatric Emergency Department Environment

David H. Rubin

> See Barkin et al: Chapter 2.

1. Which of the following statements regarding planning for a pediatric emergency department (ED) is *true?*
   A. The primary concern is to satisfy the community need for a clean health care facility.
   B. Financial planning to ensure a maximum profit margin is at the core of any planning for the establishment of a pediatric ED.
   C. The ward secretary and nurse should have private space within the pediatric ED to ensure job satisfaction.
   D. The layout planning for a pediatric ED requires input from those involved in the day-to-day treatment of children.
   E. There should be at least five cubicles for patient care in any new pediatric ED.

2. Which of the following statements regarding the establishment and formalizing of policies and procedures as the size of a pediatric ED increases is *true?*
   A. These policies may adversely affect senior staff, who may choose to leave the department.
   B. Policies and procedures may be amended only when the size of an ED increases by at least 50%.
   C. Specific staffing issues are exempted from formal policy and procedure manuals.
   D. Policies and procedures should be reviewed every 3 years.

3. The relationship between a pediatric ED and its pediatric patient population may be defined using external and internal components. Which of the following best exemplifies an *internal* component?
   A. Preexisting relationships with referring physicians.
   B. Socioeconomic status of the population.
   C. Ethnicity of the population.
   D. Attention to the emotional needs of patients.
   E. Age distribution of the population.

4. Which one of the following statements regarding ED design is *true?*
   A. The architectural design of an ED has a minor role in the delivery of health care.
   B. Separate entrances for ambulatory and ambulance patients are a high priority.
   C. Nursing stations may be private work areas to ensure effective high-quality nursing care.
   D. Physician work areas should be open and placed close to patient care areas.
   E. Nursing stations only need be within visual contact of resuscitation and trauma rooms.

5. Which one of the following statements regarding the clinical environment of the pediatric ED is *true?*
   A. Agreements and transport protocols should be developed early to provide for transport of patients with unique clinical problems.
   B. Follow-up procedures may be deferred if the patient is not critically ill.
   C. All nursing personnel require Pediatric Advanced Life Support (PALS) and Advanced Trauma Life Support (ATLS) certification before working in the pediatric ED.
   D. All radiology technicians should be PALS certified.

6. Which of the following factors may be manipulated in response to planning or assessing a pediatric ED environment?
   A. Physical space and layout.
   B. Personnel skill mix.
   C. Number of patients.
   D. Policies and procedures.
   E. All of the above.

7. Which of the following statements regarding the physical factors in a pediatric ED is *true?*
   A. Thermostatic control requires that temperatures no greater than 80° F be maintained.
   B. Severely hypothermic patients should be referred to appropriate centers for advanced care and treatment.
   C. Nurses must be able to view patients at all times, but parents may be blocked from visual access.
   D. Handwashing before performing an examination is necessary for infection control and patient comfort.

8. Which one of the following statements regarding changes in the physical arrangement of the pediatric ED is *true?*
   A. Ethnicity usually has no major impact on room size.
   B. Small differences in physical arrangements can have a positive or negative impact on staff work and morale.
   C. Privacy is not an issue in the pediatric ED.
   D. Electrical connections must be inspected monthly by appropriate staff.

9. The ability to communicate in the same subcultural language as patients is crucial for health care providers. Is this statement *true or false?*
   A. True
   B. False

10. Which of the following statements regarding training and research in the pediatric ED environment is *true?*
   A. Training of physicians in any ED should be concentrated on daytime hours with little or no night duty.
   B. Training and research in the ED must be approved by the local health department.
   C. The educational value of training has not been demonstrated to affect low-income patients.
   D. The participation of trainees in the delivery of medical care to ED patients requires awareness and sensitivity.

ANSWERS   [See Barkin et al: Chapter 2.]

1. The answer is **D,** pages 8 and 9.
   To ensure maximal program efficiency, the layout planning for a pediatric ED requires the most input from those involved in the day-to-day treatment of children. Although one of many community concerns may be a clean health care facility, it is not the primary concern of those planning a pediatric ED. The concerns of all department staff should be recognized when planning a pediatric ED. However, private space for the ward secretary and nurse usually is not possible. There is no recommendation regarding the minimum number of cubicles for inclusion in a pediatric ED.

2. The answer is **A,** page 9.
   As the volume in a pediatric ED increases, the need for formal policies and procedures may affect senior staff members. These physicians, who are familiar with a particular independent style of practice, may think of leaving the department in search of a less formal department. Specific staffing issues are not necessarily exempted from formal policy and procedure manuals. Policies and procedures should be reviewed yearly. The other choices do not apply to policy and procedures in the pediatric ED.

3. The answer is **D,** pages 8 to 11.
   The *internal* components of the pediatric population that relate to a particular pediatric ED include physical environment of the ED, attention to the emotional needs of children, educational resources for staff and patients, and training and research. The *external* components include size, age, ethnicity, socioeconomic status, general health patterns, and special problems such as managed-care expectation and preexisting relationships with referring physicians.

4. The answer is **B,** page 12.
   The architectural design of an ED has a major role in the delivery of health care. Nursing stations should be open work areas, not private work areas, to ensure effective high-quality nursing care and concentration on patient stability. Physician work areas should be placed close to patient care areas but also should be enclosed to allow private discussions. Nursing stations should be in close proximity, not just within close visual contact, of resuscitation and trauma rooms.

5. The answer is **A,** page 12.
   Follow-up procedures and policies such as reporting suspected child abuse should be established and applied to all patients who are seen in the pediatric ED. Nursing personnel should be PALS certified; however, in most institutions ATLS is recommended but not required. There is no policy regarding PALS training of radiology department technicians.

6. The answer is **E,** page 8.

   In planning or assessing a pediatric ED environment, it is important to determine who the patients are, what their health needs are, and what the department's needs are. In response to those needs, the following factors can be manipulated: physical space and layout, personnel skill mix, number of patients, and scheduling of patients.

7. The answer is **D,** page 11.

   Temperature control is an important factor easily overlooked in pediatric care. Heat lamps, warmed intravenous (IV) solutions, and heated blankets are standard equipment that should be available in EDs. There is no absolute temperature level that is required in the pediatric ED environment, but patients and staff should feel comfortable. This may be especially important in resuscitation rooms where severely hypothermic patients are treated. Other important aspects of the physical environment are attractive, soothing surroundings and close attention to the tactile aspect of pediatric care. Staff and parents should be able to see the patient.

8. The answer is **B,** page 9.

   Ethnicity may affect treatment room size. Certain ethnic groups expect three or four people to make all decisions jointly regarding a child. Small differences in physical arrangements can have a positive or negative impact on staff work and morale. A triage desk placed too high may make triage a more physically demanding job for a nurse.

9. The answer is **A, true,** page 10.

   Sociocultural compatibility of staff and patients will help avoid the unconscious violation of subgroup norms. Insensitivity to how patients interpret questions may adversely affect the collection of historical information. Furthermore, interpretation of instructions received either verbally or on discharge instructions may affect outcome. The instruction "take one of these pills three times per day" must be understood by both patient and staff member. Not only language but also ethnic and cultural practices may prevent or delay expected outcomes. Translators should be relied on to communicate accurately specific aspects of the entire patient and doctor interaction.

10. The answer is **D,** pages 11 and 12.

    There is no requirement for either daytime or nighttime exposure of trainees. It is important for trainees to appreciate the different types of patients who come to the ED at different hours of the day and night, and therefore exposure to work at all hours is advantageous. The local health department does not participate in training schedules. The educational value of training programs is potentially beneficial to all socioeconomic groups.

Injury Prevention and Control

Dawn E. Williamson

See Barkin et al: Chapter 3.

1. Which one of the following statements is *true* regarding childhood injury in the United States?
   A. It is not a major public health problem.
   B. Injury is the leading cause of death in childhood.
   C. Falls are a preponderant cause of fatal injury.
   D. Bicycles are a rare cause of nonfatal injury.
   E. Drowning is a rare cause of death in toddlers.

2. Which one of the following problems is the cause of the highest mortality rate for adolescents 15 to 19 years old?
   A. Unintentional poisonings.
   B. Injuries related to falls.
   C. Fires and burns.
   D. Firearm homicides and suicides.

3. Common causes of death from injury in children younger than 5 years old include all of the following *except:*
   A. Fires and burns.
   B. Drowning.
   C. Motor vehicle occupant injuries.
   D. Firearm homicides.

4. Which of the following statements is *true?*
   A. Motor vehicle–related trauma is not a concern in the pediatric population.
   B. Data on nonlethal injury are more complete than on fatalities.
   C. Death caused by injuries from firearms is common in children up to 19 years of age.
   D. Injuries account for 70% of deaths in those 5 to 19 years old.

5. Laws mandating the use of approved child restraint devices for infants and toddlers riding in automobiles are in effect in all states.
   A. True
   B. False

6. All of the following are strategies to prevent childhood injury *except:*
   A. Infant car seats.
   B. Apartment window guards.
   C. Childproof containers.
   D. Delayed licensing of teenage drivers.
   E. Infant cardiopulmonary resuscitation (CPR) courses.

7. Which of the following is *not* an important factor in deciding priorities for injury prevention strategies?
   A. Incidence of injury.
   B. Severity of injury.
   C. Economic impact of injury.
   D. Cost-effectiveness.
   E. Commercial support.

8. All of the following statements are true regarding the Champion Trauma Score *except:*
   A. It is an anatomically based scale.
   B. It estimates injury severity.
   C. It is based on initial vital signs and level of alertness.
   D. It can be used to compare predicted outcomes with observed ones.
   E. It can be used in evaluating trauma care systems.

9. Which one of the following statements regarding childhood injuries in the United States is *true?*
   A. They account for more deaths than all other diseases.
   B. They account for nearly 1 million ED visits each year.
   C. They account for 10% of all childhood ED visits.
   D. They cost an estimated $1 billion annually.
   E. They are not a major public health problem.

10. A child is riding a bicycle and is hit by an automobile at an intersection. The intervention most likely to prevent another child from being injured is:
    A. Educational programs promoting safer riding habits.
    B. Programs promoting use of bicycle helmets.
    C. Laws prohibiting children from riding bicycles after dark.
    D. A bicycle path avoiding traffic.
    E. Laws requiring bicycle reflectors.

11. Haddon's matrix for the analysis of injury-producing events includes all of the following *except:*
   A. Cells are used to examine the cause and solution for each injury phase.
   B. The preevent phase is when the conditions that cause the injury-producing energy transfer occur.
   C. The event phase is when energy transfer occurs.
   D. The postevent phase involves interventions to alter the long-term impact of the injury.
   E. The outlook phase involves intense research and education.

12. According to Haddon's matrix for the analysis of injury producing events:
   A. Programs promoting the use of bicycle helmets affect the event phase.
   B. Designated pediatric trauma centers involve the preevent phase.
   C. Interventions to promote safer riding habits affect the event phase.
   D. Laws prohibiting bicycles on the street after dark affect the postevent phase.
   E. Laws requiring bicycle reflectors affect the event phase.

ANSWERS   [See Barkin et al: Chapter 3.]

1. The answer is **B,** pages 15 to 17.
   Injuries are a major public health problem. They represent the leading cause of death for children in the United States. Falls are a preponderant cause of nonfatal injuries, especially in children younger than 12 years old. Bicycles are a common cause of nonfatal and fatal injury. Drowning is a common cause of death in toddlers, which reflects exposure to the hazards of childhood.

2. The answer is **D,** page 17.
   Older teenagers have injury rates much greater than other age groups. Motor vehicle occupant deaths and firearm homicides and suicides are the most common causes of injury-related death in this age group.

3. The answer is **D,** page 17.
   Patterns of injury and fatality vary by age group. In children younger than 5 years old, nonfirearm homicides (child abuse), fire and burns, and drowning cause the most deaths. This is followed closely by motor vehicle occupant injuries.

4. The answer is **C,** pages 17 and 18. Motor vehicle–related trauma is consistently the most common cause of death in childhood, followed by death from firearms. Injuries account for 40% of deaths in children 1 to 4 years old and 70% of deaths in those 5 to 19 years old. More data are available on fatal injuries than on nonfatal injuries because of reporting practices.

5. The statement is **A, true,** page 21.
   Between 1977 and 1985, all 50 states implemented laws mandating the use of approved child restraint devices.

6. The answer is **E,** pages 20 and 21.
   An infant CPR course is not an injury prevention strategy.

7. The answer is **E,** pages 19 and 20.
   Commercial support is not a factor in deciding the priorities for injury prevention strategies.

8. The answer is **A,** page 19.
   The Champion Trauma Score is the best known of the physiologically based trauma scales (Boxes 3-1 to 3-3 on pages 7 and 8).

Box 3-1
Pediatric Trauma Score

	+2	+1	−1
Size (kg)	>20	10-20	<10
Airway	Normal	Maintained	Unmaintained
Systolic blood pressure (mm Hg)	>90	50-90	<50
Central nervous system	Awake	Obtunded	Coma
Open wound	None	Minor	Major
Skeletal trauma	None	Closed	Open-Multiple

From Tepas JJ, Mollitt DL, Talbert JL, et al: *J Pediatr Surg* 22:14-18, 1987.

Box 3-2
Champion Trauma Score

Glasgow Coma Scale score	Systolic BP (mm Hg)	Respiratory rate (breaths/min)	Respiratory effort	Cap refill	Coded value
14-15					5
11-13	>89	10-24			4
8-10	70-89	25-34			3
5-7	50-69	>34		Normal	2
3-4	0-49	1-9	Normal	Delayed	1
	Pulse	None	Retractive	None	0

From Champion HR, Sacco WJ, Carnazzo AJ, et al: *Crit Care Med* 9:672-676, 1981.

Box 3-3
Revised Trauma Score

Glasgow Coma Scale score	Systolic BP (mm Hg)	Respiratory rate (breaths/min)	Coded value
13-15	>89	10-29	4
9-12	76-89	>29	3
6-8	50-75	6-9	2
4-5	1-49	1-5	1
3	0	0	0

From Champion HR, Sacco WJ, Copes WS, et al: *J Trauma* 29:623-629, 1989.

9. The answer is **A,** page 15.
   Each year nearly 16 million children are treated in EDs for injuries. Injuries represent 40% of all visits. The annual cost of childhood injury is estimated at $13.8 billion.

10. The answer is **D,** page 16.
   Interventions that demand a sustained change in behavior to be effective often fail to produce major reductions in injury rates. Interventions that require new legislative action are difficult to implement.

11. The answer is **E,** page 16.
   Haddon described a matrix that can be used to analyze events resulting in injury. The matrix has no outlook phase. All other choices are the different aspects of this theory.

12. The answer is **A,** page 16.
   In applying Haddon's matrix to bicycle crashes, the preevent phase includes interventions that change certain characteristics of the bicyclist and reduce the likelihood of a crash (i.e., safer riding habits, more visible bicycles, bicycle paths, laws changing the social or cultural environment). The event phase assumes that the crash occurs and tries to reduce the likelihood or severity of injury (i.e., helmets). The postevent phase involves access to optimal acute care and rehabilitation.

4

Emergency Medical Services for Children

Steven Lelyveld • Karen Balzanto

See Barkin et al: Chapter 4.

1. At the scene of a pediatric arrest you immediately open the airway and begin cardiopulmonary resuscitation (CPR) while a colleague calls 911. The paramedics arrive 10 minutes later and follow full advanced life support (ALS) resuscitation protocols. They bring the child to a pediatric ED. Which of the following has the greatest impact on the child's survival?
   A. Bystander CPR.
   B. Paramedic ALS resuscitation.
   C. Initial ED management.
   D. Rapid medical and surgical evaluation.
   E. Postresuscitation pediatric intensive care unit (PICU) management.

2. At a trauma scene you find a child with no external injuries and a very weak pulse. You open the airway and follow advanced trauma life support (ATLS) protocols while a colleague calls 911. The paramedics arrive 2 minutes later and institute full ALS resuscitation. They transport the child to a pediatric trauma center (PTC). Which of the following has the greatest impact on the child's survival?
   A. Paramedic ALS resuscitation.
   B. Initial ED management.
   C. Rapid trauma service intervention.
   D. Postresuscitation pediatric ED management.

3. Which of the following statements concerning the epidemiology of childhood use of emergency medical services is *true?*
   A. Approximately 10% of children transported to an ED require tertiary care.
   B. Approximately 25% of pediatric ED visits are for traumatic events.
   C. Most children seen in an ED are either younger than 2 or older than 10.
   D. Approximately 10% of all ED visits are for children.
   E. ED visits for medical complaints exceed trauma complaints at all ages.

4. The most frequent cause of death in children up to 14 years old is:
   A. Firearm-related injury.
   B. Suffocation and poisoning.
   C. Burn-related injury.
   D. Vehicle-related injury.
   E. Submersion injury.

5. A 7-year-old trauma victim is being transported on a cold, rainy day. Which of the following should be considered in the design of the ambulance?
   A. Size-appropriate intravenous (IV) equipment, endotracheal tubes, and other equipment.
   B. Passenger and health care provider restraints.
   C. Space for a parent.
   D. A connection between the passenger and driver compartments.
   E. All of the above.

6. After a vehicular accident, a 15-kg child is crying but makes eye contact. The systolic blood pressure (BP) is 80 mm Hg. The midfemur has a deformity without any break in the skin. The Pediatric Trauma Score (PTS) is:
   A. −1.
   B. 3.
   C. 6.
   D. 9.
   E. 12.

7. With the expanded availability of ALS transport, a clear improvement has been shown in the outcomes of children with:
   A. Poisoning.
   B. Status epilepticus.
   C. Vascular instability from dehydration.
   D. Vascular instability from trauma.
   E. Respiratory compromise.

8. In the training of prehospital providers (Paramedic, Emergency Medical Technician-B, Emergency Medical Technician-Intermediate, First Responder), pediatric-specific topics currently account for what proportion of the curriculum?
   A. Less than half.
   B. Approximately half.
   C. Approximately one third.
   D. Approximately one quarter.
   E. Less than one tenth.

9. As a director of emergency medical services (EMS) who is dealing with short interhospital distances, you must write protocols for children with disabilities. The best management of a child in status epilepticus with a tracheostomy tube would include:
   A. Secure the airway and contact the primary care physician.
   B. Secure the airway and transport to the closest hospital.
   C. Secure the airway and transport to an ED approved for pediatrics (EDAP).
   D. Secure the airway and transport to a pediatric critical care center (PCCC).
   E. Secure the airway and contact the health maintenance organization (HMO) for the closest affiliated hospital.

10. A clear improvement in pediatric outcomes has been shown for which field technique?
    A. Early defibrillation.
    B. Intraosseous access.
    C. Intravenous epinephrine.
    D. Early airway management.

11. The American College of Emergency Physicians (ACEP) Pediatric Prehospital Protocols and similar protocols issued by other groups affiliated with the development of EMS for Children (EMSC) were released after extensive field testing for safety and effectiveness.
    A. True
    B. False

12. The National Pediatric Trauma Registry is used principally to:
    A. Track long-term disability.
    B. Track short-term outcome.
    C. Maintain a data bank of trauma scores and ICD-9 External Cause of Injury Codes (E-codes).
    D. Evaluate protocols.
    E. Improve the quality of trauma management.

13. An enhanced 911 system (911e) improves care by:
    A. Funding additional ambulances and paramedics.
    B. Increasing the number of dispatchers.
    C. Providing dispatchers with the caller's address.
    D. Providing a two-tier response for minor or serious complaints.
    E. Providing a central registry for patients with special needs.

14. Regionalization, specialty transport, and secondary transport as part of EMSC were recommended by the 1993 Institute of Medicine Report and mandated by subsequent legislation.
    A. True
    B. False

15. An effective pediatric trauma system must include ready availability of pediatric surgeons.
    A. True
    B. False

16. A 30-kg child is responsive but speaking gibberish. The child has an 8-cm deep gash on the right arm, a deformity of the left ankle, and a systolic BP of 80 mm Hg. This child is most appropriately transported to:
    A. The closest hospital.
    B. An ED approved for pediatrics (EDAP).
    C. A pediatric trauma center (PTC).
    D. A pediatric critical care center (PCCC).
    E. The most prominent children's hospital in the state.

ANSWERS [See Barkin et al: Chapter 4.]

1. The answer is **A,** pages 25 and 26.
   Children who suffer out-of-hospital cardiopulmonary arrests have a greater than 90% death rate. Cardiac arrest in children is rarely a primary event. The best outcomes occur when prearrest respiratory or circulatory failure is recognized and treated. Bystander CPR and EMT interventions are effective in near drowning and foreign body aspiration. Early effective airway management has been shown to be the most critical step.

2. The answer is **C,** page 36.
   Approximately 80% of trauma deaths occur before admission, most with EMS personnel present. The basic principles governing resuscitation are the same for both medical and surgical problems. Initial airway management is critical. In the trauma patient with uncontrolled bleeding, no amount of fluid resuscitation will take the place of surgical intervention. In these circumstances, reliance on basic life support (BLS) techniques in the earliest phases of resuscitation is better for the patient than the delay imposed by ALS modalities other than definitive airway management. Rapid surgical intervention becomes the dominant factor in this child's ultimate survival.

3. The answer is **C,** page 25.

The ages of children who need EMS show a bimodal distribution; most are either younger than 2 or older than 10. Between 0.3% and 0.5% of children transported to an ED require tertiary care. Although children account for 25% to 30% of ED visits, they represent only 5% to 10% of ambulance runs. Approximately 50% of all visits are for traumatic events, with motor vehicle–related trauma as the leading cause in children older than 2. In younger children, fever, respiratory, and other medical complaints are preponderant.

4. The answer is **D,** page 26.

Vehicle-related injuries account for 50% of all deaths up to 14 years old and 80% of deaths between 14 and 24 years old (Table 4-1).

5. The answer is **E,** page 28.

Prehospital equipment guidelines have been developed by ACEP, American Academy of Pediatrics (AAP), and other groups involved with EMS. Lap belts and shoulder harnesses are used for sitting passengers. Chest, hip, and leg straps restrain patients on stretchers. Child safety seat restraints are available but are not part of current guidelines for ambulance design. If the clinical condition allows, it is best to let a parent comfort the child either by sitting in the ambulance or by being available through direct communication with the driver's cab.

6. The answer is **D,** pages 28, 37 to 38.

The PTS (Box 3-1 on page 7) assigns +2, +1, or -1 based on the child's size, airway patency, systolic BP, central nervous system (CNS) status, presence of open wounds, and evidence of skeletal injury. Children with a trauma score of 8 or less are best managed in a trauma center. In this case the child would receive +1 for a weight of 15 kg, +2 for a normal airway, +1 for a systolic BP of 80 mm Hg, +2 for good eye contact, +2 for no open wounds, and +1 for the closed skeletal injury for a total of 9.

TABLE 4-1   Causes of Death in Children

Causes	Age 0-14 yr	Age 14-24 yr	Total
Motor vehicle	3,400	15,000	18,900
Drowning	1,250	1,300	2,550
Fire, burns	1,200	500	1,700
Poisoning, suffocation	520	750	1,270
Firearms	230	600	830
TOTAL	6,600	18,650	25,250

Adapted from Matlack ME: Current problems in the management of pediatric trauma. In Haller JA Jr, editor: *Emergency medical services for children: report on the ninety-seventh Ross conference on pediatric research,* Columbus, Ohio, 1989, Ross Laboratories.

7. The answer is **E,** page 26. Early field airway management and ventilation have improved the outcomes of children with near drowning or respiratory complaints. Very little research has been done on the effects of prehospital management in children.

8. The answer is **E,** page 27.

Before 1994 the pediatric component of training was only 3 of 100 to 120 hours for EMTs and only 15 of 1000+ hours for paramedics. An improved pediatric curriculum for EMT-B was released in 1994. For other providers current guidelines include education in meningitis, Reye's syndrome, and other illnesses that cannot be diagnosed in the field. Trainees are not given sufficient time for directly supervised "hands-on" experience. Revision of Paramedic, EMT-I, and First Responder curricula is under way to address these deficiencies.

9. The answer is **D,** pages 34 and 35.

Contacting a primary care physician may significantly delay this child's care. Not all hospitals have the equipment or available staff to meet the needs of children. It is best for the system to identify the capabilities of affiliated health care institutions. An EDAP provides basic services and has voluntarily met minimal standards for staffing, education, equipment, and protocols for the initial stabilization of children. A PCCC has met the EDAP criteria and has additional expertise, including a pediatric intensive care unit and dedicated pediatric medical and surgical specialists. As with the trauma system, severe and complex medical management issues are best addressed in a regional fashion.

10. The answer is **D,** page 35.

Outcome studies have been performed primarily on adults. Children rarely suffer primary cardiac events. Early airway management in children with multiple trauma or near drowning is the only field technique that has been shown clearly to be critical to survival.

11. The answer is **B, false,** page 35.

The ACEP Pediatric Prehospital Protocols and similar protocols were developed based on current thinking about pathophysiology and inhospital management standards. Such protocols have not been tested to determine whether they improve the outcome in pediatric patients.

12. The answer is **E,** page 37.

The National Pediatric Trauma Registry focuses on both long-term disability and short-term outcome. With a large population-based data bank, it is a powerful quality management tool. The ultimate aim is to improve the care of pediatric trauma victims.

13. The answer is **C,** page 34.

Just as technology now can provide consumers with a caller's telephone number, 911e can locate the address of the caller. Unfortunately, many regions do not have even basic 911 service.

Box 4-1
Components of Trauma Center with
Pediatric Expertise

Full-service general/children's hospital
Institutional commitment to pediatric trauma
Organized, integrated pediatric trauma service
Responsible surgeon director
Qualified, trained physicians and nurses
Dedicated pediatric ED/ICU areas
Properly equipped OR/ED/ICU facilities
Weekly case review conference
Active quality management program
Community outreach/injury prevention programs

---

14. The answer is **B, false,** pages 24 and 25.
   The IOM report recommended that EMSC be an integral part of the existing EMS system. It further recommended that primary care, prevention, and rehabilitation be linked to EMSC as part of the comprehensive care of children. Other key components included: education of the public, training of health care providers, system planning, evaluation of outcomes, research, and governmental oversight. Subsequent governmental funding has led four fifths of the states to develop EMSC programs, not all based on geographic regionalization.

15. The answer is **B, false,** pages 38 and 39.
   Optimal pediatric trauma care requires that all components of the trauma system have special pediatric expertise (Box 4-1). Given the scarcity of pediatric surgeons, the most important requirements are that all aspects of the system function smoothly and that all health care providers have education and experience with pediatric patients.

16. The answer is **C,** page 28.
   This child has a pediatric trauma score of 6 (size +2; airway +2; BP +1; CNS +1; open wound -1; skeletal injury +1) (see Box 3-1 on page 7). Scores of 8 or less are best managed in a PTC. An EDAP voluntarily meets minimal standards for the initial stabilization of children. A PCCC has the full spectrum of pediatric medical and surgical services available. A PTC must have this availability on site at all times. Where several PCCCs exist in relatively close proximity, one may be designated the receiving hospital for pediatric trauma.

5

Interhospital Transport

David H. Rubin

See Barkin et al: Chapter 5.

1. Which of the following statements regarding advance preparation for interhospital transport is *true?*
   A. Most hospitals require that a list of receiving hospitals and phone numbers be distributed to all staff members.
   B. Pediatric code cards should be readily available to all staff members but should not be publicly displayed on walls.
   C. Pediatric Advanced Life Support (PALS) should be offered as training to Emergency Medical Technicians (EMTs).
   D. A hospital can require that payment for transport be made before the patient leaves the hospital.
2. Which of the following statements regarding ambulance personnel is *true?*
   A. All ambulance personnel are well trained in the care of children.
   B. Ambulance personnel are not usually trained or experienced in the management of the critically ill child.
   C. Ambulance personnel are routinely certified in advanced trauma care of children.
   D. Ambulance personnel may not administer cardiac medications to children.
3. Which of the following statements regarding transport of critically ill children is *true?*
   A. A specialized pediatric team is the best choice to care for critically ill children even if the team takes longer to arrive.
   B. Helicopter transport should be the highest priority for critically ill children.
   C. Insertion of endotracheal tubes and intravenous lines is easier in helicopters than in fixed-wing aircraft.
   D. Pediatric and neonatal equipment is available in most transport units.
4. A 4-year-old boy is injured in a motor vehicle accident and sustains a severe head injury. He arrives by ambulance at a local hospital with a general ED and a pediatric resident who is on rotation from the nearby university medical center. The resident feels comfortable stabilizing the patient and would like to treat the patient in the adult intensive care unit (ICU). Your recommendation is to:
   A. Stabilize the patient in the ED and wait to see if the patient's condition improves.
   B. Prepare to transfer the patient to the nearby university medical center pediatric ICU using a dedicated pediatric critical care transport team.
   C. Prepare to transfer the patient to the pediatric ICU at the nearby university medical center using any available ambulance with advanced cardiac life support capability.
   D. Transfer the patient to the ICU in the hospital and allow the pediatric resident to assume control of the patient's care.
5. All of the following activities should be initiated by the *referring hospital* to expedite transition of care to the transport team *except:*
   A. Suture all lacerations.
   B. Complete copies of all radiologic studies, including computed tomography (CT) scans, before transport.
   C. Complete consent-to-transport form.
   D. Prepare blood products for transport if needed.
6. Which of the following is a responsibility of the *referring hospital?*
   A. Appropriate level of care transport team.
   B. Verification of insurance acceptable to receiving hospital.
   C. Transcript of nursing communication between referring and receiving hospitals.
   D. Policies and procedures regarding care of critically ill patients at the receiving hospital.

7. Which of the following are important skills recommended as necessary for personnel involved in the transport of pediatric patients?
   A. Procedural and communication skills.
   B. Medical degree.
   C. Advanced degree in public health.
   D. Nursing certification.
8. Which of the following statements regarding the legal issues in pediatric transport is *true?*
   A. All legal responsibility for patient well-being rests with the referring hospital.
   B. All legal responsibility for patient care shifts to the receiving hospital after the transfer is accepted on the telephone.
   C. The referring hospital decides when to shift legal responsibility for patient care.
   D. The legal responsibility for patient care is a continuum ranging from the beginning of patient care and treatment at the referring hospital to the arrival of the patient at the receiving hospital.

9. Which of the following statements regarding inter-hospital transport is *true?*
   A. Speed of transport is a critical factor in most serious motor vehicle accidents.
   B. Speed of transport is only a critical factor for victims of multiple trauma.
   C. The receiving hospital is responsible for the mode of transport of the patient.
   D. The receiving hospital is responsible for notification of public health officials of the status of multiple-trauma patients.
10. The referring hospital is responsible for the medical integrity of the receiving hospital.
   A. True
   B. False

ANSWERS [See Barkin et al: Chapter 5.]

1. The answer is **C,** page 42.
Although a list of receiving hospitals and phone numbers should be attached to the ED telephone, it need not be distributed to all staff members. Pediatric Code Cards should be easily accessible to staff members and may be placed on the crash cart or posted on a wall. They should not be placed in a drawer with other documents. Administrative issues such as payment for transport should be addressed in predetermined contracts or protocols between two hospitals and not at the time of transport.

2. The answer is **B,** pages 28 and 42.
Although many ambulance crews are well trained and comfortable with the care of children, studies have shown that many crews require further training and may be (understandably) uncomfortable performing the transport of critically ill children. Ambulance crews are trained at many levels. (See page 28, Barkin et al for an outline of specific criteria for basic life support and advanced life support)

3. The answer is **A,** page 43.
A specialized pediatric team is the best choice to care for critically ill children even if it takes longer for the team to arrive. The level of care for these patients during transport time is the major concern. Helicopter transport is beneficial for some, but it is not always the highest priority transport vehicle. Helicopters are notoriously difficult places to perform many important procedures, especially in younger children. Only *dedicated* pediatric and neonatal transport teams carry pediatric and neonatal equipment.

4. The answer is **B,** page 43.
There are currently no standards to determine when a critical care transport team is required for a specific patient. However, "reasonable" criteria for the use of a critical care transport team include the following:
   Any patient with anticipated ICU admission on arrival at the receiving hospital.
   Any patient with the potential for significant respiratory or neurologic deterioration during transport.
   Any patient resuscitated from a life-threatening event that may recur.

5. The answer is **A,** page 43.
The patient's parents should complete the consent-to-transport form, which should specify the receiving hospital and the mode of transport. Copies of all hospital records and radiologic studies also should be prepared. The suturing of all lacerations and completion of "all necessary radiologic studies" should not delay transport and, if not serious, may be delayed until arrival at the receiving hospital. Insurance status should not determine to which hospital the patient is transferred.

6. The answer is **A,** pages 43 and 44.
The referring hospital should provide copies of all medical records, x-ray films, CT scans, and any other items that pertain to the patient before transport. The referring hospital is also responsible for choosing a mode of transport. Transcripts of nursing communications need not be included in the material submitted to the receiving hospital. However, nurses' notes regarding patient care should be part of the medical record. Policies and procedures are not part of the written material that must be provided to the receiving hospital.

7. The answer is **A,** page 44.

Personnel criteria focus on training and experience in pediatric transport rather than on educational degrees of team members. Cognitive, procedural, and communication skills are necessary for pediatric transport.

8. The answer is **D,** page 44.

Legal responsibilities during patient transport operate on a continuum. Increasing involvement in the patient's care means greater responsibility. No single hospital accepts all legal responsibility. The legal responsibility starts with the referring hospital and gradually shifts to the receiving hospital after its personnel arrive at the referring hospital for transport.

9. The answer is **B,** page 43.

The *referring* hospital is responsible for the mode of transport of the ill patient. The receiving hospital is not required to notify public health officials. No evidence has shown that speed of transfer is beneficial for any group of patients *except for victims of multiple trauma.*

10. The answer is **A, true,** page 44.

All legal responsibility lies with the referring hospital until another hospital has been contacted. All responsibility shifts to the receiving hospital once the patient arrives at the receiving hospital. Under the Omnibus Budget Reconciliation Act (OBRA), the referring hospital is considered responsible for the medical integrity of the receiving hospital.

CHAPTER

6

Pain Control, Analgesia, and Sedation

Robert Crupi

See Barkin et al: Chapter 7.

1. Which of the following opiate receptors in the central nervous system (CNS) is predominantly responsible for analgesic activity?
   A. κ Receptors.
   B. ς Receptors.
   C. μ-1 Receptors.
   D. μ-2 Receptors.
   E. γ-Aminobutyric acid (GABA) receptors.
2. Which of the following corresponds to the developmental stage of pain perception in a 2-year-old child?
   A. No understanding.
   B. Fear of painful situation.
   C. Illogical and egocentric perception.
   D. Cause and effect.
3. The major drawback of behavioral-based pain assessment scales is that they require which of the following?
   A. Training of observers.
   B. Practice by the patient.
   C. Patient cooperation.
   D. Patient who is of school age or older.
   E. Complicated formulas for scoring.
4. Which of the following sedative and analgesic agents has *not* been used successfully by transmucosal administration?
   A. Midazolam.
   B. Ketamine.
   C. Fentanyl.
   D. Butorphanol.
   E. Oxycodone.
5. Which of the following sedative agents can be reliably administered by the rectal route?
   A. Diazepam.
   B. Midazolam.
   C. Thiopental.
   D. Chloral hydrate.
   E. All of the above.

6. Rectal methohexital is *not* recommended for routine ED sedation for which of the following reasons?
   A. Poor rectal absorption.
   B. Prolonged sedation.
   C. Delayed onset of action.
   D. Risk of airway obstruction.
   E. Absence of analgesic properties.
7. Which of the following side effects is most commonly associated with ketamine?
   A. Bradycardia.
   B. Laryngospasm.
   C. Bronchospasm.
   D. Hypotension.
   E. Chest wall rigidity.
8. Which of the following is *not* a feature of conscious sedation?
   A. Minimally depressed level of consciousness.
   B. Partial loss in maintenance of an independent, patent airway.
   C. Ability to respond appropriately to physical stimulation or verbal command.
   D. Depth of sedation less than deep sedation.
   E. Required monitoring at frequent, regular intervals.
9. Which of the following is *not* associated with nonsteroidal antiinflammatory drugs (NSAIDS)?
   A. Decreased renal blood flow.
   B. Hepatic dysfunction.
   C. Irreversible platelet function inhibition.
   D. Antipyretic properties.
   E. Potent analgesic effects in renal colic.
10. Which of the following statements regarding ketorolac (Toradol) is *false?*
    A. The Food and Drug Administration approved it for those 16 years of age and older.
    B. Elimination half-life in children is similar to adults.
    C. A 60-mg dose was equivalent to 12 mg of morphine in double-blind trials.
    D. It is the only parenteral NSAID available for use in the United States.
    E. A narcotic-sparing effect has been shown in ED patients treated for sickle cell crisis.

11. Which of the following narcotic agents is classified as a "mixed" agonist-antagonist at opioid receptors?
    A. Meperidine.
    B. Fentanyl.
    C. Methadone.
    D. Nalbuphine.
    E. Hydromorphone.

12. Which of the following is the most common side effect associated with fentanyl?
    A. Hypotension.
    B. Histamine release.
    C. Facial pruritus.
    D. Bronchospasm.
    E. Myocardial depression.

13. Which of the following statements regarding the pharmacologic properties of meperidine is *false*?
    A. Intravenous (IV) administration produces tachycardia.
    B. Increased risk of seizures is associated with repeated administration.
    C. Sedative effect is enhanced in combination with hydroxyzine.
    D. Oral absorption is poor in comparison with morphine.
    E. Tremors are associated with a principal metabolite.

14. An 8-month-old girl recovering from bronchiolitis requires sedation in the ED for repair of a complex laceration. She is not in respiratory distress and has an oxygen saturation of 97% as measured by pulse oximetry on room air. Auscultation of the chest reveals bilateral scattered expiratory wheezes. Appropriate monitoring is in place. Which of the following sedative agents should you *avoid* in this setting?
    A. Fentanyl.
    B. Diazepam.
    C. Midazolam.
    D. Ketamine.
    E. Chloral hydrate.

15. Chlorpromazine induces hypotension or seizures in susceptible individuals by its ability to block which of the following receptors?
    A. β-Adrenergic receptors
    B. α-Adrenergic receptors
    C. GABA receptors
    D. μ-2 opiate receptors
    E. Histamine receptors

16. A 3-year-old boy is seen in the ED for a laceration repair and is administered midazolam intravenously for conscious sedation. He becomes extremely agitated following the successful completion of the procedure. The patient is hemodynamically stable and has an oxygen saturation of 98% as measured by pulse oximetry on room air. The most appropriate immediate course of action is:
    A. Administer an additional bolus of midazolam.
    B. Administer flumazenil.
    C. Administer an analgesic agent.
    D. Administer supplemental oxygen.
    E. Provide supportive therapy.

17. In which of the following settings would the use of ketamine be an appropriate sedative agent?
    A. Congestive heart failure.
    B. Status asthmaticus requiring endotracheal intubation.
    C. Procedures involving the posterior pharynx.
    D. Cystic fibrosis.
    E. Ocular trauma with globe penetration.

18. Which of the following statements regarding midazolam is *false*?
    A. Causes less phlebitis than diazepam when given intravenously.
    B. Nasal administration is painful.
    C. Oral route is efficacious.
    D. Rectal route has greater efficacy than nasal route.
    E. Paradoxical agitation is a side effect.

19. Which of the following is *not* included among recommendations to reduce the systemic toxicity from topical anesthesia using tetracaine (0.5%), adrenaline (epinephrine 1:1000), and cocaine (11.8%), also known as TAC?
    A. Single 3-ml or smaller dose.
    B. Avoidance of mucosal contact.
    C. Application time of less than 20 minutes.
    D. Formulation of a TAC gel.
    E. TAC with half the standard concentration of epinephrine.

20. Which of the following statements regarding the "caine" local anesthetics is *false*?
    A. Amide group includes lidocaine and bupivacaine.
    B. Buffered lidocaine has reduced efficacy.
    C. Heated lidocaine up to 42° C has reduced infiltration pain.
    D. Bupivacaine has longer duration of anesthesia than lidocaine.
    E. Addition of epinephrine should be avoided in wounds with a high risk of contamination.

21. Which of the following side effects is *not* associated with nitrous oxide?
    A. Excitement.
    B. Emesis.
    C. Opisthotonos.
    D. Hypersalivation.
    E. Lightheadedness.

22. Which of the following is the most important consideration in choosing a sedative and analgesic agent?
    A. Potency.
    B. Efficacy and safety.
    C. Avoidance of masking diagnoses.
    D. Induction of drug dependency.
    E. Ability to measure pain objectively.

ANSWERS   [See Barkin et al: Chapter 7.]

1. The answer is **C**, pages 49 and 57.
   Four types of opiate receptors have been identified in the CNS. The μ-1 receptor is predominantly responsible for analgesic activity. The μ-2 receptor produces respiratory depression and physical dependence. The receptor, located primarily in the spinal cord, causes spinal analgesia, mild sedation, and miosis. The σ receptor induces hallucinations and dysphoria. GABA receptors are not opiate receptors. Benzodiazepines exert their effects by inhibition of GABA receptors in the CNS.

2. The answer is **C**, pages 50 and 51.
   Childhood developmental levels of understanding and reaction to pain may be summarized by age. Pain assessment and control in children must take these developmental stages into account. Toddlers can localize pain and often see illness as punishment for something they have said or done. Pain perception at this stage is illogical and egocentric. Guided use of these facts for reassurance of the patient and family can improve psychologic management of pain in the ED (Table 6-1 on page 19).

3. The answer is **A**, pages 50 and 52.
   Several drawbacks limit the use of pain assessment scales in the ED. Behavioral scales require training of observers to reduce interobserver variability. Self-report scales generally require practice by a cooperative patient. Pain assessment methods are age dependent. Behavioral scales are included among methods for infant, preschool, and school-age to adult pain assessment. The CHEOPS Behavioral Scale (see Table 7-1, page 51 in Barkin et al) is used most reliably for preschool children. The CHEOPS score is easily determined by adding the score for each item listed. No studies of ED patients have systematically addressed the issues of validity and accuracy of pain scales in children.

4. The answer is **E**, pages 53 and 56.
   Transmucosal administration of sedatives and analgesics has been used successfully with midazolam, ketamine, fentanyl, and butorphanol. Oxycodone is a potent oral semisynthetic opioid narcotic with limited application for pediatric ED patients.

5. The answer is **E**, pages 53 and 57.
   Diazepam, midazolam, methohexital, thiopental, and chloral hydrate can be reliably administered by the rectal route.

6. The answer is **D**, pages 57 and 58.
   Rectal methohexital was shown to cause airway obstruction in 7% of the children in one study in which it was administered for induction of anesthesia. Oxygen desaturation was also observed in 12% of the children in one ED study of rectal methohexital. Because of the risk of airway obstruction, rectal methohexital cannot be recommended for routine ED sedation.

7. The answer is **B**, pages 56 and 58.
   Side effects of ketamine include laryngospasm, tachycardia, hypertension, vomiting, hypersalivation, nightmares, emergent reactions, and increased intracranial pressure. Ketamine induces bronchodilation. Chest wall rigidity is associated with fentanyl.

8. The answer is **B**, page 54.
   Conscious sedation is a "minimally depressed level of consciousness that retains the patient's ability to maintain a patent airway independently and continuously, and respond appropriately to physical stimulation or verbal command."* Deep sedation is a "controlled state of depressed consciousness or unconsciousness from which the patient is not easily aroused, and which may be accompanied by a partial or complete loss of protective reflexes."* Deep sedation requires continuous monitoring. Conscious sedation patients may be monitored at frequent, regular intervals.

9. The answer is **C**, page 55.
   NSAIDS produce reversible platelet function inhibition. Side effects of NSAIDS include renal and hepatic dysfunction. Ibuprofen decreases renal blood flow. Reversible renal failure has been reported in a hypovolemic child treated with ibuprofen. NSAIDS have antipyretic properties and have been demonstrated to have potent analgesic effects in renal colic.

10. The answer is **E**, page 55.
    One ED trial failed to show a narcotic-sparing effect in patients with pain from sickle cell crises. All of the other responses are true.

---

*American Academy of Pediatrics, Committee on Drugs: Guidelines for monitoring and management of pediatric patients during and after sedation for diagnostic and therapeutic procedures, *Pediatrics* 89:1110-1115, 1992.

TABLE 6-1   Developmental Sequence of Pain Perception and Reaction in Children

Age	Perception	Reaction
Newborn-6 mo	No understanding	General stress response, withdrawal, crying, physiologic response[*]
6 mo-1½ yr	Fear of painful situation	Screaming, restlessness, localization, physiologic response
1½-6 yr	Illogical and egocentric perception	Reality distortion, fantasies, poor time appreciation
7-10 yr	Cause-and-effect, understanding verbal description possible	Physiologic response
11-17 yr	Logical perception, abstraction	Deception, bravado to hide pain

[*]Physiologic response to pain is generally associated wtih tachycardia, increased arterial blood pressure, mydriasis, and diaphoresis.

11. The answer is **D,** page 56.

    "Mixed" agonist-antagonist opioids include agents such as pentazocine, nalbuphine, butorphanol, and sufentanil. Analgesia is produced by agonist action on specific (κ) receptors. The ceiling on respiratory depression occurs with antagonism of the other (μ) receptors. Meperidine, fentanyl, methadone, and hydromorphone are classified as opioid agonists.

12. The answer is **C,** pages 54 and 56.

    Fentanyl may induce facial pruritus. In one preoperative sedation trial, facial pruritus occurred in 80% of patients in the fentanyl group. Fentanyl's potency is approximately 100 times that of morphine. It is a preferred agent for patients with trauma or cardiac disease because of its ability to block nociceptive stimuli without hemodynamic compromise, histamine release, or exacerbation of bronchospasm.

13. The answer is **D,** page 56.

    Meperidine is a synthetic narcotic analgesic with few advantages over morphine. It has relatively small therapeutic range in which analgesia is achieved and above which toxicity occurs. A principal metabolite, normeperidine may produce tremors, disorientation, and seizures. There is an increased risk of seizures associated with repeated administration. Unlike other opioids, meperidine produces tachycardia when given intravenously. Its main advantage over morphine is that it is absorbed well orally. When meperidine is combined with hydroxyzine or promethazine, its sedative and possibly analgesic effects are enhanced.

14. The answer is **E,** pages 53, 56 to 58.

    Oxygen desaturation has been associated with chloral hydrate doses of 70 to 100 mg/kg when administered to wheezy infants recovering from bronchiolitis. Chloral hydrate given in a dose of 50 to 80 mg/kg also has the disadvantage of a prolonged duration of action usually lasting up to 2 or 3 hours until the patient is alert. Fentanyl does not cause histamine release or exacerbation of bronchospasm. Trials of pediatric sedation have reported diazepam or midazolam to be generally efficacious and safe. The benzodiazepine antagonist flumazenil may enhance the safety profile for sedation with benzodiazepines. Ketamine might be the most appropriate sedative agent for this patient, since it induces bronchodilation.

15. The answer is **B,** page 58.

    Chlorpromazine is a phenothiazine with sedative, amnestic, anti–motion sensation, and antihistaminic effects. Chlorpromazine induces hypotension or seizures in susceptible individuals by its ability to block α-adrenergic receptors.

16. The answer is **E,** page 57.

    Paradoxical agitation following midazolam administration is regularly reported. This disinhibition phenomenon typically follows an otherwise effective sedation experience and usually resolves within 15 minutes without specific therapy.

17. The answer is **B,** page 58.

    Ketamine has many relative contraindications. They include: upper or lower respiratory infection, procedures involving the posterior pharynx, cystic fibrosis, age younger than 3 months, head injury, increased intracranial pressure, acute glaucoma or globe penetration, uncontrolled hypertension, congestive heart failure, arterial aneurysm, allergy or previous adverse reaction to ketamine, acute intermittent porphyria, and thyrotoxicosis. Ketamine, in a dose of 1 to 1.5 mg/kg given intravenously, has been reported to be a beneficial sedative agent for endotracheal intubation in asthmatic children with respiratory failure because it is a bronchodilator.

18. The answer is **D,** page 57.

    Midazolam is a short-acting, water-soluble benzodiazepine. It may be administered by the oral, nasal, rectal, intramuscular, and IV routes. A double-blind ED sedation trial showed no differences between oral (0.5 mg/kg) and nasal (0.25 mg/kg) midazolam administration. Rectal administration of midazolam has reduced efficacy, which may be related to reduced plasma concentrations. All of the other responses are true.

19. The answer is **E,** page 60.

    Tetracaine, adrenaline, and cocaine, also known as TAC, may cause systemic toxicity after topical application for local anesthesia. Cocaine absorption has been documented after TAC application. Significant side effects associated with TAC use have included seizures and death. TAC at half its standard concentration and TAC with half the standard concentration of cocaine are also effective in providing local anesthesia and may limit systemic toxicity. All of the other responses are true.

20. The answer is **B**, pages 60 and 61.

When lidocaine is given with bicarbonate (0.1 mEq/ml; 1:10 by volume), a reduction in infiltration pain may occur by neutralizing the normally acidic pH to 7.0. Studies have shown no reduction in the efficacy of buffered lidocaine. All of the other responses are true.

21. The answer is **D**, page 59.

Side effects of nitrous oxide are generally mild and include lightheadedness, drowsiness, nausea, emesis, excitement, restlessness, and opisthotonos. Hypersalivation is not associated with nitrous oxide but is commonly associated with the use of ketamine.

22. The answer is **B**, pages 50 and 61.

When choosing sedative and analgesic agents, the pediatric emergency physician must keep in mind the dual objectives of safety and efficacy. The beneficial effects of these agents must be weighed against their expected complications and in relation to the objective of sedation and analgesia for each child. The routine use of potent sedative and analgesic agents at doses producing significant cardiorespiratory depression appears unwarranted for minor procedures such as uncomplicated laceration repair. The inability to measure pain accurately and reproducibly and the fear of masking diagnoses or inducing drug dependency have been cited as factors contributing to inadequate pain control.

Death of a Child

F. Meridith Sonnett • Peter S. Dayan

See Barkin et al: Chapter 8.

1. The most common cause of death in children older than 1 year of age is:
   A. Child abuse.
   B. Infection.
   C. Sudden infant death syndrome (SIDS).
   D. Accidents.
   E. Congenital anomalies.
2. Cardiopulmonary resuscitation (CPR) should be instituted in the field in all of the following circumstances *except:*
   A. Absence of respirations.
   B. Absence of pulse.
   C. No discernible blood pressure.
   D. Lividity.
   E. Ventricular fibrillation for longer than 20 minutes.
3. When a child has died in the ED after an unsuccessful resuscitation, you, as the physician, should:
   A. Inform the family immediately.
   B. Inform the family only after the child has been transported to the morgue.
   C. Inform the family only after notifying the medical examiner (ME) and the hospital administrator.
   D. Contact the patient relations office and have one of its representatives inform the family.
   E. Perform all necessary postmortem tests before informing the family.
4. When a child is being resuscitated in the ED, the best way to deal with the immediate family members who are in the ED is to:
   A. Discuss the need for an autopsy if the child dies.
   B. Give the family as little information as possible until the resuscitation effort is over.
   C. Wait at least 30 minutes for family members to have time to gather their thoughts and emotions before providing them with information.
   D. Provide brief, accurate, and frequently updated reports about the child's condition.

5. The most correct statement regarding organ donation in the setting of an ED is:
   A. The subject of organ donation should be broached with the child's family by any professional while resuscitation is ongoing.
   B. Only specifically designated transplant team members should discuss organ donation with the child's family.
   C. Parents wanting to discuss organ donation should be discouraged until the outcome of their child has been determined.
   D. Legislation in some states mandates that health care professionals discuss organ donation with family members.
   E. Organ donation does not apply to children younger than 1 year old.
6. Which of the following statements concerning autopsies on children is *true?*
   A. Autopsies are required on all children who die in an ED.
   B. Autopsies are required only in cases of *unexplained death.*
   C. Once the ME, or coroner, decides that an autopsy is not needed, that decision cannot be challenged.
   D. Once a death case is accepted by the ME, an autopsy is usually required.
   E. Autopsies can be performed only with parental consent.

7. The most accurate definition of a critical incident stress debriefing (CISD) is:
   A. An informal meeting that is run by a mental health professional or peer support personnel within 12 hours of a critical incident (i.e., the death of a child in the ED) and allows staff members to express their feelings in relation to the incident.
   B. A structured confidential meeting 24 to 72 hours after a critical incident that has adversely affected staff members.
   C. A formal meeting where the individual performances of those involved in the critical incident are reviewed by a panel of peers.
   D. A formal meeting with department chairpersons, hospital administrators, and the staff involved with the critical incident, which takes place within 2 to 4 hours of the critical incident.
   E. An informal meeting with the staff involved in the critical incident and experts in the field to review how to improve performance during a critical incident. Specific scenarios are described.

ANSWERS   [See Barkin et al: Chapter 8.]

1. The answer is **D,** page 71.
   In infants under 1 year of age *natural causes* are responsible for the majority of deaths. Natural causes include congenital anomalies, SIDS, infections, and prematurity. In children over the age of 1 year, accidents are the most common cause of death. Accidents include motor vehicle accidents (most commonly), drowning, smoke inhalation, burns, and falls. In urban areas, death as a result of firearms has become increasingly common in the adolescent age group.

2. The answer is **D,** page 71.
   Prehospital personnel use very specific criteria to pronounce a child dead in the field. Different protocols are used by the different emergency medical service (EMS) systems. Some EMS protocols do allow *judgment calls* on the part of the prehospital personnel. The circumstances in which the pronouncement of death is indisputable include postmortem rigidity or lividity, decapitation, decomposition, and incineration. Most EMS personnel initiate CPR in the face of apnea, absence of pulse, inability to obtain blood pressure, and cardiac arrest regardless of the length of time. Rapid transport of the critically ill or injured child is of the utmost importance.

   Transportation of a child whose prognosis is dismal also allows the family to benefit from the services that a medical facility can provide, such as offering emotional support from the staff (physicians, nurses, social workers, patient relations workers), arranging for clergy to be present if the family requests, and addressing the issue of organ transplantation.

3. The answer is **A,** page 73.
   When a child dies in the ED, the person of the *highest* professional level (usually the physician on duty in the ED and preferably the physician involved with the resuscitation) must inform the family immediately. It is important to use the words *dead* or *died* when informing the family; euphemisms are often misunderstood. Until family members are informed of the death and given the opportunity to see and hold the child, the body should not be transported anywhere and postmortem studies should not be performed. In most states the ME must be informed of all pediatric deaths that occur in the ED. This can be done after the family has been informed. Physicians should be familiar with the specific state laws.

4. The answer is **D,** pages 72 and 73.
   Giving family members accurate information as soon as possible is very important. Waiting even a few minutes for information when a child is critically ill can be unbearably long. Therefore one person in the ED should be designated to report on the child's condition every few minutes. The information should be brief but accurate, should be given in simple, understandable terms, and should not eliminate all hope but should still be realistic. Although the need for an autopsy may be an issue, this can be handled after the resuscitation effort is completed.

5. The answer is **D,** page 74.

Organ donation is a difficult issue to discuss at any time but particularly in the ED, when the events surrounding a child's death are often sudden. Parents are devastated and unprepared for this event. The issue of organ donation must be approached in a sensitive manner with the parents. Although organ donation should be discussed routinely with the family, in some states professionals in the health care setting are required by law to discuss the issue of organ donation. Some hospitals have organ donor programs, in which a team member is immediately available to discuss organ donation with the family. Each hospital should have resources available to access the appropriate agency for organ donation if the family expresses an interest. Whatever decision the family makes must be accepted and respected. There are no age limits for organ donation.

6. The answer is **D,** page 74.

When an ME accepts a case, an autopsy is usually performed. Parental consent is not required if the ME deems the autopsy necessary as in cases of trauma, unexpected death, SIDS, and suspicious or unexplained death, including suspected child abuse. The physician involved with the case may approach the family to obtain consent for an autopsy if the ME does not think an autopsy is necessary. Some families may request an autopsy because they believe that the results will tell them why their child died.

7. The answer is **B,** page 75.

The death of a child in the ED is an extremely stressful event for all those involved and often has a great emotional impact on the ED staff. Staff members need ways to ventilate their feelings, and most have adopted *informal* methods. However, when the event is extraordinarily stressful, such as in multiple casualties or the death of a staff member's child, two types of intervention are appropriate. Answer *A* describes what is known as *defusing;* it is a brief informal meeting and often negates the need for a formal *debriefing.* Debriefing, more specifically referred to as a critical incident stress debriefing, is a structured meeting with the staff members involved and a specific CISD team, which includes several mental health professionals and trained counselors. This debriefing session allows each staff member to describe the experience and provides strategies to help the staff deal appropriately with feelings. When a critical event has occurred, it is important not to place blame on any one individual or group of individuals.

8

Legal Issues

Alexandra E. Trinkoff

See Barkin et al: Chapter 10.

1. A 6-year-old girl is sitting with her parents in the ED waiting area. The parents have notified the front desk that they are waiting for their private physician to arrive at the ED to treat their daughter. Which of the following actions would be most appropriate?
   A. Allow parents and child to wait for the private physician without being seen.
   B. Triage the patient, obtain vital signs and chief complaint, and allow family to wait for a private physician in the waiting area.
   C. Triage the patient, conduct a medical screening, and report findings to the private physician.
   D. Have the patient sign in so that the ED is aware that patient is in the waiting area. Require the parents to sign the form refusing care by the ED staff.
   E. Based on provider status this patient may be treated differently as a courtesy to the private physician.

2. A 14-year-old boy comes to the ED with a severe laceration of his right arm. The wound is bleeding profusely. However, the teenager is not accompanied by an adult. All of the following statements are *true except:*
   A. Although the ED has the duty to evaluate the minor's wound, any care provider is prohibited from treating the minor without parental consent.
   B. The minor may be examined and treated if the health care professional evaluates the condition as an emergency.
   C. The minor may be treated if the minor appreciates the nature of his condition and the alternatives to and consequences of this treatment.
   D. The patient may be treated if parental consent can be obtained by phone.
   E. The patient may be treated if his 25-year-old aunt arrives with a written note from the mother and consents to treatment.

3. A 16-year-old girl comes to the ED complaining of sudden onset of right flank pain. The girl has a 2-year-old daughter whom she financially supports. Which of the following statements is *most correct?*
   A. The girl can consent for treatment for her daughter but not for herself.
   B. The girl can consent to treatment for both herself and her daughter.
   C. The girl can be examined only if her parents sign a consent to treatment.
   D. The girl may be examined during a medical screening; however, she cannot be treated unless it is a medical emergency.
   E. The girl cannot be treated without parental notification if the symptoms could be related to sexually transmitted diseases or pregnancy.

4. An unconscious 10-year-old girl arrives in the ED via ambulance. All of the following statements regarding her care are *true except:*
   A. Because the patient is unconscious and there is no parent or guardian present in the ED, consent is presumed in this probable medical emergency.
   B. The patient may be examined and resuscitated if required, but no invasive procedures may be performed without consent of a parent or a court order.
   C. The police can be notified if parents or legal guardian cannot be located.
   D. Once a parent or legal guardian has been located, physician should obtain informed consent to treat.
   E. Emergency medical service (EMS) personnel should be interviewed to obtain as much information as possible regarding circumstances surrounding the injury and the location of the family.

5. A parent comes in with a 13-year-old boy and says the son has been acting "kind of crazy" lately. By way of example, the parent says the boy has been leaving the house at night, staying out late, and running with the "wrong kind of crowd." The parent demands that the ED physician perform a drug test on the son. Which of the following statements is *incorrect?*
   A. The physician can order a drug test and provide the results to the parent, the minor, or both.
   B. The physician may refuse to do the drug test.
   C. The physician is not required to perform a drug test simply because the guardian of the minor requests it.
   D. If the adolescent refuses to have the test done, the physician cannot perform the test.
   E. If the minor refuses to have the test done, the ED staff may, if medically indicated, perform the test.
6. A mother brings in an infant who has a temperature of 105° F (40.6° C) and is limp and lethargic. After appropriate testing the ED physician determines that the child may be suffering from meningitis. The mother refuses to allow the physician to administer any antibiotics, regardless of the route. In this circumstance the physician should first:
   A. Start antibiotic intravenous therapy against the express wishes of the mother.
   B. Discharge the child against medical advice.
   C. Admit the child without starting antibiotics.
   D. Call administration for a court order to start antibiotic therapy.
   E. Call child protective services.
7. An ambulance brings an unconscious 15-year-old boy into the ED. The teenager has no identification, and his parents cannot be contacted immediately. The ED physician should do the following:
   A. Monitor the patient carefully but not conduct any invasive procedures until parental consent can be obtained.
   B. Transfer the patient to a facility that has previously treated the patient.
   C. Require the chief executive officer to sign consent forms.
   D. If required to treat the emergency, have the patient taken to surgery.
   E. Locate the guardian before treatment.
8. EMS personnel bring in a patient who has been severely beaten. Injuries include a fractured skull, a broken arm, and multiple severe contusions. As an ED physician, you have a duty to do which of the following:
   A. Report the incident to the local police department.
   B. Treat the patient if an emergency medical condition exists.
   C. Attempt to contact the parents or legal guardian as soon as possible.
   D. Document all information obtained or observed regarding the incident.
   E. All of the above.
9. A patient comes to the ED with complaints of breathing difficulty and chest pain. The decision is made to admit the patient to a floor for further observation and testing. No bed is available on the floor immediately, so the patient is placed in the hallway on a stretcher to await transport. While awaiting transport, the patient stops breathing, the mother starts screaming, and the patient is rushed back to the ED. The mother, as plaintiff, sues for malpractice on behalf of the patient. Can the mother succeed in her claim based on negligence of ED personnel?
   A. Yes, if the patient suffered damage.
   B. Yes, regardless of whether the patient suffered any damage.
   C. No, because the patient was not in the ED when the incident occurred.
   D. No, because once the decision to admit a patient has been made, the ED no longer has a duty to the patient.
   E. No, because even if the patient suffered damage, the ED personnel did not directly cause the damage.
10. A 2-year-old child is brought to the ED with a temperature of 103° F (39.4° C). The parents are insured by a health maintenance organization (HMO) that does not authorize treatment by your facility. The nurse practitioner performs triage, examining the child and taking the temperature, blood pressure, and medical history. Does this meet the facility's duty to screen the child appropriately to determine whether an emergency medical condition exists?
   A. Yes, if the child is in no apparent distress and the parents are trustworthy to return if the child's condition grows worse.
   B. Yes, if the vital signs are normal and the examination was sufficient to rule out a medical emergency.
   C. No. Simple triage is not the same as a medical screening examination.
   D. No. The patient should be further examined and treated regardless of the ability to pay.
   E. No. The examination was not conducted by a physician.
11. A 3-year-old child is brought to the ED by hearing-impaired parents. Neither parent can communicate by talking or reading lips. Which of the following best summarizes your obligations to this family?
   A. The family should be referred to a nearby facility that has sign language interpreters on staff.
   B. If possible, a sign language interpreter should be contacted to communicate with the parents.
   C. The 3-year-old child can be used as an interpreter between ED staff and the parents.
   D. A mixture of body language and informal sign language can be used to communicate with the parents.

12. On your way to work, you witness a car accident. You stop and perform emergency first aid on the passengers of one car. What best describes your liability?
    A. None, as long as you do not charge for your services.
    B. None, as long as all acts are done in good faith.
    C. Low, as long as there is an emergency and services are rendered in good faith.
    D. Low, as long as you do not charge. It is outside your practice and you have no preexisting duty to treat victim.
    E. High, if the patient's injuries are misdiagnosed and the patient suffers damages as a result.

13. The Federal Express deliverer passes out in the waiting area of your children's hospital. You render emergency services in the waiting room. What best describes *your* liability for treating this patient?
    A. You have limited liability even if you do not charge the patient for the services.
    B. You are liable for all services provided.
    C. You would be liable if you did not render services because you have a duty to the patient.
    D. You are not liable because there was an emergency.
    E. You are liable because services are rendered in a medical facility.

14. Which of the following statements regarding EMTALA (a federal statute mandating the medical examination and stabilization of patients in emergencies) is *incorrect?*
    A. Treatment is required of any emergency condition.
    B. An appropriate medical screening examination is required, including appropriate ancillary services, to determine whether an emergency medical condition exists.
    C. Admission to the hospital is required if clinically warranted.
    D. Stabilization of a medical condition is required when, in the absence of immediate medical attention, the condition could place the health of a patient in serious jeopardy or seriously impair body functions or organs.
    E. A safe and appropriate transfer to another facility is required once the patient is medically stabilized.

15. An 8-year-old boy comes to the ED with severe right arm pain caused by a fall. An x-ray film of the arm shows that the boy has a severe fracture requiring immediate surgery. However, your facility does not have any orthopedic surgeons on staff to perform the operation. Your responsibilities include all of the following *except:*
    A. Stabilizing the fracture to prevent further injury.
    B. Providing pain relief for the child.
    C. Locating an appropriately qualified orthopedic surgeon to operate on the child.
    D. Transferring the child to a facility equipped to perform this procedure.
    E. Suggesting parents arrange private transportation of the patient to another facility.

16. A 15-year-old in labor comes to the ED. The patient is in the early stages of labor. The cervix has not yet become dilated or completely effaced. Your facility does not have an obstetric service. Your duty as a physician in the ED is to:
    A. Arrange for or perform delivery of the baby in the ED.
    B. Admit the patient to the hospital and locate an obstetrician to deliver the baby.
    C. Monitor the well-being of the fetus and the mother, determine whether the patient is in imminent danger of delivering the baby, and if not, transfer the patient to another facility with an obstetric service after appropriate communication.
    D. Attempt to arrest labor and transfer the patient.

17. The patient comes in after having been bitten severely by the family dog. What best describes the responsibility to report this incident?
    A. The bite must be reported only if there is rabies in the area.
    B. The bite must be reported only if dog has been exposed to rabies.
    C. The bite need not be reported if there is no known rabies exposure.
    D. The bite need not be reported if the patient is prophylactically treated for rabies.
    E. The bite must be reported regardless of rabies exposure.

18. The police bring an 18-year-old man to the pediatric ED and demand that ED staff members conduct a body cavity search for packets of cocaine. Are you required to examine or treat the patient?
    A. Yes. Because the patient is in police custody, the patient must be examined and treated.
    B. No, because the patient denies ingesting cocaine.
    C. No. Because the man is 18, he can refuse all services.
    D. Yes. A medical screening must at least be conducted.
    E. No. The police have no authority to order treatment.

19. A mother brings her 12-year-old daughter to the ED for treatment of her severely sprained ankle. The patient's insurance covers only care at a nearby facility. Does your facility have a duty to the patient?
    A. No, because you have a right to compensation for your work.
    B. No, because a sprained ankle is not a true medical emergency.
    C. Yes. The patient must be examined to determine if an emergency exists.
    D. Yes. The patient must be examined and treated only if the insurance company agrees to pay.
    E. Yes. The patient must be treated only if the patient guarantees payment.

The next two questions involve the following scenario: While you are sitting in a restaurant, a child at a nearby table starts to choke.

20. You do nothing, and the family later finds out you are a physician. Can the family succeed in a malpractice action based on your omission?
    A. Yes, because your omission was the proximate cause of harm to the child.
    B. Yes, because the child suffered harm as a result.
    C. No, because you had no duty to the child.
    D. No, because the restaurant should have been prepared for such a situation.
    E. Yes, because by virtue of your training, you owed a duty to the child.

21. You immediately rush to the aid of the child and dislodge a piece of hot dog from the child's throat. In the process, the child sustains a broken rib, which should be considered a possible complication of the Heimlich maneuver. Can the family succeed in a malpractice action based on your involvement?
    A. Yes, because even Good Samaritans are liable for gross negligence.
    B. Yes, because your action was the proximate cause of the child's damage.
    C. No, because the injury could have been sustained elsewhere.
    D. No, because care was rendered in an emergency outside your regular practice, and there was no gross negligence.
    E. Yes, because the child was injured.

ANSWERS [See Barkin et al: Chapter 10.]

1. The answer is **C,** page 82.
   Although the patient is waiting for a private physician to evaluate her condition, this does not relieve the hospital or the physician on duty of all responsibility to her and her parents. The right of parents to refuse care for their children while waiting for their private doctor is not absolute. The decision to refuse treatment must be an informed decision. Therefore a brief medical screening, which is required by federal law, should be conducted to rule out an acute emergency. The parents may still refuse treatment, however, as long as the child is not in danger and the parents indicate a desire to wait.

2. The answer is **A,** pages 82 and 83.
   Although parental consent should be obtained before treating a minor, it is not required every time a minor is treated. For example, a minor almost always can be treated in an emergency. If life, limb, or any body function is in danger, an emergency exists. Also, in many states a minor can be treated if classified as *mature.* A mature minor, generally, is near the age of majority and is able to appreciate the nature of conditions, the alternatives, and the consequences of treatment versus nontreatment. Phone consent, although not optimal, is a substitute for a parent being present in the ED. However, two people should confirm a telephone consent. In all cases the risk of performing the test must be weighed against its benefits. The key to acting *in loco parentis* (in the place of the parent) is whether the decisions that are made are reasonable.

3. The answer is **B,** pages 83 and 84.
   Although states vary on their definition of an emancipated minor, generally minors who are financially independent, living away from home, married, or a member of the U.S. Army are considered able to make health care decisions on behalf of themselves. In many states being the primary caretaker of a child allows the mother to make decisions on behalf of herself and her child. Here, the girl financially supports her daughter, indicating a level of independence that would afford the mother emancipated minor status. As a parent, the girl can almost always consent to treat her child. However, in this scenario only the mother requires treatment. Right flank pain can be indicative of a sexually transmitted disease or pregnancy. Many states allow minors to consent to their own treatment of these conditions. If the girl meets the definition of emancipated minor in the state where she is seeking treatment, an emergency does not have to exist in order for her to be treated. However, if an emergency does exist, the patient can be treated without parental consent regardless of her being a minor.

4. The answer is **B,** page 84.
   If there is danger of harm to life, limb, or body function, the medical staff has a duty to treat the child regardless of whether a guardian has been located or a court has issued an order. Here, the girl is unconscious, indicating that delay in treatment could present a risk of danger to life, limb, or body function. Therefore the patient can be treated in an ED.

5. The answer is **D,** page 83.

The ED physician does not have a duty to perform every test requested by a layperson. Rather, the physician's license gives the physician the right to order laboratory tests if clinically warranted. Drug tests, regardless of the circumstances surrounding the request, should be performed only for medical reasons. The test can be performed whether or not the minor patient consents as long as the guardian consents to the procedure. However, an informed consent should be obtained if drawing blood or catheterizing an uncooperative patient is necessary.

6. The best answer is **A,** page 83.

If antibiotic therapy is necessary to prevent imminent danger to the life of a minor, therapy should not be withheld while awaiting a court order. In addition, the child should not be discharged from an institution simply because a parent refuses the course of treatment recommended by the physician. If the physician determines that antibiotic therapy should be started as soon as possible but that it is not critical to start immediately, the physician can admit the child without starting therapy while administration intervenes with the parents. Parents do not have the unchallenged right to withhold lifesaving therapy from their children. Even in cases where a parent's religious beliefs prevent the parent from accepting medical treatment, the courts have held that emergency medical treatment can be given over parental objections.

7. The answer is **D,** page 84.

If required, even invasive procedures can be performed without consent in an emergency. Consent to treat is presumed in this case because the minor is unconscious. If a parent or legal guardian is not available, having hospital personnel sign consent forms will not obviate the hospital from liability. Also, although the ED physician should treat the emergency immediately, there is no reason that a guardian cannot be located simultaneously.

8. The answer is **E,** pages 84 and 85.

Both penetrating and nonpenetrating injuries resulting from acts of violence or criminal activity must be reported to the police. Injuries in this case could also be the result of child abuse and may also have to be reported to child protective services. If a child's condition is a medical emergency, meaning that the condition threatens the life, limb, or any body function of the minor, treatment as an emergency is presumed even without parental consent.

9. The answer is **A,** pages 90 and 91.

For the mother to win her claim based on medical negligence, she must show: (a) that the ED had a duty to the patient, (b) that the ED breached that duty, (c) that the patient suffered damages, and (d) that the alleged breach proximately caused the patient's damages. Here, regardless of the ED's decision to admit, the patient is the ED's responsibility until the patient is transferred. Therefore, by not monitoring the patient more closely or recognizing how ill the patient was, the ED breached that duty. As long as the patient suffered damage (and stopping breathing can be considered damage) and that injury can be connected to the ED's failure to monitor the child more closely, the mother could win the malpractice action.

10. The answer is **B,** page 88.

Although EMTALA requires that qualified personnel conduct the medical screening examination, it does not specifically require the examination to be conducted by a physician. As long as the nurse practitioner is acting within the scope of licensure and all patients are treated similarly, the nurse practitioner may be authorized to conduct the medical screening examination. The examination must be detailed enough to rule out a medical emergency, and answer B states it was. The examination went beyond mere triage, so the fact that it occurred during triage is not significant.

11. The answer is **B,** page 85.

If possible, a sign language interpreter should be called in. The Americans with Disabilities Act requires hospitals that accept federal funds to be accessible to patients with disabilities. The hospital is required to make reasonable accommodation to a patient with a disability. Here, the patient is not disabled, but the parents, as the legal guardians of the patient, must also be accommodated. The patient should never be referred to another facility based on disability. This can be construed as discrimination on the basis of disability. Moreover, although the emergency physician and department are under no obligation to provide a sign language interpreter for all cases, if possible, one should be obtained. An exchange of written communication can substitute for sign language translation.

12. The answer is **D,** pages 85 and 86.

Good Samaritan statutes generally provide immunity from malpractice actions for physicians and others who provide service in an emergency situation. Usually, to fall within the statutory immunity: (a) assistance must be rendered free of charge, (b) there is an emergency circumstance, (c) care is provided outside the physician's usual practice, and (d) there is no preexisting duty to the patient. The physician's services must be rendered in good faith and without gross negligence.

13. The answer is **A,** pages 85 and 86.

    The rendering of services (a) free of charge, (b) in an emergency, (c) outside of the physician's usual practice, and (d) by a physician with no duty to treat the patient is covered by most Good Samaritan statutes. Here, the Federal Express deliverer, an adult, loses consciousness in the hospital. The only question is whether because services are rendered in a medical facility, this is outside the physician's usual practice. Because the patient did not intentionally seek services, the services were not rendered in the ED, and the physician usually treats children, aiding this patient can be considered outside the physician's usual practice.

14. The answer is **A,** pages 87 to 90.

    EMTALA specifically requires a facility to provide a medical screening examination, stabilizing treatment, or appropriate and safe transfer of the patient. EMTALA does not require treatment of any emergency condition. If an emergency exists, the facility is required to provide further medical examination and such treatment that may be required to stabilize a medical condition within the staff and facilities available at the hospital. Therefore the facility is not responsible to operate if there are no surgeons on staff.

15. The answer is **E,** pages 87 to 90.

    EMTALA requires the hospital to provide an appropriate medical screening examination within the capability of the hospital's ED to determine whether an emergency condition exists. If an emergency condition is determined to exist, as it does here, the hospital must either: (a) provide staff and facilities to further examine and treat the patient so as to stabilize the medical condition, or (b) transfer the individual to another medical facility that can treat the emergency medical condition. EMTALA does not require the hospital to provide staff to treat every conceivable medical emergency. Here, the ED physician should stabilize the patient as best as possible and arrange for transportation of the patient to another facility appropriately equipped to deal with the emergency. The ED is not required to transfer all patients. However, in this case, the arm could be only temporarily stabilized.

16. The answer is **C,** pages 87 to 90.

    If the facility does not have an obstetric service, the facility may and should transfer the pregnant woman who is having contractions to another hospital before delivery if there is adequate time to do so safely. If, however, there is inadequate time to transfer her, or the transfer poses a threat to the health or safety of the woman or unborn child, the delivery of the child and placenta may have to be performed at the facility. In this case the facility should have an emergency vehicle waiting to transfer the mother and newborn child to an appropriate facility for postbirth care. The first facility is under an obligation to stabilize the patient, which means that no material deterioration of the condition is likely within reasonable medical probability to result from or occur during the transfer of the patient from the first facility to the receiving facility.

17. The answer is **E,** page 84.

    Most jurisdictions require that severe dog bites be reported regardless of rabies exposures. Although rabies is one concern, control of savage animals is also a great public concern. Reporting of other animal bites, including those of raccoons, skunks, bats, and rodents, also is required in most jurisdictions.

18. The answer is **D,** page 87.

    Although the patient is 18 years old, an attempt must be made to examine him to determine if an emergency exists. The staff also must determine if the patient is competent. If competent, the patient could refuse further treatment. However, if the patient purposely or inadvertently ingested cocaine, he may not be competent to consent to or refuse treatment. Therefore ED staff must at a minimum examine the patient. However, the ED staff must remember that the man is a patient regardless of police activity. If there is no medical reason for further treatment or examination, the police cannot demand that further treatment be given. For the physician to be able to examine the patient best, the police should be asked to leave.

19. The answer is **C,** pages 87 and 88.

    EMTALA requires only that a facility's staff stabilize and treat a medical emergency. An emergency medical condition is defined in the statue as "a medical condition manifesting itself by acute symptoms of sufficient severity such that the absence of immediate medical attention could reasonably expect it to result in placing the health of the individual in serious jeopardy." If the employee performing the medical screening rules out a medical emergency, the hospital may transfer the patient to another facility or advise the patient to seek care elsewhere.

20. The answer is **C,** pages 90 and 91.

    While a physician working in an ED owes a duty to all patients who come to the ED, the physician does not owe a duty to all people at all times. Therefore the omission was not a breach of any duty or the proximate cause of any harm.

21. The answer is **D,** pages 85 and 86.

    Care rendered in an emergency situation outside a physician's usual practice is usually granted immunity from lawsuits under local Good Samaritan laws. Here, you had no preexisting duty to the patient. Care was rendered free of charge outside the usual practice. These factors indicate that you were indeed acting as a Good Samaritan.

Respiratory Distress and Failure

Javier Sanchez

See Barkin et al: Chapter 11.

1. A 6-week-old infant comes to the ED with signs of respiratory distress. Which of the following findings would be consistent with impending respiratory failure?
   A. Bilateral basilar rales.
   B. A respiratory rate of 45 breaths per minute.
   C. Audible grunting.
   D. Wheezing auscultated at the axillae.
   E. Acrocyanosis.
2. A 14-month-old infant comes to the ED with cyanosis, tachypnea, and altered mental status. Which of the following findings most supports the decision to intubate the child's trachea immediately?
   A. Arterial blood gas measurement showing a pH of 7.25.
   B. Pulse oximetry reading of 87% on room air.
   C. $Paco_2$ of 56 mm Hg.
   D. Clinical assessment revealing the presence of respiratory failure.
   E. Pao_2 of 56 mm Hg.
3. An unconscious 15-year-old boy is brought to the ED because of massive facial trauma and bleeding. The patient was punched and kicked by four other boys and is in respiratory distress. Which of the following is the best method of securing his airway?
   A. Placement of a nasopharyngeal airway.
   B. Blind nasotracheal intubation.
   C. Placement of an oropharyngeal airway.
   D. Cricothyroidotomy
   E. Bag-valve ventilation.
4. Which of the following physical findings is seen only with lower airway disease?
   A. Audible grunting.
   B. Inspiratory stridor.
   C. Tachypnea.
   D. Rales.
   E. Cyanosis.
5. A 6-week-old infant is brought to the ED. The mother is concerned that her baby "is not right." Which of the following sets of vital signs would reflect impending respiratory distress, failure, and shock in a 6-week-old infant?
   A. Respiratory rate 60 bpm
      Heart rate 160 bpm
      Blood pressure (systolic) 75 mm Hg
   B. Respiratory rate 50 bpm
      Heart rate 150 bpm
      Blood pressure (systolic) 75 mm Hg
   C. Respiratory rate 80 bpm
      Heart rate 180 bpm
      Blood pressure (systolic) 60 mm Hg
   D. Respiratory rate 45 bpm
      Heart rate 130 bpm
      Blood pressure (systolic) 80 mm Hg
   E. Respiratory rate 30 bpm
      Heart rate 100 bpm
      Blood pressure (systolic) 70 mm Hg
6. In the patient described in question 5, which of the following is the best immediate therapeutic option after positioning the head, administering oxygen by mask, and giving fluids?
   A. Placement of an oral airway.
   B. Placement of a head box with Fio_2 of 50%.
   C. Placement of nasal prongs with oxygen flow rate of 6 L/min.
   D. Intubation of the child's trachea.
   E. Performance of a cricothyroidotomy.
7. A 5-year-old known asthmatic arrives in the ED in acute distress. The patient has marked tachypnea, subcostal retractions, and diffuse wheezing bilaterally. Which method of oxygen delivery will deliver the highest possible concentration of oxygen?
   A. Nasal cannulae.
   B. Face tent.
   C. Nonrebreathing O_2 mask.
   D. Venturi mask.

8. You have just intubated the trachea of a 6-month-old infant. Which of the following *best* demonstrates the correct placement of an endotracheal tube (ET)?
   A. Presence of bilateral breath sounds over the chest and abdomen.
   B. Condensation in the ET.
   C. Slight improvement in O_2 saturation.
   D. Assessment of end-tidal CO_2.
   E. Chest wall movement.

9. Three hours later, while receiving mechanical ventilation, the child described in question 8 acutely deteriorates. Which of the following would be the *least* helpful in the management of this child?
   A. Suction the ET.
   B. Obtain an arterial blood gas.
   C. Obtain a chest x-ray.
   D. Auscultate both lung fields.
   E. Ask the respiratory therapy team to evaluate the equipment.

10. Infants are more susceptible than adults to respiratory emergencies because of which of the following?
   A. Greater resistance in lower airways.
   B. Large tongue, small mandible, and soft epiglottis.
   C. More compliant, less stable chest wall.
   D. Higher metabolic requirements.
   E. All of the above.

For questions 11 to 14, match the following artificial airways and the appropriate clinical scenario.
   A. Oropharyngeal airway.
   B. Nasopharyngeal airway.
   C. Both.
   D. Neither.

11. _____ Indicated in conscious or semiconscious patients.
12. _____ Prevents the soft tissue of the oropharynx from collapsing.
13. _____ May be used with bag-valve-mask (BVM) ventilation.
14. _____ Prevents intubated patients from biting and occluding the ET.

15. A 3-year-old child is brought to the ED after the parents noticed that he was coughing while playing with a toy made of small pieces. The child is having some difficulty breathing, and stridor is noted. Which of the following is indicated at this time?
   A. Four hard back blows.
   B. A finger sweep of the child's mouth.
   C. Nasotracheal intubation.
   D. Abdominal thrusts.
   E. Administration of nebulized racemic epinephrine.

16. Pulse oximetry can be accurately used to monitor patients with all of the following conditions *except:*
   A. Hypoxemia.
   B. Carbon monoxide poisoning.
   C. Sickle cell disease.
   D. Cystic fibrosis.
   E. Cyanotic heart disease.

17. Which of the following clinical conditions is not an indication for intubation?
   A. Hypoventilation.
   B. Loss of protective airway reflexes.
   C. Severe bronchospasm.
   D. Metabolic alkalosis.
   E. Pulmonary toilet.

ANSWERS   [See Barkin et al: Chapter 11.]

1. The answer is **C,** page 97.
   The presence of grunting is considered an ominous sign of impending respiratory failure. The presence of tachypnea, rales, wheezing, and cyanosis is consistent with a diagnosis of bronchiolitis. Bronchiolitis is the most common cause of respiratory distress and failure in children younger than 1 year old.

2. The answer is **D,** page 100.
   The decision to intubate and secure the airway is usually based on clinical findings, response to oxygen administration, and laboratory findings. A child with altered mental status and cyanosis has significant tissue hypoxia. Clinical assessment revealing respiratory failure should prompt immediate treatment designed to provide adequate ventilatory support. Obtaining radiographic or laboratory studies would only delay such a decision.

3. The answer is **D,** page 100.
   Patients with severe facial or airway trauma require cricothyroidotomy or tracheostomy to secure the airway. Orotracheal and nasotracheal intubation is quite difficult and is relatively contraindicated in most patients with significant facial trauma.

4. The answer is **D,** page 97.
   Rales, wheezing, and rhonchi are consistent with lower airway pathology. Upper airway causes of respiratory distress are produced by partial obstruction. They have been described as stridor, stertor (snoring), or gurgling.

TABLE 9-1   Vital Signs by Age

Age	Respirations (breaths per min)	Pulse (beats per min)	Blood pressure (systolic: mm Hg)
Newborn	30-60	100-160	50-70
1-6 wks	30-60	100-160	70-95
6 mon	25-40	90-140	80-100
1 yr	20-40	90-130	80-100
3 yrs	20-30	80-120	80-110
6 yrs	12-25	70-110	80-110
10 yrs	12-20	60-90	90-120

TABLE 9-2   Available O_2 Delivery Systems

Device	Room air entrainment	Concentration of O_2	Flow needed
Simple mask	Yes	30%-60%	6-10 L/min
Partial rebreather	Yes	50%-60%	10-12 L/min
Non-rebreather	No	Up to 95%	10-12 L/min
Venturi mask	Yes	Variable but predictable	Variable
Face tent/shield	Yes	Up to 40%	10-15 L/min
Oxygen hood	No	80%-90%	10-15 L/min
Oxygen tent	Yes	30%-50%	10-15 L/min
Nasal cannula	Yes	Variable	Up to 4 L/min

Box 9-1
Indications for Intubation

Acute respiratory failure
- Po_2 <60 mm Hg or Sao_2 <93% or Fio_2 >0.6 (sea level)
- Pco_2 >50 mm Hg (acutely)
- Apnea
- Hypoventilation

Airway protection
- Neurologic dysfunction (seizure, ingestion, coma)
- Loss of protective airway reflexes (gagging, coughing)
- Inability to control copious secretions (CHF, ARDS, infection)
- Upper airway obstruction, airway edema, trauma
- Ingestion
- Airway edema, trauma, burns

Decrease the work of breathing
- Hemodynamic instability
- Metabolic acidosis
- Severe bronchospasm

Therapeutic intervention
- Hyperventilation for increased ICP
- Emergency drug administration with no vascular access
- Pulmonary toilet

---

5. The answer is **C,** page 97.
   The upper and lower limits for respiratory rate, heart rate, and blood pressure are listed in the table below. In the child presented in the scenario, a respiratory rate of 80 breaths per minute, heart rate of 180 beats per minute, and blood pressure of 60 mm Hg (systolic) would be consistent with a diagnosis of respiratory distress, failure, and shock (Table 9-1).

6. The answer is **D,** pages 96 and 97.
   The infant described is in shock. This places an increased metabolic demand on the infant. The infant's trachea should be intubated to allow for a decreased work of breathing, which is contributing to the state of shock. The infant will not tolerate an oral airway, and a head box and nasal prongs are not appropriate in this case. The infant does not require a surgical airway (i.e., cricothyroidotomy).

7. The answer is **C,** pages 98 and 99.
   A nonrebreathing mask can deliver up to 95% O_2. Nasal cannulae and Venturi masks can deliver variable concentrations of oxygen. Face tents can deliver up to 40% oxygen. It is also important to remember that the most effective delivery system is the one the child will tolerate (Table 9-2).

8. The answer is **D,** page 100.
   Signs associated with successful endotracheal intubation are visualization of the ET passing through the vocal cords, condensation in the ET, clinical improvement in the patient, chest wall movement, and symmetric breath sounds over both lung fields. The color change or specific wave pattern associated with the use of an end-tidal CO_2 device is a confirmation test. It is the most accurate and rapid method that reflects successful endotracheal intubation. Changes in oxygen saturation by pulse oximetry significantly lag behind information obtained from a CO_2 capnometer.

9. The answer is **B,** page 103.
   Obtaining an arterial blood gas will confirm the deterioration, not the cause. Deterioration of a child on a respirator can be remembered with the mnemonic *DOPE*:

   Dislodged tube: can be assessed by auscultating both lung fields.
   Obstructed tube: requiring suctioning.
   Pneumothorax: confirmed by x-ray.
   Equipment failure: requiring assessment by appropriate personnel.

10. The answer is **E,** page 96.

All of the factors noted in this question contribute to infants being more susceptible to respiratory emergencies. Infants are susceptible because of the (a) increased physical work of breathing, which increases oxygen consumption, and (b) smaller airway, which produces increased resistance to airflow, especially when traumatized or inflamed. The effect of airway edema is that 1 mm of edema in the normal infant trachea decreases the cross-sectional area by 75% and increases resistance sixteenfold.

Answers for questions 11 to 14 come from page 98 in Barkin et al.

11. **B**
12. **C**
13. **C**
14. **A**

Oropharyngeal airways are used in unconscious patients. Nasopharyngeal airways are better tolerated in conscious patients. They both keep the soft tissues of the oropharynx from collapsing against the posterior pharyngeal wall. They may both be used in concert with BVM ventilation. Oropharyngeal airways are used in intubated patients to prevent biting of the tube.

15. The answer is **D,** page 101.

The child is conscious, so stand behind the patient and place your hands in the midline about the level of the abdomen. One hand should be made into a fist and pressure exerted into the patient's abdomen with a quick upward motion and repeated until the foreign body is dislodged or 10 maneuvers have been completed. Back blows are used in infants. Intubation is not warranted in this alert, responsive child. Nebulized racemic epinephrine is not indicated, and blind finger sweeps should *not* be performed in a conscious child. However, blind finger sweeps are recommended if the child becomes unconscious.

16. The answer is **B,** page 99.

Pulse oximetry can be used to monitor patients with all of the conditions noted except for carbon monoxide poisoning. In addition, it does not reflect oxygen saturation when methemoglobinemia is present.

17. The answer is **D,** page 100.

Common indications for intubations are summarized on page 100. Metabolic alkalosis, as seen in pyloric stenosis, rarely results in respiratory compromise (Box 9-1).

◆
10
◆

Cardiopulmonary Resuscitation

Michael A. Mojica • *Deborah A. Levine*

> See Barkin et al: Chapter 12.

1. Which of the following statements about the pediatric airway is *false?*
   A. The glottic opening is more cephalad and anterior in the neck of a child.
   B. An infant has a short, stiff epiglottis.
   C. The narrowest portion of the airway is below the glottic opening at the level of the cricoid cartilage.
   D. The tongue is relatively large.
   E. Hyperextension of the head may more easily occlude the child's airway.

2. An 8-month-old infant comes to the ED with a 3-day history of cough, runny nose, and fever to 102° F (38.9° C). She is sitting in her father's lap crying. Assessment reveals a respiratory rate (RR) of 60 breaths per minute with mild intercostal retractions. Her color is pink. She has good aeration with a prolonged expiratory phase. No stridor or grunting is heard. How would you describe her breathing status?
   A. Normal breathing.
   B. Respiratory distress.
   C. Early respiratory failure.
   D. Complete respiratory arrest.
   E. Cardiopulmonary arrest, absence of respiratory effort.

3. Appropriate management for the patient in question 2, after determination of pulse oximetry and monitoring, would include:
   A. Keep the patient with the parent, provide oxygen as tolerated, and reassess.
   B. Provide oxygen as tolerated, reassess, and lay the patient flat on a stretcher.
   C. Provide bag-valve-mask (BVM) ventilation with 100% Fio_2 and lay the patient flat on a stretcher.
   D. Perform endotracheal intubation and lay the patient flat on a stretcher.
   E. Initiate a sequence of five back blows and five chest thrusts.

4. A 4-year-old child fell from the top of a playground slide. She is unresponsive and cyanotic without spontaneous respiratory effort. The first step in managing this child's airway would be:
   A. Needle cricothyrotomy.
   B. Five abdominal thrusts.
   C. Jaw thrust maneuver with in-line cervical immobilization.
   D. Head tilt–chin lift maneuver with in-line cervical traction.
   E. Endotracheal intubation using a rapid sequence induction.

5. The 4-year-old child in question 4 requires intubation. The ideal appropriate equipment for this child would include:
   A. 3.0 endotracheal tube (ET) with a straight no. 1 laryngoscope blade.
   B. 4.0 ET with a curved no. 1 laryngoscope blade.
   C. 5.0 ET with a straight no. 2 laryngoscope blade.
   D. 6.0 ET with a curved no. 2 laryngoscope blade.
   E. 7.0 ET with a straight no. 3 laryngoscope blade.

6. Endotracheal intubation is *not* indicated for which of the following:
   A. Control and protection of the airway.
   B. Prolonged mechanical ventilation.
   C. Tension pneumothorax.
   D. Hyperventilation of the patient with a head injury.
   E. Improved oxygen delivery and ventilation.

7. Which circulatory finding is the hallmark of the diagnosis of late (decompensated) shock?
   A. Capillary refill of 4 seconds.
   B. Altered mental status.
   C. Depressed anterior fontanelle.
   D. Hypotension.
   E. Absent distal pulses.

8. An alert, 8-month-old infant has a history of diarrhea. She appears pale and has an RR of 45 breaths per minute, a strong central pulse at a rate of 180 beats per minute, and a systolic blood pressure of 85 mm Hg. Her extremities are cool and mottled and have a capillary refill time of 4 seconds. What would best describe her circulatory status?
   A. Normal circulatory status.
   B. Early (compensated) shock caused by hypovolemia.
   C. Early (compensated) shock caused by supraventricular tachycardia.
   D. Late (decompensated) shock caused by hypovolemia.
   E. Late (decompensated) shock caused by supraventricular tachycardia.

9. Appropriate initial management for the child described in question 8 would include which of the following?
   A. Initiation of an appropriate regimen of oral rehydration therapy.
   B. Placement of an intraosseous line, fluid bolus of 20 ml/kg of normal saline.
   C. Synchronous cardioversion 0.5 joule/kg.
   D. Placement of an intravenous (IV) line, fluid bolus of 20 ml/kg of normal saline.
   E. Placement of an IV line, adenosine 0.1 mg/kg IV.

10. A 5-year-old child involved in a motor vehicle accident has spontaneous respirations but is lethargic. The heart rate (HR) is 160 beats per minute, and blood pressure (BP) is 60/45 mm Hg. The abdomen is tense, distended, and ecchymotic. A trauma surgeon is consulted and calls for an operating room to be readied. Despite 60 ml/kg of normal saline, BP does not improve. The next step in fluid resuscitation of the child would include which of the following?
   A. O-negative whole blood 10 ml/kg.
   B. O-negative packed red blood cells 10 ml/kg.
   C. Normal saline bolus 20 ml/kg.
   D. 5% albumin 10 ml/kg.
   E. Epinephrine 0.1 µg/kg/min IV infusion.

11. A 6-month-old infant is brought to the ED apneic with an HR of 40 beats per minute and a systolic BP of 50 mm Hg. Initial rates of ventilation and chest compressions for this patient include which of the following?
   A. Ventilation: 20 breaths/minute, chest compression: 100/min or more.
   B. Ventilation: 12 breaths/min, chest compression: 80/min.
   C. Ventilation: 40 breaths/min, chest compression: 120/min.
   D. Ventilation: 10 breaths/min, chest compression: 60/min or more.
   E. Ventilation: 60 breaths/min, chest compression: 140/min.

12. The 6-month-old patient in question 11 is adequately oxygenated and ventilated, and chest compressions are initiated. An initial dose of epinephrine is given intravenously, resulting in a transient rise in BP and HR. A repeat dose of epinephrine would include which of the following?
   A. 0.1 mg/kg of the 1:1000 solution IV.
   B. 0.01 mg/kg of the 1:10,000 solution IV.
   C. 0.01 mg/kg of the 1:1000 solution endotracheally.
   D. 0.2 mg/kg of the 1:10,000 solution IV.
   E. 10 µg/kg/min IV infusion.

13. A 3-month-old infant with a 1-day history of irritability and decreased feeding has the following vital signs: HR 45 beats per minute, systolic BP 70 mm Hg. The patient is intubated with no change in vital signs. The capillary refill time is 4 seconds. After administering oxygen, your next step would be:
   A. Observation.
   B. Chest compressions at 100/min.
   C. Epinephrine 0.01 mg/kg of the 1:10,000 solution IV.
   D. Epinephrine 0.1 mg/kg of the 1:1000 solution endotracheally.
   E. Atropine 0.02 mg/kg IV.

14. A 12-year-old child comes to the ED without spontaneous respirations and pulseless. ECG reveals a wide complex tachycardia. Initial management should be:
   A. Defibrillation: 2 joules/kg.
   B. Synchronous cardioversion: 2 joules/kg.
   C. Defibrillation: 0.5 joule/kg.
   D. Epinephrine 0.01 mg/kg of the 1:10,000 solution IV.
   E. Lidocaine 1 mg/kg IV.

15. The patient in question 14 fails to respond to the initial intervention. Subsequent management of this patient would include which of the following?
   A. Defibrillation: 4 joules/kg.
   B. Epinephrine 0.01 mg/kg of 1:10,000 solution.
   C. Synchronous cardioversion: 0.5 joule/kg.
   D. Defibrillation: 2 joules/kg.
   E. Lidocaine 1 mg/kg.

16. A 10-year-old child falls from a tree and is brought to the ED apneic and pulseless. After successful intubation and ventilation the cardiac monitor reveals a narrow complex at a rate of 110 beats per minute without detectable pulses. Management of this patient's circulatory status could include all of the following *except*:
   A. Epinephrine 0.01 mg/kg IV of 1:10,000 solution.
   B. Atropine 0.02 mg/kg.
   C. Obtain IV access, fluid bolus of 20 ml/kg of normal saline.
   D. Needle thoracentesis.
   E. Pericardiocentesis.

17. A 2-month-old infant is found unresponsive in his crib. Assessment reveals an apneic and pulseless infant with the rhythm strip demonstrating asystole confirmed in two leads. After establishing effective ventilations and chest compressions, the initial treatment of choice after oxygen and positioning the head should include which of the following?
    A. Epinephrine 0.01 mg/kg of 1:1000 solution endotracheally.
    B. Defibrillation 2 joules/kg.
    C. Lidocaine 1 mg/kg.
    D. Cardioversion 0.5 joule/kg.
    E. Epinephrine 0.01 mg/kg of 1:10,000 solution IV.

18. A 3-month-old infant is brought in to the ED with a 1-day history of poor eating and rapid breathing. The child is pale with a pulse of 300 beats per minute, BP 50/35 mm Hg. He is found on respiratory examination to have rales, hepatomegaly, and very weak distal pulses. ECG reveals a narrow complex tachycardia at 300. Initial management of this child would be:
    A. Administer adenosine 0.01 mg/kg.
    B. Administer a fluid bolus of normal saline 20 ml/kg.
    C. Synchronous cardioversion 0.5 joule/kg.
    D. Synchronous cardioversion 2 joules/kg.
    E. Administer lidocaine 1 mg/kg via an endotracheal tube.

19. All of the following are true of adenosine *except:*
    A. May be used for unstable supraventricular tachycardia if IV line is in place.
    B. Metabolized rapidly by red blood cells.
    C. Produces a transient heart block.
    D. Given with an initial dose of 0.1 mg/kg.
    E. May be given via endotracheal tube.

20. A 3-kg infant in severe cardiorespiratory compromise caused by bradycardia is being oxygenated and ventilated successfully. Epinephrine is given without response. The correct IV dose of atropine for this patient is:
    A. 0.06 mg
    B. 0.1 mg
    C. 0.5 mg
    D. 1 mg
    E. 2 mg

21. CaCl 10% is indicated for which of the following?
    A. Hypomagnesemia.
    B. Asystole.
    C. Bradycardia.
    D. Hyperkalemia.
    E. β-Blocker overdose.

22. Sodium bicarbonate is indicated for which of the following scenarios:
    A. A 15-year-old who ingested a tricyclic antidepressant with a widened QRS.
    B. A 10-year-old in status asthmaticus with arterial blood gas (ABG) findings of pH 7.24, Pco_2 62, Po_2 75.
    C. A 2-year-old with a witnessed cardiopulmonary arrest 5 minutes ago.
    D. A 5-year-old with acute diarrhea in early hypovolemic shock.
    E. A 6-month-old in cardiogenic shock with a K^+ of 3 mEq/L.

23. A 1-year-old infant is found unresponsive in bed. Assisted ventilation and intravascular access are initiated. The bedside glucose test reveals a glucose level of 20 mg/dl. Initial IV management should include:
    A. D25 2 ml/kg (0.5 g/kg)
    B. D25 8 ml/kg (2 g/kg)
    C. D10 2 ml/kg (0.2 g/kg)
    D. D50 4 ml/kg (2 g/kg)
    E. D5 ⅓ NS at 40 ml qh for 1 hour (0.2 g/kg)

24. A 1-month-old infant comes to the ED with a pulse of 180 beats per minute and BP 50/35 mm Hg. A liver edge is palpable to the umbilicus. Skin is mottled and cool with weak distal pulses. Chest x-ray examination reveals cardiomegaly. During the administration of 20 ml/kg of Ringer's lactate, respirations become labored and rales are heard at both bases. The next step in the management of this patient would be:
    A. Sodium bicarbonate 1 mEq/kg IV.
    B. Repeat fluid bolus 20 ml/kg.
    C. Dopamine 5 to 10 μg/kg/min IV infusion.
    D. Synchronous cardioversion 0.5 joule/kg.
    E. Epinephrine 0.01 mg/kg of the 1:10,000 solution IV.

25. Identify the medication infusion with the correct primary indication:
    A. Isoproterenol—hypertensive crisis.
    B. Dobutamine—normotensive cardiogenic shock.
    C. Nitroprusside—ventricular fibrillation.
    D. Epinephrine—decompensated hypovolemic shock.
    E. Lidocaine—bradycardia associated with severe cardiorespiratory compromise.

ANSWERS   [See Barkin et al: Chapter 12.]

1. The answer is **B**, pages 105 and 106.
   An infant has a relatively large and floppy epiglottis. Airway visualization is generally best achieved using a straight laryngoscope blade to lift the epiglottis away from the airway. All other statements are true.

2. The answer is **B**, page 105.
   Respiratory distress may be characterized by tachypnea and increased work of breathing and may be associated with a change in color or mental status and decreased or abnormal breath sounds (Fig. 10-1).

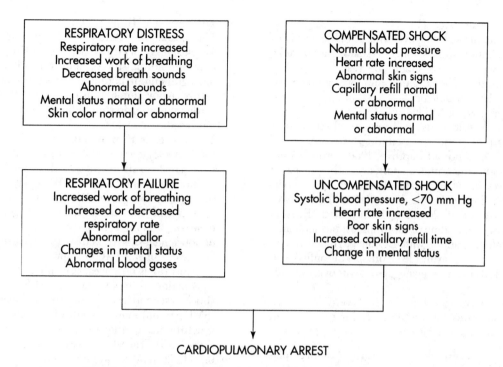

FIG. 10-1 Pathway to cardiopulmonary arrest in the pediatric patient.

3. The answer is **A,** page 105.

The infant or child in respiratory distress should be maintained in a position of comfort with a caregiver, and oxygen should be delivered as tolerated. The patient should be placed on a cardiac and oxygen saturation monitor and reassessed frequently. Specific therapy may be initiated. If the patient is in respiratory failure, the patient should be removed from the caregiver, and effective ventilation initiated. This infant did not manifest any historical or clinical signs suggesting an indication for foreign body–obstructed airway maneuvers.

4. The answer is **C,** page 105.

The initial step in managing the airway in the traumatized child is to open the airway with the jaw thrust maneuver while maintaining the cervical spine in a neutral position. Because this is a case involving trauma, the cervical spine must be protected and the head tilt should not be used.

5. The answer is **C,** page 106.

The correct ET size may be approximated by using the Broselow tape, matching the diameter of the child's fifth finger, or using the following formula: ET tube internal diameter (ID) = [Age (years)/4] + 4. A straight laryngoscope blade is generally used in infants and young children. The correct length of the laryngoscope blade may be measured from the patient's gum or tooth line to the glottic opening.

6. The answer is **C,** page 106.

Endotracheal intubation is indicated for the following: airway control and protection; those who need prolonged mechanical ventilation; patients who have suspected increased intracranial pressure and who require hyperventilation; and improved oxygenation and ventilation. Tension pneumothorax is managed in an emergency with a needle thoracentesis followed by a tube thoracostomy. Positive-pressure ventilation may worsen the course of tension pneumothorax.

7. The answer is **D,** page 105.

Shock is defined as inadequate tissue perfusion. Signs of decreased central organ perfusion such as a decrease in or absence of central pulse or an altered mental status may be present. Changes in distal perfusion are present, such as changes in the character of distal pulses, skin color, skin temperature, and capillary refill. Compensatory mechanisms such as tachycardia and vasoconstriction maintain BP in a normal range during early (compensated) shock. Hypotension is a late and often precipitous finding, and it defines late (decompensated) shock in the pediatric population.

8. The answer is **B,** page 105.

Early (compensated) shock is defined by a normal BP. Tachycardia and signs of poor distal perfusion such as absence of or decrease in distal pulses, changes in skin color or temperature, and a prolonged capillary refill are also present. The history of diarrhea and HR of 180 beats per minute are most suggestive of hypovolemic shock.

9. The answer is **D,** page 111.
Management of early hypovolemic shock consists of fluid resuscitation with isotonic crystalloid at 20 ml/kg IV. Intraosseous access should be reserved for late (decompensated) shock, cardiopulmonary arrest, or urgent medication delivery.

10. The answer is **B,** page 111.
The child described is in traumatic hypovolemic shock. Despite initial resuscitation with crystalloid fluids, vital signs do not improve. Blood products are indicated for the trauma patient with persistent decompensated hypovolemic (hemorrhagic) shock. Packed red blood cells at a dose of 10 ml/kg or whole blood at a dose of 20 ml/kg is indicated. Further boluses of normal saline or albumin are not indicated for the trauma patient with significant blood loss if blood products are available. Epinephrine infusion is not indicated for the management of hypovolemic shock.

11. The answer is **A,** page 108.
The correct rates of rescue breathing and chest compressions are listed below:

	Ventilation	Chest Compressions
Neonate	40-60/min	120/min
Infant	20/min	100/min or more
Child	20/min	100/min
Adult	12/min	80-100/min

12. The answer is **B,** page 109, Fig. 12-7.
The drug of choice for *unstable bradycardia* is epinephrine. The initial dose of IV or intraosseous epinephrine is 0.01 mg/kg of the 1:10,000 solution. Subsequent IV or intraosseous epinephrine doses are the same as the initial dose and can be repeated every 3 to 5 minutes. Endotracheal epinephrine dosage is 0.1 mg/kg of the 1:1000 solution. The higher IV dose of epinephrine is *not* indicated in the treatment of bradycardia. However, it is used in the protocol for *asystole* and *ventricular fibrillation.* The correct epinephrine infusion rate is 0.05 to 1 µg/kg/min.

13. The answer is **B,** page 109.
Chest compressions are indicated for a patient in shock with an HR less than 80 beats per minute (infant) and less than 60 beats per minute (child) after securing an airway. Immediate pharmacologic management of bradycardia is reserved for patients manifesting signs of severe cardiorespiratory compromise, such as poor perfusion, hypotension, or respiratory difficulty.

14. The answer is **A,** pages 109 and 110.
Pulseless ventricular tachycardia is a nonperfusing rhythm that is managed immediately with defibrillation at an energy level of 2 joules/kg.

15. The answer is **A,** pages 109 and 110.
If an initial defibrillation attempt at an energy level of 2 joules/kg is unsuccessful, a second and third attempt at 4 joules/kg should follow. Pharmacologic management with epinephrine, lidocaine, or bretylium may be required if initial attempts at defibrillation are unsuccessful.

16. The answer is **B,** page 109.
The circulatory status of this patient is described as pulseless electrical activity (PEA). Epinephrine may be administered, and the identification and management of potentially treatable causes such as severe hypovolemia, tension pneumothorax, and pericardial tamponade should be initiated. Atropine is not indicated.

17. The answer is **E,** page 110.
Pharmacologic management of asystolic cardiopulmonary arrest consists primarily of epinephrine. Initial IV or intraosseous dosage is 0.01 mg/kg of the 1:10,000 solution. Subsequent IV or intraosseous doses of epinephrine may be given at 10 times the standard dose or 0.1 mg/kg of the 1:1000 solution. Initial endotracheal dosage is also 10 times the standard or 0.1 mg/kg of the 1:1000 solution.

18. The answer is **C,** pages 111 and 112.
This patient is in congestive heart failure (cardiogenic shock) secondary to supraventricular tachycardia (SVT). Initial management of *unstable* SVT includes synchronous cardioversion at 0.5 joule/kg. Alternatively, if IV access is readily available, adenosine 0.1 mg/kg may be administered.

19. The answer is **E,** page 112.
Adenosine is the drug of choice for SVT. It is indicated for unstable SVT when IV or intraosseous access is already established. Adenosine has a half-life of 10 seconds. It produces a transient atrioventricular block that terminates the reentry rhythm. The dose is 0.1 mg/kg up to a maximum of 12 mg. Adenosine cannot be administered via the endotracheal route.

20. The answer is **B,** page 115.
Atropine is indicated for symptomatic bradycardia at a dose of 0.02 mg/kg via the IV or intraosseous route. A minimum dose of 0.1 mg is recommended because of an association of paradoxical bradycardia with lower doses. Although optimal endotracheal dosage is unknown, a dose of two to three times the standard dosage is often recommended. The maximum dose is 0.5 mg for an infant and 1 mg for a child.

21. The answer is **D,** page 115.
Calcium is indicated only for documented hypocalcemia, hyperkalemia, hypermagnesemia, and calcium channel blocker overdose. Calcium is available as a chloride (10%) at a dose of 0.2 ml/kg. Calcium is not indicated for asystole, bradycardia, or β-blocker overdose.

22. The answer is **A,** page 115.
Sodium bicarbonate is indicated only for documented severe metabolic acidosis with adequate ventilation, for prolonged arrest, or for serum alkalinization for treatment of hyperkalemia or tricyclic antidepressant overdose. Sodium carbonate may worsen respiratory acidosis if inadequate ventilation exists, may cause intracellular acidosis and worsen cardiac contractility, and will cause intracellular shifts, worsening a hypokalemic state.

23. The answer is **A,** page 115.
Hypoglycemia is managed by the administration of dextrose at a dose of 0.5 to 1 g/kg. This can be achieved as follows:

D50	1 to 2 ml/kg
D25	2 to 4 ml/kg
D10	5 to 10 ml/kg
D5	20 to 40 ml/kg

A rapid bolus of a D25 solution is most often recommended for hypoglycemic children. D10 is recommended for neonatal hypoglycemia (page 202 in Barkin et al).

24. The answer is **C,** page 116.
The infant described is in cardiogenic shock. This patient's clinical status deteriorated after initial fluid resuscitation. Dopamine infusion is indicated for patients with poor myocardial and peripheral perfusion. Sodium bicarbonate, additional fluid therapy, cardioversion, or epinephrine is not indicated.

25. The answer is **B,** pages 115 and 116.
Dobutamine is indicated for patients with normotensive cardiogenic shock. It acts as a positive inotrope but causes peripheral vasodilation, which can produce hypotension. Isoproterenol is indicated for hemodynamically significant bradycardia caused by heart block unresponsive to atropine. Nitroprusside is a potent vasodilator used in the treatment of severe hypertension and heart failure unresponsive to diuretic therapy. Epinephrine infusion is indicated for symptomatic bradycardia, hypotension unresponsive to fluid therapy, and cardiopulmonary arrest. Lidocaine infusion is used to treat ventricular dysrhythmias.

CHAPTER

11

Shock

Jessica C. Foltin

See Barkin et al: Chapter 13.

1. Which of the following is *true* regarding scalp vein cannulation?
   A. The overlying skin should not be shaved.
   B. A tourniquet, preferably a rubber band, should be applied at the midface region.
   C. A catheter should be inserted into the most proximal portion of the vein and advanced caudally.
   D. The tourniquet should not be removed before a flush solution is infused. If the proximal scalp blanches, this indicates correct catheter placement.

2. Which of the following statements regarding central vein catheterization is *true?*
   A. Flow rate is indirectly proportional to the catheter gauge.
   B. Flow rate is directly related to catheter length.
   C. Complications are rare.
   D. Local anesthetics are not necessary.
   E. As the radius of the catheter increases, the resistance to flow decreases by the fourth power of the change in the radius.

3. Which of the following statements is *true* regarding venous anatomy?
   A. The femoral vein lies 25 to 50 mm lateral to the femoral artery in most children.
   B. In the pulseless patient the femoral artery can be approximated at a point four fifths of the way from the symphysis pubis to the anterior iliac crest.
   C. The external jugular vein is least visible when the child is in Trendelenburg's position.
   D. The external jugular vein is an ideal location for placement of a guidewire or longer catheter.
   E. The right subclavian vein is more commonly cannulated than the left because the pleural cap is usually lower on the right side.

4. Which of the following is *true* regarding vascular access approaches to the internal jugular vein?
   A. A triangle should be visualized using the bellies of the sternal and clavicular branches of the sterno-cleidomastoid muscle with the sternum creating the base of the triangle.
   B. For the medial approach the needle is inserted into the apex of the triangle, mentioned in answer A, at a 45-degree angle aimed at the ipsilateral nipple.
   C. If unsuccessful, the needle should be withdrawn to a subcutaneous level and redirected more medially.
   D. For the posterior approach, the needle is inserted at the lateral end of the sternocleidomastoid muscle and directed toward the ipsilateral nipple.
   E. The anterior approach to the internal jugular is the simplest approach with the lowest complication rate in children.

5. Which one of the following is *true* regarding intraosseous needle insertion?
   A. In the child younger than 12 years, long bone marrow contains spacious venous sinusoids that conduct medications and fluids into the venous system.
   B. The preferred site in infants and children is the distal tibia.
   C. The sternum is an ideal location for intraosseous needle placement.
   D. A point two finger-breadths below the tibial tuberosity should be chosen for insertion.
   E. Not all resuscitative medications are amenable to intraosseous infusion.

6. A 3-year-old boy comes to the ED with a 3-day history of persistent vomiting and diarrhea. He appears lethargic with a heart rate (HR) of 165 beats per minute, respiratory rate (RR) of 40 breaths per minute, blood pressure (BP) of 80/50 mm Hg, and temperature of 97.8° F. The most likely type of shock in this clinical scenario is:
   A. Hypovolemic shock.
   B. Cardiogenic shock.
   C. Distributive shock.
   D. Septic shock.
   E. Neurogenic shock.

7. Which of the following is *true* regarding management of a patient in septic shock?
   A. Children in shock should not be intubated electively.
   B. Physiologic indications for intubation include an arterial oxygen tension (Pao_2) less than 90 mm Hg with an Fio_2 greater than 0.5.
   C. The most common complication in the intubated child is endotracheal tube kinking.
   D. Optimal positive end-expiratory pressure (PEEP) is associated with decreased intrapulmonary shunting and maximal lung compliance.

8. Which of the following statements is *incorrect* regarding hypovolemic shock?
   A. Hypovolemic shock is the most common type of shock encountered in the pediatric population.
   B. A normal blood pressure may be observed in children with mild to moderate hypovolemic shock.
   C. The initial management of hypovolemic shock should be 20 ml/kg fluid boluses followed by inotropes.
   D. In patients with sepsis, third spacing will protect against hypovolemic shock.
   E. Reduced renal perfusion in shock leads to renal sodium and water retention.

9. Which of the following statements is *incorrect* regarding sepsis and septic shock?
   A. Confirmation of infection with positive blood cultures is not necessary.
   B. The immunocompromised patient frequently develops sepsis from normal bacterial flora.
   C. Myocardial function is normal in patients with septic shock.
   D. Systemic vascular resistance is decreased.
   E. Patient survival has been linked to development of compensatory ventricular dilation.

10. Signs of hypovolemic shock include all of the following *except:*
    A. Tachycardia.
    B. Peripheral vasoconstriction.
    C. Warm extremities.
    D. Delayed capillary refill.
    E. Oliguria.

11. Which of the following statements regarding physical examination and laboratory parameters in hypovolemic shock is *true?*
    A. Capillary refill of greater than 3 seconds indicates a 5% fluid deficit.
    B. The cardiac silhouette is typically large on chest radiograph.
    C. Hypotension is observed as an early sign of significant intravascular fluid loss.
    D. Clinically significant dehydration is associated with weight loss.
    E. A greater compromise in systemic perfusion is seen in the young child compared with the adolescent for a fluid loss of 5% to 7%.

12. Which of the following is *true* regarding volume loss?
    A. Hypernatremic dehydration results when the sodium deficit is greater than the free water deficit.
    B. Hypotension is not observed in patients with hypernatremic dehydration until approximately 25% of body weight is lost.
    C. Acute blood loss usually produces circulatory compromise when 15% to 20% of intravascular volume is lost.
    D. Tachycardia and peripheral vasodilatation is often the only evidence of hemorrhage in the pediatric trauma patient.
    E. Hypotonic dehydration is associated with a proportionally greater loss of water than sodium.

13. Which of the following statements regarding cardiogenic shock is *correct?*
    A. The child with cardiogenic shock shows inadequate perfusion only if inadequate intravascular volume exists.
    B. In cardiogenic shock, adrenergic compensatory mechanisms fail to divert blood flow from the kidneys, gut, and skin to maintain blood flow to heart and brain.
    C. The cardiac silhouette is usually normal in size on chest radiograph.
    D. Signs of cardiogenic shock are often identical to signs of tamponade.
    E. Echocardiography should be used to rule out cardiac tamponade.

14. Reliable early signs of septic shock in a child include which of the following:
    A. Irritability.
    B. Increased serum lactate.
    C. Tachypnea.
    D. Mottled skin.
    E. All of the above.

15. Which of the following statements is *incorrect* regarding ancillary tests?
    A. Lactic acidosis is not a sensitive indicator of inadequate systemic perfusion.
    B. The arterial blood gas is useful to evaluate both ventilation and oxygenation.
    C. The hemoglobin and hematocrit may be artificially normal in the face of an acute decrease in intravascular volume.
    D. A chest radiograph should be performed to check cardiac size and exclude pneumonia, pneumothorax, and pulmonary edema.
    E. Hematologic evaluation is necessary if nontraumatic hemorrhage or disseminated intravascular coagulation (DIC) is apparent.

16. Intubation should be considered for which of the following:
    A. Apnea.
    B. Airway obstruction or a potential for obstruction (e.g., facial burns).
    C. Hypoxia.
    D. Hypoventilation and hypercarbia.
    E. All of the above.

ANSWERS   [See Barkin et al: Chapter 13.]

1. The answer is **C,** page 148.
   The overlying skin may require shaving to improve access. The tourniquet, a rubber band, should be placed at the level of the forehead. A catheter should be inserted into the most proximal portion of the vein and advanced caudally. The tourniquet requires removal before flushing, and if the proximal scalp blanches, this indicates possible arterial placement.

2. The answer is **E,** page 148.
   The flow rate is directly proportional to catheter gauge and indirectly proportional to catheter length. Complications of central venous pressure (CVP) placement may include pneumothoracic events and should be anticipated. Local anesthetics should be provided.

3. The answer is **E,** page 148.
   The femoral vein lies medial to the femoral artery. The femoral artery is midway between the anterior iliac crest and the symphysis pubis. The external jugular is best visualized when the infant is in Trendelenburg's position. Because of the large number of valves and the tortuosity of this vessel, it is sometimes difficult to advance a guidewire or longer catheter through the length of the external jugular vein. Because the pleural cap is lower on the right, the right subclavian vein is more often chosen for cannulation.

4. The answer is **B,** page 149.
   The bellies of the sternal and clavicular branches of the sternocleidomastoid muscle form a triangle. The clavicle forms the base of this triangle. All reattempts should be made more laterally, and all needle punctures should be made lateral to the carotid artery pulse. The anterior approach to the vessel is difficult in children and has a higher complication rate. In the posterior approach the needle is directed toward the sternal notch, whereas in the medial approach the needle is directed toward the ipsilateral nipple.

5. The answer is **D,** page 152.
   In the child younger than 5 years these spacious venous sinusoids provide access to the venous system. The preferred site in infants and children is the proximal tibia. The sternum should be avoided as an intraosseous needle site because its use increases the potential for accidental full-thickness puncture. Also, a sternal needle may interfere with cardiopulmonary resuscitation (CPR) efforts. A point two fingerbreadths below the tibial tuberosity is ideal for insertion.

6. The answer is **A,** page 123.
   Shock caused by inadequate intravascular volume relative to the vascular space is known as hypovolemic shock. Shock from impaired myocardial function is termed cardiogenic. Shock associated with inappropriate distribution of blood flow and increased capillary permeability is distributive; septic shock is the best example of this form. Neurogenic shock should be considered in the pediatric trauma victim with spinal cord injury if hypotension persists despite adequate volume resuscitation.

7. The answer is **D,** pages 103 and 133.
   Children in shock should be intubated electively before further deterioration complicates management. Physiologic indications for intubation include Pao_2 less than 50 mm Hg at Fio_2 greater than 0.5 or $Paco_2$ greater than 50 mm Hg (unless chronic or compensatory for metabolic alkalosis). **DOPE** is a mnemonic device used for the complications of endotracheal intubation, which include: tube **D**isplacement, tube **O**bstruction, **P**neumothorax, or **E**quipment failure. Optimal PEEP is the minimal PEEP required to allow maximal oxygen delivery.

8. The answer is **D,** page 123.
   Hypovolemic shock is the most common type of shock in the pediatric population. It is defined as shock associated with a reduction in intravascular volume relative to the vascular space. In patients with sepsis, vasodilatation or third spacing may lead to a relative hypovolemia. It is recommended that up to three fluid boluses be administered in hypovolemic shock before the use of pressor agents.

9. The answer is **C,** page 126.
   Myocardial function is abnormal in patients with sepsis. Early in the septic process, ventricular dilatation may occur and ventricular ejection fraction may fall as low as 20%. The compensatory ventricular response during sepsis is an increase in ventricular compliance. As long as intravascular volume remains adequate, the compliant ventricle may be able to maintain a reduced but adequate stroke volume in the face of a reduced ejection fraction through dilation with an increase in ventricular end-diastolic volume. This dilation, coupled with an increase in heart rate and a fall in systemic vascular resistance, typically results in a cardiac output that is much higher than normal. The likelihood of patient survival has been linked to ventricular dilation. When the septic condition is treated effectively, cardiac output, heart rate, and ventricular compliance return to normal, usually within 24 hours.

10. The answer is **C,** page 127.
    The clinical signs observed in the child with hypovolemic shock are those of inadequate systemic perfusion associated with intravascular fluid loss or redistribution. The child demonstrates tachycardia, peripheral vasoconstriction, cool extremities, delayed capillary refill, and oliguria.

11. The answer is **D,** page 127.
    A capillary refill time of more than 3 seconds is associated with a fluid deficit of more than 10%. The cardiac silhouette in hypovolemic shock is typically small. Hypotension is observed as a late sign of significant fluid loss. Clinically significant dehydration is associated with weight loss. Because body water constitutes a smaller percentage of body weight in older children and adults than in young children, a compromise in systemic perfusion is observed in the adolescent once the fluid equivalent of 5% to 7% of body weight is lost acutely.

12. The answer is **C**, page 128.

Hypernatremic dehydration results when free water deficit is greater than the sodium deficit. Because of a shift of free water into the intravascular space in the child who is hypernatremic, a compromise in systemic perfusion will not develop until severe dehydration is present (more than 15% of body weight). Acute blood loss leads to compromised perfusion at 15% to 20% loss, and vasoconstriction and tachycardia may be the only evidence of hemorrhage. Hypotonic dehydration is associated with a greater loss of sodium than water.

13. The answer is **E**, page 129.

The child with cardiogenic shock shows signs of inadequate systemic perfusion despite adequate intravascular volume. Adrenergic mechanisms typically divert blood flow to the heart and brain. Pulmonary edema and an enlarged cardiac silhouette are typically noted on chest radiograph. Signs of *decreased* cardiac output and shock are often identical to signs of tamponade, which should be ruled out using echocardiography.

14. The answer is **E**, page 132.

Since children tend to develop hypotension late in the course of any type of shock, other findings such as irritability, tachypnea, and mottled skin should prompt an early recognition of septic shock.

15. The answer is **A**, page 132.

Lactic acidosis may be the most sensitive indicator of inadequate perfusion. Arterial blood gas analysis is extremely useful, but hemoglobin and hematocrit may be artificially normal unless volume resuscitation with any fluid other than whole blood has occurred.

16. The answer is **E**, page 133.

Children in shock should be intubated electively before respiratory deterioration or arrest complicates shock management. Intubation should be considered in children with respiratory arrest or apnea, airway obstruction, hypoxemia, hypoventilation, hypercarbia, or increased intracranial pressure.

CHAPTER

12

Dysrhythmias

Edward E. Conway, Jr.

See Barkin et al: Chapter 14

1. Which of the following cardiac dysrhythmias is *not* associated with an underlying cardiac abnormality?
   A. Multifocal premature ventricular contractions.
   B. Premature ventricular contraction (PVC) couplets.
   C. PVCs that increase during exercise.
   D. Premature atrial contractions.

2. Which of the following abnormalities is *not* associated with PVCs?
   A. Hypoxemia.
   B. Metabolic acidosis.
   C. Hypoglycemia.
   D. Hypokalemia.
   E. Hypernatremia.

3. A 6-month-old boy comes to the ED with a history of poor feeding and breathing quickly. The infant is alert and awake and appears in mild respiratory distress with acrocyanosis. He had a ventricular septal defect repaired 2 months ago and is not taking any cardiac medications. His electrocardiogram (ECG) is depicted in Fig. 12-1.
   Which of the following interventions is most appropriate at this time?
   A. Intravenous (IV) administration of verapamil 0.1 mg/kg.
   B. Asynchronous cardioversion with 4 watt-sec/kg.
   C. Rapid IV administration of adenosine 100 µg/kg.
   D. IV administration of digoxin 10 µg/kg.
   E. IV administration of magnesium sulfate 25 mg/kg.

4. A 14-year-old athletic girl complains of tightness in her chest. Which one of the following is the most likely cause of her discomfort?
   A. Ventricular tachycardia.
   B. PVCs.
   C. Costochondritis.
   D. Pneumomediastinum.
   E. Atrial flutter.

5. All of the following statements concerning adenosine are *true except:*
   A. It must be given slowly.
   B. The site of action is at the AV node.
   C. Its half-life is measured in seconds.
   D. Side effects include chest pain and hypotension.
   E. It should not be used in patients with sick sinus syndrome.

6. You are evaluating a 7-year-old in the ED and ask the nurse to initiate cardiac monitoring, which shows that the heart rate is 260 beats per minute. You, however, palpate a femoral pulse of 130 beats per minute. Which of the following best explains this finding?
   A. Improper lead placement.
   B. Muscle twitching.
   C. Loose electronic connections.
   D. Improperly set sensitivity.

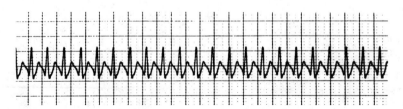

FIG. 12-1

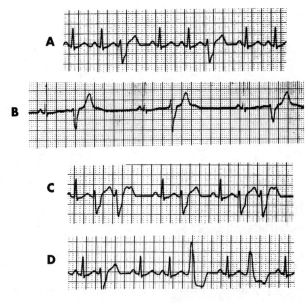

FIG. 12-2

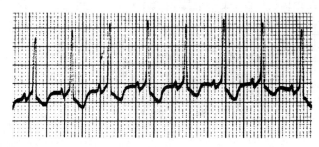

FIG. 12-3

For questions 7, 8, 9, and 10, match the four ECGs of Fig. 12-2 with the proper description. Each answer may be used only once.

7. Ventricular bigeminy. _____

8. Ventricular couplet. _____

9. Multiform ventricular premature beats. _____

10. Unifocal premature ventricular beats. _____

11. The ECG in Fig. 12-3 is obtained from a 2-month-old infant following cardioversion for a heart rate of 280 beats per minute. Which of the following findings would be atypical for this infant?
    A. Diaphoresis.
    B. Tachypnea.
    C. Grunting.
    D. Irritability.
    E. Syncope.

12. The most likely diagnosis for the infant described in question 11 is which of the following?
    A. Ventricular tachycardia.
    B. Atrial flutter.
    C. Atrial fibrillation.
    D. Congenital complete heart block.
    E. Wolff-Parkinson-White (WPW) syndrome.

13. What is the most common cause of the dysrhythmia shown in Fig. 12-4 on page 46?
    A. Drug ingestion.
    B. Repair of congenital heart disease.
    C. Viral infection.
    D. Myocardial tumor.

14. Which of the following interventions would *not* be useful in treating the dysrhythmia depicted in question 13?
    A. Synchronized cardioversion.
    B. Digoxin.
    C. Quinidine.
    D. Amiodarone.
    E. Verapamil.

15. A 14-year-old boy with a history of sensorineural hearing loss is brought to the ED complaining of palpitations after being frightened during a Halloween walk. According to his friends, he "passed out" for several minutes. An ECG is obtained and shown in Fig. 12-5 on page 46. The patient is hemodynamically stable, but the dysrhythmia shown in Fig. 12-5 continues to recur. Which of the following is the best therapeutic option to take next?
    A. IV infusion of lidocaine 1 mg/kg.
    B. IV magnesium sulfate 25 mg/kg.
    C. Epinephrine 0.1 mg/kg intravenously.
    D. IV bolus of lidocaine 1 mg/kg followed by an infusion of 20 µg/kg/min.
    E. Verapamil 0.1 mg/kg intravenously.

16. A 5-month-old infant brought to the ED is not eating well, according to his grandmother. The triage nurse reports that the "heart sounds funny," and she obtains an ECG, which is shown in Fig. 12-6 on page 46.
    Which of the following statements concerning this scenario is *false*?
    A. There may be an associated congenital heart defect.
    B. The infant's mother may have systemic lupus erythematosus.
    C. All children with this rhythm are symptomatic and require therapy.
    D. The rhythm may respond to atropine and isoproterenol.
    E. Transcutaneous pacing may be required.

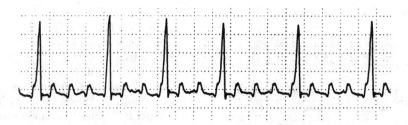

FIG. 12-4

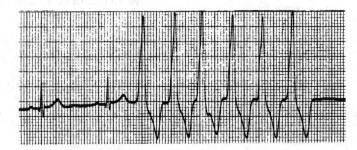

FIG. 12-5

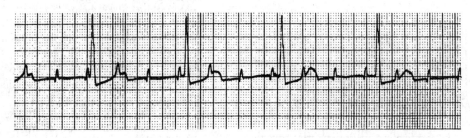

FIG. 12-6

ANSWERS [See Barkin et al: Chapter 14, pages 156-165.]

1. The answer is **D**, pages 158 and 159.

   PVCs result from either premature depolarization of a ventricular focus or reentry. They are not uncommon in infants and children, and in the presence of a structurally and functionally normal heart, they are benign. PVCs that appear in couplets, that increase with exercise, or that appear as multiform all suggest an underlying cardiac abnormality. Premature atrial contractions arise from a premature depolarization of an atrial focus. They are seen commonly in infants and are usually benign (Fig. 12-7 on page 47).

2. The answer is **E**, page 159.

   PVCs may be caused by hypoxia, acidosis, hypoglycemia, hypokalemia, hyperkalemia, and certain medications, such as digitalis, sympathomimetics, and phenothiazines. Cardiac abnormalities associated with PVCs include prolonged QT syndrome, cardiomyopathy, myocarditis, postoperative cardiac surgery, mitral valve prolapse, and cardiac tumors.

3. The answer is **C**, pages 159 and 161.

   The ECG demonstrates supraventricular tachycardia (SVT), and the infant is in mild distress. Thus the therapeutic option for stable SVT would be the rapid administration of 100 µg/kg of adenosine. (*See answer to question 5.*)

4. The answer is **C**, page 631.

   Chest pain in adolescents, unlike in adults, generally has a benign connotation. Chest wall or musculoskeletal pain is the most common diagnosis; most often, trauma or overuse is the cause of the pain. Costochondritis (Tietze's syndrome) is a disease of unknown origin causing a nonsuppurative inflammation of the costochondral junction.

5. The answer is **A**, pages 160 and 161.

   Adenosine is an endogenous nucleotide with a half-life of seconds. As a result of this, it must be pushed rapidly and at the most proximate site of the IV line to the patient. It causes a temporary block at the AV node and interrupts any reentry circuit that involves the AV node. Adenosine should be used cautiously in patients with asthma, since it may cause bronchospasm. Chest pain, flushing, and a slight decrease in blood pressure are also possible side effects.

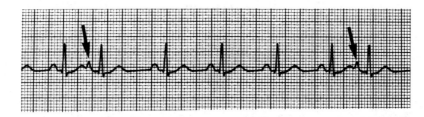

FIG. 12-7 Atrial premature beat. Note that QRS is similar, but P wave is different in the premature beat (2 and 7) compared with the regular sinus beats.

6. The answer is **D,** page 156.

   Potential artifacts may be caused by muscle twitching, alternating current, electric interference from nearby electronic equipment, and loose electric connections. The heart rate may be determined by palpating a central or peripheral pulse, from the cardiac monitor, or by analyzing a paper ECG recording. If the sensitivity on the monitor is improperly set, the heart rate may appear to be doubled because the T waves are tall and are counted as R waves, or it may underestimate the heart rate if the R wave is small.

7. The answer is **B,** page 159.

   Ventricular bigeminy is a regularly irregular rhythm in which every other beat is a premature ventricular contraction.

8. The answer is **C,** page 159.

   A couplet is defined as two consecutive PVCs.

9. The answer is **D,** page 159.

   PVCs that have the same shape in the same lead are referred to as uniform, whereas those with varying shapes are called multiform.

10. The answer is **A,** page 159.

    Uniform PVC with a different configuration from the normally conducted beats. A PVC is usually followed by a compensatory pause that may be full (i.e., the sum of the RR beats surrounding the PVC is equal to twice the normal RR interval) or partial.

11. The answer is **E,** page 158.

    The ECG demonstrates Wolff-Parkinson-White (WPW) syndrome, and signs and symptoms of SVT include those of congestive heart failure and low cardiac output. The vast majority of patients with SVT are uncomfortable but clinically stable.

12. The answer is **E,** pages 158 and 160.

    The ECG demonstrates WPW syndrome. There is a short PR interval (0.04 sec), a δ wave is present, and a wide QRS (0.12 sec) is noted. SVT is the most common symptomatic pediatric dysrhythmia and may be associated with a reentry circuit associated with a WPW conduction disturbance (bypass tract).

13. The answer is **B,** pages 161 and 162.

    The ECG demonstrates atrial flutter, which is an atrial dysrhythmia without involvement of the AV node that is thought to be caused by local reentry. In the fetus and young infant, atrial flutter can occur without associated heart defects, whereas most older children with flutter have an underlying heart abnormality. One series demonstrated that 61% of patients with atrial flutter had repaired congenital heart disease.

14. The answer is **E,** pages 161 and 162.

    Atrial flutter is very responsive to electrical synchronized cardioversion. Clinical improvement may be obtained by producing a higher degree of AV block with digoxin. Other medications include quinidine and amiodarone. Calcium channel blockers are not indicated in the treatment of atrial flutter.

15. The answer is **D,** pages 162 and 163.

    The ECG demonstrates ventricular tachycardia (VT). Prolonged QT interval with sudden death associated with deafness occurs in Jervell and Lange-Nielsen syndrome, and there is another form of congenital prolonged QT syndrome called Romano-Ward, which is not associated with deafness. VT in this disorder is often induced by increased sympathetic stimulation and emotional stress, such as fright or startling noises. The lengthening of the QT interval is thought to be of neural origin. Management of stable VT begins with the ABCs and is followed by administration of IV lidocaine followed by a continuous infusion. The hemodynamically unstable patient should receive a lidocaine bolus and then have DC cardioversion performed using 0.5 to 2 watt-sec/kg of energy.

16. The answer is **C,** page 164.

    The ECG demonstrates complete heart block (CHB). Many children with CHB are asymptomatic. However, symptoms may include easy fatigability, shortness of breath, syncope, and presyncope. CHB may be associated with congenital heart disease and with maternal lupus. Symptomatic children respond to atropine and isoproterenol, and transcutaneous pacing may be helpful in temporizing the situation while plans for transvenous pacing are arranged.

CHAPTER 13

Fluid and Electrolyte Balance

Gary B. Zuckerman

See Barkin et al: Chapter 15.

1. The most common cause of insensible water loss is:
   A. Diarrhea.
   B. Tachypnea.
   C. Hemorrhage.
   D. Fever.
   E. Polyuria.

2. Which of the following statements regarding fluid and electrolyte balance is *true?*
   A. The total body water percentage of the body weight increases with increasing age.
   B. Insensible water losses (ml/kg/24 hr) decrease with increasing age.
   C. The extracellular fluid compartment percentage of the body weight increases dramatically from birth to 1 year of age, then decreases with increasing age.
   D. Weight (kg) to body surface area (m^2) ratio decreases with increasing age.
   E. Maintenance water requirements for fecal and urinary water loss (ml/kg/24 hr) increase with age.

3. A 3-year-old boy comes to the ED with a 2-day history of tachypnea. The rest of the history is unremarkable. Physical examination shows that the child is well developed and well nourished. His vital signs are: pulse 100 beats per minute, respiratory rate (RR) 35 breaths per minute, temperature 99.5° F (37.5° C), and blood pressure (BP) 110/70 mm Hg. He has no flaring, retractions, grunting, wheezes, rales, or rhonchi. The rest of his examination is unremarkable.

   Laboratory examination reveals the following information: arterial blood gas in room air (ABG): pH 7.20, PCO_2 30 mm Hg, PO_2 110 mm Hg, O_2 saturation 100%.

   Serum electrolytes: Na 135 mEq/L, K 4.0 mEq/L, Cl 112 mEq/L, HCO_3 16 mEq/L, blood urea nitrogen (BUN) 10 mg/dl, creatinine 0.2 mg/dl, glucose 120 mg/dl. Chest radiograph: normal.

   The most likely cause of this child's tachypnea is:
   A. Renal tubular acidosis.
   B. Bacterial pneumonia.
   C. Ibuprofen intoxication.
   D. Diabetic ketoacidosis.
   E. Respiratory syncytial viral pneumonia.

4. A 2-year-old girl is unconscious after ingesting a large amount of her grandmother's diazepam (Valium). Her ABG reveals: pH 7.24, PCO_2 60 mm Hg, PO_2 80 mm Hg. The most appropriate management for the patient's acidemia is:
   A. Intravenous (IV) administration of sodium bicarbonate 1 mEq/kg.
   B. IV administration of 0.9% saline solution 20 ml/kg.
   C. Endotracheal intubation and mechanical ventilation.
   D. IV administration of naloxone 0.01 mg/kg.
   E. IV administration of acetazolamide (Diamox) 5 mg/kg/24 hr.

5. A 10-year-old diabetic girl has diabetic ketoacidosis. Laboratory examination reveals the following results: Na 126 mEq/L, K 4.0 mEq/L, Cl 100 mEq/L, HCO_3 11 mEq/L, BUN 38 mg/dl, creatinine 1 mg/dl, glucose 1000 mg/dl. The most likely cause of the patient's hyponatremia is:
   A. Syndrome of inappropriate antidiuretic hormone secretion.
   B. Iatrogenic water intoxication.
   C. Sodium wasting nephropathy.
   D. Pseudohyponatremia.
   E. Gastroenteritis.

6. A 5-month-old infant comes to the ED with a 1-day history of poor breast milk intake. Weight yesterday at a well baby visit was 7 kg. Today the child weighs 6 kg. On physical examination the vital signs are: pulse 190 beats per minute, RR 40 breaths per minute, BP 60/25 mm Hg, and temperature 98.6° F (37° C). Her extremities are cool and mottled. She has thready distal pulses, and the capillary refill time is greater than 4 seconds. Laboratory findings include: serum Na^+ 162 mEq/L, K^+ 4.5 mEq/L, HCO_3^+ 13 mEq/L. Which of the following is true regarding immediate fluid management for this patient?

   A. The entire fluid deficit and maintenance requirement should be given slowly and evenly over 48 hours to prevent cerebral swelling.

   B. Half of the fluid deficit should be replaced over 8 hours, and the remaining fluid deficit should be replaced over the next 16 hours.

   C. Rapid fluid boluses should be avoided to prevent cerebral swelling.

   D. A 20-ml/kg bolus infusion of 0.9% saline should be given rapidly, and the child should then be reassessed.

   E. A dopamine infusion is indicated to augment the blood pressure without causing cerebral swelling.

7. A 16-year-old girl with anorexia nervosa comes to the ED after ingesting a large quantity of furosemide and oral laxatives. She is noted on physical examination to have marked muscle weakness and abdominal distension. Her electrocardiogram (ECG) demonstrates bradycardia with absent T waves and U waves. Appropriate management of this patient includes:

   A. Polystyrene sulfonate (Kayexalate), 1 gm/kg/dose.

   B. Calcium chloride (10%), 0.2 ml/kg IV bolus.

   C. 3% saline solution, 4 ml/kg IV over 10 minutes.

   D. Lidocaine, 1 mg/kg IV over 5 minutes.

   E. Potassium chloride, 0.2 to 0.3 mEq/kg/hr IV infusion.

8. A 12-year-old boy with chronic renal failure and a history of noncompliance with dialysis appointments comes to the ED in shock. An ECG reveals a widened QRS complex and bradycardia. The most appropriate management for this child is:

   A. Calcium chloride (10%), 0.2 ml/kg IV bolus.

   B. Magnesium sulfate, 25 mg/kg IV bolus.

   C. Acetazolamide, 5 mg/kg IV infusion.

   D. Mannitol, 1 g/kg IV infusion.

9. A 9-month-old girl is brought to the ED after having seizures at home. Her parents are strict vegetarians who have never fed her any meat or dairy products. On physical examination she is noted to have joint swelling of the ankles and wrists. When a tourniquet is applied to her arm for obtaining IV access, she is noted to have carpal pedal spasm. The most appropriate management for this child is:

   A. Furosemide, 1 mg/kg IV infusion.

   B. 0.9% saline solution, 20 ml/kg IV bolus.

   C. Polystyrene sulfonate, 1 g/kg/dose.

   D. Calcium gluconate (10%), 1 ml/kg IV infusion.

   E. Bumetanide, 0.5 mg IV infusion.

10. Hypomagnesemia is associated with:

    A. Hypokalemia.

    B. Hypernatremia.

    C. Hyponatremia.

    D. Hypercalcemia

    E. Hyperkalemia.

11. A 16-month-old boy comes to the ED with a 2-day history of vomiting and diarrhea. Three days earlier the child weighed 33 lb at a well child visit. The child is noted to be lethargic. He is tachycardic (180 beats per minute) and hypotensive (60/32 mm Hg). His eyeballs are sunken and glassy. His mucous membranes are very dry, and no tears are noted when he cries. Skin pinch retraction is absent, and his capillary refill time is 4 seconds. He has not urinated in 6 hours. The child's fluid deficit is closest to:

    A. 50 ml.

    B. 100 ml.

    C. 500 ml.

    D. 1500 ml.

    E. 2250 ml.

12. Which of the following statements is true regarding laboratory studies and fluid and electrolyte abnormalities?

    A. The serum sodium determines osmolar classification of dehydration.

    B. The serum sodium predicts the degree of fluid deficit.

    C. The serum sodium determines total body water content.

    D. The serum creatinine reflects hydration status.

    E. BUN is a sensitive measure for hydration status.

13. A 2-month-old infant comes to the ED with a 3-day history of vomiting, diarrhea, and poor breast milk intake. The child is lethargic. Her heart rate is 195 beats per minute, and her BP is 80/50 mm Hg. Her fontanelle is sunken, and mucous membranes are very dry. Her extremities are cool and mottled, and her capillary refill time is greater than 3 seconds. No urine is obtained after the patient's bladder is catheterized. Multiple attempts at obtaining IV access are unsuccessful. The most appropriate management for this child is:

    A. Nasogastric rehydration.

    B. Femoral venous cutdown.

    C. Intraosseous needle placement.

    D. Saphenous venous cutdown.

    E. Scalp vein catheterization.

14. Which of the following is the most accurate for measuring continuous urine production in a severely dehydrated child during the early phase of fluid resuscitation?

    A. Urine bag.

    B. Condom catheter.

    C. Weighing diapers.

    D. Intermittent bladder catheter.

    E. Indwelling urinary catheter.

15. A 6-month-old boy with vomiting and diarrhea comes to the ED. For his maintenance fluid requirement he is given a 5% dextrose and 0.45% saline solution with 20 mEq/L potassium chloride intravenously at a rate of 30 ml/hr for 24 hours. Which of the following statements is true regarding the IV maintenance solution?
    A. It will provide the patient with twice the maintenance water requirement.
    B. The patient will receive more than twice his maintenance sodium requirement.
    C. The patient will not receive enough sodium to fulfill his maintenance sodium requirement.
    D. The patient is not receiving his maintenance potassium requirement.
    E. The patient will receive more than twice his maintenance potassium requirement.

16. A 13-month-old girl with a 2-day history of vomiting, diarrhea, and poor oral intake comes to the ED dehydrated. On physical examination she is noted to be irritable. Her heart rate is 170 beats per minute, and her BP is 100/68 mm Hg. Her eyes are sunken, and her fontanelle is flat. Her mucous membranes are dry. Capillary refill is 2 to 3 seconds. She weighed 17 kg at a well child clinic visit 3 days ago. Today she weighs 15.3 kg. The patient's combined deficit and 24-hour maintenance fluid requirement is:
    A. 1350 ml.
    B. 2200 ml.
    C. 3050 ml.
    D. 4000 ml.
    E. 5000 ml.

17. Which of the following would make a patient a poor candidate for enteral rehydration therapy?
    A. Circulatory collapse.
    B. Viral enteritis.
    C. Bacterial enteritis.
    D. Parasitic enteritis.
    E. Oliguria.

18. A 1-year-old infant with vomiting and diarrhea is undergoing oral rehydration for dehydration. The fluid deficit is accurately assessed as 50 ml/kg, and a standard oral rehydration protocol is being initiated. The child vomits twice during the first hour of therapy. The child has no signs of hemodynamic instability. Assuming the child's deficit and maintenance fluid requirements have been accurately assessed and the correct fluid and electrolyte solutions are being administered, which of the following would be an appropriate intervention?
    A. Prochlorperazine (Compazine), 2 mg IV infusion.
    B. Decrease feeding aliquots in 5 to 10 ml aliquots.
    C. Diphenhydramine (Benadryl), 1 mg/kg IV infusion.
    D. Hydroxyzine (Atarax, Vistaril), 0.5 mg/kg IV infusion.
    E. Trimethobenzamide (Tigan) suppository, 100 mg per rectum.

19. A 2-week-old infant comes to the ED with a 1-day history of poor breast milk intake. Weight yesterday at a well baby visit was 4 kg. Today the child weighs 3.4 kg. The child is found to have isotonic dehydration. Oral rehydration therapy is attempted, and the child's entire fluid deficit and 12-hour maintenance fluid requirements are given over 12 hours. The WHO rehydration solution is used for both the deficit and maintenance fluid requirements. Which of the following statements is true?
    A. The infant is at risk for becoming hypernatremic.
    B. The infant is at risk for becoming hyponatremic.
    C. The infant is at risk for becoming hypokalemic.
    D. The infant is at risk for becoming hypercalcemic.
    E. The solution is appropriate for the patient's deficit and maintenance fluid and electrolyte requirements.

20. Which of the following statements regarding discharge management of dehydrated children is true?
    A. Clear liquids as a discharge diet decrease vomiting.
    B. Breastfeeding should be deferred for 3 days following resolution of symptoms.
    C. Resumption of feedings, if tolerated, results in the resolution of diarrhea.
    D. Rice-based clear liquid diets will prevent protein starvation.
    E. Discharge follow-up is rarely necessary in a successfully rehydrated patient.

ANSWERS   [See Barkin et al: Chapter 15.]

1. The answer is **D**, page 166.

    The three main routes of water loss in children are urinary, fecal, and insensible water losses. Insensible water losses range from 10 to 40 ml/kg/24 hr. Insensible water losses include water converted in metabolic reactions, water lost through the respiratory tract, and water lost through evaporation from skin. Increased metabolic rates will increase water use and insensible water loss. The most common cause of increased insensible water loss is fever, which may elevate the daily fluid requirements by 7 ml/kg/24 hr for each degree rise in temperature above $37.2°$ C ($99°$ F). Tachypnea, which will increase insensible water loss through the respiratory tract, is not the most common cause of insensible water loss. Diarrhea, hemorrhage, and polyuria, which may account for marked total body water deficits, are not in themselves causes of insensible water loss.

2. The answer is **B**, pages 166-167, Tables 15-1 and 15-2.

    Insensible water losses (ml/kg/24 hr) are highest in infancy and decrease with increasing age because of the higher metabolic rates found in infants, which likewise decrease with increasing age. The percentages of body weight made up by the total body water, extracellular fluid compartment, and intracellular fluid compartment decrease with increasing age. Weight (kg) to body surface area (m^2) ratio increases with increasing age. Maintenance water requirements for urinary, fecal, and insensible water loss decrease with age.

3. The answer is **A**, pages 168 and 180, Table 15-8.

    The patient is tachypneic because he is trying to compensate for a metabolic acidosis (HCO_3 16 mEq/L) by producing a respiratory alkalosis (Pco_2 30 mm Hg). The metabolic acidosis has caused an acidemia (pH 7.20), defined as an abnormally low pH occurring in the blood. The anion gap is normal (11 mEq/L). The anion gap is calculated using the following equation:

    $$\text{Anion gap} = (Na^+ + K^+) \text{ mEq} - (Cl^- + HCO_3^-) \text{ mEq}$$

    The normal anion gap is 8 to 12 mEq/L. The gap is normal in disease conditions such as diarrhea or renal tubular acidosis in which the metabolic acidosis results from a loss of bicarbonate ion through the gastrointestinal tract or the kidneys. An elevated anion gap acidosis occurs with excess production of organic acids. A useful mnemonic for remembering entities that produce a large anion gap with a metabolic acidosis is **MUDPILES**: **m**ethanol, **u**remia, **d**iabetic ketoacidosis, **p**araldehyde, **i**soniazid, **i**buprofen, **i**nhalants (H_2S, CN, CO), or **i**ron overdose, **l**actic acidosis, **e**thanol or **e**thylene glycol, and **s**alicylates, **s**tarvation, or **s**olvents (benzene or toluene). The patient's history, physical examination, chest radiograph, and ABG make the possibility of pulmonary disease (bacterial or viral pneumonia) as a cause of his tachypnea unlikely.

4. The answer is **C**, pages 168 to 170.

    This patient is in acute respiratory failure secondary to benzodiazepine-induced respiratory depression. She has an uncompensated acute respiratory acidosis resulting in acidemia. Primary respiratory acidosis results from alveolar hypoventilation and carbon dioxide retention. As the carbon dioxide level increases, carbonic acid is produced and the pH falls. Treatment of acute primary respiratory acidosis is correction of the underlying cause of the ventilation problem. Primary respiratory acidosis is never corrected by administration of bicarbonate. IV fluid resuscitation with isotonic solutions is indicated in acidoses because of impaired perfusion. Naloxone is an opiate antagonist and has no role in benzodiazepine intoxication. Acetazolamide is a carbonic anhydrase inhibitor that is occasionally used for severe metabolic alkalosis. Although not included as a choice in this question, the use of flumazenil in patients with acute benzodiazepine overdose should be considered.

5. The answer is **D**, pages 170 to 172.

    Pseudohyponatremia occurs when the serum sodium concentration is low but the serum osmolality is normal or elevated. In these cases another solute has replaced the sodium ion to maintain serum osmolality. Pseudohyponatremia may occur with severe hyperlipidemia, hyperglycemia, and mannitol or urea administration. In hyperglycemic states the serum sodium level may fall 1.6 mEq/L for each 100-mg/dl rise in the serum glucose level. The actual sodium concentration may be calculated from the following equation:

    True [Na^+(mEq/L)] =
    {[(Glucose {mg/dl} − 100 mg/dl] ÷ 100 mg/dl] × 1.6 mEq/L}
    + [Serum Na^+ mEq/L]

    When correcting for the patient's hyperglycemia, her actual sodium is 140 mEq/L. The syndrome of inappropriate antidiuretic hormone secretion and iatrogenic water intoxication both result in hyponatremia secondary to an excess of free water. Both are complications associated with diabetic ketoacidosis and may cause true hyponatremia. In either case the true serum sodium concentration would be less than 135 mEq/L when corrected for hyperglycemia. Gastroenteritis may result in hyponatremia, especially if the patient receives a hypotonic solution for rehydration. The hyponatremia noted in cerebral salt wasting results from a natriuresis in patients with intracranial pathology.

6. The answer is **D,** pages 172 and 184 to 185.
   This patient is in a late stage of hypovolemic shock. She requires rapid administration of isotonic fluid boluses (0.9% saline or Ringer's lactate solution). Once the shock phase is corrected, the child would then undergo ensuing fluid resuscitation in which the fluid and deficit requirements would be given evenly over 48 hours. Cerebral swelling is a known complication of hypertonic dehydration states when a patient's serum osmolality is corrected too rapidly and water follows a concentration gradient into the relatively hyperosmolar brain cells. When a patient is in shock, however, rapid restoration of the patient's intravascular volume is essential. There is no role for dopamine or any pressor in hypovolemic shock.

7. The answer is **E,** pages 173 and 174.
   Diuretic and laxative abuse can result in marked potassium loss from the urinary and gastrointestinal tracts. This patient has physical findings (skeletal muscle weakness, ileus) and ECG evidence of marked, severe hypokalemia. If hypokalemia is associated with life-threatening dysrhythmias, potassium may be given intravenously at 0.2 to 0.3 mEq/kg/hr. If the serum potassium level is only slightly depressed and the patient is not vomiting, an oral potassium suspension of 0.2 to 0.3 mEq/kg may be attempted.

8. The answer is **A,** pages 173 to 175.
   Hyperkalemia produces muscle weakness, fatigue, depressed deep tendon reflexes, paralysis, and confusion. Prominent peaked T waves may be seen on ECG, and in severe cases a widened QRS complex and bradycardia. Complete loss of QRS morphology and the appearance of a sine wave pattern may appear in patients with severe potassium toxicity. Urinary excretion of potassium commonly is decreased or absent in pediatric patients with renal failure and can be a cause of severe potassium toxicity. Potassium supplementation is the most frequent cause of hyperkalemia in adults. Certain drugs, including digitalis, succinylcholine, spironolactone, and cyclosporine, can raise serum potassium levels. Other causes of hyperkalemia include acidosis, insulin deficiency, hyperosmolality, β-receptor blockade, strenuous exercise, hypoaldosteronism, or aldosterone resistance. Treatment of life-threatening hyperkalemia includes cardiac monitoring, vascular access, calcium chloride (10%) 0.2 ml/kg IV bolus, dextrose 0.5 to 1 g/kg IV followed by 1 unit of regular insulin for every 4 g of glucose infused, sodium bicarbonate 0.5 to 1 mEq/kg, albuterol nebulization, and polystyrene sulfonate. Magnesium sulfate supplementation is a treatment for hypokalemia, and mannitol is associated with hyperkalemia secondary to hyperosmolality. Acetazolamide causes metabolic acidosis, which could increase serum potassium levels.

9. The answer is **D,** pages 175 and 176.
   The patient has seizures, carpal pedal spasm (Trousseau's sign), and skeletal findings of rickets. These findings are manifestations of severe hypocalcemia. Hypocalcemia may result from dietary deficiencies of either calcium or vitamin D. In addition, defects in any portion of vitamin D metabolism or activity will decrease ionized calcium level. Other causes of hypocalcemia are anticonvulsant therapy, malabsorption syndromes, lack of sunlight exposure, hyperphosphatemia, pancreatitis, and hypomagnesemia. Emergency treatment of hypocalcemia consists of prompt calcium replacement with 0.5 to 1 ml/kg of a 10% solution of calcium gluconate or 0.2 ml/kg of a 10% solution of calcium chloride administered over approximately 5 minutes. Saline boluses and loop diuretics such as furosemide and bumetanide are treatments for hypercalcemia and will worsen the patient's hypocalcemia. Polystyrene sulfonate is a treatment for hyperkalemia.

10. The answer is **A,** pages 173 to 175.
    Hypomagnesemia results from either increased renal excretion or decreased gastrointestinal absorption of magnesium. Diuretics, chronic stress, and hyperadrenergic states are primary causes of renal magnesium loss. Malabsorption and increased gastrointestinal loss are frequent causes of total body magnesium depletion. Hypomagnesemia may be a cause of refractory hypokalemia and hypocalcemia.

11. The answer is **E,** pages 178 and 179.
    The patient has signs of 15% dehydration or a fluid deficit of 150 ml/kg. The child's weight before illness was 15 kg. Therefore his fluid deficit can be calculated as (150 ml/kg) × (15 kg) = 2250 ml.

12. The answer is **A,** pages 178 to 180.
    The overlap of signs and symptoms in different electrolyte abnormalities is so great that clinical differentiation may not be possible and laboratory data may be necessary to identify the specific electrolyte abnormality. The serum sodium determines osmolar classification of dehydration. It does not predict the degree of fluid deficit, nor does it determine total body water content. The serum creatinine reflects renal function and not hydration status. The blood urea nitrogen (BUN) as an isolated measurement is not a sensitive test for hydration status but in conjunction with an elevated BUN/creatinine ratio, decreased urine output, and high urine osmolality, it may indicate dehydration.

13. The answer is **C,** pages 180 and 181.
    Although this child is normotensive, she is in shock and requires rapid parenteral fluid resuscitation. Oral or nasogastric rehydration will not rapidly correct the shock state. In children who are in shock, time should not be wasted on extended searches for peripheral veins or cutdowns. If vascular access cannot be readily accomplished in these children, an intraosseous needle should be placed.

14. The answer is **E,** page 181.

Continuous monitoring of severely dehydrated children is necessary during the early resuscitation phase. In addition to frequent vital signs, such patients should be monitored for urine production. All of the listed methods provide information on urine production, but the indwelling urinary catheter is the most accurate for measuring continuous urine production.

15. The answer is **B,** pages 167 and 182.

The child correctly received his 24-hour maintenance water requirement, which was 720 ml. The 0.45% saline solution contained 77 mEq/L of sodium. In 24 hours the patient received 55.4 mEq of sodium chloride, which amounted to 7.7 mEq/kg/day of sodium. The normal maintenance sodium requirement is 3 mEq/kg/day. The infant therefore received more than twice his normal daily sodium maintenance requirement. The solution provided the child with 14.4 mEq of potassium chloride, which amounted to 2 mEq/kg/day of potassium. This is the normal maintenance potassium requirement (Table 13-1).

16. The answer is **C,** pages 167 and 181 to 184.

The patient has lost 1.7 kg, which is a 10% reduction in total body weight, assumed to be water loss. The physical findings correlate with a fluid deficit of 10%. This amounts to a fluid deficit of 100 ml/kg or 1700 ml. Her 24-hour maintenance fluid requirement is 1350 ml. Therefore her combined deficit and 24-hour maintenance fluid requirement is 1700 ml (deficit) plus 1350 ml (24-hour maintenance requirement), which equals 3050 ml.

TABLE 13-1 Composition of Common Parenteral Fluids (mEq/L)

Fluid	Na$^+$	K$^+$	Cl$^-$	HCO$_3$$^-$
D5W	0	0	0	0
0.9% NS	154	0	154	0
0.45% NS	77	0	77	0
0.2% NS	34	0	34	0
3% NS	513	0	513	0
Lactated Ringer's (LR)	130	4	109	28°
25% Albumin	140	0	110	0
Plasmanate (5% albumin)	110	2	50	0

°Contained as lactate but converts to bicarbonate when circulated through the liver. This may assist in the correction of metabolic acidosis and limit the patient's chloride load.

17. The answer is **A,** pages 184 to 188.

Failure of enteral feedings may be due to circulatory collapse, increasing fluid deficits, intractable vomiting, clinical deterioration, or failure to achieve clinical rehydration within 8 hours. Oliguria is a sign of dehydration and a predictor of enteral rehydration therapy failure. The cause of enteritis is not a predictor for success or failure of enteral therapy.

18. The answer is **B,** pages 185 to 187.

Small amounts of vomiting are not a contraindication to enteral therapy. If vomiting occurs, the quantity of enteral feeding can be reduced in 5- to 10-ml aliquots. Losses caused by ongoing diarrhea or vomiting can be replaced enterally. Antiemetic medications are contraindicated in children younger than 2 years of age and are associated with side effects and complications.

19. The answer is **A,** pages 166 to 167 and 185 to 188.

The two accepted oral rehydration solutions (WHO and Rehydralate) have high sodium contents. They are appropriate for replacing fluid deficits in cases of dehydration. They contain too much sodium to be used for maintenance fluid requirements in infants. The patient has lost 0.6 kg in 24 hours, which is assumed to be water. This represents a 15% or 150 ml/kg isotonic fluid deficit. The fluid deficit requirement for this child is 600 ml. The child's maintenance fluid requirement is 400 ml/24 hr. In 12 hours the child will receive the entire fluid deficit (600 ml) and half of the 24-hour maintenance requirement (200 ml), totaling 800 ml of fluid. The WHO solution contains 2.5 g/dl glucose, 90 mEq/L sodium, 20 mEq/L potassium, 80 mEq/L chloride, and 30 mEq/L bicarbonate. After 12 hours the child will receive 72 mEq of sodium (18 mEq/kg) and 16 mEq of potassium (4 mEq/kg). A 2-week-old infant receiving six times her 24-hour sodium requirement in 12 hours is at risk for hypernatremia.

20. The answer is **C,** page 188.

Disposition of children with dehydration must be individualized. Discharge management of dehydrated children should encourage oral fluid intake. Clear liquids as a discharge diet should be limited, since they do not decrease vomiting or diarrhea and lead only to protein starvation. Rice-based clear liquid diets may be used and have been shown to decrease diarrhea volume, but they should not replace the resumption of normal feedings. Resumption of feedings if tolerated results in the resolution of diarrhea and return to normal caloric balance. In breastfed infants prompt resumption of feeding is recommended. Any child requiring rehydration therapy should have some form of follow-up arranged at the time of discharge.

Blood Products

Lewis P. Singer

See Barkin et al: Chapter 16.

1. An immunocompromised school-aged child comes to the ED with epistaxis. A complete blood cell count (CBC) reveals a hemoglobin level of 6 g/dl and a platelet count of 6000/mm^3. Prothrombin and partial thromboplastin times are normal. The patient should be transfused with which of the following blood products?
   A. Whole blood.
   B. Packed red blood cells and platelets.
   C. DDAVP.
   D. Fresh frozen plasma.
   E. Irradiated blood products.

2. An 8-year-old child with acute lymphocytic leukemia is admitted to the hospital for a blood transfusion. The child is afebrile and has a heart rate (HR) of 80 beats per minute, a respiratory rate (RR) of 18 breaths per minute, and a blood pressure (BP) of 90/50 mm Hg. Four hours after the transfusion tachypnea, rales, and cyanosis develop. A chest radiograph reveals a ground-glass appearance. Which of the following is *not* consistent with this presentation?
   A. Congestive heart failure.
   B. Adult respiratory distress syndrome.
   C. Leukoagglutinin-associated reaction.
   D. ABO incompatibility.

3. A 6-year-old boy is struck by a bus. On examination at the ED he has moderate abdominal distension. The child requires 6 units of packed red blood cells to stabilize his vital signs for transport to the operating room. All of the following occur as a result of the blood transfusions *except:*
   A. Respiratory acidosis.
   B. Metabolic alkalosis.
   C. Hypothermia.
   D. Cardiac dysrhythmias.
   E. Hypocalcemia.

4. A 3-year-old obese child comes to the ED with a hemoglobin level of 5 g/dl. His HR is 100 beats per minute and BP is 90/60 mm Hg. Which of the following is *not* an explanation for relatively stable vital signs?
   A. Oxygen-hemoglobin dissociation curve shifted to the left.
   B. Increased 2,3-diphosphoglycerate (DPG).
   C. Increased blood volume.
   D. Increased cardiac output.
   E. Hemoglobin with decreased affinity for oxygen.

5. Which of the following is the primary treatment goal for patients who have acute blood loss?
   A. Whole blood transfusion.
   B. Fresh frozen plasma infusion.
   C. Packed red blood cell transfusion.
   D. Restoration of blood volume.
   E. Exchange transfusion with packed red blood cells and 5% albumin.

6. One should consider red blood cell transfusion when blood loss exceeds which of the following volumes in a patient who had a previously normal hemoglobin?
   A. 10% blood volume.
   B. 20% blood volume.
   C. 30% blood volume.
   D. 40% blood volume.
   E. 50% blood volume.

7. Which of the following is the relative blood volume of a 3-year-old patient who weighs 15 kg?
   A. 1500 ml.
   B. 1400 ml.
   C. 1100 ml.
   D. 900 ml.
   E. 700 ml.

8. Thrombocytopenia in patients with idiopathic thrombocytopenic purpura is due to which of the following conditions?
   A. Decreased production of platelets.
   B. Increased peripheral destruction of platelets.
   C. Thrombasthenia.
   D. Prostaglandin inhibition.
   E. Chronic salicylate use.

9. RhoGAM is indicated after infusion of platelets from an Rh-positive donor to an Rh-negative patient because:
   A. The Rh antigen is on platelets from Rh-positive donors.
   B. The plasma contains some red cells.
   C. The plasma contains B cells sensitized against the Rh antigen.
   D. Platelets from all donors induce Rh sensitization.
   E. The plasma contains white blood cells that will sensitize the Rh-negative patient.

10. The most effective way to correct hypofibrinogenemia is to infuse which of the following blood products?
    A. Platelets.
    B. Fresh frozen plasma.
    C. Factor VIII concentrate.
    D. Cryoprecipitate.
    E. Whole blood.

11. Donor blood is *not* screened for which of the following infectious diseases?
    A. Hepatitis A.
    B. Hepatitis B.
    C. Hepatitis C.
    D. HIV.
    E. Syphilis.

12. The universal donor for fresh frozen plasma for a patient with unknown blood type is:
    A. O-negative.
    B. O-positive.
    C. AB-negative.
    D. AB-positive.
    E. Any plasma.

13. The universal donor for packed red blood cells for a patient with unknown blood type is:
    A. AB-positive.
    B. AB-negative.
    C. O-positive.
    D. O-negative.
    E. Any packed red blood cells.

14. Blood stored for long periods of time (i.e., 3 weeks) usually has a potassium concentration of:
    A. 3 mEq/L.
    B. 7 mEq/L.
    C. 15 mEq/L.
    D. 40 mEq/L.
    E. 60 mEq/L.

15. Delayed transfusion reactions usually occur in alloimmunized patients. Which of the following antigen systems do *not* cause the delayed transfusion reaction?
    A. Rh.
    B. ABO.
    C. Duffy.
    D. Kell.
    E. Kidd.

ANSWERS [See Barkin et al: Chapter 16.]

1. The answer is **E,** page 191.
   All blood products contain detectable numbers of viable white blood cells, which may cause graft-versus-host disease. Irradiated blood products should therefore be used in immunosuppressed individuals to minimize the occurrence of graft-versus-host disease. Platelets are usually indicated if bleeding is associated with thrombocytopenia. Prophylactic platelet transfusions are controversial if platelet counts are higher than 10,000/mm^3.

2. The answer is **D,** page 194.
   Donor blood can contain antibodies against human leukocyte antigen (HLA) or granulocyte-specific antigens. This can lead to intravascular leukostasis and can cause fever, neutropenia, and respiratory distress. Pulmonary edema may develop from the resultant capillary leak. A ground-glass appearance on a chest radiograph is consistent with early pulmonary edema from any cause. ABO transfusion reactions usually lead to hemolytic anemia.

3. The answer is **A,** page 194.
   Citrate is the anticoagulant in packed red blood cells. Citrate is metabolized to bicarbonate in the liver and is responsible for the metabolic alkalosis that often develops after massive transfusions. It can also bind to calcium and cause hypocalcemia. Massive transfusions can also lead to hypothermia and induce cardiac dysrhythmias if the blood is not adequately warmed before transfusion.

4. The answer is **A,** page 190.
   Chronic cardiovascular compensation is the result of increased cardiac output, increased or normal blood volume, and increased levels of 2,3-DPG, which decreases the affinity of hemoglobin for oxygen. The oxygen-hemoglobin curve is shifted to the right.

5. The answer is **D,** page 190.
   Restoration of intravascular volume is the primary treatment goal of a patient who has acute blood loss.

6. The answer is **C,** page 190.
   Red cell transfusion is usually considered when blood loss exceeds 30% of the circulating blood volume.

7. The answer is **C,** page 191.
   Blood volume can be estimated from the patient's weight at 70 to 80 ml blood volume per kilogram.

8. The answer is **B,** page 191.
   Idiopathic thrombocytopenic purpura is usually a self-limited disorder following a viral illness and is due to immune destruction.

9. The answer is **B,** page 192.
   The Rh antigen is only on red blood cells. Sufficient red cells exist in the plasma of platelets to cause Rh sensitization in an Rh-negative individual. This is especially a concern for women of childbearing age. Sensitization of an Rh-negative woman may cause fetal demise if the fetus is Rh-negative.

10. The answer is **D,** page 192.

Each bag of cryoprecipitate contains between 100 and 200 mg of fibrinogen and is the most efficient way of increasing the serum fibrinogen. Fresh frozen plasma contains fibrinogen, but in significantly small concentrations.

11. The answer is **A,** page 194.

Donor blood is routinely screened for hepatitis B and C, HIV, and syphilis. Some institutions also screen with a serum glutamic oxaloacetic transaminase (SGOT) and serum glutamic pyruvic transaminase (SGPT).

12. The answer is **D,** page 193.

The universal donor would be AB-positive so that the plasma would not have any anti-A, anti-B, or anti-Rh antibodies.

13. The answer is **D,** page 193.

The universal donor would be O-negative so that there would be no ABO and Rh incompatibilities.

14. The answer is **B,** page 194.

The usual potassium concentration in old packed red blood cells is 7 mEq/L, which is only potentially toxic to patients with renal failure.

15. The answer is **B,** page 193.

Delayed transfusion reactions are usually directed against Rh, Kidd, Duffy, Kell, and MNSS system antigens.

Newborn Resuscitation and Acute Distress in the Neonate and Postnatal Period

Adolfo Grieg • *David H. Rubin*

See Barkin et al: Chapters 17 and 18.

1. Which one of the following statements regarding the Apgar score is *true?*
   A. It determines long-term outcome of the newborn.
   B. It correlates closely with acid-base disturbance at birth.
   C. It suggests a sequential, physiologically appropriate approach to resuscitation.
   D. It focuses the attention of the health care provider on the physiologic status of the newborn.

2. The components of the Apgar score include respiratory effort, heart rate (HR), color, reflex, irritability, and which of the following?
   A. Temperature.
   B. Muscle tone.
   C. Blood pressure (BP).
   D. Respiratory rate (RR).

3. A newborn infant is seen in the ED after a home delivery. During the pregnancy the mother was told that the baby could have trouble breathing at birth. The physical examination reveals cyanosis, tachypnea, and a scaphoid abdomen. Which of the following is the most appropriate procedure?
   A. Placement of a nasogastric tube and intubation of the trachea.
   B. Initiation of cardiopulmonary resuscitation (CPR) with bag-mask ventilation.
   C. A complete sepsis evaluation, including a spinal tap.
   D. An immediate echocardiogram for suspected congenital heart disease.

4. Unique anatomical characteristics of all newborns include short necks, propensity toward obstruction on flexion and extension, and:
   A. Narrowed nasal passageways.
   B. Enlarged tonsils.
   C. Relative macroglossia.
   D. Enlarged turbinates.

5. The resuscitation of newborns should follow a specific sequential, ordered approach. Which of the following sequential events best reflects this protocol?
   A. Anticipation, assessment, airway, breathing, circulation, and drugs.
   B. Airway, anticipation, chest compressions, inotropes, exposure.
   C. Bag-mask ventilation, chest compressions, drugs.
   D. Temperature control, assessment, drugs, breathing bag (Ambu-bag).

6. A newborn is delivered and appears depressed. You bring the baby to a radiant warmer, dry thoroughly, remove the wet liner, position the baby, and then:
   A. Check HR and administer CPR if pulse is less than 100 beats per minute.
   B. Suction the nose, then mouth, and observe for respiratory effort.
   C. Suction the mouth, then nose, then provide tactile stimulation.
   D. Provide tactile stimulation and observe for respiratory effort.

7. A pregnant woman is seen in the ED with ruptured membranes. She has meconium-stained amniotic fluid. Upon delivery of this infant you should:
   A. Suction the oropharynx at the perineum and, after delivery, stimulate the infant to breathe.
   B. Suction the oropharynx at the perineum and provide bag-mask ventilation.
   C. Suction the oropharynx at the perineum and bring the infant to the radiant warmer; if the infant is depressed, intubate the trachea and suction the trachea.
   D. Bring the infant immediately to the radiant warmer, stimulate breathing, and if no response occurs, intubate and suction the trachea.

8. To properly position an infant for bag-valve-mask (BVM) resuscitation, you should:
   A. Place the fingertips under the chin in order to position the mandible anteriorly.
   B. Place the head and neck in the midline, slightly extended.
   C. Perform a chin lift and jaw thrust maneuver.
   D. Use an oropharyngeal airway to maintain an open airway.

9. The most important procedure to perform to prevent meconium aspiration is:
   A. Intubation and suctioning of the trachea.
   B. Cesarean section and immediate removal of the newborn.
   C. Suctioning of the oropharynx before delivery of the thorax.
   D. Lavage of gastrointestinal contents while at the radiant warmer.

10. Which of the following best reflects the adequacy of bag-mask ventilation in a neonate?
    A. Breath sounds.
    B. Mental status.
    C. Color.
    D. Heart rate (HR).

11. A full-term infant is born to a mother who had late decelerations before delivery. As a result, she is given general anesthetic, and a cesarean section is performed. The child is born depressed, and bag-mask ventilation is initiated. If there is no improvement in the child's condition, how long should bag-mask ventilation be continued before attempting to intubate the trachea?
    A. 60 seconds.
    B. 30 to 45 seconds.
    C. 15 to 30 seconds.
    D. Bag-mask ventilation is always sufficient; intubation is not indicated.

12. To inflate a depressed infant's lungs adequately in the delivery room, the initial breaths applied via bag mask or bag endotracheal tube (ET) should be:
    A. No greater than 15 cm H_2O pressure and no longer than 2 seconds.
    B. 20 to 40 cm H_2O pressure and held for 3 to 5 seconds.
    C. 55 cm H_2O and held for 2 seconds.
    D. 20 to 40 cm H_2O pressure and given at rate of 40 breaths per minute.

13. When you are attempting to resuscitate a depressed infant, the first priority to reverse bradycardia is:
    A. Administer epinephrine 1:10,000 0.1 ml/kg intravenously (IV).
    B. Administer atropine 0.01 to 0.03 ml/kg IV.
    C. Begin chest compressions at 140 compressions per minute.
    D. Provide adequate ventilation and oxygenation.

14. An infant is delivered at home by emergency medical service (EMS) and is immediately noted to be meconium-stained and depressed. EMS immediately intubates and suctions the child's trachea. Meconium is not recovered from the trachea, but the child remains depressed. The infant arrives in the ED with an HR of 60 beats per minute. EMS informs you that ventilation has been performed for 1 minute. You assess ET placement, and it seems properly placed. What procedure should be followed next?
    A. Initiate chest compressions at a rate of 120 breaths per minute.
    B. Reintubate the trachea and place on a high-frequency ventilator.
    C. Start a peripheral IV line and administer epinephrine 0.1 ml/kg of a 1:10,000 solution.
    D. Administer atropine 0.01 ml/kg via ET.

15. If the patient described in question 14 does not respond to your chosen procedure, what procedure should you consider next?
    A. Perform chest compressions at a rate of 120 breaths per minute.
    B. Place an umbilical venous catheter and administer epinephrine 0.1 ml/kg of a 1:10,000 solution.
    C. Administer sodium bicarbonate 2 mEq/kg IV.
    D. Administer atropine 0.03 ml/kg IV.

16. An infant is seen in the ED 1 day after a home delivery. The mother gives a history of gestational diabetes. She states that she found it extremely difficult to keep track of her blood sugar level and found the diet very restrictive. The child appears large and weighs 4500 g. While examining the infant you note some tremulousness. The most important initial procedure in this child should be:
    A. Determine hematocrit.
    B. Measure serum magnesium level.
    C. Measure serum calcium level.
    D. Measure serum glucose level using a reagent strip (Dextrostix).

17. The infant described in question 16 remains tremulous, and you decide to place a peripheral IV line. Which of the following is the next most appropriate step?
    A. Administer calcium gluconate 10% at 2 ml/kg over 5 min.
    B. Administer 25% dextrose at 5-ml/kg bolus.
    C. Administer 10% dextrose at 3 ml/kg.
    D. Initiate an infusion of 10% dextrose at 4 to 8 ml/kg/min.

18. Which of the following statements concerning fetal asphyxia is *true?*
    A. An Apgar score less than 5 is the best indicator of fetal asphyxia.
    B. An umbilical cord blood gas value correlates directly with the Apgar score.
    C. An umbilical cord blood gas is the best indicator of fetal asphyxia.
    D. Fetal asphyxia infrequently affects other major organ systems.

19. A 4-day-old neonate is seen in the ED because of poor feeding and pale skin color. The mother states that her delivery was uneventful, and no immediate postnatal complications were noted. Physical examination reveals respiratory distress and bilateral rales on auscultation. There is a hyperactive precordium, and poor peripheral pulses are noted in all extremities. Hepatomegaly is noted on palpation. All of the following are appropriate in the management of this child *except:*
    A. Obtain an electrocardiogram (ECG).
    B. Obtain a chest radiograph.
    C. Administer furosemide.
    D. Administer 10 ml/kg packed red blood cells.

20. A 26-week gestational age baby is delivered in the ED. On examination the baby is noted to be cyanotic and bradycardic and to have retractions. After performing intubation and beginning mechanical ventilation, the next step in the management of this baby is:
    A. Place the baby under a radiant warmer.
    B. Administer IV calcium chloride.
    C. Assure adequate symmetric lung expansion.
    D. Avoid excessive stimulation or manipulation.
    E. Obtain chest radiograph to evaluate for air bronchograms.

21. A 1-hour-old neonate is brought to the ED after being delivered at home. The parents state that the infant appears blue and purses his lips while quiet, but turns pink when he cries. The diagnosis of this infant can be confirmed by:
    A. Chest radiograph.
    B. Arterial blood gas (ABG) performed simultaneously from right upper and lower extremities.
    C. Hyperoxia test.
    D. Inability to pass a size 5 French feeding tube through each nostril.

22. A mother is brought to the ED after being found in a drug den with an infant who was just delivered. EMS states that mother is a known heroin abuser. The child was found to have an HR of 90 beats per minute with little respiratory effort. Bag-mask ventilation was provided to the child until arrival in ED. Appropriate management of this child should include:
    A. Immediate administration of IV naloxone 0.1 ml/kg.
    B. Support of ventilation until spontaneous ventilation is achieved.
    C. Administration of phenobarbital.
    D. Administration of flumazenil.

23. A cyanotic 1-week-old infant is brought to the ED for evaluation. He appears comfortable with a quiet precordium and no apparent respiratory distress. Which of the following procedures would be the most important to determine the etiology of the cyanosis?
    A. Chest radiograph.
    B. ABG determination while breathing room air and while breathing 100% oxygen.
    C. Hemoglobin electrophoresis.
    D. An ECG.

24. An infant is seen in the ED with jitteriness and poor feeding. The total serum calcium level is 6.5 mg/dl. Hypocalcemia may be seen in all of the following conditions *except:*
    A. Infant of diabetic mother.
    B. Early administration of cow's milk.
    C. Hypermagnesemia.
    D. Maternal hyperparathyroidism.
    E. Birth asphyxia.

25. A 3-day-old infant comes in with a history of bilious vomiting. Which of the following radiologic evaluations would best confirm the diagnosis in this infant?
    A. Flat and upright radiograph of the abdomen.
    B. Barium enema.
    C. Upper gastrointestinal series with small bowel follow-through.
    D. Computed tomography (CT) scan of the abdomen.

26. A 2-kg full-term neonate was delivered to a mother with severe preeclampsia. The Apgar scores were 8 and 9 at 1 and 5 minutes, respectively. The baby appears wasted with little subcutaneous fat, but is active and in no distress. However, some jitteriness is observed. Dextrostix testing found a glucose level less than 20 mg/dl. The most likely cause of the infant's hypoglycemia is:
    A. Insulin-secreting tumor.
    B. Bacterial sepsis.
    C. TORCH infection.
    D. Decreased glycogen storage.
    E. Glycogen storage disease.

27. A 6-hour-old full-term infant has pallor. The delivery was uneventful and maternal history unremarkable. Vital signs are normal. The only pertinent physical finding is pallor; the hematocrit is 25%. What is the appropriate study to determine a diagnosis in this infant?
    A. Kleihauer-Betke test.
    B. Bone marrow aspiration.
    C. Coombs' test.
    D. Evaluation of the peripheral smear.

28. A 3-day-old infant is brought to the ED with seizures. The infant had an unremarkable delivery and postnatal course. The first laboratory examination that should be performed in this child is:
    A. CT scan.
    B. Liver function studies.
    C. Dextrostix.
    D. Electroencephalogram.
    E. Arterial blood gas (ABG).

29. A full-term 3-kg infant is delivered at home and is brought to the ED 6 days later because of fever and a rash. The mother states that she has a rash in her vaginal area. On examination the infant has petechiae, jaundice, hepatomegaly, a vesicular rash, and a temperature of 101.4° F (38.6° C). The platelet count is 19,000/mm^3. Which of the following will support the correct diagnosis in this newborn?
    A. Urine culture for cytomegalovirus (CMV).
    B. Spinal fluid examination.
    C. Giemsa stain of skin scrapings.
    D. Rubella titers.

30. A 4-day-old infant has a history of decreased urine output, a pink coloration noted in the diaper, and a decreased appetite. Pregnancy was complicated by maternal diabetes. Which of the following laboratory investigations would be the most immediately helpful in the management of this patient?
    A. Serum blood urea nitrogen (BUN) level.
    B. Serum creatinine level.
    C. Measurement of urine output.
    D. Serum potassium determination.

31. A 32 weeks' gestation infant is seen in the ED soon after his discharge from the neonatal intensive care unit. The parents state that the infant was on a monitor and medication for apnea while in the hospital, but was discharged home just with a monitor. They heard the alarm sound, but when they arrived at the infant's bedside, all appeared well. The most likely etiology for the alarm sounding in this case is:
    A. Hypothermia.
    B. Prone positioning.
    C. Loose leads on the apnea monitor.
    D. Hypercalcemia.

32. The most common bacterial agent known to cause pneumonia in the first month of life is:
    A. *Staphylococcus aureus.*
    B. *Chlamydia trachomatis.*
    C. Group B *Streptococcus.*
    D. *Ureaplasma urealyticum.*

33. An infant is delivered at home and is brought to the ED. Paramedics state that the delivery was uneventful. The Apgar scores were 9 and 9 at 1 and 5 minutes, respectively. The baby is well developed with an RR of 50 breaths per minute. Capillary refill time is less than 2 seconds, and there are strong distal pulses. On auscultation the baby has slightly diminished breath sounds on the right and a pulse oximeter reading of 92%. All of the following would be appropriate therapeutic options *except:*
    A. Transillumination of the chest.
    B. ABG determination.
    C. Chest radiograph.
    D. Aspiration of the right hemithorax by needle thoracostomy.

34. A newborn is seen in the ED. She was delivered to a 35-year-old gravida 3 para 2 mother who states that there was profuse vaginal bleeding during pregnancy. Physical examination reveals a pale, limp child with prolonged capillary refill. Which of the following choices for fluid resuscitation would *not* be an appropriate choice in this infant?
    A. 0.9% sodium chloride.
    B. 10% dextrose solution.
    C. O-negative blood.
    D. Residual placental blood.
    E. 5% albumin.

35. Which of the following is the first normal physiologic response to fetal asphyxia?
    A. Decreased adrenal blood flow.
    B. Initial increase in cardiac output followed by decrease in cardiac output.
    C. Decreased cardiac output.
    D. Decreased cerebral blood flow.
    E. Increased renal perfusion.

36. A full-term infant is delivered by cesarean section because of failure of labor to progress. The infant is noted to have a lumbar meningomyelocele. Which of the following should be performed immediately?
    A. Lumbar puncture.
    B. Serum electrolyte determination.
    C. Cover the meningomyelocele with sterile gauze moistened with saline.
    D. CT scan of the brain and spinal cord.
    E. Determination of α-fetoprotein level.

37. A former 28-week premature infant who is now 3 months corrected age is brought to the ED with respiratory distress. The infant is receiving home oxygen therapy, theophylline, and diuretics. Physical examination reveals an infant in moderate respiratory distress. Rales, wheezing, and retractions are present. All of the following will be helpful in managing this infant *except:*
    A. Chest radiograph.
    B. Recent weight.
    C. Group B streptococcal antigen determination.
    D. Furosemide 1 ml/kg intravenously.
    E. Trial of nebulized β-agonists.

38. A 29-year-old gravida 1 para 0 mother is in active labor with a 30-week gestational pregnancy and is expected to be brought to the ED. All of the following equipment will be helpful *except:*
    A. Radiant warmer.
    B. Laryngoscope with a curved blade.
    C. 3.0-mm ET.
    D. Suction apparatus.
    E. Umbilical vein insertion tray.

39. A 2-day-old newborn is brought to the ED. The patient is pale and lethargic, and the HR is 80 beats per minute. CPR is immediately initiated, and adequate ventilation is provided using 100% oxygen. At reevaluation the HR is still 80 beats per minute. Which of the following is the next appropriate intervention?
    A. Atropine 0.01 ml/kg intramuscularly.
    B. NaHCO$_3$ 2 mEq/kg IV.
    C. 10 ml/kg 0.9% sodium chloride IV.
    D. Epinephrine (1:10,000) 0.01 ml/kg IV.

40. A 2.9-kg boy is delivered by emergency cesarean section. He has a history of abruptio placentae and poor fetal tracings. The infant's trachea is intubated. The baby is pale and mottled, and blood pressure is 45/28 mm Hg. Apgar scores are 3 at 1 minute and 5 at 5 minutes. The next step in treatment is:
    A. Perform a femoral cutdown and infuse 20 ml/kg 0.9% sodium chloride.
    B. Give epinephrine 0.01 ml/kg via the ET to increase BP.
    C. Perform umbilical venous catheterization and infuse 10 ml/kg 0.9% sodium chloride.
    D. Administer sodium bicarbonate 2 mEq/kg IV.
    E. Administer a dopamine infusion at 10 μg/kg/min.

41. A full-term neonate is delivered by emergency cesarean section for failure of labor to progress. The mother had received meperidine 2 hours before delivery. At delivery the infant is lethargic with lack of respiratory effort. The patient's trachea is intubated, but there is no change in color despite positive-pressure ventilation with 100% oxygen. Which of the following interventions is *incorrect?*
    A. Auscultate the axilla for equal breath sounds.
    B. Visually check for correct ET position.
    C. Inflate the lungs with 15 cm H_2O of peak pressure.
    D. Give naloxone 0.01 ml/kg endotracheally.
    E. Ventilate at 24 breaths/min.

42. A 16-year-old is seen in the ED in active labor. EMS reports meconium staining of the amniotic fluid. The initial step in the management of this infant following delivery includes which of the following?
    A. Stimulate and initiate positive-pressure ventilation.
    B. Intubate the trachea and suction.
    C. Suction the oropharynx at delivery of the head.
    D. If no meconium is recovered from the posterior pharynx, intubation is not required.
    E. Administer positive-pressure ventilation and surfactant.

43. A full-term infant has petechiae scattered over the entire body. The patient is well developed and in no distress. The infant's platelet count is 11,000/mm^3. Which one of the following tests would *not* be helpful in the diagnosis of thrombocytopenia?
    A. Maternal platelet count.
    B. Maternal PLA-1 antigen.
    C. Presence of neonatal giant hemangioma on physical examination.
    D. CMV culture.
    E. Coombs' test.

ANSWERS [See Barkin et al: Chapters 17 and 18.]

1. The answer is **D,** page 197.
   The Apgar score focuses the attention of the health care provider on the status of the newborn. The score neither correlates closely with the degree of acid-base disturbance at birth nor intuitively suggests a sequential physiologically appropriate approach to resuscitative efforts.
2. The answer is **B,** page 198.
   The components of the Apgar score are HR, respirations, muscle tone, reflex, irritability, and color (Table 15-1.)
3. The answer is **A,** page 198.
   A scaphoid abdomen suggests a diaphragmatic hernia, which is most appropriately treated with intubation of the trachea and nasogastric tube insertion. These babies may suffer massive gastric distention or perforation if hyperventilated with a bag and mask.

4. The answer is **C,** page 198.
   Anatomically, all newborns have a short neck, relative macroglossia, and a tendency toward airway obstruction when the neck is overly extended or flexed. Furthermore, the respiratory system of the newborn is fluid-filled in utero and must be cleared to initiate effective respirations. The airway may be further compromised by aspiration of meconium.
5. The answer is **A,** page 198.
   The ABCs of neonatal resuscitation include: A: anticipation, assessment, airway; B: breathing; C: circulation; D: drugs; E: extras, evaluation.
6. The answer is **C,** page 199.
   This is the proper sequence to use in resuscitation as in the *Textbook of Neonatal Resuscitation,* published in 1994 by the American Heart Association. Most infants respond to simple resuscitative measures such as warming, drying, suctioning, and tactile stimulation. Advanced resuscitation procedures include ventilation, chest compressions, and medications.
7. The answer is **C,** page 199.
   This is the recommended sequence to use with a child born through meconium-stained fluid. There is controversy regarding the need to intubate nondepressed, meconium-stained infants.

TABLE 15-1 Apgar Score

Sign	Score		
	0	1	2
Heart rate	Absent	Slow (<100/min)	>100/min
Respirations	Absent	Slow, irregular	Good; crying
Muscle tone	Limp	Some flexion	Active motion
Reflex irritability	No response	Grimace	Vigorous
Color	Blue or pale	Acrocyanosis	Completely pink

8. The answer is **B**, page 200.

The best method to achieve adequate airway patency in a newborn is to place the head and neck in the midline and slightly extended. Placing the fingertips under the chin to position the mandible anteriorly (as in the adult) is not recommended because pressure on the tissues in the submental triangle results in airway occlusion.

9. The answer is **C**, pages 198 and 199.

The proper approach to the child with meconium staining of the amniotic fluid and potential meconium aspiration is to provide fetal monitoring, suctioning of the oropharynx before delivery of the thorax, and tracheal intubation with suctioning when thick particulate meconium is observed.

10. The answer is **D**, page 200.

Proper assessment of the adequacy of ventilation is the key to successful BVM ventilation. In all infants the HR is a monitor of the adequacy of ventilation. Breath sounds also are useful.

11. The answer is **C**, page 200.

If there is no rapid improvement in HR after 30 to 45 seconds of *adequate* bag-mask ventilation, intubation of the trachea is indicated. The correct ET size can be estimated from birth weight (Figure 15-1).

12. The answer is **B**, page 201.

To provide optimal initiation of ventilation in depressed infants, inflate the lungs gradually to a peak pressure of 20 to 40 cm H_2O for 3 to 5 seconds once or twice and then inflate at an average rate of 40 breaths per minute using a prolonged inflation period.

13. The answer is **D**, page 201.

In the depressed newborn, the first priority is providing adequate oxygenation and ventilation. The ventilation reverses the reflex bradycardia that accompanies hypoxia. This problem should be addressed first in any resuscitation.

14. The answer is **A**, page 201.

If bradycardia continues for more than 30 to 60 seconds after adequate ventilation, including intubation, cardiac massage should be initiated.

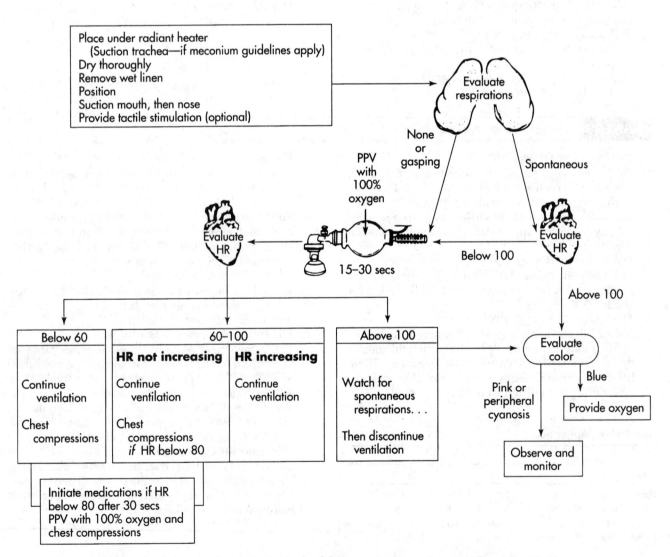

FIG. 15-1 Overview of resuscitation in the delivery room. (From American Heart Association: *Textbook of neonatal resuscitation*, Washington, DC, 1994, The Association.)

15. The answer is **B**, pages 201 and 202.
    If maintenance of the airway is achieved and CPR fails, administration of medications becomes necessary. Administration via an umbilical venous line is an effective method. Although not a choice in this question, endotracheal administration of epinephrine could also be considered.

16. The answer is **D**, page 212.
    This scenario depicts a typical case of postdelivery hypoglycemia developing in the infant of a diabetic mother because of hyperinsulinemia in response to poor maternal glucose control.

17. The answer is **C**, page 212.
    The treatment of *symptomatic* neonatal hypoglycemia includes the immediate administration by an IV line of 0.25 to 0.5 g/kg of glucose. This can be accomplished by giving 3 to 5 ml/kg of a 10% dextrose solution.

18. The answer is **C**, page 202.
    The umbilical cord blood gas is generally accepted as the best indicator of fetal asphyxia, although it correlates poorly with the Apgar score. The Apgar score does not correlate well with acid-base disturbance or with the degree of asphyxia.

19. The answer is **D**, page 210.
    The patient described in the scenario is in congestive heart failure. Blood products are not indicated in the patient with congestive heart failure who is not anemic. An ECG would provide supporting data for a possible anatomic location of the heart lesion. The most common causes of congestive heart failure in neonates are (in order of frequency) hypoplastic left ventricle, coarctation of the aorta, ventricular septal defect, truncus arteriosus, endocardial cushion defect, aortic stenosis, patent ductus arteriosus, and arteriovenous malformations. The management of congestive heart failure in the neonate includes oxygen and other ventilatory support, IV access, and administration of a diuretic (such as furosemide 1 ml/kg IV) and an inotropic agent. Consideration should also be given in this age group to the possibility of maintaining the patency of the ductus arteriosus. Continuous infusion of prostaglandin E_1 may be lifesaving.

20. The answer is **C**, pages 200 and 201.
    Once intubation has been performed, adequate symmetric expansion of the lungs must be demonstrated. The ET must also be secured to prevent its entry into the mainstem bronchi or its accidental removal.

21. The answer is **D**, pages 208 and 811.
    This is a typical case of a newborn with choanal atresia. Neonates, as obligate nasal breathers, are unable to breathe and feed effectively when nasal obstruction is present. Inability to pass size 5 French feeding tube into each nostril is the standard for diagnosis.

22. The answer is **B**, page 209.
    Naloxone should be administered only to infants with respiratory depression from *acute* suspected narcotic exposure and *not* to all infants exposed to narcotics. The infant whose mother abused narcotics *chronically* is less likely to have respiratory depression, and naloxone may precipitate drug-induced withdrawal seizure. Thus, if an infant with chronic exposure has respiratory depression, support of ventilation is the treatment of choice.

23. The answer is **B**, page 211.
    The most important test to confirm a diagnosis of cyanotic heart disease is a comparison of the arterial Pao_2 while the patient breathes room air and while the patient breathes 100% oxygen (hyperoxia test). The Pao_2 rises above 100 mm Hg in the infant with primary pulmonary disease but remains below this level in the infant with cyanotic heart disease.

24. The answer is **C**, pages 211 and 212.
    Hypocalcemia can be seen during the first 24 hours of life, primarily in premature infants. Other causes include infants with birth asphyxia and diabetic mothers. Late onset neonatal hypocalcemia can be due to maternal hyperparathyroidism or hypomagnesemia.

25. The answer is **B**, page 213.
    Bilious vomiting in a neonate should be assumed to be a volvulus caused by malrotation until proved otherwise. A contrast enema using air or barium should precede all upper gastrointestinal studies.

26. The answer is **D**, page 212.
    Hypoglycemia is defined as a whole blood glucose value of less than 30 mg/dl or a plasma glucose level less than 35 mg/dl in the first 3 days of life in a term newborn. Hypoglycemia develops in small-for-gestational-age infants and premature infants as a result of decreased glycogen stores. The treatment of neonatal hypoglycemia is 0.25 to 0.5 g/kg of glucose given intravenously. After this initial bolus an IV infusion should be initiated with 10% glucose at 4 ml/kg/hr.

27. The answer is **D**, pages 213 and 214.
    The easiest and most informative test of those listed in this question is the examination of the peripheral smear. This can yield information regarding red blood cell size and hemoglobin concentration. The most common etiology of anemia in the neonate is acute blood loss.

28. The answer is **C**, page 219.
    Neonatal seizures have a variety of causes. Metabolic causes (e.g., hypoglycemia, hyponatremia, hypernatremia, hypocalcemia) are among the most common and easily treatable. The other tests listed may be warranted but are not necessary in an emergency. Other causes of neonatal seizures include asphyxia and birth trauma, intracranial hemorrhage, developmental brain disorder, and meningitis.

29. The answer is **C,** page 217.

The vesicular rash described and the other physical signs suggest a diagnosis of herpes (HSV-2), which could be diagnosed by a Giemsa stain of scrapings from the lesions. Infants with HSV-2 almost always acquire the virus at time of delivery from the mother who has an active genital herpes lesion. The virus has an incubation period of 2 to 40 days (mean = 6 days).

30. The answer is **A,** page 219.

Acute renal failure in the newborn is suspected when the urine output falls to less than 0.5 ml/kg/hr or if the BUN level is greater than 20 mg/dl. The serum creatinine may also rise. However, in the first few days of life the serum creatinine reflects the mother's level and may be falsely elevated in the neonate. Hyperkalemia is a late finding in severe acute renal failure. The history of maternal diabetes raises the possibility of renal vein thrombosis as a cause of this newborn's renal failure.

31. The answer is **C,** page 220.

When the apnea monitor alarm goes off and the child is well, loose leads on the apnea monitor are a frequent cause. Another cause may be that the HR is drifting below the set limits in an asymptomatic child. Other causes to consider are sepsis, hypoglycemia, and seizure activity.

32. The answer is **C,** page 221.

Pneumonia in the first month of life is caused by a pathogen acquired either during the birth process or postnatally, or by aspiration of orogastric contents. The most common bacterial cause of pneumonia in the first month of life is group B *Streptococcus*. Viral agents such as respiratory syncytial virus, CMV, and HSV-2 may also cause pneumonia.

33. The answer is **D,** page 221.

In a child with only mild symptoms and no evidence of hypotension, aspiration of a pneumothorax may not be indicated. If a child were severely symptomatic and experiencing hypotension, an immediate needle aspiration would be indicated.

34. The answer is **B,** page 201.

D10 would not be an appropriate choice in a hypovolemic patient to improve volume status. Volume expansion should be administered in 10-ml/kg increments to infants with clinically evident volume contraction, followed by reassessment. Choices for volume expansion in the neonate include normal saline solution, plasmanate, residual placental blood, O-negative blood, or maternal blood.

35. The answer is **B,** page 205.

In acute fetal asphyxia, cardiac output is initially maintained and a diving reflex ensues to provide blood to adrenal glands, brain, and heart. This reflex leads to diminished blood flow to skin, kidneys, and intestines.

36. The answer is **C,** page 218.

Meningomyelocele occurs in 1 in 500 births. Macrocephaly may prevent vaginal delivery. Prenatal diagnosis can be accomplished by obtaining an α-fetoprotein level and confirmed by a screening ultrasonography. Associated complications may include Arnold-Chiari malformation, hydrocephalus, and lack of sphincter tone and lower extremity movement. Seizures are not associated with meningomyelocele. It is imperative that the area be covered with saline-soaked gauze to prevent fluid losses and infection.

37. The answer is **C,** page 220.

The infant has bronchopulmonary dysplasia, a chronic lung disorder of low–birth weight infants. Many infants are discharged home receiving oxygen, as well as bronchodilators and diuretics. Group B streptococcal infection is a common cause of respiratory distress in the first month of life.

38. The answer is **B,** pages 197 and 198.

A 30 weeks' gestation infant should weigh approximately 1200 g, and based on this weight, an ET size 2.5 to 3.0 should be used. A straight, not a curved, blade should be used to intubate the premature infant's trachea.

39. The answer is **D,** pages 201 and 202.

Medication should be administered if the HR falls below 100 beats per minute after adequate ventilation with 100% oxygen and cardiac massage. The appropriate concentration and dosage of epinephrine is 0.01 ml/kg (1:10,000) given intravenously (Table 15-2).

40. The answer is **C,** page 201.

The patient's poor capillary refill, decreased blood pressure, and skin mottling are signs and symptoms of hypovolemia. Initial treatment should consist of umbilical catheter placement and infusion of an appropriate volume expander, which may include normal saline, 5% albumin, residual placental blood, or O-negative blood.

TABLE 15-2   Drug Therapy for Resuscitating the Newborn

Drug (how supplied)	Dosage	Route	Amount
Epinephrine (1:10,000)	0.01 mg/kg	IV, ET	0.1 ml/kg
Sodium bicarbonate 4.2% (0.5 mEq/ml)	1-2 mEq/kg	IV	2-4 ml/kg
Naloxone (1 mg/ml)	0.1 mg/kg	IV, IM, ET	0.1 ml/kg
Atropine (0.1 mg/ml)	0.01-0.03 mg/kg	IV, IM, ET	0.1-0.3 ml/kg (minimum 0.1 mg/dose)

IV, Intravenous; *IM,* intramuscular; *ET,* endotracheal.

41. The answer is **C,** pages 200 and 201.

Proper documentation of ET placement is of paramount importance. The patient was delivered by cesarean section with subsequent lack of the vaginal squeeze, which increases the amount of lung fluid to be absorbed. Initial breaths administered by positive-pressure ventilation have to be approximately 20 to 40 cm H_2O to expand the collapsed alveoli and overcome the increased lung fluid. The mother received meperidine, which can lead to neonatal depression.

42. The answer is **C,** pages 198 to 200.

Thick particulate meconium staining of the amniotic fluid requires aggressive management. Suctioning of the oropharynx before delivery of the thorax is mandatory, followed by tracheal intubation if particulate meconium is observed.

43. The answer is **E,** page 214.

Initial steps in the evaluation of neonatal thrombocytopenia include determination of maternal platelet count and presence of PLA-1 antigen. Neonatal giant hemangioma can cause entrapment of platelets. TORCH infection may cause thrombocytopenia. Coombs' test will not be helpful in evaluating thrombocytopenia.

16

Approach to Multiple Trauma

Diane M. Sixsmith

See Barkin et al: Chapter 19.

1. The leading cause of injury death among children less than 19 years of age is:
   A. Motor vehicle–pedestrian accident.
   B. Burns.
   C. Suicide.
   D. Motor vehicle occupant accident.
   E. Assault.
2. The majority of pediatric trauma deaths occur:
   A. In community hospitals that are not trauma centers.
   B. Immediately following the injury or accident.
   C. Because of inadequate resuscitation in the ED.
   D. Following prolonged resuscitation and surgery.
   E. Because of inadequate or delayed prehospital care.
3. The usual cause of early death (within hours of injury) in trauma is:
   A. Major internal hemorrhage.
   B. Multiple organ failure.
   C. Cardiac dysrhythmia.
   D. Brainstem herniation.
   E. Electrolyte imbalance.
4. Among injury severity scoring systems the Pediatric Trauma Score (PTS):
   A. Has fewer components to score than the CRAMS scale (**c**irculation, **r**espiration, **a**bdomen, **m**otor, and **s**peech) and is thus easier to calculate.
   B. Was field-tested first in adult trauma patients to test its predictive validity.
   C. Is calculated by assigning a numerical value to Glasgow Coma Scale, systolic blood pressure, and respiratory rate (RR).
   D. Is a better predictor for ED disposition than the Revised Trauma Score.

5. A 6-year-old boy riding a bicycle is struck by a car going 30 miles per hour as it jumps the curb. The boy is brought into the ED immobilized on a long board with a cervical collar. His systolic blood pressure is 100 mm Hg, RR is 26 breaths per minute, and heart rate (HR) is 120 beats per minute. His airway is clear, and his capillary refill time is normal. His eyes are open; he is moving all extremities, is agitated and moaning, and does not answer when you ask him his name. His abdomen is soft. The test most likely to provide information for diagnosis and immediate management is:
   A. A complete blood count (CBC).
   B. An arterial blood gas (ABG) measurement.
   C. A computed tomographic (CT) scan of the head.
   D. A CT scan of the abdomen.
   E. A pelvic x-ray film.
6. Which of the following injuries increases the risk of mortality in children?
   A. Head injury.
   B. Cervical spine fracture.
   C. Major skeletal trauma.
   D. Lacerated liver.
   E. Postoperative complications.
7. An 8-year-old girl is struck by an automobile as she runs out into the street to catch a ball. She would be most likely to sustain which of the following injuries?
   A. A fractured pelvis, a parietal skull fracture, and a C2 fracture.
   B. A C7 fracture, a fractured shoulder, and a lacerated liver.
   C. A ruptured spleen, a fractured femur, and a frontal lobe contusion.
   D. A fractured pelvis, bilateral ankle fractures, and a ruptured bladder.
   E. An occipital skull fracture, a fractured humerus, and a fractured pelvis.

8. The patient described in question 7 is responsive only to painful stimuli. Her PTS is 4. Immediate initial management would be:
   A. Supplemental oxygen, immobilization of the cervical spine, endotracheal intubation, and intravenous (IV) access.
   B. Supplemental oxygen by face mask, IV access, and typing and cross matching for 2 units of whole blood.
   C. Supplemental oxygen with an oropharyngeal airway, IV access, and immobilization of the cervical spine.
   D. Immobilization of the cervical spine, an oropharyngeal airway, and CBC.
   E. An oropharyngeal airway, IV access, and a CT scan of the head and pelvis.

9. For optimal management of a pediatric trauma patient, the members of the trauma team should include, at minimum:
   A. A physician in charge, a respiratory therapist for airway management, a documentation nurse, and two other health care professionals.
   B. A physician in charge, a second physician who manages the airway with the assistance of a respiratory therapist, two other physicians, and a nurse for documentation.
   C. A physician in charge, a second physician who manages the airway, two other physicians or experienced health professionals, a documentation nurse, and two or more bedside nurses.
   D. A pediatric surgeon, a charge nurse, two additional health care professionals experienced in trauma, and a respiratory therapist.
   E. A physician in charge, a pediatric surgeon, two additional physicians, a documentation nurse, and two or more bedside nurses.

10. A 14-year-old boy has sustained a stab wound to the left posterior subscapular area in an argument on the basketball court. He is brought into the ED by the police. He is pale and agitated. His systolic blood pressure is 80 mm Hg, RR is 30 breaths per minute, and pulse is weak with a rate of 130 beats per minute. He has decreased breath sounds on the left, and his trachea is deviated to the right. Immediate management sequence would be:
   A. 100% oxygen by nonrebreather, placement of a chest tube in the left fifth intercostal space, midaxillary line, and establishing IV access.
   B. Endotracheal intubation, establishment of IV access, and rapid infusion of 1 L of lactated Ringer's solution.
   C. Endotracheal intubation, establishment of IV access, and portable chest radiograph.
   D. 100% oxygen by nonrebreather, establishment of IV access, and a portable chest radiograph.
   E. Needle decompression in the second left intercostal space in the midclavicular line, endotracheal intubation, and establishment of IV access.

11. If the patient described in question 10 improves with the initial treatment, the next step is:
    A. Obtain a CT scan of the lung.
    B. Call the thoracic surgeon to manage the stab wound.
    C. Administer 2 units of type-specific blood.
    D. Obtain an ABG.
    E. Examine for other injuries.

12. A 2-year-old boy has fallen from a second-story window onto the sidewalk below. He is brought in immobilized with a cervical collar. His eyes are closed and do not open. He grimaces and withdraws from painful stimuli. His systolic blood pressure is 60 mm Hg, HR is 140 beats per minute, and RR is 36 breaths per minute, which are noisy with bloody secretions around the mouth and tongue. Immediate management sequence should be:
    A. Endotracheal intubation, establishment of IV access, and infusion of 250 ml of Ringer's lactate solution.
    B. Endotracheal intubation, establishment of IV access, withholding of fluids until extent of head injury has been assessed, and obtaining a portable cervical and chest radiograph.
    C. Endotracheal intubation, intraosseous cannulation, and infusion of 250 ml D5 ½ normal saline.
    D. Cricothyrotomy, establishment of IV access, and infusion of 250 ml of Ringer's lactate solution.
    E. Suctioning and positioning of the airway, supplemental oxygen by face mask, and establishment of IV access.

13. The child's systolic blood pressure in question 12 remains at 50 to 60 mm Hg after the treatment chosen. Which of the following best explains this finding?
    A. Head injury with impending herniation.
    B. Pericardial tamponade.
    C. Multiple fractures.
    D. Ongoing blood loss with insufficient volume replacement.
    E. Persistent hypoxia.

14. A 7-year-old girl is an unrestrained backseat passenger in a multivehicle accident in which another person died at the scene. She is brought into the ED on a long board with a cervical collar in place, oxygen by nasal cannula at 4 L/min, and normal saline infusing in an antecubital vein. Her systolic blood pressure is 95 mm Hg, HR is 105 beats per minute, and RR is 20 breaths per minute. She is alert, moving all extremities, and is able to respond on command and tell you her name and where she goes to school. Capillary refill time is 1 second. Which of the following steps is the most important in the management of this patient?
    A. Perform a secondary survey.
    B. Call the trauma team.
    C. Order x-ray films of the chest and cervical spine.
    D. Type and crossmatch for 2 units of blood.
    E. Stabilize the airway with rapid sequence intubation.

15. The child described in question 14 has persistent upper abdominal tenderness. Systolic blood pressure is now 100 mm Hg, HR is 105 beats per minute, and RR is 20 breaths per minute. Which of the following is the next appropriate step in the evaluation of this patient?
    A. Exploratory laparotomy.
    B. ACT scan of the abdomen with contrast.
    C. Diagnostic peritoneal lavage.
    D. A CT scan of the abdomen without contrast.
    E. Flat and upright x-ray film of the abdomen.

16. A 14-year-old boy apparently has been accidentally shot in the abdomen with a small caliber gun by a friend. He is brought in by ambulance pale, confused, and diaphoretic. His systolic blood pressure is 75 mm Hg, HR 125 beats per minute, and RR 24 breaths per minute. He has a 14-gauge catheter in his antecubital fossa and has received almost 1 L of normal saline before arrival. There is no obvious hemorrhaging. Management of this child's airway is best obtained by:
    A. 10 to 12 L oxygen by nonrebreather face mask.
    B. Nasal intubation.
    C. Endotracheal intubation with rapid sequence induction, using midazolam and a neuromuscular blocking agent.
    D. Endotracheal intubation with rapid sequence induction using only midazolam.
    E. Assisted ventilation with a bag-valve mask (BVM).

17. The best initial method for evaluation and management of the abdominal gunshot wound in the child described in question 16 is:
    A. Abdominal plain film radiograph.
    B. Diagnostic peritoneal lavage.
    C. CT scan of the abdomen.
    D. Exploratory laparotomy.

18. Which of the following issues in training prehospital personnel about field management of pediatric trauma is the most important after administration of oxygen, immobilization of the neck, and attention to hemorrhage?
    A. Attaining skill in IV access.
    B. Getting the compromised child to the ED as soon as possible.
    C. Knowing fluid administration rates for pediatric patients.
    D. Attaining skill in pediatric endotracheal intubation.
    E. Stabilizing the pediatric patient before transport.

19. Videotaped trauma resuscitations:
    A. Are an important part of the medical record that should be saved along with the patient's other medical records.
    B. Are an important continuous quality improvement tool that can be used for credentialing trauma surgeons.
    C. Should have a protocol for their use that includes destroying them after their review or after a set period of time.
    D. Violate patient confidentiality and cannot be viewed without prior patient or parent permission.
    E. Are an important method of quality assessment but present significant medicolegal issues, which limit their usage.

20. Rapid sequence induction for intubation:
    A. Includes pretreatment with pancuronium before vecuronium administration.
    B. Is contraindicated in patients with head injury.
    C. Should not be performed in patients who are agitated.
    D. Requires preoxygenation for 4 to 5 minutes by a nonrebreather mask without positive pressure.
    E. Is preferentially performed with sodium thiopental to reduce the muscle fasciculation associated with succinylcholine.

21. When the physician is performing rapid sequence induction, the first step is to:
    A. Evaluate the patient's airway anatomy.
    B. Administer neuromuscular blockade followed by sedation.
    C. Perform the Sellick maneuver.
    D. Administer sedation followed by neuromuscular blockade.

22. A 10-year-old boy was pinned between a truck and a wall. On arrival in the ED, he is confused and agitated with a barely palpable femoral pulse, tachycardic at 150 beats per minute, with grunting respirations. He has apparently sustained massive crush injuries to his abdomen, pelvis, and femur. To intubate this patient, which of the following agents should *not* be used?
    A. Midazolam.
    B. Diazepam.
    C. Ketamine.
    D. Thiopental.
    E. Lorazepam.

23. After the airway of the child described in question 22 is secured, the optimal next step should include which one of the following?
    A. Insert two large-bore IV lines, infuse a liter of Ringer's lactate solution as fast as possible, and request O-negative blood.
    B. Notify the operating room that the patient is on the way for exploratory surgery.
    C. Insert two large-bore IV lines, and type and crossmatch for 4 units of donor-specific blood.
    D. Insert two 22-gauge large-bore IV lines, and apply medical antishock trousers (MAST).
    E. Insert a central venous line and infuse Ringer's lactate solution until the central venous pressure approaches 5 mm H_2O.

24. Parents have accompanied their son to the hospital in the ambulance. The charge nurse tells you they are begging to come in to see their son. The child is not improving with treatment, and you believe the prognosis is poor. The best way to manage this situation is to:
   A. Call the hospital chaplain and ask him to prepare the parents for the possibility of the child's death.
   B. Go out to the waiting area and carefully explain to the parents what is going on and what further treatments and procedures are anticipated.
   C. Have the charge nurse explain to the parents that it is still too early to know the prognosis and that someone will be out to talk to them when the child's condition is more stable.
   D. Have the pediatric social worker stay with the parents and explain to them the usual procedures in this situation.

25. In the multiply injured patient, along with initial assessment and control of the airway, it is imperative to immediately address:
   A. Internal hemorrhage.
   B. Severely angulated fractures.
   C. A depressed level of consciousness.
   D. An obvious skull fracture.
   E. Immobilization of the cervical spine.

ANSWERS   [See Barkin et al: Chapter 19.]

1. The answer is **D,** page 223.
   Injury is the leading cause of death in children above 9 months of age in the United States. Motor vehicle occupant injuries are the leading cause of injury death, causing 47% of all injury deaths.

2. The answer is **B,** page 223.
   Mortality in trauma has a trimodal distribution with more than 50% of trauma deaths occurring immediately after the injury, usually at the scene, because of fatal injuries such as decapitation, ventricular rupture, or brainstem herniation. Early deaths are those that occur within hours of injury and represent about 30% of trauma deaths.

3. The answer is **A,** page 224.
   The usual cause of early death is major internal hemorrhage. Trauma education and trauma centers focusing on early detection and treatment can help to decrease deaths in this category.

4. The answer is **D,** page 224.
   Injury severity scoring systems have been developed both to predict ultimate outcome and to assist in triage decisions. The PTS is a better predictor for ED disposition while the Revised Trauma Score is a predictor of injury severity (see Chapter 4, question 6). The CRAMS score is used for field triage.

5. The answer is **C,** pages 224 and 225.
   This child has a Pediatric Glasgow Coma Score of 11, which suggests a moderate neurologic defect. In the presence of a normal blood pressure and only mildly elevated HR and RR, circulatory or respiratory decompensation is not the cause of this child's altered mental status. Hence, neither a CBC nor a blood gas study (while part of the overall workup) is likely to provide meaningful information. A CT scan of the abdomen or pelvic films may be required later, but the most important immediate diagnostic consideration is establishing the presence or absence of a head injury.

6. The answer is **A,** page 224.
   Both adults and children with head injuries have an increased risk of mortality. The head is involved in 80% of multiple injuries, and 30% of childhood injury deaths result from a head injury.

7. The answer is **C,** page 226.
   When a child pedestrian is struck by a motor vehicle, a common injury pattern is a fractured femur, a chest or upper abdominal injury, and a head injury. This is called Waddell's triad and arises from the child's leg hitting the car bumper and the child being thrown onto the hood of the car and then thrown to the street, resulting in a contralateral head injury.

8. The answer is **A,** page 230.
   Early intubation is necessary if a child is neurologically impaired to secure the airway, prevent aspiration, and maintain adequate ventilation. Supplemental oxygen by mask or an oral airway is insufficient if the respiratory drive might become or already is impaired. In addition, venous access for fluid administration must be established immediately to support circulation. The mechanism of injury in this child makes it necessary to evaluate for cervical spine fracture as soon as possible.

9. The answer is **C,** page 227.
   A trauma team should always have a designated physician in charge who is experienced in the management of trauma. The presence of other physicians is needed to manage the airway and assist with procedures. A documentation nurse records the events as they take place, while other nurses are necessary for the multiple tasks that are needed in any trauma resuscitation. A pediatric surgeon is not mandatory if the other physician team members have experience in trauma.

10. The answer is **A,** pages 228 and 231.

Although a needle in the second intercostal space anteriorly could be both diagnostic and therapeutic in this boy, the physical findings leave little doubt as to the presence of a tension pneumothorax. Management has to be immediate and aggressive to prevent further deterioration. The definitive procedure, then, for this patient, who also needs to be assessed for a hemothorax, is a chest tube. If the patient improves after relief of pneumothorax, intubation may not be needed.

11. The answer is **E,** page 231.

After the initial A (Airway), B (Breathing), C (Circulation), and D (Disability assessment), next comes E (Exposure), which means remove all clothing and examine for other injuries. Stab wounds can often be multiple, or there can be other associated problems.

12. The answer is **A,** page 230.

Because of his compromised neurologic status, this child needs his airway secured with endotracheal intubation. He is obviously volume depleted as well and needs volume expansion as soon as possible. Volume is not withheld from head-injured patients if they are in shock. Hypotonic fluids are *not* appropriate for patients who are in shock or who have a head injury.

13. The answer is **D,** page 225.

Closed head injury is not a primary cause of shock in children, and major internal hemorrhage should be suspected if the patient is hypotensive and tachycardic.

14. The answer is **A,** page 232.

Although this patient was in a serious accident with the potential for serious injury, her vital signs and primary survey are normal. Since her condition apparently is stable, she can be evaluated for other injuries before any diagnostic or therapeutic maneuvers are performed.

15. The answer is **B,** page 233.

With the potential for and suspicion of an intraabdominal injury, this patient needs to have further evaluation. Since her condition is stable, a CT scan of the abdomen with contrast provides more information and is less invasive than a diagnostic peritoneal lavage. Flat and upright x-ray films of the abdomen are not helpful in this patient.

16. The answer is **C,** page 235.

Since this patient is in shock and needs stabilization of his airway with maintenance of ventilation, and since he is agitated and confused, rapid sequence induction with sedation and paralysis is best. Nasal intubation is difficult and may be traumatic in an agitated patient, and assisted ventilation with a BVM is also difficult, unreliable, and unable to be maintained for any length of time.

17. The answer is **D,** pages 229 and 233.

Because of the almost certain damage to intraabdominal organs from a gunshot wound, an exploratory laparotomy is mandatory. In the presence of shock, the definitive care is in the operating room and should not be delayed by diagnostic testing.

18. The answer is **B,** page 227.

Skill levels in pediatric prehospital care vary with locale and resources available. Since prehospital care providers usually have less experience with pediatric patients than with adults, they need to get children to definitive care in EDs as soon as possible and not waste time on the scene attempting to perform maneuvers with which they may be less familiar.

19. The answer is **C,** page 227.

Continuous quality improvement in trauma involves regular interdisciplinary case conferences, chart reviews, morbidity and mortality reviews, and videotapes of actual trauma resuscitations so that trauma team members later have the opportunity to critique performance. Since videotapes are only a quality improvement tool and are in no way a substitute for the medical records, they should be destroyed at an appropriate interval after they have fulfilled the purpose for which they were made.

20. The answer is **D,** page 235.

Preoxygenation for 3 to 5 minutes provides a reserve of oxygen if any delays in ET placement occur. Prior treatment with pancuronium eliminates fasciculations associated with succinylcholine and the concomitant rise in intracranial, intraocular, and intragastric pressure but has no effect on the release of potassium from cells in patients with burn or crush injuries.

21. The answer is **A,** page 235.

Before administration of any medications for rapid sequence induction, the patient's airway must be evaluated to ensure that there are no anatomic or other abnormalities that may prevent successful intubation. The next steps are preoxygenation, sedation, muscle relaxation, and intubation.

22. The answer is **D,** page 234.

The physical examination and vital signs of this patient suggest shock secondary to significant volume loss. Because of his agitation, it is best to intubate this patient with the rapid induction technique, sedating him before paralysis and intubation. Of the available sedative agents, it is best to avoid thiopental because of its potential for worsening hypotension and perfusion.

23. The answer is **A,** page 231.

This patient has hypovolemic shock with loss of approximately 35% to 40% of his blood volume. Per Advanced Trauma Life Support guidelines, he requires blood for resuscitation in addition to crystalloid. His altered mental status and barely palpable pulse suggest incipient arrest. Hence, he needs rapid volume replacement. Since type-specific blood is usually not available for 10 to 15 minutes, O-negative blood should be requested. It is, however, reserved for those patients in profound shock.

24. The answer is **B,** page 225.

Since parents have responsibility for a child's well-being and have the decision-making role for the child, it is important to keep them informed of events taking place. Their level of trust and cooperation is likely to be greater if they are involved as early as possible. There is no substitute for the actual physician in charge discussing the child's condition. The parents will not perceive chaplains, social workers, or nurses as having the same level of knowledge about their child's injuries or prognosis. However, actually permitting them to be with their child during the emergency treatment is impractical, frightening, and anxiety producing.

25. The answer is **E,** page 229.

The cervical spine has a high risk for injury because of the large head of the child and the flexible, weak neck muscles. Keeping the cervical spine immobilized while the airway is being controlled is important to prevent further damage to a potentially injured spine.

Head Trauma

Diane M. Sixsmith

See Barkin et al: Chapter 20.

1. Which of the following statements concerning "primary brain injury" is *correct*?
   A. Refers to the ischemic damage that occurs to brain tissue during hypotension.
   B. Can arise from acceleration/deceleration injuries.
   C. Results in neuron death because of systemic hypoperfusion.
   D. Is defined as global damage caused by respiratory or cardiac arrest.
   E. Is a result of cerebral hypometabolism.
2. Which of the following has *not* been implicated in neuronal death following brain injury?
   A. Systemic acidosis.
   B. Extracellular calcium accumulation.
   C. Cerebral temperature elevation.
   D. Oxygen-derived free radicals.
   E. Increase in glutamate levels.
3. Which of the following statements concerning autoregulatory capacity of cerebral blood flow is *true*?
   A. Is adversely affected with secondary brain injury but not primary brain injury.
   B. Is immature in infants and young children.
   C. Depends primarily on vasogenic mechanisms.
   D. Is affected primarily by small changes in arterial Pao_2.
4. The first compensatory mechanism to counteract increased intracranial volume in the younger child is:
   A. A displacement of cerebrospinal fluid (CSF) from the cranium into the dural sac of the spinal cord.
   B. Localized decrease in cerebral blood flow.
   C. Decrease in intracranial pressure.
   D. Reopening of sutures that are not fused.
   E. Collapse of the ventricles.
5. Uncal herniation has a progression of symptoms in the following order, from earlier to later:
   A. Decerebrate posturing, bilateral pupillary dilatation, bradycardia.
   B. Pupillary dilatation with preservation of light reflex, bradycardia, decerebrate posturing.
   C. Unilateral pupillary dilatation, decerebrate posturing, bilateral pupillary dilatation.
   D. Loss of light reflex, unilateral pupillary dilatation, decerebrate posturing.
   E. Systemic hypertension, unilateral pupillary dilatation, decerebrate posturing.
6. Which of the following is the most frequent cause of head injury in preschool children?
   A. Falls.
   B. Motor vehicle occupant accidents.
   C. Motor vehicle–pedestrian accidents.
   D. Bicycle injuries.
   E. Child abuse.
7. Although children are more vulnerable to head injury than adults, they tend to have better outcomes because:
   A. The mechanisms of head injury in childhood are less severe.
   B. Children have greater skull bone density.
   C. The pediatric brain has a higher water content.
   D. The pediatric brain has inherent plasticity.
   E. The pediatric brain is less susceptible to shear injuries.

Use the following scenario to answer questions 8 through 11:

A 3-month-old boy is brought in by his baby-sitter with a chief complaint of vomiting, poor feeding, and decreased responsiveness. She states that he seemed to be vomiting his feeding 4 hours earlier, and then after a brief period of crying, fell asleep. He had a normal birth and has had normal development. On examination the baby is found to open his eyes, cry, and withdraw his arms and legs only to painful stimuli. Otherwise, he is obtunded. The systolic blood pressure (BP) is 100 mm Hg, the heart rate (HR) is 120 beats per minute, the respiratory rate (RR) is 30 breaths per minute and unlabored, and the temperature is 99.5° F (37.5° C).

8. All of the following are appropriate in the management of this child *except:*
   A. Request a computed tomographic (CT) scan of the brain.
   B. Obtain further history.
   C. Order a complete blood count (CBC) and electrolytes.
   D. Perform an immediate lumbar puncture.
   E. Perform a detailed neurologic examination.

9. The pediatric Glasgow Coma Score of this child is:
   A. 11 and indicates severe injury.
   B. 5 and indicates minor injury.
   C. 9 and indicates moderate injury.
   D. 6 and indicates severe injury.
   E. 13 and indicates severe injury.

10. The patient's systolic BP progressively drops to 60 mm Hg, HR decreases to 78 beats per minute, and there is decerebrate posturing. Pupils are dilated and unresponsive. The next step in management is:
    A. 150 ml of lactated Ringer's solution rapidly infused.
    B. Serial neurologic examinations.
    C. Rapid sequence induction and endotracheal intubation.
    D. Skull x-rays.
    E. Transfusion with 150 ml of packed red blood cells.

11. Based on the CT scan shown in Fig. 17-1, the most likely diagnosis of this child is:
    A. Subdural hemorrhage.
    B. Parietal skull fracture.
    C. Cortical cyst.
    D. Hypoxic encephalomalacia.
    E. Epidural hematoma.

12. A 10-year-old girl comes to the ED 4 hours after having fallen while skating. She hit the back of her head on the sidewalk. There was no loss of consciousness. She is complaining now of a severe headache with nausea, no vomiting, and no visual disturbances. Vital signs are BP 100/60 mm Hg, HR 80 beats per minute, RR 18 breaths per minute, and temperature 98.6° F (37° C). Physical and neurologic examinations are normal. The findings of a noncontrast CT scan of the brain are normal. The best management of this patient would be:
    A. Obtain a magnetic resonance imaging (MRI) scan.
    B. Admit for observation.
    C. Measure the hemoglobin level.
    D. Obtain a skull radiograph.
    E. Reassure the patient and her parents.

13. Which of the following statements concerning posttraumatic seizures is correct?
    A. Occur in 5% of patients within the week after injury.
    B. Carry a poor prognosis if they occur immediately after injury.
    C. Will occur in 30% of all head-injured children sometime within the first year after injury.
    D. Occur most commonly in patients with concussion.
    E. Should immediately raise the suspicion of increased intracranial pressure.

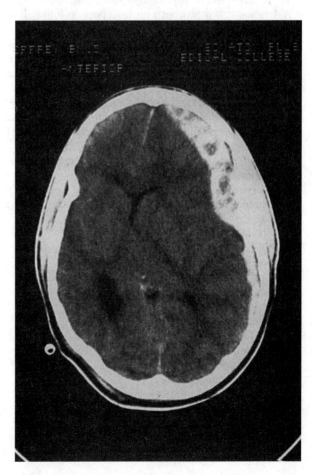

FIG. 17-1

14. A 7-year-old boy is brought to the ED by his mother because he is complaining of a headache every morning before he goes to school. He has also been difficult to manage at home and at school, and his teacher is complaining that he is not paying attention or completing his schoolwork. He was evaluated in the ED for injuries 5 days earlier when he was struck by a car traveling 10 mph and hit his head on the ground. At that time, cervical spine and left femur x-rays, CT scan of the brain, CBC, and urinalysis were normal. In light of this history, which of the following is *true?*
    A. There is probably an undiagnosed structural lesion of the brain.
    B. MRI is warranted.
    C. The mother should be reassured that the symptoms are benign and will most likely resolve within a few weeks.
    D. Lumbar puncture should be performed.

15. Which of the following statements concerning MRI is *true?*
    A. It is the procedure of choice to evaluate a child with an acute head injury.
    B. It is less sensitive than noncontrast CT scans for detecting nonhemorrhagic lesions.
    C. It must be performed on all head-injured children who have persistent symptoms.
    D. It is the definitive procedure to identify diffuse axonal injury.
    E. It has fewer complications than noncontrast CT.

16. A 4-year-old boy has been hit by a pop-up foul ball at a professional baseball game. He had loss of consciousness for a minute or two, but then became awake and alert. He is brought to the ED immobilized on a long board, with a cervical collar. He is unresponsive, and his right pupil is slightly larger than his left. He has a boggy swollen area over his right ear. His systolic BP is 95 mm Hg, his HR is 100 beats per minute, and his RR is 22 breaths per minute. The best management step to take next is:
    A. Rapid sequence induction and endotracheal intubation.
    B. Cervical spine x-ray.
    C. Noncontrast CT scan.
    D. Oral airway and 100% oxygen by mask.
    E. Intravenous (IV) mannitol.

17. A skull x-ray for the patient described in question 16:
    A. Should be done before CT.
    B. Has no place in the evaluation of this child.
    C. Should be done only on neurosurgical request.
    D. Is not diagnostic in children younger than 2 because of large suture spaces.

18. The CT scan shown in Fig. 17-2 was obtained from the patient described in question 16. It is most consistent with a (an):
    A. Subdural hematoma.
    B. Subarachnoid hemorrhage.
    C. Cerebral contusion.
    D. Epidural hematoma.

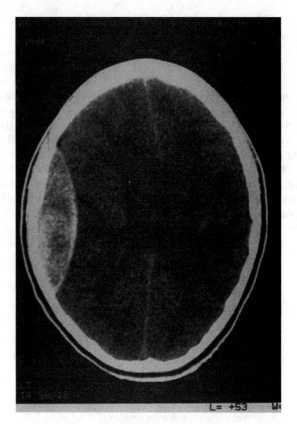

FIG. 17-2

19. Considering the mechanism of injury and findings on examination of the patient in question 16, the definitive management for this patient is most likely to be:
    A. Neurosurgical intervention.
    B. Dexamethasone (Decadron) and mannitol.
    C. Observation.
    D. Serial neurologic examinations and a repeat CT scan in 24 hours.
    E. Intracranial pressure monitoring.

20. A 15-year-old boy is brought to the ED on a long board, with a cervical collar in place after being knocked down on the basketball court and hitting his head. Observers did not note loss of consciousness, but they did state that the patient appeared dazed and confused for several minutes after the event. In the ED the patient is amnesic about the few minutes immediately after the fall. His neurologic examination and cervical spine x-ray are normal. The best management of this patient would be:
    A. Admit for observation.
    B. Obtain an MRI.
    C. Perform serial neurologic examinations in the ED for 4 hours and then discharge home if stable.
    D. Obtain a skull x-ray.

21. Which of the following is the most commonly seen pediatric skull fracture?
    A. Depressed fracture of the occiput.
    B. Linear fracture of the parietal bone.
    C. Linear fracture of the occipital bone.
    D. Stellate fracture of the parietal bone.
    E. Depressed fracture of the parietal bone.

22. Which one of the following statements concerning a "growing fracture" is *true?*
    A. Occurs in adolescents during a rapid growth spurt.
    B. Occurs in children younger than 2 who have had significant head trauma.
    C. Occurs in children younger than 2 with no or minor history of trauma.
    D. Heals without incident and rarely requires neurosurgical intervention.
    E. Is the name for a benign anatomic variant in infants with large suture lines.

23. A 13-year-old girl hit the back of her head when she fell on the street while in-line skating. She had transient loss of consciousness. She comes to the ED 6 hours later complaining of headache, tenderness at the injury site, and a runny nose. Her vital signs and neurologic examination are normal. She has clear fluid from her nose on examination, and bruising and tenderness behind her ears and at her occiput. The best pharmacologic approach to this injury is:
    A. A broad-spectrum antibiotic orally for 5 days.
    B. Mannitol and dexamethasone (Decadron).
    C. IV ceftriaxone.
    D. Acetaminophen for analgesia as needed.
    E. Phenytoin.

24. The management of the patient described in question 23 includes which one of the following?
    A. Neurosurgical consultation and immediate surgery.
    B. Neurosurgical consultation and symptomatic care.
    C. Discharge from the ED with neurosurgical follow-up in 72 hours.
    D. Discharge from the ED with instructions to return if symptoms worsen.
    E. Admission to the intensive care unit (ICU).

25. Which one of the following statements concerning intracranial hemorrhages in the newborn is *true?*
    A. Are usually subarachnoid and asymptomatic.
    B. Are usually intracerebral and symptomatic.
    C. Are usually intracerebral and asymptomatic.
    D. Are usually subarachnoid and symptomatic.

26. Rapid sequence induction for endotracheal intubation in children less than 5 years of age with significant head injury requires the following sequence of drugs:
    A. Atropine, midazolam, vecuronium, succinylcholine.
    B. Atropine, lidocaine, thiopental, vecuronium.
    C. Lidocaine, midazolam, vecuronium, succinylcholine.
    D. Lidocaine, vecuronium, succinylcholine.
    E. Midazolam, lidocaine, vecuronium.

27. The best indication of insufficient central nervous system perfusion and oxygenation is:
    A. Pupillary size.
    B. Level of consciousness.
    C. Pulse oximetry reading of 97%.
    D. Lack of neurologic findings.
    E. Tachycardia.

ANSWERS   [See Barkin et al: Chapter 20.]

1. The answer is **B,** page 236.
   Primary brain injury occurs at the moment of impact, either by penetration of a foreign body or by nonimpact shear forces that occur during acceleration/deceleration injuries. Secondary brain injury results from hypoxia, ischemia, or other results of cerebral hypometabolism.

2. The answer is **B,** page 236.
   Neuronal death after brain injury is a complex of poorly understood mechanisms at the cellular level, including dysfunction of the ion pumps; intracellular accumulation of calcium, sodium, and chloride; intracellular swelling; glutamate accumulation; and release of phospholipids, oxygen-derived free radicals, thromboxanes, and leukotrienes. Systemic acidosis may enhance neuronal damage during the reperfusion phase.

3. The answer is **B,** page 237.
   Autoregulation of cerebral blood flow depends on interacting neurogenic, vasogenic, and myogenic mechanisms. It is exquisitely sensitive to arterial Pa_{CO_2} and is immature in infants and young children. It does not depend on mean arterial pressure.

4. The answer is **A,** page 237.
   Initial increases in intracranial pressure are compensated by displacement of CSF. This is followed by collapse of the ventricles, widening of sutures if they are not fused, and ultimately a decrease in cerebral blood flow.

5. The answer is **C,** page 237.
   The earliest sign of uncal herniation is depression of the level of consciousness followed by unilateral pupillary dilatation because of compression of the third cranial nerve against the temporal lobe. Decerebrate posturing and bilateral pupillary dilatation occur in turn as pressure increases further. Systemic hypertension and bradycardia are terminal signs, part of "Cushing's triad," which occurs late and carries an ominous prognosis.

6. The answer is **A,** page 237.
   Falls account for the greatest incidence of head injury in preschool children, while in school-age children and adolescents, head injury is likely to be caused by sports-related injuries or motor vehicle accidents.

7. The answer is **D,** page 238.

Children's outcomes are better because of the inherent plasticity of the brain tissue. In actuality their injuries tend to be more severe for a number of reasons, including their larger proportionate head size and, hence, greater vulnerability. Because their brains are softer with a higher water content, they are also more susceptible to acceleration/deceleration injuries.

8. The answer is **D,** page 238.

The patient's presentation is not consistent with the history, in that symptoms are of relatively recent onset with no precipitating factors such as history of infection or developmental problems. Considering the marked depression in consciousness, child abuse or injury has to be assumed until proven otherwise. Although all the other steps listed in this child's management must also be accomplished, obtaining more history is very important. Lumbar puncture should not be performed on patients with suspected intracranial injury until a CT scan is performed.

9. The answer is **C,** page 240.

This child gets 2 for eye opening, 4 for best motor response, and 3 for best verbal response. Scores of 8 to 12 indicate moderate injury; less than 8 suggests severe injury (Table 17-1).

10. The answer is **C,** pages 242 and 243.

The worsening neurologic status of this child, as evidenced by unresponsive pupils, bradycardia, and decerebrate posturing, indicates rapidly rising intracranial pressure, which demands emergency intervention and stabilization of the airway. Intubation is necessary to hyperventilate to decrease intracranial pressure. In this child the decrease in systolic BP may be due to a large epidural hematoma, but it may also be secondary to impending herniation. Hence, airway management is the critical first maneuver.

11. The answer is **A,** page 249.

The CT scan shows subdural hemorrhage, which is a typical finding in the shaken baby syndrome, consistent with this child's presentation and vague history.

12. The answer is **E,** page 240.

The symptoms of this girl are typical for trauma-induced migraine, which resolves spontaneously and responds well to β-blockers. In the absence of neurologic findings and with a normal CT scan, this child can be managed conservatively without further intervention.

13. The answer is **A,** page 241.

Posttraumatic seizures will occur within the first week in 5% of children hospitalized with head injury and after the first week in another 5%. A seizure immediately after injury has no prognostic significance.

14. The answer is **C,** page 241.

This child's symptoms are characteristic of "posttraumatic" or "postconcussive" syndrome. Most children recover normally, and symptoms may be related to anxiety of the parents or a preexisting, undiagnosed attention deficit disorder.

TABLE 17-1   Pediatric Glasgow Coma Score (PGCS)

Glasgow Coma Score	Pediatric modification	
Eye opening	**Eye opening**	
≥1 year	*0-1 year*	
4 Spontaneously	Spontaneously	
3 To verbal command	To shout	
2 To pain	To pain	
1 No response	No response	
Best motor response	**Best motor response**	
≥1 year	*0-1 year*	
6 Obeys command		
5 Localizes pain	Localizes pain	
4 Flexion withdrawal	Flexion withdrawal	
3 Flexion abnormal (decorticate)	Flexion abnormal (decorticate)	
2 Extension (decerebrate)	Extension (decerebrate)	
1 No response	No response	
Best verbal response	**Best verbal response**	
>5 years	*2-5 years*	*0-2 years*
5 Oriented and converses	Appropriate words and phrases	Cries appropriately, smiles, coos
4 Disoriented and converses	Inappropriate words	Cries
3 Inappropriate words	Cries/screams	Inappropriate crying/screaming
2 Incomprehensible sounds	Grunts	Grunts
1 No response	No response	No response

PGCS is the sum of individual scores from eye opening, best verbal response, and best motor response. PGCS of 13 to 15 indicates mild head injury; PGCS of 8 to 12 indicates moderate head injury; PGCS of <8 indicates severe head injury.

15. The answer is **D**, pages 241 and 242.

Although MRI is the procedure of choice for diagnosing diffuse axonal injury and is more sensitive than CT for nonhemorrhagic lesions, it is a lengthier procedure and is more difficult to arrange for an unstable patient. Hence, it is practically more difficult and more expensive for the routine evaluation of head-injured patients, in which CT is still the initial imaging study of choice. As question 14 demonstrates, not all patients with persistent symptoms require further testing.

16. The answer is **A**, page 242.

Unconscious and with a PGCS of less than or equal to 8, this child appears to have a moderate injury and requires airway management and stabilization. There is no indication for IV mannitol, and an oral airway is not a reliable method of controlling ventilation. CT and cervical spine films are of course necessary but can be performed after initial stabilization.

17. The answer is **B**, page 247.

CT scanning is the appropriate test to eliminate the possibility of an intracerebral injury.

18. The answer is **D**, page 249.

The CT scan displays the typical finding seen in an epidural hematoma (right parietal).

19. The answer is **A**, page 248.

The mechanism of injury and the findings on neurologic examination suggest a skull fracture and an epidural hematoma. Hence, neurosurgical operative intervention will be necessary. Mannitol may be indicated, but only as a temporizing measure for elevation of intracranial pressure if hyperventilation fails. Dexamethasone (Decadron) is not indicated in trauma.

20. The answer is **C**, page 245.

The patient's presentation is typical for a concussion. Since there was no true loss of consciousness and neurologic examination is normal, there is low risk for injury.

21. The answer is **B**, page 246.

Linear skull fractures comprise 75% of fractures in children, and the parietal bone is the most common site.

22. The answer is **B**, page 247.

The "growing fracture" in children younger than 2 years of age who are experiencing rapid brain growth results from significant trauma that produces a fracture with a dural tear. In the postinjury period the rapid brain growth can result in a leptomeningeal cyst that requires neurosurgical intervention.

23. The answer is **D**, page 248.

Most basal skull fractures can be treated conservatively. No clear evidence has been presented that prophylactic antibiotics reduce the risk of infection, and they may favor the growth of resistant organisms.

24. The answer is **B**, page 248.

Management of basal skull fractures is neurosurgical consultation and symptomatic care. Frequently, no treatment is required.

25. The answer is **A**, page 248.

Intracranial hemorrhages in the newborn are usually due to birth trauma. Since the bleeding is of venous origin, they are frequently asymptomatic and are located in the subarachnoid space.

26. The answer is **B**, page 234.

Atropine is necessary to reduce the likelihood of bradycardia, followed by lidocaine to suppress the cough reflex and reduce intracranial pressure. This is followed by sedation with thiopental and then paralysis with vecuronium.

27. The answer is **B**, page 238.

The best indication of insufficient perfusion and oxygenation in the brain is level of consciousness. An increase in pupillary size or focal neurologic findings may be indicative of increased intracranial pressure. Pulse oximetry and vital signs are not specific for brain perfusion.

CHAPTER 18

Facial Trauma

Peter S. Dayan • F. Meridith Sonnett

See Barkin et al: Chapter 21.

1. A 5-year-old boy sustained extensive midfacial injury after an MVA. His respiratory rate (RR) is 8 breaths per minute, and breaths are regular but shallow. The oxygen saturation is 92% with 5 L of oxygen delivered by face mask. The anesthesiologist states that it will be difficult to obtain a good mask seal with a bag-valve-mask (BVM). The most appropriate next step is to:
   A. Perform immediate cricothyrotomy.
   B. Nasally intubate the patient.
   C. Perform rapid sequence intubation.
   D. Attempt oral intubation with in-line cervical spine traction.
   E. Perform immediate tracheostomy in the operating room.

2. A 4-year-old boy has a 2-week history of foul-smelling nasal discharge. Physical examination reveals a temperature of 38.2° C, mucopurulent discharge only from the right naris, and tenderness over the right maxillary sinus. The patient is too uncooperative for a nasal visual examination. You would:
   A. Prescribe a 2-week course of antibiotics.
   B. Prescribe antibiotics and a nasal decongestant.
   C. Confirm the diagnosis of sinusitis with a radiograph before prescribing antibiotics.
   D. Perform rhinoscopy or consult an otorhinolaryngologist to rule out a foreign body.
   E. Perform rhinoscopy or consult an otorhinolaryngologist to rule out a foreign body, and prescribe antibiotics.

3. A 5-year-old child sustained a laceration to the forehead during a fall. There was no loss of consciousness, and the child is alert and neurologically intact, with no step-off noted on forehead palpation. You are going to use topical LAT (lidocaine, adrenaline, tetracaine) gel for anesthesia. Compared to a topical TAC (tetracaine, adrenaline, and cocaine) solution, LAT gel:
   A. Can be used on mucosal surfaces.
   B. Can be used on the pinna.
   C. Is more cost effective.
   D. Provides greater analgesia.
   E. Needs to be held in place longer.

4. A 15-year-old girl was hit in the right eye with a softball. She is noted to have periorbital ecchymosis on the right side, a small subconjunctival hemorrhage, bloody discharge from her right naris, and hypesthesia below her right eye. Extraocular movement is intact. Plain radiographs of the orbit are negative. The appropriate next step would be to:
   A. Obtain a computed tomographic (CT) scan of the orbit.
   B. Obtain a head CT scan for possible basilar skull fracture.
   C. Discharge the patient to home with evaluation by a maxillofacial surgeon if diplopia develops.
   D. Obtain plain radiographs to evaluate for a nasal fracture.
   E. Reassure the patient that no significant injury has occurred.

5. An 18-year-old man is intubated and hemodynamically stabilized after being thrown from his motorcycle. He has obvious midfacial injuries. A head CT scan shows a basilar skull fracture. On CT evaluation of his face, he has a fracture through the lower third of his maxilla, palate, and pterygoid plates on the right and complete separation of the facial bones from the cranium on the left. According to the LeFort classification for maxillary fractures, this patient has a:
   A. LeFort I fracture on the right and LeFort II fracture on the left.
   B. LeFort I fracture on the left and LeFort II fracture on the right.
   C. LeFort III fracture on the right and LeFort I fracture on the left.
   D. LeFort I fracture on the right and LeFort III fracture on the left.
   E. LeFort II fracture on the left and LeFort III fracture on the right.

6. A 6-year-old girl sustained nasal trauma during a fall from her bunk bed. She has marked nasal swelling and ecchymosis. Rhinoscopy reveals a boggy, pink mass emanating from her left septal wall, obstructing the nasal passage. The next step is to:
   A. Obtain plain radiographs to document a nasal fracture before treatment.
   B. Perform needle aspiration of the mass.
   C. Perform incision and drainage of the mass.
   D. Ensure ear, nose, and throat (ENT) follow-up within 3 days to reevaluate the nose.
   E. Prescribe antibiotics to prevent infection and obtain ENT follow-up within 2 days.

7. A 10-year-old boy sustained a 0.5-cm laceration to his right eyelid margin during a skating accident. He has a completely normal eye examination and a negative fluorescein test. The next step would be to:
   A. Obtain an orbital CT scan to evaluate for orbital injury.
   B. Suture the wound with 6-0 absorbable sutures under conscious sedation.
   C. Suture the wound with 6-0 nonabsorbable sutures under conscious sedation.
   D. Obtain an ophthalmologist consult to examine the eye and suture the wound.
   E. Use local anesthesia to better evaluate the wound

8. A 5-year-old girl has a chin laceration after falling while running. The laceration is 2 cm long and gaping. She has no facial asymmetry, sublingual hematoma, trismus, or malocclusion. She has an enamel fracture of her upper lateral incisor. The area of her mandible laceration is tender, but no crepitus or step-off is palpated. There is no tenderness at the mandibular condyles. The most appropriate management would be to:
   A. Suture the chin laceration and arrange dental follow-up.
   B. Suture the chin laceration and get an immediate dental consultation.
   C. Obtain mandibular radiographs, suture the chin only if the x-rays are negative, and get an immediate dental consult.
   D. Obtain mandibular radiographs, suture the chin only if the x-rays are negative, and arrange dental follow-up.
   E. Suture the chin laceration and not arrange a dental follow-up.

9. A 16-year-old girl felt immediate pain after something flew into her left eye as she was riding her bicycle behind a car. She now has pain in that eye with a small subconjunctival hemorrhage. The pupil has a normal shape, and visual acuity is equal in both eyes. No obvious foreign bodies are noted on inspection of the eye and after eyelid eversion. Dilute fluorescein instillation reveals no evidence of a corneal abrasion. The next most appropriate step is to:
   A. Instill 1 drop of 5% homatropine into the injured eye and arrange ophthalmology follow-up within 48 hours.
   B. Instill 2 drops of 0.5% proparacaine into the injured eye and observe for resolution of symptoms.
   C. Instill one drop of 5% homatropine into the injured eye, prescribe topical antibiotics, and arrange ophthalmology follow-up within 48 hours.
   D. Prescribe 1 drop of topical 0.5% proparacaine every 6 hours for 2 days.
   E. Obtain an ophthalmology consult.

10. A 17-year-old boy comes to the ED after being hit in the right eye with a shovel. He has vomited several times since the incident. The right eye is swollen shut, but gentle lid retraction reveals bloody chemosis. Visual acuity in the right eye is 20/200 (left 20/30) with an afferent pupillary light defect. The most important next step is to:
    A. Place a soft pressure patch over the injured eye.
    B. Give the patient antiemetics and nothing by mouth.
    C. Instill 1 drop of 5% homatropine and 0.5% proparacaine in the injured eye.
    D. Obtain an orbital CT scan and an ophthalmology consult.
    E. Place a shield over the eye.

11. A 16-year-old boy comes to the ED after an unknown liquid has been sprayed into both eyes. At home he had irrigated his eyes with tap water for 20 minutes. He says he feels slight pain in the right eye more than in the left. The most important next step is to:
    A. Obtain an immediate ophthalmology consult for an assumed chemical injury.
    B. Apply an antibiotic ointment to prevent superinfection and discharge the patient.
    C. Instill one drop of a cycloplegic to facilitate slit-lamp examination.
    D. Irrigate each eye concurrently with 1 L of normal saline.
    E. Irrigate the right eye with 1 L of normal saline.

12. A 15-year-old girl was fighting with her 12-year-old sister. Both sustained corneal abrasions. No foreign bodies are noted in the eye, and visual acuity is normal. The 15-year-old was wearing her contact lenses and has subsequently removed them. Management of corneal abrasions in both contact lens and non–contact lens wearers may include all the following *except*:
    A. Semipressure patching.
    B. Topical antibiotics.
    C. Cycloplegia.
    D. One drop of topical anesthetic in the ED.

13. A teenage boy sneaks up behind a friend and rubs "super glue" in her eye. The 15-year-old friend now cannot open her eye and feels pain. In the ED an attempt to separate the lids gently is unsuccessful. The most appropriate next step is to:
    A. Apply sustained traction to the lids.
    B. Apply moist saline solution compresses for 24 hours.
    C. Apply Neosporin ophthalmic ointment to the lids for 24 hours.
    D. Obtain an ophthalmology consult.

14. A 14-year-old girl comes to the ED 2 days after being in a fight. The only injury is a markedly swollen and ecchymotic right ear with a blue, boggy auricular mass noted on examination. There is no Battle's sign (discoloration over the skin of the mastoid region of the skull) or "raccoon eyes"; the tympanic membrane is intact without hemotympanum; and hearing is normal. The definitive therapy for this patient is to:
    A. Incise and drain the auricular hematoma.
    B. Aspirate the blood from the auricular hematoma.
    C. Apply ice for 24 hours.
    D. Apply a pressure dressing and follow up in 24 hours.
    E. Apply ice, antibiotic ointment, and a pressure dressing.

15. A 4-year-old boy sustained a laceration to his left ear helix 2 days ago. He had two 5-0 absorbable sutures placed through the cartilage and five 6-0 nonabsorbable sutures placed through the skin. He now comes to the ED with redness, swelling, and pain over the suture site. You would:
    A. Start oral antibiotics and arrange follow-up within 24 hours.
    B. Remove the sutures, start oral antibiotics, and arrange for follow-up within 24 hours.
    C. Discharge home with instructions for warm soaks to the ear four to six times daily and arrange for follow-up within 24 hours.
    D. Remove the sutures, administer intravenous (IV) antibiotics, and admit to the hospital.
    E. Consult a plastic surgeon and discharge to home if the surgeon believes it is just local cellulitis.

16. An 18-year-old man is hit in the face with a baseball bat. On examination, he is alert and interactive with marked swelling, ecchymosis, tenderness, and crepitus along the lateral aspect of his right orbital rim. He has a lateral subconjunctival hemorrhage of the right eye and tenderness on intraoral palpation of his zygomatic arch. The best radiographic study would be a:
    A. Waters' (occipitomental) view.
    B. Towne view.
    C. CT scan (coronal and axial views).
    D. Submentovertex (jug-handle) view.
    E. Caldwell (posteroanterior) view.

17. A 17-year-old boy was punched in the jaw. He has swelling and tenderness to palpation of the right mandibular body. There is no intraoral swelling, sublingual hematoma, trismus, malocclusion, mandibular shift, dental trauma, or facial asymmetry. Plain radiographs are negative, and the patient is able to eat without difficulty. The next step would be to:
    A. Obtain a CT scan of the mandible.
    B. Obtain a maxillofacial surgery consult.
    C. Place the patient on a soft diet and arrange follow-up within 24 hours.
    D. Discharge the patient to home with the diagnosis of chin contusion.
    E. Obtain a Waters' view for clarification.

18. A 5-year-old girl inserted a stick in her ear and now has a small amount of blood coming from the canal. A perforation of the tympanic membrane with a small, lateral flap is noted. Hearing is normal. Weber's test for sensorineural hearing deficit is negative. Cranial nerve function is intact bilaterally. No vertigo or nystagmus is elicited with pneumatic otoscopy. The most appropriate management would be to:
    A. Obtain an immediate ENT consult for a possible perilymphatic fistula.
    B. Reassure the parents that the perforation will heal without any intervention and with no consequences.
    C. Refer the patient to ENT within a few days.
    D. Tell the parents that if the perforation does not heal within 2 to 3 weeks, the child will need an ENT evaluation.
    E. Prescribe topical antibiotics to prevent infection.

19. A 17-year-old assault victim had his face repeatedly hit against a fire hydrant. In the ED he is awake and alert with obvious facial injuries. He has some oral bleeding but appears able to maintain his airway. Cervical spine radiographs are negative. To differentiate the possible types of LeFort maxilla fractures sustained, you would:
    A. Attempt to mobilize the palate.
    B. Palpate for localized crepitus.
    C. Evaluate extraocular movements.
    D. Assess the patient for an open bite.
    E. Assess mandible mobility.

20. A 10-year-old boy tripped and hit his teeth on a marble counter. He is noted to have isolated dental injuries to his central and lateral upper incisors. The teeth are not fractured, intruded, extruded, or mobile. Both teeth are painful on biting down and are tender to percussion. The most likely diagnosis and its treatment would be:
    A. Subluxated incisors, referral to a dentist.
    B. Periodontal ligament or cementum injury, immediate dentistry consult.
    C. Concussion, no specific follow-up.
    D. Concussion, referral for next available dental follow-up.
    E. Root and pulp injury, dental follow-up within 24 hours.

21. A 4-year-old girl comes to the ED at midnight after sustaining a crown fracture to her lateral upper incisor. The tooth is not mobile, intruded, or extruded. A small amount of blood is noted from the distal end of the fractured tooth. The blood is easily wiped off, leaving a pinpoint red dot at the center of the fracture. The most appropriate management of this patient would be to:
    A. Obtain an immediate dental consultation.
    B. Arrange for dental follow-up within 24 hours.
    C. Prescribe antibiotics for prophylaxis and arrange for dental follow-up within 24 hours.
    D. Reassure the parents and arrange for the next possible dental follow-up.
    E. Place a temporary splint on the tooth and arrange for follow-up in the morning.

22. A 12-year-old boy comes to the ED 50 minutes after falling while running. He has avulsed his upper central incisor, which he is carrying in his hand. The dental resident, who was called from triage, is unavailable for 2½ hours. The appropriate management would be to:
    A. Replace the tooth in its socket and call another dentist for rapid consultation.
    B. Place the tooth in Hanks Balanced Salt Solution or a dental fluoride solution and wait for the dentist.
    C. Place the tooth in Hanks Balanced Salt Solution or a dental fluoride solution and call another dentist for more rapid consultation.
    D. Have the child hold the tooth under his tongue and wait for the dentist.
    E. Scrub the root and crown of the tooth, replace the tooth in its socket, and call another dentist for more rapid consultation.

23. A 10-year-old boy hit his upper canine on a metal railing. The tooth is not fractured or displaced but is laterally mobile 2 mm. The appropriate next step is to:
    A. Obtain immediate consultation for splinting.
    B. Arrange for follow-up within 24 hours.
    C. Arrange for the next possible dental appointment and reassure the parents that the tooth will stabilize without splinting.
    D. Tell the parents that a dental referral is unnecessary, since no long-term consequences will result from the injury.
    E. Prescribe prophylactic antibiotics.

24. A 4½-year-old boy fell 20 minutes ago, avulsed his right upper central incisor, and sustained a nongaping lip laceration crossing his vermilion border. In the ED you would:
    A. Replace the tooth in its socket, obtain an immediate dental consult, and suture the lip laceration.
    B. Place the tooth in Hanks Balanced Salt Solution, obtain an immediate dental consult, and suture the lip laceration.
    C. Replace the tooth in its socket, obtain an immediate dental consult, and allow the lip laceration to heal by secondary intention.
    D. Only suture the lip laceration.

25. A 4-year-old sustained a 0.5-cm laceration through the middle third of her tongue, not all the way through, but 0.5-cm deep with minimal blood oozing from the wound. You would:
    A. Suture the tongue with absorbable sutures.
    B. Suture the tongue with nonabsorbable sutures.
    C. Discharge the patient on a bland diet.
    D. Admit the patient for IV fluids.
    E. Prepare the patient for conscious sedation or general anesthesia to repair the wound.

26. A 2-year-old girl bit on an electrical cord in her house and sustained a burn to the commissure and vermilion border of the lip. No bleeding is evident, and the patient is playing and taking a bottle in the ED. Appropriate management would be to:
    A. Obtain an ECG.
    B. Analyze the urine for possible myoglobinuria.
    C. Start IV fluids at two times maintenance.
    D. Admit the patient to the hospital for early surgical management.
    E. Discharge the patient to home with close surgical follow-up.

27. A 4-year-old boy has a 70% intruded right upper incisor after a fall. Appropriate management would be to:
    A. Obtain an immediate dental consultation.
    B. Prescribe oral antibiotics and allow the tooth to reerupt over time.
    C. Extract the tooth if it does not reerupt within 3 to 4 weeks.
    D. Obtain the next available dental appointment.
    E. Obtain a panoramic view of the teeth to rule out fracture and discharge home with dental follow-up if the results are negative.

28. A 15-year-old boy is hit above the nose and right eye with a metal pipe. He has a flattened broad nasal bridge, and the distance between his right and left medial canthi is greater than the distance from the medial to the lateral canthus. The most likely diagnosis is:
    A. A nasal fracture.
    B. A nasoethmoidal fracture.
    C. A supraorbital fracture.
    D. A blow-out fracture of the orbital floor.
    E. A nasal contusion.

29. A 5-year-old girl fell and injured her nose. She has significant swelling, but no septal hematoma or difficulty breathing is evident. The most important next step in management is:
    A. Arrange for follow-up within 3 to 4 days with a plastic surgeon or ENT surgeon.
    B. Obtain nasal radiographs.
    C. Obtain a nasal CT to evaluate for deformity.
    D. Arrange for follow-up within 1 to 2 weeks with a plastic surgeon or ENT surgeon.

1. The answer is **D,** page 253.
   The ABCDs of trauma take precedence over specific management of the facial injury. The extensive facial trauma, however, will make airway management difficult. Oral intubation should be the initial management of this patient. It would be preferable to intubate the patient in the operating room if one is immediately available because cricothyrotomy will be needed if intubation fails. If intubation is done in the ED, the cricothyrotomy tray should be open, and the equipment must be checked and ready. Paralysis during rapid sequence intubation should be avoided if a good mask seal is difficult to attain, but sedation should be used. Nasal intubation is often difficult and may result in cranial penetration if there is a cribriform plate fracture. Cervical spine motion must be minimized during intubation as concomitant cervical spine injury is seen with facial trauma.

2. The answer is **E,** page 259.
   The patient has a history of unilateral symptoms consistent with a nasal foreign body. Examination may be difficult in the young child. Adequate restraint is imperative, and sedation may be necessary. A head lamp will free the hands for manipulation of the nasal speculum. Suctioning secretions and applying a topical anesthetic and vasoconstrictor will improve visualization. If the foreign body is not easily removed or not visualized but suspected, an ENT consult is appropriate. One complication of a nasal foreign body is sinusitis, which requires antibiotics. This diagnosis is likely in the question scenario.

3. The answer is **C,** page 257.
   LAT gel is more cost effective than TAC solution and negates the use of a controlled substance, cocaine. The thick gel provides the potential benefit of less anesthetic runoff compared with the solution. LAT and TAC provide approximately equal analgesia, although some patients need additional infiltration of lidocaine after either topical preparation. LAT and TAC both contain epinephrine and are contraindicated in areas of end-vascular supply such as the pinna. LAT and TAC are contraindicated on or near mucosal membranes. Absorption of TAC across mucosal membranes probably has led to at least two deaths. Although no deaths have been reported with LAT, it is less time tested and contains potent anesthetics with potential systemic side effects if absorbed.

4. The answer is **A,** page 260.
   The scenario clearly points to the diagnosis of an infraorbital floor (blow-out) fracture with injury to the infraorbital nerve, producing midfacial hypesthesia and blood in the sinus draining through the nose. A CT scan should be ordered because the clinical findings are so suggestive of fracture, and plain films may be negative or difficult to interpret. A maxillofacial surgery consult also would be appropriate. In patients with infraorbital floor fractures, diplopia on upward gaze may develop days after the injury as swelling resolves and entrapment of the inferior rectus muscle occurs.

5. The answer is **D,** page 262.
   The LeFort classification categorizes maxillary fractures by their horizontal level. A LeFort I fracture goes through the lower third of the maxilla, palate, and pterygoid plates. A LeFort II fracture occurs through the nasal bones, orbital floor, and pterygoid plates into the pterygomaxillary fossa. When a LeFort II fracture extends through the zygomatic arches, it results in complete separation of the facial bones from the cranium and is then called a LeFort III fracture. LeFort fractures are unusual in childhood, result from significant forces, and are commonly associated with basilar skull fractures. Different LeFort fractures may be noted on the two sides of the face. As always, management of the ABCDs of trauma takes precedence over specific fracture management (Fig. 18-1).

6. The answer is **C,** page 263.
   The patient described probably has a septal hematoma. The hematoma may be associated with a nasal fracture, but radiographs may be falsely negative or falsely positive and do not change acute management of the hematoma. The septal hematoma must be evacuated immediately. If blood is allowed to remain under pressure, it will disrupt blood supply to the nasal cartilage with consequent risk of an infected hematoma, chondritis, and nasal deformity from cartilage necrosis. The procedure of choice is incision and drainage, which probably will necessitate conscious sedation or general anesthesia. Antibiotics are recommended after incision and drainage to prevent potential infection.

7. The answer is **D,** page 266.
   All lacerations to the eyelid margins should be evaluated and managed by an ophthalmologist. Precise apposition of the lid margins must be obtained to prevent eyelid deformities that would leave the cornea exposed. The specialist also evaluates for possible globe penetration. If globe injury is suspected, a CT scan may be ordered. Other eyelid lacerations for which an ophthalmologist should be consulted include lacerations of the medial eyelid where lacrimal drainage occurs and the upper lateral upper third of the eyelid where the lacrimal duct runs, and lacerations associated with ptosis (possible levator palpebrae injury).

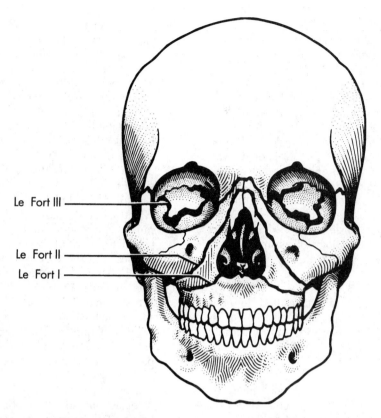

FIG. 18-1 LeFort classification of maxillary fractures. LeFort I: palate facial dysjunction. LeFort II: pyramidal dysjunction. LeFort III: craniofacial dysjunction.

8. The answer is **A,** pages 262 and 282.

This patient has an uncomplicated chin laceration. The examination of the mandible does not indicate a high likelihood of associated fracture. An x-ray therefore is not indicated. The patient also has an Ellis class I tooth fracture, which needs only dental follow-up to smooth the edges of the tooth.

9. The answer is **E,** page 267.

The mechanism of action suggests a high-velocity foreign body was propelled from a car tire into the patient's eye. Although no foreign body is visible, the pain and subconjunctival hemorrhage cannot be explained by a simple corneal abrasion because the dilute fluorescein test is negative. This patient may have a small, retained foreign body with a self-sealing corneal laceration. Patients with corneal lacerations may have a positive Seidel (direct, concentrated fluorescein) test or an irregularly shaped pupil because of prolapse of the iris, but neither finding is 100% sensitive. Without an obvious explanation for the patient's continued signs and symptoms, an ophthalmology consult with slit-lamp examination is appropriate. Proparacaine should never be prescribed for outpatient use and, in the question scenario, may mask the symptoms of a potentially significant injury. One drop of 5% homatropine is useful to relieve the pain associated with corneal abrasions by paralyzing the iris and ciliary body for 12 to 24 hours.

10. The answer is **E,** page 270.

The patient has signs and symptoms of a scleral rupture (open globe). Any pressure to the eye, such as with a pressure patch, is contraindicated because it may lead to orbital content extrusion. A hard shield should immediately be placed over the eye. Other management considerations in a patient with scleral rupture follow the mnemonic "SANTA": **S**hield, **A**ntiemetic (if indicated), **N**PO, **T**etanus immunization (if indicated), and **A**ntibiotics (after consultation). An immediate consult is obviously necessary. This patient should receive antiemetics to decrease the risk of further ocular injury resulting from the vomiting.

11. The answer is **D,** page 272.

Immediate eye irrigation is essential for good outcome after chemical injury. The patient was correct to initially irrigate his eyes at home. However, even when irrigation has been initiated outside the hospital, if the patient has any symptoms in the ED, the affected eye(s) should be irrigated immediately with 1 L of normal saline. As long as irrigation is not delayed, a quick test of initial visual acuity can be performed and a drop of proparacaine instilled into the affected eye before irrigation. After initial irrigation the conjunctival pH should be checked. If the pH is not 7.4, irrigation is continued. After irrigation a thorough eye examination should be completed, including visual acuity and fluorescein testing. An ophthalmologist must be consulted if any sign of ocular injury is present.

12. The answer is **A,** pages 267 and 269.

Treatment for corneal abrasions includes topical antibiotics, cycloplegia, 1 drop of topical anesthetic (e.g., 0.5% proparacaine) in the ED, and semipressure patching (if the patient is not wearing contact lenses). Topical anesthetic is not prescribed for outpatient use because it can be toxic to the corneal epithelium. Patients wearing contact lenses should not have their eyes patched because of an increased risk of infection after patching. Most texts state that all patients with corneal abrasions should have ophthalmology follow-up. This is especially important for corneal abrasions involving central vision because scarring, although unusual, can lead to prolonged visual disturbance. All patients with corneal abrasions who wear contact lenses should have ophthalmology follow-up within 24 hours because of the risk of rapidly progressive infection.

13. The answer is **D,** page 273.

An ophthalmologist should be consulted for this patient because of potential globe involvement as evidenced by mechanism (surprise injury without time to close the eye) and complaint of pain, which suggest a corneal injury. Without likely globe involvement, as when someone rubs their lid while using "super glue," separation of the lids can usually be achieved by applying moist saline compresses or Neosporin ophthalmic ointment for 24 hours.

14. The answer is **A,** page 275.

Auricular hematomas must be evacuated because, like a nasal septal hematoma, the accumulated blood may interrupt blood supply to the cartilage. This will cause necrosis of the existing auricular cartilage and formation of abnormal and excessive cartilage. The end result is a physical deformity, cauliflower ear. Needle aspiration may be attempted but will not evacuate all the blood if it has already clotted. Our patient comes in 2 days after injury with likely clot formation. Incision and clot evacuation is followed by the application of antibiotic ointment and a pressure dressing. Follow-up should be arranged within 24 hours.

15. The answer is **D,** page 275.

The patient's case is suggestive of a chondritis and not a simple cellulitis. Without prompt IV therapy, this is often a rapidly progressive infection with loss of ear cartilage. *Pseudomonas aeruginosa* causes 95% of cases, with *Staphylococcus* grown concomitantly in 50% of cases. Admission to the hospital, administration of IV antibiotics, removal of the sutures, and plastic surgery evaluation are all important components of the patient's care.

16. The answer is **C,** page 260.

Controversy exists over the study of choice for facial trauma. Although plain films are generally adequate to rule out a mandible fracture, CT scanning is believed to be more sensitive for other facial fractures. A CT scan is often recommended as the initial study when there is a high suspicion of fracture, especially for periorbital fractures. The patient in the scenario has a high likelihood of a zygoma/periorbital fracture and should undergo CT. The Waters view evaluates the midface (including the periorbital rims and maxillary sinuses) and is considered the single most informative view of all facial plain radiographs. The Towne view is effective to diagnose fractures of the mandibular ramus and condyles. The submentovertex view is useful to show the zygomatic arches and paranasal sinuses, and the Caldwell view helps to evaluate the frontal bones and paranasal sinuses.

17. The answer is **D,** page 262.

When a mandible fracture is suspected, radiographs should include an anteroposterior (AP), right and left lateral oblique, and a Towne view. Plain films are generally sufficient to rule out a fracture. Except for pain and swelling, the patient has no significant findings for a mandibular fracture.

18. The answer is **C,** page 276.

After a traumatic perforation of the tympanic membrane, if the membrane appears folded medially or laterally, ENT referral is necessary to unfold the flap. Failure to unfold the flap may result in improper healing with risk of cholesteatoma formation. A cholesteatoma may also develop after a tympanic membrane perforation even if no flap is evident. A perforation without a flap that does not heal spontaneously within 2 to 3 weeks should be evaluated by an ENT specialist. The patient should be informed to keep the ear dry.

19. The answer is **A,** page 262.

The examiner can assess the likely level of a LeFort fracture by grasping the anterior maxillary arch (avoid placing pressure on the teeth) and attempting to move the maxilla forward and backward. If a LeFort I fracture is present, the hard palate will move but not the nose or orbits. Evidence for a LeFort II fracture includes movement of the palate and nose. The patient has sustained a LeFort III fracture when movement of the palate, nose, and orbits occurs. Obviously, airway management is of primary concern before diagnostic examination for specific fracture type.

20. The answer is **D,** page 280.

A concussion is among the most benign of dental injuries. The tooth is not mobile, displaced, or fractured. Management is the same for primary and permanent teeth and includes analgesia and parental reassurance. Dental follow-up within a few days is recommended to assess for resolution and any unusual complications.

21. The answer is **A,** page 282.

The red dot in the middle of the fracture is blood and indicates an Ellis class III injury to the pulp, necessitating immediate dental evaluation. This is true for primary or permanent teeth. If the pulp is exposed for more than 6 hours, a pulp infection may develop. The dentist is likely to place a calcium hydroxide coating over the tooth or perform root canal surgery.

22. The answer is **A,** page 281.

All avulsions of a *permanent* tooth require immediate dental consultation. The goal is to preserve the tooth's viability. Viability depends on the amount of injury to the periodontal ligament and the amount of extraoral time. If extraoral time is less than 1 hour, the tooth should be replanted. If more than 1 hour has elapsed since avulsion, the tooth should be placed in a liquid medium such as Hanks Balanced Salt Solution. Never scrub the root of the tooth, but excess debris can be sponged away gently. Although replacing the tooth in its socket is the best method to preserve its viability, it is best to obtain rapid dental evaluation because the tooth may not be properly replaced. The dentist is likely to splint the tooth in place, prescribe antibiotics, and arrange for close follow-up.

23. The answer is **B,** page 278.

The child has sustained a subluxation injury to his tooth. Management may be simple observation or splinting, depending on the degree of mobility. Mobility in this scenario is moderate. Immediate consultation is unnecessary, but dental evaluation within 24 hours is recommended because of the potential for pulp necrosis.

24. The answer is **D,** pages 280 and 258.

All lip lacerations across the vermilion border need careful suturing for best cosmetic outcome. The first stitch should approximate the vermilion border exactly. Primary teeth should never be replanted after avulsion because of the risk of pulp necrosis with injury to the underlying permanent tooth. Referral to a dentist is needed only if other injuries are suspected. If a tooth is avulsed and unable to be found, one must assess whether the tooth is imbedded in a laceration (e.g., tongue laceration), was intruded rather than avulsed, or has been aspirated. Radiographs should be used for clarification.

25. The answer is **C,** page 258.

Tongue lacerations most often do not need to be sutured. Tongue lacerations that may need to be sutured include lacerations that significantly distort normal anatomy, are through both outer layers, are half the diameter of the tongue's width, involve the tip, or bleed excessively. If the tongue needs to be sutured, sedation is often necessary. Absorbable sutures are used for closure.

26. The answer is **E,** page 257.

Parents should be made aware that oral electrical burns might be complicated by bleeding from the labial artery within the first 2 weeks after injury and scarring, microstomia, and disruption of the vermilion border chronically. It is unusual, however, for the patient to sustain injury other than local injury as the electrical energy is dissipated at the point of contact. Present recommendations are to treat conservatively, with delayed surgical revision as needed. Patients can be discharged if they are able to tolerate liquids but must have close surgical follow-up.

27. The answer is **A,** page 279.

Any patient with an intruded tooth should be evaluated by a dentist. This patient should see the dentist *immediately* because the tooth is intruded more than 50% of its crown length. The dentist may need to extract the primary tooth so as not to endanger the development of the permanent tooth bud. The dentist may obtain a panoramic view of the teeth to assess for underlying fracture or impingement of the intruded tooth upon the permanent dentition (see Table 21-3, page 279 in Barkin et al.)

28. The answer is **B,** page 263.

The clinical findings suggest a nasoethmoidal fracture involving the nasal and lacrimal bones and ethmoid labyrinth. These fractures of the medial orbital wall result in increased intercanthal distance because of disruption of the medial canthal ligament. The fracture is suggested by tenderness and bone movement when pressure is applied at the medial canthus. If this fracture is suspected, a CT scan is the study of choice because plain radiographs may be misread as negative.

29. The answer is **A,** page 263.

Patients with a possible nasal fracture can most often be discharged with early follow-up. Children should have follow-up sooner than adults because of rapid healing. Reduction of a displaced fracture will be more difficult in a child if more than a week has elapsed since injury. Radiographs are not imperative at first because they do not change management. If significant breathing difficulty or a septal hematoma is evident, acute management is necessary.

19

Neck and Spinal Cord Trauma

Francisco A. Medina

See Barkin et al: Chapter 22.

1. Which of the following statements regarding normal cervical spine soft tissue widths and body measurement in a 2-year-old is *true?*
   A. A predental space of 6 mm.
   B. A 3-mm subluxation of the anterior aspect of the spinous process anterior to the posterior cervical line
   C. A prevertebral soft tissue space at C2 of 9 mm.
   D. A prevertebral soft tissue space between C6 and the trachea of 12 mm.

2. Which of the following statements best describes cervical spine pseudosubluxation?
   A. The anterior aspect of the spinous process of C2 is subluxated up to 4 mm
      anterior or posterior to the posterior cervical line.
   B. An excess laxity of the transverse ligament in children so that the predental
      space is widened compared to adults.
   C. Pseudosubluxation of C2 occurs anterior to C3 by up to 3 mm in up to 40% of children less than 8 years of age.
   D. Prevertebral soft tissue depth is affected by phases of respiration, swallowing, and flexion.

3. Which of the following statements best describes the differences between adult and pediatric cervical spine anatomy?
   A. Children generally manifest adult patterns of cervical spine injuries at 6 years of age.
   B. The most common cervical spine fracture in children less than 8 years of age occurs at the atlantoaxial region.
   C. The child's hypermobile upper cervical spine decreases the risk of injury from acceleration and torsion forces.
   D. The pediatric cervical spine is less susceptible to torsional forces and angular momentum.

4. You are evaluating a 5-year-old pedestrian struck by a car. She does not complain of pain or tenderness, and the physical examination is normal. When reviewing the cervical spine series, you note a lucent horizontal line at the base of the dens on the odontoid view with no other abnormalities noted on x-ray. Which is the most likely diagnosis?
   A. A type 1 (involving the apex of the dens) fracture of the odontoid.
   B. A Jefferson fracture.
   C. An unstable cervical spine fracture.
   D. An epiphyseal growth plate.
   E. A compression fracture.

5. Atlantoaxial instability can be found in patients with:
   A. Down's syndrome
   B. Juvenile rheumatoid arthritis.
   C. Morquio's disease.
   D. All of the above.

6. Which of the following statements best describes the unique features of the *pediatric* cervical spine compared with the adult cervical spine?
   A. Has more diagonally oriented articular surfaces.
   B. Ligamentous attachments are weaker than the bony elements.
   C. In the very young the C3-C4 vertebral bodies are often wedged because of the ossification process.
   D. In children without a history of trauma, the absence of lordosis and absence of flexion curvature are common.
   E. The most common fracture is that of the atlas.

7. Which of the following statements best describes SCIWORA: Spinal Cord Injury Without Radiologic Abnormality?
   A. It occurs less frequently in children under 8 years of age.
   B. It accounts for 5% of pediatric cervical spine injuries.
   C. Transient symptoms of paresthesias, weakness, and burning sensation down the spine related to neck movement are rarely noted.
   D. Neurologic deficits usually appear immediately.
   E. A history of paresthesias may be the only clinical finding.

8. Which of the following radiologic views are the minimum required for an adequate assessment of a patient's cervical spine?
   A. Cross-table lateral cervical spine, anteroposterior, and open mouth odontoid views.
   B. Complete portable cross-table lateral cervical spine view.
   C. Portable cross-table lateral, open mouth odontoid, and flexion-extension views.
   D. Portable anteroposterior, open mouth odontoid, and oblique views.
   E. None of the above.

9. Which of the following best describes a Jefferson fracture?
   A. It is produced by a hyperextension force.
   B. A fracture of the posterior arch of C1.
   C. A fracture of the vertebral body of C1 with disruption of the bony fragments.
   D. A burst fracture of the anterior or posterior arch of C1 with lateral displacement.

10. A 5-year-old girl not wearing a helmet falls from her bicycle. An Emergency Medical Service (EMS) crew evaluates and transports her to your ED without immobilization. What clinical signs and symptoms will determine whether immobilization of the spine is necessary?
    A. Head trauma with undetermined duration of loss of consciousness and normal physical examination.
    B. Neck trauma, with mild headache, vomiting, and normal physical examination.
    C. Head trauma with brief loss of consciousness and a clinical displaced femur fracture in severe pain.
    D. Mild facial trauma with vomiting, headache, and neck pain.
    E. All of the above.

11. A 12-year-old boy was an unrestrained front seat passenger in a car involved in a front end collision. The car sustained significant damage. The boy was up and walking around at the scene and was brought to the ED by a bystander. At present he is sitting in a chair in triage and complains only of some vague back pain. Which of the following is the next most appropriate step?
    A. Have him sit in a position of comfort until you perform an evaluation.
    B. Immobilize his spine until you can evaluate him.
    C. Send him to radiology in a wheelchair for a cervical spine series before further evaluation.
    D. Send him to radiology with spine immobilization for a computed tomographic (CT) scan before further evaluation.
    E. Assess whether the patient can move his neck in all directions.

12. Which of the following best describes "hangman's fracture"?
    A. Usually a fracture of C3-C4.
    B. A stable fracture.
    C. Associated with severe hyperextension of the spine.
    D. Bilateral cervical spine pedicle fracture.
    E. Usually a fracture of the posterior pedicles of C7.

13. The anterior cord syndrome would be suggested by the absence of:
    A. Proprioception.
    B. Vibratory sensation.
    C. Pain.
    D. Motion.

14. A 5-year-old boy was struck by a car while riding his bicycle. The child was found unconscious by EMS. Cardiopulmonary resuscitation (CPR) and spinal immobilization were initiated, but the patient was unresponsive on arrival at the ED. Clinical findings suggestive of a transection of the descending fibers of the spinal cord in this patient would be:
    A. Increased patellar reflexes.
    B. Absence of perirectal sensation and wink.
    C. Increased rectal tone.
    D. Increased bulbocavernosus reflex.
    E. Increased muscle tone.

15. A 9-year-old boy is seen in the ED after he was struck by a car. He received 20 ml/kg of crystalloid in the ED. He cannot move his lower and upper extremities. Portable cross-table lateral radiographs of his C-spine are normal. Which of the following clinical findings would suggest spinal shock in this child?
    A. Blood pressure (BP) 90/60 mm Hg, pulse (P) 160 beats per minute, warm skin.
    B. BP 70/30 mm Hg, P 150 bpm, cold, clammy skin.
    C. BP 90/60 mm Hg, P 100 bpm, cold skin, and oliguria.
    D. BP 80/50 mm Hg, P 100 bpm, oliguria, and cold clammy skin.
    E. BP 70/30 mm Hg, P 80 bpm, warm skin.

16. The treatment of acute spinal injury should include which one of the following?
    A. Methylprednisolone, initial dose of 1 mg/kg intravenous (IV) over 15 min.
    B. Tomography of the spine to rule out hematoma.
    C. Surgery of the spine if reduction is refractory to traction.
    D. Naloxone given within the first 48 hours.

17. A 6-month-old infant was ejected from his stroller when it was struck by a car. On physical examination, you note that he cries and flexes and withdraws his lower extremities in response to stimulation. From these findings you can conclude:
    A. That there is no paralysis of his lower extremities.
    B. That there is no spinal cord injury.
    C. That a cervical spine injury is likely.
    D. Very little, because these movements can be seen in infants with paralyzed limbs.
    E. That a lumbosacral cord injury is likely.

18. Which of the following clinical findings is seen in the anterior cord syndrome?
    A. A loss of vibration below the lesion.
    B. A loss of pain and temperature above the lesion.
    C. A loss of proprioception above the lesion.
    D. A loss of motor function below the lesion.
    E. A loss of kinesthesia and touch below the lesion.

19. A 12-year-old girl suffered a penetrating injury to the neck during an assault. What clinical signs will make you suspect a cord hemisection (Brown-Séquard's syndrome)?
    A. Ipsilateral increment of pain.
    B. Ipsilateral loss of pain and temperature.
    C. Bilateral loss of motor function.
    D. Ipsilateral distal loss of motor function and proprioception.

20. The initial portable radiographs during stabilization of a 3-month-old hypotensive multiple trauma patient should include which of the following?
    A. Cross-table lateral cervical spine, AP view of the cervical spine and chest.
    B. Three views of the cervical spine, AP pelvis and chest.
    C. Cross-table lateral and AP cervical spine, with open mouth odontoid view.
    D. Cross-table lateral of the cervical spine.
    E. Chest and AP view of the pelvis.

21. A 7-year-old child sustains a blunt injury to the neck. A thorough neurologic examination should be performed in this patient to eliminate the possibility of which of the following injuries?
    A. Ophthalmic nerve injury.
    B. Glossopharyngeal nerve injury.
    C. Facial nerve injury.
    D. Injury to the recurrent laryngeal branch of the vagus nerve.
    E. Brain injury from direct trauma.

22. Which of the following radiographic studies is the most useful in visualizing the lower cervical vertebral bodies in a newborn if you do not see C7 on the lateral film?
    A. Diver's view.
    B. Tomograms.
    C. Swimmer's view.
    D. Oblique views.
    E. AP view.

23. A 1-year-old infant is seen in the ED after a high-speed motor vehicle accident. The patient sustained multiple trauma. In the ED the patient is immobilized, with breathing characterized as extremely shallow. The child has no midfacial injuries. Which of the following best describes the preferred technique of endotracheal intubation in this patient?
    A. Blind nasotracheal intubation.
    B. Oral tracheal intubation without medications.
    C. Oral tracheal intubation with in-line stabilization using rapid sequence intubation technique if required.
    D. Blind nasotracheal intubation with the use of a rapid sequence technique.
    E. Nasotracheal intubation with Magill forceps and temporary neck and head immobilization by an assistant and no medications.

24. You are evaluating a 10-year-old boy with neck pain after he has sustained a flexion-axial loading injury during football practice. His cervical spine plain films are equivocal. You feel compelled to rule out a cervical spine fracture or dislocation. The best study to do is:
    A. Magnetic resonance imaging (MRI).
    B. Myelogram.
    C. CT scan.
    D. Tomography.
    E. Ultrasound.

ANSWERS   [See Barkin et al: Chapter 22.]

1. The answer is **D**, pages 299 to 302.
   In reviewing a portable cross-table lateral cervical spine x-ray view, attention must be paid to the prevertebral space. Normal *prevertebral space distances* have been defined as:
   > Equal or less than 7 mm in children and adults anterior to C2.
   > Equal or less than 5 mm or 40% of the AP diameter of C3-C4 vertebral. bodies, anterior to C3-C4 in children and adults.
   > Less than 14 mm in children younger than 15 and equal to or less than 22 mm in adults between C6 and the trachea.
   The width of the prevertebral soft tissue may change with respiration, crying, and flexion or extension of the neck. The presence of air in the prevertebral space is a sign of rupture of the airway or esophagus.

2. The answer is **C**, page 299.
   Pseudosubluxation of C2 occurs anterior to C3 up to 3 mm in as many as 40% of children less than 8 years of age. This is not a normal variant in older age groups. C2-C3 subluxation alone in a 5-year-old child is not suggestive of a hangman's fracture.

3. The answer is **B**, pages 292 and 293.
   The most common cervical spine lesions in children less than 8 years of age are centered in the atlantoaxial region because of the increased flexibility of this anatomic area. The child's hypermobile upper cervical spine increases, not decreases, the risk of injury from acceleration and torsion forces.

4. The answer is **D**, pages 290 and 293.
   The axis (C2) has five primary ossification centers. An epiphyseal growth plate separates the odontoid from the axis; this disappears between 3 and 7 years of age. Before closure it appears as a lucent horizontal line. A Jefferson fracture is a burst fracture of the anterior or posterior arches of C1.

5. The answer is **D,** page 300.

Inflammatory disorders can affect the dens and the transverse ligament behind it. Patients with Down's syndrome, Morquio's disease, or rheumatoid arthritis commonly demonstrate laxity of the transverse ligament and instability at the atlantoaxial level.

6. The answer is **C,** pages 287 to 293.

The pediatric spine exhibits incomplete ossification, epiphyseal growth plates, synchondroses, hypermobility, and several normal and congenital variations. Younger children tend to sustain avulsions or epiphyseal separations rather than true fracture. The most common cervical spine lesion in children less than 8 years of age remains centered in the atlantoaxial region and includes odontoid fractures, atlantoaxial dislocation or subluxation, and hyperextension fractures of the axis.

7. The answer is **E,** pages 302 and 303.

SCIWORA is more common in children. The incidence varies between 4% and 66% of SCI accompanied by an incidence of complete cord injury of 40% to 55%. SCIWORA is a diagnosis of exclusion that should be made only after occult fractures and ligament and disk damage have been ruled out with CT scans, flexion-extension views, and myelography. MRI is usually necessary to rule out spinal cord compression. It generally does not show abnormality immediately after the injury but reveals atrophy of the spinal cord 1 to 3 months after the injury. SCIWORA tends to involve the cervical cord and is associated with a poor prognosis. Neurologic deficits may not appear until hours or days after the injury.

8. The answer is **A,** pages 297 to 302.

Using the "minimal" cervical spine series includes portable cross-table lateral cervical spine, open mouth odontoid, and anteroposterior views. Evaluations based on a single portable cross-table lateral view are not completely reliable.

9. The answer is **D,** page 293.

A Jefferson fracture is produced by a vertical compression force transmitted through the occipital condyles to the superior articular surfaces of the lateral masses of the atlas. This type of fracture may be seen in football players.

10. The answer is **E,** page 298.

In spinal cord injury, immobilization is the first step in treatment and prevention of exacerbation of any injury of the central nervous system. History and physical examination abnormalities are not always available and may be difficult to obtain in the emergency setting.

11. The answer is **B,** pages 310 to 314.

All patients with a history of significant injury, evidence of neurologic impairment, or radiologic evidence of abnormalities should be treated in the ED with the presumption that they have mechanically and neurologically unstable injuries. About 15% to 20% of patients with spine or spinal cord trauma may initially be able to walk after an accident. Although ambulatory at the scene, this patient should be immobilized pending a thorough evaluation. Radiologic studies should not be performed until the patient is evaluated, and appropriate workup and intervention are initiated.

12. The answer is **C,** page 293.

Extension can cause compression and subsequent fracture of the posterior neural arch of C1 or the pedicles of C2 as a result of the weight of the heavy occiput. This is known as a hangman's fracture.

13. The answer is **D,** page 296.

The anterior cord injury is marked by contusion of the anterior cord or laceration or thrombosis of the anterior spinal artery. Such patients have complete paralysis and hyperalgesia. It commonly occurs with flexion or vertical compression injuries.

14. The answer is **B,** pages 294 to 297.

A gross motor examination of the extremities must determine spontaneous and purposeful movements. Muscle tone is usually flaccid as a result of lower neuron lesions or spinal shock. The absence of rectal tone implies only a 2% to 3% chance of partial or complete recovery. The absence of a bulbocavernosus reflex indicates the presence of spinal shock.

15. The answer is **E,** page 295.

Spinal shock may accompany injury. Flaccid paralysis, areflexia, priapism, and sensory loss distal to the lesion are noted with impaired temperature control. Choice E demonstrates hypotension, bradycardia, and temperature instability characteristic of spinal shock.

16. The answer is **C,** page 312.

When possible, closed reduction and external bracing are the treatment of choice. Surgical decompression may be indicated with acute neurologic deterioration, penetrating injuries of the spinal cord, inability to achieve a closed reduction, or presence of a foreign body in the spinal canal. It also may be necessary for potentially unstable injuries. High-dose methylprednisolone 30 mg/kg beginning within 8 hours of injury, followed by an infusion of 5.4 mg/kg/hour for 23 hours is recommended to improve neurologic function.

17. The answer is **D,** page 294.

Evaluating infants for spinal cord injury is difficult. It is important to know that mass flexion withdrawal movements in response to stimulation may occur in infants with paralyzed limbs. This movement can be indistinguishable from normal movement.

18. The answer is **D,** page 296.

Anterior cord injury is marked by contusion to the anterior cord or laceration or thrombosis of the anterior spinal artery. Such patients have complete paralysis and hyperalgesia with preservation of touch and proprioception.

19. The answer is **D,** page 297.

Penetrating injuries may produce a cord hemisection that presents as Brown-Séquard's syndrome, with ipsilateral motor, proprioception, and light-touch deficits; contralateral pain; and temperature impairment.

20. The answer is **B,** pages 297 to 303.

In a hypotensive trauma patient, the cervical spine must be cleared. A cross-table lateral film is not sufficient to detect possible injuries. Chest x-ray and AP pelvic films should also be obtained to eliminate the chest and pelvis as possible sources of the shock.

21. The answer is **D,** page 308.

Blunt trauma to the neck can cause life-threatening injuries and may be less obvious. Stridor or alteration in phonation may be seen with injury to the vagus nerve, or specifically to the recurrent laryngeal branch.

22. The answer is **A,** page 299.

The swimmer's view (transaxillary view) may be helpful in visualizing the lower cervical spine if not visualized on the initial lateral film.

23. The answer is **C,** pages 310 and 311.

Determination of the safest technique for endotracheal intubation in pediatric patients with suspected cervical spine injury is controversial. Although nasotracheal intubation is classically used, its benefits have not been clearly documented; nor is it easily achieved in younger children, in whom it may be contraindicated. The use of a rapid sequence induction-intubation technique may provide the advantages of a smooth oral intubation without mobilization of the neck in a combative child.

24. The answer is **C,** page 297.

There are a number of radiologic modalities available to further evaluate a cervical spine injury. CT scan is excellent for evaluating bony injuries like fractures or dislocations. MRI is superior in demonstrating spinal cord injury, as well as differentiating extramedullary from intramedullary lesions. Tomography has largely been replaced by CT. Myelography is rarely necessary, although it can be helpful when clinical signs of cord compression, neurologic deficit, or deterioration are not explained by other studies. Ultrasound is not used in the evaluation of cervical spine injuries.

20

Thoracic Trauma

Anju Tejani • *Jeffrey S. Fine* • *George L. Foltin*

See Barkin et al: Chapter 23.

1. A 14-year-old girl sustains a stab wound to the left side of the chest. She arrives at the ED with heart rate (HR) 140 beats per minute, respiratory rate (RR) 45 breaths per minute, blood pressure (BP) 70/30 mm Hg. Appropriate management of this injury includes all of the following *except:*
   A. Fluid resuscitation.
   B. Oxygen administration.
   C. Wound debridement.
   D. Left thoracostomy.
   E. Medical antishock trousers (MAST).

2. A 7-year-old boy involved in a fight is kicked in the right side of his chest. He has mild palpable tenderness over the fourth and fifth ribs, no respiratory compromise, and no evidence of other injuries on physical examination. A chest radiograph confirms fractures of the fourth and fifth ribs. The appropriate management for this injury is:
   A. Ibuprofen.
   B. Strapping the chest wall.
   C. Epidural anesthesia.
   D. Intercostal nerve block.
   E. Transcutaneous electrical nerve stimulation.

3. A 14-year-old boy sustains a blast injury to the right side of the chest and arrives in the ED intubated, with a large sucking chest wound. What would be the most appropriate management for this patient?
   A. Right thoracostomy.
   B. Occlude the wound on three sides only.
   C. Right thoracostomy and occlude the wound on three sides only.
   D. Right thoracostomy and occlude the wound on all four sides.
   E. Urgent thoracotomy for repair of the chest wall.

4. Clinical signs suggesting acute cardiac tamponade include all of the following *except:*
   A. Hypotension.
   B. Muffled heart sounds.
   C. Pulsus paradoxus.
   D. Distended neck veins.
   E. Electrical alternans.

5. A 7-year-old boy was brought to the ED after being shot in the left side of his chest. You suspect esophageal injury because of blood-tinged gastric aspirate. The appropriate diagnostic strategy would be:
   A. Esophagoscopy alone.
   B. Barium swallow followed by esophagoscopy.
   C. Gastrografin swallow, barium swallow, and esophagoscopy.
   D. Barium swallow, Gastrografin swallow, and esophagoscopy.
   E. Gastrografin swallow and esophagoscopy.

6. A 16-year-old boy was struck by a car and pinned against a wall. He was then transported to the ED, where he has an HR 160 beats per minute, RR 45 breaths per minute, BP 70/palpable. He appears pale and in severe respiratory distress. On examination bowel sounds are heard over the left side of the chest. The abdomen is diffusely tender with some bruising over the right flank. All of the following would be appropriate in the initial management of this teenager *except:*
   A. Mechanical ventilation.
   B. Fluid resuscitation.
   C. MAST.
   D. Nasogastric tube placement.
   E. Bladder catheterization.

7. A 10-year-old boy was struck by a car while crossing the street. On arrival at the ED he is obtunded, with an HR 140 beats per minute, RR 40 breaths per minute, BP 70/palpable. On examination the patient has good air entry bilaterally; the abdomen is distended and tense; and the neurologic examination is nonfocal. Lateral cervical spine x-ray is normal. Chest x-ray reveals a small right pneumothorax. The patient needs to go to the operating room for exploratory laparotomy. Which must be done before mechanical ventilation?
   A. Head computed tomographic (CT) scan.
   B. Anteroposterior (AP) and open mouth cervical spine x-rays.
   C. Right thoracostomy.
   D. Needle thoracentesis.
   E. Central line placement.

8. An 11-year-old boy involved in a motor vehicle collision was found to have fractures of the lower ribs (9, 10, and 11) on the left side. An abdominal CT scan revealed a subcapsular splenic hematoma. The patient is complaining of severe pain at the site of the rib fractures and has shallow breathing. What would be the most appropriate treatment for the pain?
   A. Strapping of the chest wall.
   B. Morphine.
   C. Acetaminophen.
   D. Intercostal nerve block.
   E. Ibuprofen.

9. An 8-year-old boy is brought to the ED after being struck by a car. On arrival he has an HR 140 beats per minute, RR 35 breaths per minute, BP 70/20 mm Hg. Each of the following choices could explain this child's shock *except:*
   A. Liver laceration.
   B. Cardiac tamponade.
   C. Hemothorax.
   D. Tension pneumothorax.
   E. Subdural hematoma.

10. A 14-year-old girl is brought to the ED after a fall from a three-story building. On examination she is in severe respiratory distress and has subcutaneous emphysema and decreased air entry over the left lung field. After the patient is intubated, a chest tube is inserted on the left, which has a persistent massive air leak, and the child's respiratory status does not improve. What would be the next appropriate step after ensuring there is no equipment failure?
   A. Insert another thoracostomy tube on the left side.
   B. Insert a thoracostomy tube on the right side.
   C. Reintubate the patient.
   D. Perform bronchoscopy.
   E. Perform pericardiocentesis.

11. A 12-year-old boy with a gunshot wound to the left side of the chest has an HR 180 beats per minute, RR 50 breaths per minute, BP 70/palpable with very weak pulses. The patient is intubated and being appropriately ventilated. A few minutes into the resuscitation the patient becomes pulseless. The next step would be:
   A. Epinephrine.
   B. Pericardiocentesis.
   C. Bilateral thoracostomy tubes.
   D. Blood transfusion.
   E. Open thoracotomy.

12. A 9-year-old boy was hit with a baseball over the sternum. He comes to the ED 2 hours later complaining of chest pain. He has an HR 120 beats per minute, RR 30 breaths per minute, and BP 90/50 mm Hg. He has equal breaths sounds bilaterally. Bruising is noted over the midsternum. ECG recording of patient is shown in Figure 20-1. What is the best test to confirm the diagnosis?
   A. Chest radiograph.
   B. Cardiac enzymes.
   C. Echocardiography.
   D. Thoracic CT scan.
   E. Electrocardiography.

13. In children, which of the following injuries are most commonly associated with falls from a height?
   A. Abdominal injury, rib fractures, and pelvic fractures.
   B. Extremity fractures, abdominal injury, and pulmonary contusion.
   C. Head injury, multiple lower extremity fractures, and chest wall trauma.
   D. Femur fracture and thoracic and intraabdominal injuries.
   E. Diaphragmatic injuries and Chance fracture.

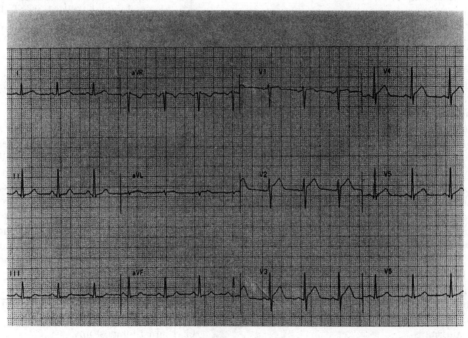

FIG. 20-1

14. A 5-year-old boy who was riding his bicycle was hit by a truck and thrown against a wire fence. The patient arrives in the ED markedly cyanotic, with inspiratory gurgling, subcutaneous emphysema, and severe retractions. The most likely explanation for his condition is:
    A. Cardiac tamponade.
    B. Tension pneumothorax.
    C. Pulmonary contusion.
    D. Laryngeal transection.
    E. Tracheobronchial rupture.
15. What other injury is commonly associated with the injury described in question 14?
    A. Rib fractures.
    B. Myocardial contusion.
    C. Rupture of great vessels.
    D. Cervical fracture.
    E. Esophageal rupture.
16. A 16-year-old boy is brought to the ED after a high-speed motor vehicle collision. His chest x-ray is shown in Figure 20-2. All the following are true about this condition *except:*
    A. It may be treated with pericardiocentesis and observation.
    B. It is more common with penetrating trauma than blunt trauma.
    C. Cardiovascular collapse may develop rapidly if not treated.
    D. Patients usually have muffled heart sounds and tachycardia.
    E. Patients must go to the operating room for definitive management.

17. The most common complication of myocardial contusion is:
    A. Papillary muscle tear.
    B. Ventricular tachydysrhythmia.
    C. Rupture of the ventricular wall.
    D. Complete heart block
    E. Endocardial aneurysm formation.
18. A 12-year-old girl involved in a high-speed motor vehicle collision sustains a large subdural hematoma. She has equal air entry bilaterally, and her abdomen is not distended. She is taken to the operating room for evacuation of the subdural hematoma after a negative peritoneal lavage. The initial chest radiograph was negative. A few minutes after the surgery begins, her condition deteriorates. Her HR is 140 beats per minute, BP 70/20 mm Hg. The therapy that would most likely improve the patient's condition is:
    A. Blood transfusion.
    B. Needle thoracentesis.
    C. Surgical hemostasis.
    D. Epinephrine.
    E. Hyperventilation.
19. A 10-year-old girl is brought to the ED after sustaining a stab wound at the level of the right nipple in the midclavicular line. She is in severe respiratory distress and has decreased air entry over the right lung field. A right thoracostomy tube is placed that initially drains 350 ml of blood and that continues to produce bloody drainage for the subsequent hour. What is the most likely explanation for her deterioration?
    A. Hemothorax.
    B. Tension pneumothorax.
    C. Cardiac tamponade.
    D. Intraabdominal bleeding.
    E. Vena cava rupture.

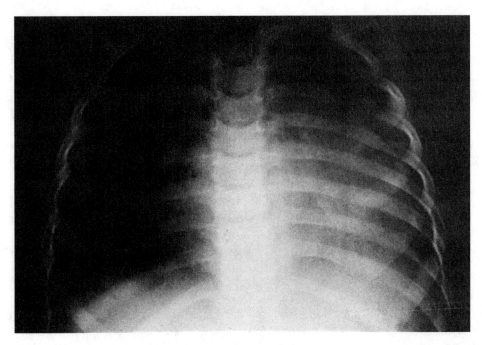

FIG. 20-2

20. Which statement regarding insertion of a thoracostomy tube is *true?*
   A. The preferred position is at the fifth intercostal space at the posterior axillary line.
   B. The tube should traverse the lower border of the upper rib to prevent damage to the neurovascular bundle.
   C. The tube should traverse the upper border of the lower rib to prevent damage to the neurovascular bundle.
   D. An initial drainage of 4 to 5 ml/kg of blood indicates need for urgent thoracotomy.

21. Complications of pericardiocentesis include all of the following *except:*
   A. Cardiac dysrhythmia.
   B. Coronary artery laceration.
   C. Diaphragmatic perforation.
   D. Splenic laceration.
   E. Pericardial tamponade.

22. A 15-year-old boy is brought to the ED after a high-speed motor vehicle collision. Which of the following vital signs would be most indicative of cardiac tamponade?
   A. HR 40 bpm, RR 40 bpm, BP 70/40 mm Hg (inspiration and expiration).
   B. HR 40 bpm, apneic, BP 60/palpable (inspiration and expiration).
   C. HR 140 bpm, RR 45 bpm, BP 75/35 mm Hg (inspiration), 90/40 mm Hg (expiration).
   D. HR 140 bpm, RR 40 bpm, BP 100/50 mm Hg (inspiration), 105/70 mm Hg (expiration).
   E. HR 150 bpm, RR 50 bpm, BP 100/45 mm Hg (inspiration), 90/50 mm Hg (expiration).

23. A 6-year-old boy involved in a motor vehicle collision is transferred to your ED. On arrival the patient is tachypneic and has retractions. His chest radiograph is shown in Fig. 20-3. Which of the following blood gas results would best correlate with this patient's condition?
   A. pH 7.50, Pao_2 85, $Paco_2$ 30, HCO_3 18.
   B. pH 7.32, Pao_2 60, $Paco_2$ 40, HCO_3 18.
   C. pH 7.24, Pao_2 40, $Paco_2$ 60, HCO_3 18.
   D. pH 7.30, Pao_2 92, $Paco_2$ 50, HCO_3 20.
   E. pH 7.20, Pao_2 75, $Paco_2$ 20, HCO_3 10.

24. A 5-year-old boy has a 2-cm stab wound in the midaxillary line, just below the level of the left nipple. On arrival at the ED he has an HR 100 beats per minute, RR 24 breaths per minute, BP 96/50 mm Hg. Chest radiograph and abdominal CT scan are normal. Which of the following would be best to rule out a diaphragmatic injury?
   A. Peritoneal lavage.
   B. Thoracotomy.
   C. Thoracic CT scan.
   D. Laparoscopy.
   E. Abdominal ultrasound.

25. A 2-year-old girl involved in a high-speed motor vehicle collision was trapped between the front and rear passenger seats. She is brought to the ED disoriented and in mild respiratory distress. On examination she has cyanosis of the face and upper extremities and subconjunctival and retinal hemorrhages. After adequate ventilation is ensured, the most appropriate diagnostic test would be:
   A. Peritoneal lavage.
   B. Esophagoscopy.
   C. Echocardiography.
   D. Thoracic CT scan.
   E. Aortography.

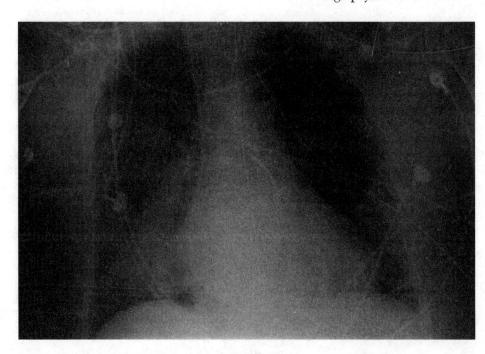

FIG. 20-3

26. All of the following injuries are frequently associated with the condition described in question 25 *except:*
    A. Flail chest.
    B. Pulmonary contusion.
    C. Cardiac tamponade.
    D. Liver laceration.
    E. Spinal fractures.

27. A 5-year-old child is brought to the ED after a motor vehicle collision. The child underwent a full trauma evaluation, including thoracic and abdominal CT scans with intravenous (IV) and oral contrast, and cervical spine x-rays. Which of the following injuries may not have been adequately evaluated by the above investigations?
    A. Pulmonary contusion.
    B. Subcapsular splenic hematoma.
    C. Diaphragmatic injury.
    D. Pulmonary laceration.
    E. Perforated ileum.

28. A 9-year-old boy comes to the ED complaining of epigastric pain that had been worsening for 1 week. He was involved in a motor vehicle collision 1 year ago in which he had sustained a pulmonary contusion. Which of the following conditions would most likely be responsible for his current pain?
    A. Esophageal stricture.
    B. Papillary muscle rupture.
    C. Diaphragmatic hernia.
    D. Pleural adhesions.
    E. Myocardial contusion.

29. Which of the following statements about thoracic trauma in young children is *true?*
    A. A mobile mediastinum allows children to compensate for increases in intrathoracic pressure.
    B. The elasticity of the thoracic cage results in an increased incidence of rib fractures in children.
    C. Children's intercostal muscles are well developed and can adequately compensate for diaphragmatic injury.
    D. The elasticity of the chest wall in children results in increased incidence of pulmonary contusion as compared with adults.
    E. Decreased oxygen consumption improves children's ability to cope with respiratory compromise for longer periods of time than adults.

30. Complications of thoracostomy tube placement include all of the following *except:*
    A. Pulmonary laceration.
    B. Splenic injury.
    C. Bronchopulmonary fistula.
    D. Pleural-cutaneous fistula.
    E. Infection.

31. Jugular venous dilatation may not accompany tension pneumothorax when associated with which of the following injuries?
    A. Subdural hematoma.
    B. Laryngeal transection
    C. Pulmonary contusion.
    D. Hemoperitoneum.
    E. Flail chest.

32. A 3-year-old girl is brought to your ED after a *low-speed* motor vehicle collision. Her vital signs are HR 130 beats per minute, RR 24 breaths per minute, BP 90/70 mm Hg. An AP chest x-ray done as part of the initial trauma evaluation shows a widened mediastinum. The most likely cause for this finding is:
    A. Pneumothorax.
    B. Aortic dissection.
    C. Esophageal rupture.
    D. Radiologic artifact
    E. Cardiac tamponade.

33. Which other finding on chest radiograph would indicate the need for further investigation?
    A. Elevation of the left mainstem bronchus.
    B. Shift of the trachea to the right.
    C. Shift of the esophagus to the left.
    D. Presence of an aorticopulmonary window.
    E. Elevation of the right hemidiaphragm.

34. A 13-year-old boy is seen in the ED after being struck by a van. On examination he has an HR 120 beats per minute, RR 45 breaths per minute, BP 100/60 mm Hg. He has dullness to percussion and decreased air entry over the right side of the chest. The most likely diagnosis is:
    A. Cardiac tamponade.
    B. Myocardial contusion.
    C. Pneumothorax.
    D. Hemothorax.
    E. Diaphragmatic rupture.

35. Chest CT scan is *least* helpful in making the diagnosis of:
    A. Diaphragmatic rupture.
    B. Aortic rupture.
    C. Esophageal injury.
    D. Pulmonary contusion.
    E. Hemothorax.

36. Thoracotomy in the ED is indicated in which of the following instances:
    A. Blunt chest trauma with pneumothorax.
    B. Penetrating chest trauma with hemothorax.
    C. Penetrating chest trauma with asystole.
    D. Diaphragmatic rupture with herniation of intestinal contents.
    E. Aortic dissection with intraabdominal hemorrhage.

37. In children less than 3 years of age, most rib fractures are a result of:
    A. Motor vehicle collision.
    B. Child abuse.
    C. Metabolic diseases.
    D. Falls.
    E. Connective tissue diseases.

38. A 6-year-old boy involved in a motor vehicle collision sustains a large hemothorax. Which of the following statements about treatment of this condition is true?
    A. Large collections of blood should be drained rapidly to alleviate respiratory compromise.
    B. Small to moderate collections of blood may not require drainage if the patient is asymptomatic.
    C. Thoracotomy is necessary to ensure complete drainage of blood.
    D. Empyema is a common complication in large collections of blood.
    E. Incomplete drainage of blood can result in fibrothorax and restrictive lung disease.

ANSWERS [See Barkin et al: Chapter 23.]

1. The answer is **E**, page 330.
   The use of MAST is contraindicated in patients with thoracic trauma, especially penetrating trauma, even though the patient is hypotensive. The rate of bleeding may be seriously accelerated by an increase in afterload, which occurs with the application of the MAST. All other choices would be appropriate in a patient with thoracic trauma.

2. The answer is **A**, pages 329 and 330.
   Rib fractures are not as common in children as in adults. Most fractures occur at the posterolateral aspects of the middle and lower ribs. In contrast to the adult, children rarely experience enough discomfort to cause splinting or atelectasis. Nonsteroidal antiinflammatory agents may be used as first-line therapy for mild pain. Strapping of the chest wall is not recommended. For patients with more severe pain, resulting in splinting and pulmonary compromise, intercostal nerve block and epidural analgesia may be used. Transcutaneous electrical nerve stimulator is not indicated in management of acute pain.

3. The answer is **D**, page 326.
   Open pneumothorax occurs when there is a communication between the pleural cavity and the atmosphere as seen with large-knife, gunshot, or blast injuries. Definitive therapy is placement of a thoracostomy tube at a site remote from the wound and complete occlusion of the wound. Occlusive dressing on three sides may be used as a temporizing measure in the field. For wounds larger than the patient's airway, complete collapse of the lung occurs, resulting in mediastinal flutter in children (side-to-side movement of the child's mobile mediastinum). In addition to thoracostomy and complete occlusion, these large wounds may require thoracotomy for wound debridement and closure.

4. The answer is **E**, pages 326 and 327.
   Cardiac tamponade occurs more commonly secondary to penetrating thoracic trauma, especially stab wounds. Clinical signs include muffled heart sounds, hypotension, distended neck veins (Beck's triad), and tachycardia. In severe cases, pulsus paradoxus may occur. Electrical alternans (defined as voltage shifts in magnitude of alternate beats seen on the ECG tracing) is not seen with acute tamponade. It is seen in conditions such as myocarditis, pericarditis with effusion, and digitalis toxicity.

5. The answer is **C**, page 329.
   Esophageal injury is uncommon in children. However, if not recognized early, it can rapidly progress to mediastinitis, sepsis, and death. The mortality rate from esophageal injury is 5% if the injury is diagnosed within 24 hours, and it increases to 75% if the injury is diagnosed after 24 hours. Mediastinal crunch (Hamman's sign) is rarely heard in children. A chest radiograph may show pneumomediastinum. A patient suspected of esophageal injury should first undergo a Gastrografin swallow because if there is a significant tear, the extravasated material will be absorbed. If the Gastrografin swallow is negative, it is followed by a barium swallow, which is more sensitive in identifying small leaks. If both are negative, the patient should then have esophagoscopy. This further decreases the risk of missing any injury.

6. The answer is **C**, page 328.
   In a patient with diaphragmatic injury, precipitous deterioration can occur with use of the abdominal portion of the MAST. The resulting increase in intraabdominal pressure further pushes abdominal contents into the thorax and causes increased respiratory compromise. All of the other maneuvers would be appropriate in this patient.

7. The answer is **C,** page 326.

In a patient who is going to need positive-pressure ventilation, a thoracostomy tube must be inserted for even a small pneumothorax to prevent the development of a tension pneumothorax. All of the other choices are not essential before intubation and mechanical ventilation if a patient needs to go to the operating room immediately. For instance, a cervical collar may be left on until after surgery, or an intraoperative intracranial pressure monitor may be inserted. Needle thoracentesis is only a temporizing measure to treat tension pneumothorax, and air could reaccumulate during positive-pressure ventilation. Central line placement need not be performed before mechanical ventilation.

8. The answer is **D,** pages 329 and 330.

Intercostal nerve block or epidural anesthetic are effective treatments for severe pain associated with rib fractures that result in splinting and respiratory compromise. Acetaminophen and ibuprofen would not be effective therapy for severe pain. Some surgeons believe that parental therapy with an opioid analgesic agent might mask abdominal pain that would be a warning sign of significant injury. In this case, the intercostal nerve block would relieve the pain associated with the fracture, but not mask pain related to intraabdominal injury, or alter the patient's mental status.

9. The answer is **E,** pages 326 and 327.

In children, subdural hematomas do not usually cause blood loss sufficient to produce hypovolemic shock. Both hemothorax and liver laceration can result in significant blood loss and hypovolemia. Cardiac tamponade and tension pneumothorax both lead to a decrease in the venous return.

10. The answer is **D,** page 328.

In this patient no lung expansion occurred after thoracostomy, and there was a massive air leak from the thoracostomy tube. In such cases the practitioner must suspect a tracheobronchial disruption. These injuries are potentially lethal, and diagnosis is made via bronchoscopy (preferably rigid bronchoscopy). Smaller injuries require tube thoracostomy and supportive care. Severe injuries with associated vascular damage require thoracotomy for definitive repair.

11. The answer is **E,** page 324.

Open thoracotomy is the treatment of choice in patients with penetrating trauma who had vital signs and then lost them during resuscitation. It allows the practitioner to open the pericardium to relieve cardiac tamponade; to administer open cardiac massage; to provide temporizing treatment of injuries such as perforation of the heart and bleeding of lung or hilum; to provide direct occlusion of the thoracic aorta; and to place a large-bore catheter into the right atrium for fluid resuscitation. The procedure can be lifesaving in these patients.

12. The answer is **C,** pages 328.

The ECG findings are consistent with myocardial contusion. The abnormalities include ST and T wave changes. Furthermore atrial and ventricular dysrhythmias may be seen with this problem. Cardiac enzymes will be elevated with myocardial contusion, and a creatine phosphokinase-MB (CPK-MB) ratio of 5% or greater suggests the diagnosis. Confirmation of the diagnosis is achieved by echocardiography. Multiple gated acquisition (MUGA) scans may be used to obtain additional information.

13. The answer is **C,** page 319.

Head injury, lower extremity fractures, and chest wall trauma are frequently found in children with falls from a height. The other patterns of injury unique to childhood are (1) the "lap-belt" complex, consisting of blow-out injuries of the diaphragm or small bowel and lumbar spine fractures (Chance fractures), and (2) "Waddell's triad," occurring in small children struck by an automobile, resulting in femur fracture and head and abdominal trauma.

14. The answer is **D,** page 325.

Injury to the larynx and trachea usually occurs after direct trauma or rapid deceleration against stretched wire or clothesline. Complete anatomic obstruction of the upper airway in a child is very unusual. The posterior displacement of the tongue is the most common cause of airway obstruction in trauma patients. All the choices can cause respiratory distress, but inspiratory gurgling is characteristically seen with upper airway obstruction. Subcutaneous emphysema in addition to laryngeal transection may be seen with tension pneumothorax and tracheobronchial rupture. Emergency endotracheal intubation should be attempted before going to a surgical airway. A fiberoptic laryngoscope may be used for better visualization.

15. The answer is **D,** page 325.

Hangman's fracture is frequently associated with laryngeal transection secondary to the mechanism of injury. Management of these patients should always include cervical spine immobilization.

16. The answer is **A,** page 326.

The x-ray demonstrates enlargement of the cardiac silhouette consistent with cardiac tamponade. Patients with cardiac tamponade commonly have sustained stab injuries, since those with gunshot wounds usually die before arrival at the hospital. Tamponade is a rare sequela of blunt trauma. Patients may have tachycardia, hypotension, muffled heart sounds, pulsus paradoxus, and distended neck veins, although distended neck veins may not be present in a hypovolemic patient. Once the condition is diagnosed the patient must be taken to the operating room for definitive repair. Pericardiocentesis is used as a temporizing measure before the patient is taken to surgery.

17. The answer is **B,** page 328.

Myocardial contusion is uncommon in children. It usually occurs secondary to direct blunt forces applied to the chest. Patients have chest pain and other nonspecific symptoms. Investigations to aid in the diagnosis are ECG, cardiac enzymes, and echocardiography. The most frequent complication is ventricular tachydysrhythmia. The other choices are all known complications but are uncommon. Management of these patients includes observation in a monitored setting and treatment of dysrhythmias if they occur.

18. The answer is **B,** page 326.

In a victim of multiple trauma, tension pneumothorax should be suspected when a patient's condition suddenly deteriorates, even though initial x-ray findings are negative. This is especially true when deterioration occurs after positive-pressure ventilation is initiated. In such instances needle thoracentesis would be lifesaving.

19. The answer is **A,** page 326.

Blood in the pleural space can tamponade bleeding from the lung parenchyma or the hilum. Rapid evacuation of a massive hemothorax may result in severe rebleeding. Therefore blood must be evacuated slowly by intermittent clamping and unclamping of the chest tube.

20. The answer is **C,** page 324.

The preferred position for thoracostomy tube placement in a trauma patient is the fifth intercostal space (level of the nipple) between the anterior and midaxillary line. The neurovascular bundle lies in a groove along the lower border of the rib; therefore the tube should traverse the upper border of the lower rib to avoid damage to these structures. The tube should be directed posteriorly and superiorly. Initial drainage of more than 10 to 15 ml/kg or continuing drainage of more than 2 to 4 ml/kg indicates significant bleeding and the need for thoracotomy to control the bleeding. Drainage of bile indicates diaphragmatic rupture with eventration of abdominal contents into the chest cavity. A chest radiograph must always be obtained to confirm position of the tube and lung reexpansion.

21. The answer is **D,** page 327.

Various acute and long-term complications can occur with pericardiocentesis. Acute complications include myocardial penetration, arrhythmias, hemopericardium, pneumothorax, coronary artery laceration, and diaphragmatic perforation. Delayed complications include pericardial-peritoneal or pericardial-cutaneous fistula, pneumothorax, local infection, and pericardial tamponade.

22. The answer is **C,** page 327.

The definition of pulsus paradoxus is a fall in systolic BP of more than 10 mm Hg when measured in inspiration as compared with expiration. In addition to cardiac tamponade, it may be seen in cases of severe asthma, COPD, pulmonary edema, and tension pneumothorax when an increase in the intrathoracic pressure during inspiration results in decreased venous return to the heart.

23. The answer is **B,** page 327.

The chest radiograph shows pulmonary contusion, which is the most frequently observed chest injury in children. Loss of alveolar capillary integrity and transudation of fluid result in intrapulmonary shunting, ventilation-perfusion abnormalities, and hypoxemia. The clinical picture is similar to adult respiratory distress syndrome (ARDS). Arterial blood gas analysis shows hypoxemia, although mild hypercarbia can be seen. Treatment depends on severity. Mild cases need only supportive care and close observation. In more severe cases the mainstays of therapy are positive-pressure ventilation with positive end expiratory pressure (PEEP), avoiding overhydration, and prevention of secondary pneumonia. It is important to note that the initial chest x-ray may be negative even with significant injury. Thoracic CT scan is more sensitive for early detection of pulmonary contusion. Choice C is incorrect because the results noted are not physiologic. The pH should be lower given the $Paco_2$ and the HCO_3.

24. The answer is **D,** page 330.

Laparoscopy is the best method for ruling out diaphragmatic injuries. Chest radiograph and peritoneal lavage may be negative even in the presence of injury, especially after penetrating trauma. Thoracic CT scan or abdominal ultrasound may also miss small tears not associated with displacement of abdominal contents. Thoracotomy would be indicated only for operative repair of a severe intrathoracic injury such as bronchopulmonary disruption.

25. The answer is **D,** page 330.

This patient has findings typical for traumatic asphyxia. This is a rare but striking phenomenon that occurs when a sudden increase in intrathoracic pressure associated with compression of the chest is transmitted through the valveless veins of the head and upper extremities, resulting in rupture of capillaries. Petechial hemorrhages of the conjunctiva, retina, and skin of the upper extremities and face are seen. Similar hemorrhages occur in the brain, resulting in transient neurologic findings. The prognosis is good in most cases, with symptoms resolving over the course of several days as the hemorrhages are reabsorbed. However, because of the severity of forces applied to the chest, a diligent search must be made for intrathoracic and intraabdominal injuries such as rib fractures, pulmonary contusion, and liver injury. Thus thoracic CT scan would yield the most information about underlying chest and abdominal trauma.

26. The answer is **C,** page 330.

Cardiac tamponade is rarely associated with this type of injury. Flail chest, rib fractures, pulmonary contusion, intraabdominal trauma (especially liver laceration), and spinal fractures are frequently associated with traumatic asphyxia.

27. The answer is **C,** page 328.

Although most diaphragmatic injuries secondary to blunt trauma are large tears with resultant eventration of abdominal contents into the chest cavity, some small tears may be missed on chest radiograph, as well as CT scan of the abdomen or chest. All the listed injuries should be adequately evaluated by these tests.

28. The answer is **C,** page 328.

Unrecognized small diaphragmatic tears later can lead to diaphragmatic hernia and bowel strangulation. Therefore some traumatologists recommend routine exploration by laparoscopy, especially with penetrating trauma, or if there is a suspicion of injury and other investigations are negative.

29. The answer is **D,** page 319.

Certain anatomic and physiologic characteristics are the reasons for differences in patterns of thoracic trauma and the responses to it in children as compared with adults. The elastic chest wall allows kinetic energy to be transmitted to the underlying parenchyma, resulting in a higher incidence of pulmonary contusion and a lower incidence of rib fractures. Even small increases in intrathoracic pressure on one side of the chest can cause a shift of the mediastinum, which can further compromise respiratory and cardiac function. Children's intercostal muscles are poorly developed, which leads to early fatigue. Ventilation may be further compromised by impaired diaphragmatic excursion caused by gastric distention from aerophagia, commonly seen in pediatric patients. Children also have an increased oxygen consumption and decreased functional residual capacity, making them more susceptible to hypoxia.

30. The answer is **C,** page 334.

Immediate complications of thoracostomy tube placement include local bleeding, pulmonary contusion or laceration, pneumothorax or hemothorax, infection, bronchopleural or pleurocutaneous fistula and diaphragmatic, splenic, or hepatic injury. Bronchopulmonary fistula is not seen with this procedure.

31. The answer is **D,** page 326.

Increase in intrathoracic pressure results in decreased venous return to the heart and venous congestion (especially in head and upper extremity veins) manifesting as distended jugular veins. However, if the patient is hypovolemic (as in a patient with hemoperitoneum), this sign will not be present. The other answers are not associated with hypovolemia.

32. The answer is **D,** page 328.

Rupture of the aorta or aortic dissection is very rare in children. Early on, vital signs may be stable, however, even in the face of aortic dissection. It is seen with *severe deceleration events* (high-speed collision, fall from extreme heights). The most common site of injury is at the level of the attachment of the ligamentum arteriosum. In this scenario, with a low-risk mechanism of injury, the abnormality seen on the chest radiograph is most likely to be an artifact of an AP film obtained for an uncooperative crying child.

33. The answer is **B,** page 328.

Other findings that suggest true aortic injury are depression of the left mainstem bronchus, shift of the trachea and esophagus to the right, loss of the aorticopulmonary window, and blurring of the aortic knob secondary to formation of expanding hematoma around the injured aorta. Tracking of blood along the pleura results in the apical cap sign.

34. The answer is **D,** page 326.

Hemothorax after blunt trauma and gunshot wounds is usually caused by bleeding from lung parenchyma. With stab wounds, hemothorax results from damage to intercostal vessels. The characteristic findings are respiratory distress, decreased air entry on the side of the hemothorax with shift of the trachea to the opposite side, and dullness to percussion. In pneumothorax, signs are similar except the lung field is hyperresonant to percussion. With cardiac tamponade and myocardial contusion, air entry should be equal on both sides. With diaphragmatic rupture, bowel sounds may be heard over the chest. However, if air entry is decreased secondary to eventration of abdominal contents, the chest should be resonant to percussion.

35. The answer is **A,** pages 322 and 323.

A patient with diaphragmatic rupture may not show any abnormalities on chest CT scan if the tear is small and no abdominal contents have been displaced into the chest cavity. Esophageal injury will be suspected because of air in the mediastinum, although further investigation will be required to confirm the diagnosis. In aortic rupture a widened mediastinum is seen, even though aortography must be done before repair. CT scan is sensitive and specific for both pulmonary contusion and hemothorax.

36. The answer is **C,** page 324.

Of the choices given, the only one that requires emergency thoracotomy in the ED is a patient with penetrating trauma who had measurable vital signs and then loses them during resuscitation. In choices A, B, and D, thoracotomy is not specifically indicated. For children with abdominal bleeding, cross-clamping of the distal thoracic aorta has largely been abandoned because of persistent bleeding from multiple collaterals. Other indications might be in a patient with pericardial tamponade, especially when associated with penetrating trauma, or a patient with a massive air leak from a bronchial tear requiring clamping of the damaged bronchus.

37. The answer is **A,** pages 318 and 329.
    Rib fractures are usually a result of blunt trauma, most frequently related to motor vehicle collisions. However, it is important to think about child abuse when the history is inconsistent with the physical examination, and chest radiograph reveals multiple fractures in different stages of healing. Metabolic problems such as rickets and connective tissue disorders such as osteogenesis imperfecta are uncommon causes of rib fractures.

38. The answer is **E,** pages 326 and 329.
    Hemothorax is a collection of blood in the pleural space. Bleeding occurs from the lung parenchyma or the intercostal or internal mammary vessels. Most authorities recommend that all collections be completely drained to minimize the risk of infection of the residual blood and the development of fibrothorax and restrictive lung disease. Thoracotomy is necessary only when thoracostomy placement is unsuccessful in draining the blood collection. Large collections should be drained slowly because there is risk of significant rebleeding if done rapidly. Empyema is not the most common complication seen.

21

Abdominal Trauma

Anthony J. Ciorciari

See Barkin et al: Chapter 24.

1. Which of the following statements regarding pediatric abdominal trauma is correct?
   A. Most children with major abdominal trauma require operative intervention.
   B. Inadequate resuscitation remains the leading cause of preventable death.
   C. Of children admitted to a pediatric trauma center, 25% have documented abdominal injuries.
   D. Abdominal trauma is a major cause of traumatic death in childhood.
   E. Abdominal injury occurs in approximately 50% of all children with fatal injuries.

2. Compared with an adult, a child has:
   A. Proportionately smaller solid viscera.
   B. More rigid ribs.
   C. A bladder that is located more intraabdominally.
   D. Less protuberant abdomen.
   E. More abdominal muscle fat.

3. A 6-year-old boy is seen in the ED after sustaining blunt abdominal trauma. On examination you notice a large, firm, and tender suprapubic mass. There is no blood at the child's meatus. The next step in the management of this patient is:
   A. Order a computed tomographic (CT) scan of the abdomen.
   B. Order a pelvic radiograph
   C. Insert a Foley catheter.
   D. Insert a nasogastric tube.
   E. Prepare for diagnostic peritoneal lavage.

4. Which type of shock is most common in the child with serious abdominal injury?
   A. Hemorrhagic.
   B. Septic.
   C. Obstructive.
   D. Distributive.
   E. Neurogenic.

5. Which of the following is *least* frequently injured in blunt abdominal trauma?
   A. Liver.
   B. Spleen.
   C. Kidneys.
   D. Gastrointestinal tract.
   E. Pancreas.

6. Which of the following is the *most* likely to be injured in penetrating abdominal trauma?
   A. Liver.
   B. Spleen.
   C. Kidneys.
   D. Gastrointestinal tract.
   E. Pancreas.

7. Which of the following statements regarding pediatric abdominal trauma is *true*?
   A. Urban centers have a lower incidence of penetrating trauma when compared with the national average.
   B. Knives are the most lethal agent of injury.
   C. In children 13 years of age or older, 40% of penetrating injuries are from knives or handguns.
   D. Penetrating injury in a preschooler is more likely to be caused by accidental impalement by objects such as scissors or fences.
   E. Blunt trauma has a higher mortality than penetrating trauma.

8. A 7-year-old girl comes to the ED after being hit by a car. She has a noticeable left femur fracture. Her vital signs reveal a pulse of 180 beats per minute and thready and a blood pressure (BP) of 70/40 mm Hg. She responds to verbal stimuli. Her breaths are equal on both sides, and her oxygen saturation is 100%. Her skin is pale and clammy. You have started fluid resuscitation. Of the following, the next best step in management is:
   A. Direct admittance of the patient to the pediatric intensive care unit (ICU).
   B. Abdominal ultrasound.
   C. Diagnostic peritoneal lavage.
   D. CT scan of the head.
   E. Intubation of the patient's trachea and use of positive-pressure ventilation.

9. Which of the following statements is *correct* regarding injuries from motor vehicle accidents for pediatric vehicle occupants or pedestrians?
   A. Abdominal trauma is the most common type of injury.
   B. The abdomen is the most frequent site of significant blood loss.
   C. The most likely segment of the spine damaged in a lap-belt injury is the sacral portion.
   D. Disruption of the diaphragm is common in lap-belt injuries.
   E. A higher fraction of serious injury occurs outside the passenger compartment.

10. Which of the following statements regarding bicycle injury is correct?
   A. Abdominal trauma is the most lethal type of injury.
   B. Chance-type spinal fractures occur approximately 30% of the time.
   C. Kidney and intestinal injury is rare.
   D. The handlebar can cause a pancreatic contusion.
   E. Diaphragmatic injury occurs in more than 50% of seriously injured children.

11. A 3-year-old boy fell from a height of 8 feet. The *most* likely location of his injury would be his:
   A. Head.
   B. Chest.
   C. Abdomen.
   D. Pelvis.
   E. Lumbar spine.

12. Which of the following findings on physical examination would suggest a genitourinary injury?
   A. Gross blood at the rectum.
   B. Periumbilical ecchymosis.
   C. Decreased rectal tone.
   D. High-riding prostate.
   E. Priapism.

13. Which of the following laboratory tests is the most important to obtain during the initial resuscitation of a child with abdominal trauma?
   A. Type and crossmatch.
   B. Complete blood count (CBC).
   C. Platelet count.
   D. Electrolytes.
   E. Liver enzymes.

14. Which of the following abdominal radiograph findings would suggest abdominal injury?
   A. Absence of air in the stomach.
   B. Visualization of the psoas shadow.
   C. Air in the rectum.
   D. Inferiorly displaced transverse colon.
   E. Ability to visualize the kidneys.

15. Which of the following modalities is the best way to diagnose an intramural duodenal hematoma?
   A. Ultrasound.
   B. Abdominal radiograph.
   C. CT scan with oral barium.
   D. Diagnostic peritoneal lavage.
   E. Nuclear scan.

16. A 12-year-old boy comes into the ED after being hit in the lower back with a baseball bat. He is hemodynamically stable. He has an ecchymotic area over his left lower back. His abdomen is soft and not tender. The prostate examination is normal, and there is no blood at the meatus. His initial blood work reveals a hematocrit value of 45%. His urine reveals 50 red blood cells/high-power field (RBCs/HPF). Of the following, your next management decision should be to:
   A. Order a retrograde urethrogram.
   B. Discharge after 4 hours of observation.
   C. Admit to the pediatric ICU.
   D. Perform a diagnostic peritoneal lavage.
   E. Order an intravenous (IV) urogram.

17. When evaluating blunt abdominal trauma with a diagnostic peritoneal lavage, what is the RBC cutoff point between a positive and a negative result?
   A. 1,000 RBCs/mm^3.
   B. 5,000 RBCs/mm^3.
   C. 10,000 RBCs/mm^3.
   D. 50,000 RBCs/mm^3.
   E. 100,000 RBCs/mm^3.

18. Which of the following effluent findings on diagnostic peritoneal lavage would constitute a negative or indeterminate finding?
   A. Stool.
   B. Bile.
   C. 700 WBCs/mm^3.
   D. Amylase level of 100 IU/L.
   E. Alkaline phosphatase level of 10 IU/L.

19. You are caring for a 13-year-old girl who fell off a bike going at a rapid speed. She arrived alert with a pulse of 130 beats per minute and a BP of 110/80 mm Hg. Her abdomen was diffusely tender. Initial resuscitation with 20 ml/kg of crystalloid solution brought her pulse to 110 beats per minute and her BP to 130/80 mm Hg. Her chest radiograph reveals no pneumohemothorax; however, there is evidence of air under her diaphragm. Your next management decision should be to:
   A. Perform diagnostic peritoneal lavage.
   B. Transfer to the operating room.
   C. Admit to the pediatric ICU.
   D. Continue stabilization in the ED.
   E. Order a CT scan of the abdomen.

20. You are caring for a 16-year-old boy who fell off a moving motorcycle. On admission his pulse was 110 beats per minute and his BP was 110/70 mm Hg. He complains of right upper quadrant pain, and that location is tender. After 20 ml/kg of crystalloid solution, his pulse is 100 beats per minute and his BP is 120/70 mm Hg. A CT scan of the abdomen reveals a subcapsular liver hematoma. Your next management decision should be to:
   A. Transfuse with whole blood.
   B. Admit to the pediatric ICU.
   C. Transfer to the operating room.
   D. Perform a diagnostic peritoneal lavage.
   E. Order measurement of amylase and lipase concentrations.

21. Which of the following statements regarding splenic injury is correct?
    A. Nonoperative management is more successful than it is for hepatic injury.
    B. Strict bed rest for 2 to 3 days is recommended in nonoperative situations.
    C. Postsplenectomy infections are uncommon.
    D. At least 90% of the splenic mass should be salvaged to maintain its function.
    E. Vaccine for *Streptococcus pneumoniae* should be given 1 month after surgery.

22. A 7-year-old boy comes to the ED for evaluation of abdominal pain. His mother states that 4 days ago, he fell from the top bunk of a bunk bed and landed on a toy truck. Since then, he has been complaining of abdominal pain. However, today he appears much worse. He is lethargic with a thready pulse of 180 beats per minute and a BP of 70 mm Hg by palpation. His skin is cool and clammy. A portable upright chest and abdominal radiograph shows no free air under the diaphragm and a nonobstructive bowel gas pattern. His urine shows no evidence of microscopic hematuria. You suspect the injury to be a:
    A. Rebleed from a renal laceration.
    B. Traumatic pancreatitis.
    C. Rupture of a splenic hematoma.
    D. Complication of a duodenal hematoma.
    E. Liver contusion.

23. You are examining an 8-year-old boy who fell out of a window approximately 15 feet. In your initial examination, the pelvis is unstable and there is blood at the meatus. Your next step in the evaluation of possible urethral injury is:
    A. IV urogram.
    B. Foley catheter.
    C. Pelvic ultrasound.
    D. Retrograde urethrogram.
    E. An RBC count for the meatal blood.

24. The one proven indication for the use of the pneumatic antishock garment is:
    A. Immobilization of a femur fracture.
    B. Control of abdominal bleeding.
    C. Reversal of distributive shock.
    D. Immobilization of pelvic fractures.
    E. Control of bleeding from renal injury.

25. A 10-year-old boy is seen in the ED with a gunshot wound to the abdomen after a drive-by shooting. He is alert and crying. His pulse is 130 beats per minute with BP 100/70 mm Hg. On examination there is a single wound just above the umbilicus. The bullet cannot be palpated. There is no exit wound. Disposition at this time should be to the:
    A. Operating room.
    B. Pediatric ICU.
    C. Observation area of the ED.
    D. Angiography suite.
    E. Nuclear scan suite.

26. A 12-year-old girl comes into the ED after being hit by a car. She is alert and is complaining about pain in her lower abdomen. Her pulse is 160 beats per minute and thready; her BP is 80/50 mm Hg. She has equal breath sounds, and her oxygen saturation is 99%. Her pelvic radiograph reveals a pelvic fracture. An open diagnostic peritoneal lavage is performed, the results of which are negative. After the administration of 40 ml/kg of crystalloid solution, her vital signs and examination remain the same. Your next management decision should be to:
    A. Order a CT scan of the abdomen.
    B. Admit to the pediatric ICU.
    C. Obtain pelvic angiography.
    D. Transfer to the operating room.
    E. Continue stabilization in the ED.

27. Treatment of simple traumatic pancreatitis includes all of the following *except:*
    A. IV antibiotics.
    B. Bed rest.
    C. Nasogastric decompression.
    D. IV fluids.
    E. Bowel rest.

ANSWERS [See Barkin et al: Chapter 24.]

1. The answer is **B,** page 335.
   Inadequate resuscitation remains the leading cause of preventable death. Approximately 8% of children admitted to pediatric trauma centers have documented abdominal trauma. Fewer than 15% of children with major abdominal trauma need surgical intervention, with the minority secondary to blunt trauma. Head and thoracic injuries are the major causes of pediatric death; abdominal injury occurs in approximately 22% of children with fatal injuries.

2. The answer is **C,** page 335.
   Compared with adults, children have proportionally larger solid viscera, less rigid ribs and muscle fat, and a more protuberant abdomen. In small children the bladder is an intraabdominal structure, which leaves it more vulnerable to injury in abdominal trauma.

3. The answer is **C,** page 335.
   When presented with a child, status postabdominal trauma, who has a large, tender suprapubic mass, the first step in evaluation is to rule out a distended bladder causing the problem. Keep in mind that blood at the meatus and a high-riding boggy prostate are considered contraindications for catheter placement. In that situation a retrograde urethrogram would be the correct management decision.

4. The answer is **A,** page 336.
   Of all the types of shock, hemorrhagic shock is the one most likely for a child who has suffered serious abdominal trauma. In children, tachycardia may be your first, or only, evidence of a hypoperfusion state.

5. The answer is **E,** page 337.
   According to the National Pediatric Trauma Registry the frequency of injury to intraabdominal organs in blunt abdominal trauma is as follows: spleen, 30%; liver, 28%; kidneys, 28%; gastrointestinal tract, 14%; and pancreas, 3%. (Refer to Table 24-4, page 337 in Barkin et al.)

6. The answer is **D,** page 337.
   According to the National Pediatric Trauma Registry the frequency of injury to intraabdominal organs in penetrating abdominal trauma is as follows: gastrointestinal tract, 40%; liver, 27%; kidneys, 10%; spleen 9%; and pancreas 6%. (Refer to Table 24-4, page 337 in Barkin et al.)

7. The answer is **D,** pages 336 and 337.
   Examination of statistics from urban centers reveals a higher percentage of penetrating trauma when compared with the national average. Penetrating trauma carries the highest mortality rate, with the firearm the most lethal agent of injury. In fact, 75% of penetrating injuries to children older than 13 years of age involve knives or firearms. However, in children younger than 13 years of age, penetrating injury is more likely to be caused by accidental impalement on objects such as scissors or fences.

8. The answer is **C,** pages 337 and 338.
   Motor vehicle accidents can cause a specific injury pattern known as Waddell's triad, which consists of closed head injury, intraabdominal injury, and midshaft femur fracture. It is unwise to attribute hypovolemic shock to a single femur fracture. Therefore one must rule out the abdomen as a source of bleeding. Diagnostic peritoneal lavage would be the procedure of choice, since the child is not stable enough to go for a CT scan of the abdomen.

9. The answer is **B,** page 338.
   Although the most frequent site of significant blood loss in children involved in motor vehicle accidents is the abdomen, head injury by far is the most common and most lethal. Lap-belt injuries are associated with Chance-type fractures of the lumbar spine. Disruption of the diaphragm occurs, but this type of injury is rare.

10. The answer is **D,** pages 339 and 340.
    The most lethal injury caused by bicycle trauma is head injury. Abdominal injuries that are associated with bicycle trauma, including handlebar injuries, include lacerations to the kidney, spleen, and liver; pancreatic contusion; duodenal hematoma; and rupture of the intestines or common bile duct. Diaphragmatic and flexion-distraction lumbar injury can occur, but again, not close to the frequency of other major abdominal organs. Duodenal hematomas may be evidenced as bilious vomiting and abdominal pain several days following handlebar injury.

11. The answer is **A,** pages 341 and 342.
    The greater mass of the head in relation to the rest of the body usually leads to a headfirst fall. Thus falls from heights of 5 to 10 feet commonly result in head injury. However, as the height of fall increases, so does the likelihood of abdominal injury.

12. The answer is **D,** page 343.
    The presence of genitourinary injury is suggested by pelvic fractures, including the pubic bones or rami; hematuria; bloody urethral discharge; inability to void; and a boggy, high-riding prostate.

13. The answer is **A,** page 343.
    Of all the laboratory tests that are acquired in a resuscitation, none is more critical than the type and crossmatch. All other tests, including the CBC, are of limited value in the initial phase of care. The rule is that if you have enough blood for only one tube, send it for a type and crossmatch.

14. The answer is **D,** page 344.
    Abdominal radiographs are not very sensitive in predicting the extent of abdominal trauma. However, the following findings suggest abdominal injury: gastric dilatation, medially displaced lateral stomach border, inferiorly displaced transverse colon, ground-glass appearance of the abdominal cavity, blurring of the psoas shadows, associated lower rib fractures, signs of ileus, and pneumoperitoneum.

15. The answer is **C,** page 344.
    An intramural duodenal hematoma is more accurately diagnosed with a CT scan with oral barium contrast. If you suspect GI perforation, a water-soluble contrast medium should be used.

16. The answer is **E,** pages 344 and 345.
    IV urography is still indicated when isolated renal trauma is suspected. If the physician thinks there may be other solid or hollow abdominal injury (which is not suggested in the question), a CT scan of the abdomen with oral and IV contrast would be a better choice. Although the adult literature suggests that 50 or fewer RBCs/HPF is rarely associated with significant renal abnormality, pediatric studies suggest using 20 RBCs/HPF as the cutoff to ensure identification of congenital urinary tract anomalies as well. (Refer to Fig. 25-1, page 356 in Barkin et al.)

17. The answer is **E,** page 345.
    The cutoff point agreed on by most pediatricians and surgeons for a positive diagnostic peritoneal lavage is 100,000 RBCs/mm^3. Lower than 20,000 RBCs/mm^3 should be considered a negative tap. Levels between 20,000 to 100,000 RBCs/mm^3 are considered equivocal, and the test may have to be repeated sometime during the resuscitation.

18. The answer is **D,** page 345.
    Evidence of stool or bile in the effluent from a diagnostic peritoneal lavage would be considered a positive finding. The following are also considered indirect evidence of bowel injury: white blood cell count greater than 500/mm^3, amylase concentration greater than 175 IU/L, or an alkaline phosphatase level of greater than 6 IU/L.

19. The answer is **B,** page 346.
    Indications for emergency operation include radiographic evidence of pneumoperitoneum. No other diagnostic tests are needed to confirm this management decision.

20. The answer is **B,** page 347.

    With the patient's stable vital signs, nonoperative management is usually safe and would be indicated for subcapsular liver hematomas. Children with liver injuries who are not in hypovolemic shock rarely require surgical intervention.

21. The answer is **A,** page 348.

    Nonoperative management of splenic injuries is more successful than it is for liver injuries because there is a better likelihood of spontaneous cessation of bleeding. In nonoperative situations, strict bed rest should be prescribed for 7 to 10 days. The incidence of postsplenectomy infections is considerable. Approximately 50% of the splenic mass must be salvaged to continue to perform its function. When splenectomy, partial or complete, is anticipated or performed, *S. pneumoniae* vaccine should be administered as soon as possible.

22. The answer is **C,** page 348.

    Splenic lacerations that have ceased active bleeding can leak or rupture, usually between the third to fifth day after the initial incident. Duodenal hematomas, which can also develop days from the incident, may cause both intestinal obstruction (not evident with this patient) and traumatic pancreatitis (if the Vater's ampulla is involved). Rebleeding from a renal laceration would be unlikely without macroscopic or microscopic hematuria.

23. The answer is **D,** page 349.

    When a urethral injury is considered, the diagnostic test of choice is a retrograde urethrogram. If, on the other hand, a ureter or bladder injury is suspected, an excretory urogram should be ordered. A Foley catheter should not be placed when the physical examination suggests possible urethral injury without first ruling out such injury through diagnostic testing.

24. The answer is **D,** page 350.

    The only proven beneficial use of the pneumatic antishock garment (PASG) or the military (medical) antishock trousers (MAST) is for the stabilization and immobilization of pelvic fractures. Stabilization of the pelvis in most situations leads to improved hemorrhage control.

25. The answer is **A,** page 350.

    All gunshot wounds to the abdomen that on examination are thought to have invaded the peritoneum (approximately 85% of all gunshot wounds) should be evaluated surgically in the operating room.

26. The answer is **C,** page 350.

    When an uncontrolled retroperitoneal bleed secondary to a pelvic fracture is suspected, selective pelvic angiography would be the correct management decision. An abdominal source of bleeding should be ruled out through diagnostic peritoneal lavage, which in this situation should be performed open because of the presence of pelvic injury. Peritoneal lavage should be performed above the umbilicus in the presence of a suspected pelvic fracture. This is suggested to avoid false positive results.

27. The answer is **A,** pages 348 and 349.

    IV antibiotics are not indicated, nor are they beneficial, in situations of simple traumatic pancreatitis.

22

Genitourinary Trauma

Ruby F. Rivera • *Ndidi Nwokorie*

See Barkin et al: Chapter 25.

---

1. A 14-year-old boy is hit on the right flank while playing football. His vital signs are stable. Abdominal computed tomography (CT) and intravenous pyelography (IVP) show laceration of the left kidney extending into the perirenal fat but not the collecting systems. The grade of this renal injury is:
   A. Grade I.
   B. Grade II.
   C. Grade III
   D. Grade IV.
   E. Grade V.

2. Management of the renal injury in question 1 should include:
   A. Observation.
   B. Exploration only.
   C. Exploration and nephrectomy.
   D. Antibiotic prophylaxis.
   E. Angiography.

3. A 4-year-old boy pedestrian crossing a street is hit by a car. He is awake, alert, and the vital signs are stable. Physical examination reveals abdominal distension and tenderness and right flank tenderness. A rectal examination reveals stool that is guaiac positive. Urinalysis shows 40 red blood cells/high-power field (RBCs/HPF). The diagnostic test of choice is:
   A. Ultrasound.
   B. IVP.
   C. CT scan of the abdomen.
   D. Angiography.
   E. Radionuclide scan.

4. A 15-year-old boy is brought to the ED by Emergency Medical Service (EMS) after sustaining a stab wound on the left abdomen during an altercation. His vital signs remain unstable despite efforts at stabilization. Physical examination reveals abdominal distension and tenderness. His stool is guaiac positive, and urinalysis shows 50 RBCs/HPF. Before exploratory laparotomy is performed, a rapid informative study that may be done in the ED or operating room to delineate renal injury would be:
   A. CT scan of the abdomen.
   B. Angiography.
   C. Limited IVP.
   D. Ultrasound.
   E. Radionuclide scan.

5. A 5-year-old girl is seen in the ED after she fell off monkey bars. Her vital signs are stable. All of the following findings are reasons for genitourinary (GU) radiologic evaluation except:
   A. Pelvic fracture.
   B. Presence of flank ecchymosis (Grey Turner's sign).
   C. Gross hematuria.
   D. Presence of periumbilical ecchymosis (Cullen's sign).
   E. Urinalysis with 15 RBCs/HPF.

6. An 8-year-old girl is struck by a truck while on her bicycle. Her vital signs are stable. Physical examination reveals diffuse abdominal tenderness and guarding and lower rib pain on the left side. A chest x-ray and plain film of the abdomen are completed. Which of the following findings on x-ray may indicate an underlying renal injury?
   A. Clearly seen psoas shadows.
   B. Large bowel distension.
   C. Spinal transverse process fractures.
   D. Abnormal spine curvature (convex to side of injury).

7. A 17-year-old adolescent sustains a laceration on his penis while jumping over a spiked fence. Physical examination reveals a 2-cm-deep laceration on the inferior aspect of the penile shaft, penile swelling, and ecchymosis. The patient is unable to void when asked for a urine specimen. Before the laceration is repaired, which of the following radiologic evaluations should be completed?
   A. Insertion of Foley catheter.
   B. Urethrogram.
   C. IVP.

8. A 6-year-old girl sustains a straddle injury from the bar of her brother's bicycle. She has voided since the accident without signs of hematuria. Physical examination reveals a large vulvar hematoma. Management of this patient includes *all* of the following *except:*
   A. Incision and evacuation of the clot.
   B. Antibiotic prophylaxis.
   C. Sitz baths followed by ice packs.
   D. Pelvic x-ray.
   E. Cystourethrogram.

9. A 10-year-old boy who is a victim of a drive-by shooting sustains a gunshot wound to the left upper abdomen. CT scan of the abdomen shows extravasation of contrast with no evidence of injury to the renal parenchyma and no further opacification of the ureter distal to the level of the injury. Which of the following statements is true?
   A. Symptoms of ureteral injury are generally absent immediately after the injury.
   B. Hematuria is a reliable sign.
   C. CT scan is the diagnostic test of choice.
   D. Blunt trauma is the most common external mechanism resulting in ureteral injury.
   E. ED management of ureteral injury includes placement of a suprapubic catheter.

10. A 6-year-old girl is the restrained front seat passenger involved in a motor vehicle accident. On examination there are signs of pelvic instability, and she refuses to void. After initial stabilization the most important diagnostic study is:
    A. A plain film of the abdomen.
    B. A radionuclide scan.
    C. An IVP followed by a urethrogram.
    D. A cystourethrogram followed by an IVP.
    E. A contrast CT scan.

11. A 3-year-old boy fell 25 feet while climbing a tree. He shows signs of pelvic instability. After stabilization you obtain the study in Fig. 22-1. The most appropriate management for this injury is:
    A. Observation alone.
    B. Surgical repair with assurance of adequate vesical drainage.
    C. Suprapubic drainage alone for 7 to 14 days.
    D. Drainage with Foley catheter for 7 to 14 days.
    E. Suprapubic drainage followed by surgical repair at a later date.

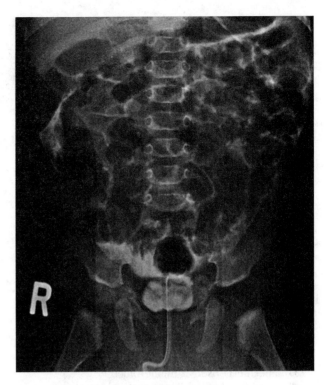

FIG. 22-1

12. A 5-year-old girl was struck by a car as she was crossing the street. She sustained multiple injuries, including a pelvic fracture. She is most likely to have associated GU injuries if she fractured which section of her pelvis?
    A. The iliac wing.
    B. The anterior arch.
    C. The pelvic ring, forming a stable fracture.
    D. The posterior arch.
    E. The acetabulum.

13. A 10-year-old boy is the unrestrained passenger in a high-speed motor vehicle accident. All of the following are *contraindications* for a Foley catheter *except:*
    A. Ecchymosis of the penis.
    B. A high-riding prostate.
    C. Blood at the urethral meatus.
    D. Gross hematuria.
    E. Ecchymosis of the scrotum.

14. A 17-year-old boy is involved in a motorcycle accident. He is brought to your ED with complaints of scrotal pain and nausea. On examination you find an empty right hemiscrotum. Which of the following best describes this patient's injury?
    A. He has sustained a right testicular torsion.
    B. He has a right testicular rupture.
    C. He sustained a right testicular dislocation.
    D. He is intermittently experiencing testicular torsion of the right testes.

15. The most likely management for the patient described in question 14 is:
    A. Surgical reduction and bilateral orchiopexy.
    B. Orchiectomy and contralateral orchiopexy.
    C. Excision of the necrotic seminiferous tubules and repair of the torn tunica albuginea.
    D. Surgical evaluation and anatomic replacement of the testis if closed reduction is unsuccessful.
    E. Close follow-up of patient until there is complete resolution of symptoms.

16. A 15-year-old boy sustained a straddle injury and now complains of severe groin pain. On examination his scrotum is extremely swollen, red, and tender. The most appropriate immediate management includes:
    A. Pelvic radiograph.
    B. Ultrasound evaluation of the scrotum.
    C. Radionuclide scan of the testis.
    D. Retrograde urethrogram.
    E. Immediate surgical exploration.

17. An 8-year-old boy falls off the diving board and strikes his groin against the edge of the board. All of the following statements regarding this injury are true *except*:
    A. Penile lacerations may be sutured after adequate anesthesia using a penile block.
    B. Associated bladder and urethral injuries are common.
    C. In the presence of marked penile swelling and ecchymosis, a urethrogram is indicated.
    D. Soft tissue injuries of the perineum commonly involve the penis, requiring surgical debridement and often skin grafting.

18. A 7-year-old boy sustains a straddle injury while playing on monkey bars. He refuses to void in the ED. On examination there is blood on the urethral meatus. The most appropriate study to obtain is:
    A. Voiding cystourethrogram.
    B. Retrograde urethrogram.
    C. IVP followed by a cystourethrogram.
    D. CT scan with contrast.
    E. Urinalysis.

19. A 5-year-old boy slipped and fell on his back while walking on an icy sidewalk. Physical examination reveals mild tenderness over the right flank; no ecchymosis or redness is noted. The spine is not tender and has full range of motion. Urinalysis shows 15 RBCs/HPF. Which of the following would be appropriate in management of this patient?
    A. CT scan of the abdomen.
    B. Ultrasound.
    C. Admittance for observation.
    D. Observation in the ED for 4 hours.
    E. IVP.

ANSWERS   [See Barkin et al: Chapter 25.]

1. The answer is **C,** pages 355 to 357.
   Renal injuries are classified as follows (Fig. 22-2 on page 109): grade I—small, subcapsular, and nonexpanding contusions or hematomas that may be associated with hematuria; grade II—hematomas confined to the retroperitoneum and lacerations less than 1 cm deep that do not result in urinary extravasation; grade III—lacerations into the perirenal fat greater than 1 cm deep, but not penetrating the collecting system and having no urinary extravasation; grade IV—deep lacerations into the collecting system, and renal vascular injury with contained hemorrhage; grade V—shattered or fractured kidney and renal pedicle injuries.

2. The answer is **A,** page 360.
   Management of grades I, II, and III renal injuries is conservative without operative intervention. Generally, all of these patients do well and do not have long-term complications. Immediate surgery is indicated for hemodynamic instability, renal pedicle injury, and expanding retroperitoneal or pulsatile hematoma; surgery may be indicated for laceration of the kidney with extensive extravasation.

3. The answer is **C,** page 358.
   CT scan of the abdomen is the diagnostic test of choice in the detection of renal injury in the stable pediatric trauma patient who may have multiple injuries. It is highly accurate and can delineate intraabdominal, retroperitoneal, and pelvic injuries simultaneously. If renal injury alone is suspected, IVP would be adequate.

4. The answer is **C,** pages 358 and 359.
   For situations in which the patient must be taken to the operating room for other injuries, a limited IVP may be helpful in demonstrating the presence of two functioning kidneys. The procedure may be performed in the ED or operating room, depending on the stability of the patient.

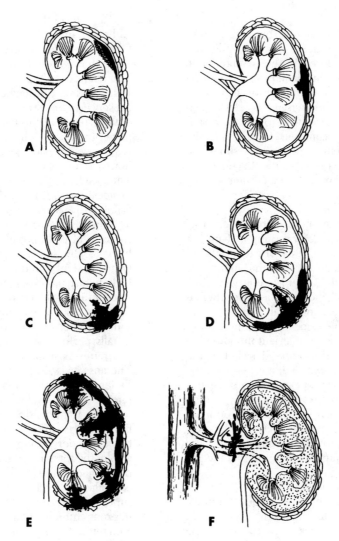

FIG. 22-2 Grading of renal injury.

5. The answer is **E,** pages 357 and 358.

Radiographic evaluation of the kidney should be undertaken when the following factors are present: hematuria of less than 20 RBCs/HPF; microscopic hematuria with shock; gross hematuria, penetrating trauma to the abdomen, physical findings consistent with renal trauma; *and a significant mechanism that warrants GU tract evaluation.* Signs and symptoms of renal trauma may be specific or subtle. Flank pain, tenderness, hematoma (Grey Turner's sign), or periumbilical ecchymosis (Cullen's sign) may indicate urologic trauma or retroperitoneal hemorrhage. Pelvic fractures are often associated with GU injury.

6. The answer is **C,** page 359.

Lower rib fractures can be associated with GU injury. Abdominal flat plate or scout radiographs should be made before contrast studies of the GU tract. Findings such as loss of psoas shadows (retroperitoneal blood), abnormal spinal curvature (concave to the side of injury), and lower rib or transverse process fractures may be clues to underlying renal injury.

7. The answer is **B,** page 365.

Patients with penile lacerations may have injured the urethra. If marked penile swelling, ecchymosis, or meatal blood is present or the patient is unable to void, a urethrogram is indicated, as is a urologic consult.

8. The answer is **E**, page 366.
   Straddle injuries from the bar of a bicycle or other object that strikes the perineal area generally are minor. Occasionally, the force is severe enough to cause a vulvar hematoma. Small hematomas can be managed by ice packs alone. Large or expanding vulvar hematomas should be incised, the clot evacuated, and the area packed loosely. Prophylactic broad-spectrum antibiotics are recommended as well as sitz baths followed by ice packs. A pelvic x-ray should be obtained to look for fractures. If a patient is unable to void, a urethrogram followed by a cystogram may be warranted.

9. The answer is **A**, page 360.
   Penetrating trauma is the most common external mechanism resulting in ureteral injury. Gunshot wounds are the primary agent in more than 90% of cases. Signs and symptoms of ureteral injury are generally absent immediately after the injury. As time passes, nonspecific complaints such as fever, hematuria, ileus, or flank or abdominal pain develop. Hematuria is an unreliable sign; it occurs in at most two thirds of patients but may be absent in more than 40% of patients with ureteral injury. The IVP is the diagnostic test of choice. However, if it is negative, the clinician must consider surgical exploration if there is a high index of suspicion of ureteral injury. Evaluation of the integrity of the ureter by CT scan is difficult; surgical exploration of the ureter may be the only reliable way to detect injury. ED management of the patient with ureteral injury focuses on therapy for associated life-threatening injury.

10. The answer is **D**, pages 361 to 363.
    Blunt trauma is the cause of most bladder injuries. While 80% of bladder injuries with rupture are associated with pelvic fractures, only 19% of pelvic fractures are associated with bladder injury. Thus in a patient with possible pelvic fracture, it is important to obtain a cystogram to assess the integrity of the bladder. This should be followed by an IVP to assess the kidneys and ureter. Urethral injury is unlikely in females.

11. The answer is **B**, page 363.
    Fig. 22-1 on page 107 shows intraperitoneal bladder rupture with extravasation of contrast into the peritoneal cavity and under the liver. Patients with this type of bladder rupture are managed surgically; the bladder is repaired, and adequate vesical drainage ensured. Patients with bladder contusions are allowed to void spontaneously and are closely monitored by a urologist. Others with contusions and associated injuries, or those with small extraperitoneal ruptures, can be managed by urethral or suprapubic drainage for 7 to 14 days. Those with large extraperitoneal rupture with extravasation may require surgical debridement of bone spicule from a pelvic fracture and repair of the bladder laceration.

12. The answer is **B**, page 367.
    Although any pelvic fracture may be associated with GU tract injury, most significant GU injuries are associated with anterior arch fractures of the pelvis.

13. The answer is **D**, page 364.
    Foley catheter placement is contraindicated in the presence of urethral injury. Signs of urethral injury include blood at the meatus, ecchymosis of the penis or scrotum, or a high-riding prostate. Gross hematuria is not a contraindication because it may occur with injury to any part of the GU tract.

14. The answer is **C**, page 365.
    Dislocation of the testis occurs when a testicle is forcibly displaced from its anatomic position, usually as a result of a high-speed motorcycle accident or, in the case of children, as a result of a forcible upward blow to the scrotum, such as in straddle injuries. Other testicular injuries that may result from trauma include testicular torsion or rupture. In both cases the scrotum is markedly swollen, erythematous, and tender. The testis is palpated within the scrotum. Ultrasound of the scrotum followed by a testicular scan is usually performed to evaluate the testis when torsion or rupture is suspected.

15. The answer is **D**, page 365.
    Patients with dislocation of the testis undergo surgical intervention to evaluate the integrity of the testis and to place it into normal anatomic position if closed reduction is unsuccessful. Patients with testicular torsion undergo surgical exploration. If the testis is viable, the torsion is reduced, and bilateral orchiopexy performed. If the testicle is necrotic, orchiectomy and contralateral orchiopexy are performed. Testicular rupture is repaired by excision of the necrotic seminiferous tubules and suturing of the torn tunica albuginea. Orchiectomy may be necessary in 6% to 30% of patients with testicular rupture.

16. The answer is **B**, page 365.
    Patients with significant blunt trauma to the testis first require evaluation by ultrasound, followed by radionuclide imaging. A number of case reports have shown ultrasonography to be accurate in distinguishing between hematoceles and abscesses from testicular rupture.

17. The answer is **D**, page 365.
    Complications arising from circumcision are the most common cause of injury to the penis. Other causes include falls, sports injuries, direct blows to the perineum, zipper entrapment of the foreskin, and tourniquet injuries. The large majority of penile injuries are minor abrasions and can be managed expectantly.

18. The answer is **B,** page 364.

Blood at the meatus is an indication of possible urethral injury, which must be excluded before passage of a Foley catheter through the urethra. Passage of a catheter through an injured urethra may convert a partial tear into a complete tear. Retrograde urethrogram is the radiologic method of choice for diagnosis of urethral injury in the pediatric trauma patient. Extravasation indicates a partial tear if contrast medium is seen in the bladder and a complete tear if no medium is seen in the bladder.

19. The answer is **D,** page 360.

Patients with minor amounts of hematuria and minor mechanism of injury may be sent home after a period of observation. All patients should be reevaluated within 24 hours if they have any degree of hematuria or did not undergo a diagnostic evaluation for hematuria during the ED visit. If the hematuria persists, IVP should be performed to look for structural or functional abnormalities.

Foreign Bodies of the Gastrointestinal Tract and Airway

Shari L. Platt • Lucia J. Santiago

See Barkin et al: Chapter 26.

1. A 2-year-old boy is seen in the pediatric ED for evaluation of a choking episode after being found playing with his mother's sewing box. He is alert and playful. Vital signs are stable. Which of the following statements concerning the chest radiograph in Fig. 23-1 on page 113 is *true?*
   A. A button is in the esophagus.
   B. A button is in the trachea.
   C. A button is on the child's shirt.
   D. The exact location of the button cannot be determined.
   E. A barium swallow must be performed.

2. A lateral chest radiograph (Fig. 23-2 on page 114) in the same patient described in question 1 shows which of the following?
   A. A button in the esophagus.
   B. A button in the trachea.
   C. A button on the child's shirt.
   D. A button at the cricopharyngeus.
   E. A button in the stomach.

3. The child remains stable and asymptomatic. The next step in the management of the child described in question 1 is:
   A. Perform the Heimlich procedure.
   B. Discharge to home and instruct parents to check the stool for the button.
   C. Administer glucagon and repeat the x-ray in 6 hours.
   D. Observe the patient and repeat the x-ray in 6 hours.
   E. Remove the button in the operating room (OR) via endoscopy.

4. You choose to admit the child and repeat the x-ray in 12 hours. The child remains stable. The x-ray at this time is shown in Fig. 23-3 on page 114. Your management at this time is:
   A. Discharge to home, since the child remains stable.
   B. Administer glucagon and repeat the x-ray in 6 hours.
   C. Remove the button via esophageal bougienage.
   D. Remove the button in the OR via balloon catheter.
   E. Remove the button in the OR via endoscopy.

5. A 3-year-old female comes to the pediatric ED with acute onset of stridor. She had been eating cereal. She has no medical problems, and her immunizations are up to date. She has no pertinent history of choking or gagging. A foreign body in the esophagus should be suspected because:
   A. She is immunized for *Haemophilus influenzae* type B, so epiglottitis is unlikely.
   B. Less than 50% of these patients have a history of a witnessed event.
   C. Foreign body ingestion is more common in females than in males.
   D. Food impaction is a common cause of esophageal obstruction in children.
   E. Esophageal foreign body is unlikely; it rarely causes airway-related symptoms.

6. The diagnosis of foreign body aspiration in toddlers is often missed because:
   A. It requires a high index of suspicion, often despite a negative history.
   B. It is always asymptomatic in children.
   C. It is more common in the older child.
   D. Food tends to be radiolucent on x-ray.
   E. Respiratory illnesses are more commonly seen in this age group.

7. A 3-year-old girl has swallowed a nickel while playing with her sister. The most likely location of impaction is at the level of the:
   A. Cricopharyngeus.
   B. Aortic arch.
   C. Gastroesophageal junction.
   D. Stomach.
   E. Pylorus.

8. A 2½-year-old boy comes to the pediatric ED in mild respiratory distress with wheezing and tachypnea. He choked on a peanut a week ago but has been asymptomatic until today. A chest x-ray reveals mild atelectasis on the right. The next best step in management is:
   A. Observation and antibiotic therapy.
   B. Observation and bronchodilator therapy.
   C. Lateral decubitus x-rays.
   D. Bronchoscopy in the OR.

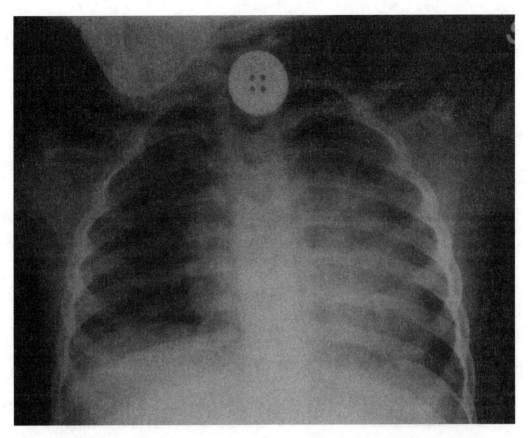

FIG. 23-1   Radiograph of a 3-year-old boy obtained for evaluation of a choking episode.

9. A 3½-year-old girl comes to the pediatric ED with a complaint of sore throat and refusal to swallow. She is drooling. She can speak but is in mild respiratory distress. Her mother suspects that she swallowed a plastic toy airplane. Chest x-ray is normal. The next best step in management is:
   A. Barium swallow.
   B. Direct visualization by endoscopy in the OR.
   C. Xeroradiography.
   D. Computed tomographic (CT) scan.
   E. Balloon catheter removal procedure.

10. Which statement best applies to foreign body ingestion in children?
    A. The incidence is more common in boys than in girls.
    B. Children have obvious symptoms of gastrointestinal (GI) obstruction.
    C. Objects in the esophagus rarely pass spontaneously into the stomach.
    D. Coins are the most common type of foreign body in children.
    E. Esophageal perforation is a common complication.

11. In the hands of a skilled technician, balloon catheter removal of an esophageal foreign body is safe and efficacious for:
    A. Removal of a "jack" at the cricopharyngeus.
    B. Removal of a coin at the aortic knob.
    C. Removal of multiple coins in the esophagus.
    D. Removal of a coin lodged for 3 days.
    E. Removal of a coin in an uncooperative 6-year-old.

12. A 2-year-old boy comes to the pediatric ED after swallowing a silver dollar. He is happy and asymptomatic. A chest x-ray is normal, and the coin is seen in the stomach. The mother is hysterical and insists on immediate removal of the coin. You tell her:
    A. That you agree, and call for the endoscopist.
    B. That you recommend admission.
    C. That you recommend observation.
    D. That you recommend taking a laxative.
    E. To check the stool and return if the coin is not retrieved in 72 hours.

13. The child in question 12 returns to the pediatric ED 1 week later. He now has bilious vomiting, abdominal distension, and pain. You are concerned about:
    A. Obstruction at the splenic flexure.
    B. Obstruction at the ileocecal junction.
    C. Perforation in the ascending colon.
    D. Lead intoxication from absorption of the coin in the GI tract.
    E. Perforation in the descending colon.

14. Regarding complications of esophageal foreign bodies, all of the following are true *except:*
    A. Less than 1% result in perforation.
    B. Complications usually occur more than 24 hours after impaction.
    C. Complications include retropharyngeal abscess and mediastinitis.
    D. Patients suffering from complications may have cardiorespiratory compromise.
    E. Children with esophageal perforation caused by foreign body ingestion may be asymptomatic.

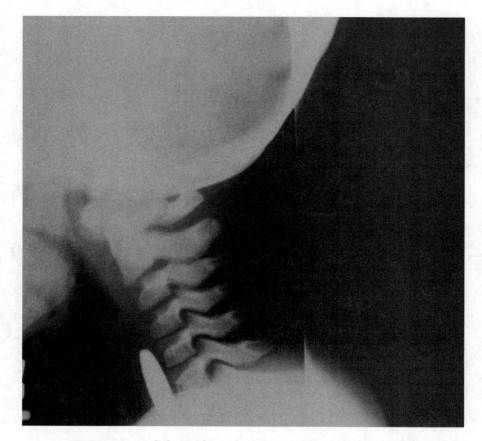

FIG. 23-2   Lateral chest radiograph of the same patient as in Fig. 23-1.

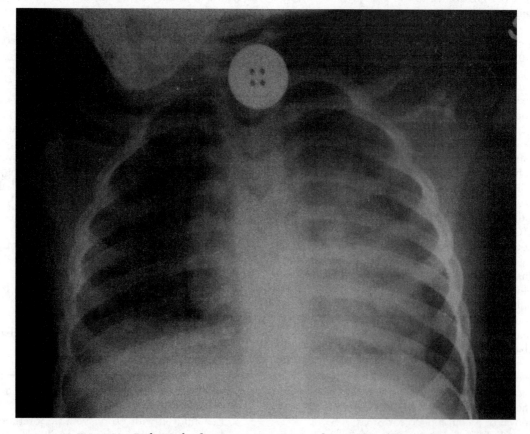

FIG. 23-3   Radiograph of patient in Figs. 23-1 and 23-2 taken 12 hours later.

15. An 18-month-old infant ingests a hearing aid battery. A chest radiograph reveals the battery in the upper third of the esophagus. Appropriate management would include:
    A. Follow-up radiograph in 12 hours.
    B. Magnet tube removal technique.
    C. Esophageal bougienage.
    D. Rigid endoscopy under general anesthetic.
    E. Discharge with follow-up in 24 hours.

16. An asymptomatic 2-year-old girl ingested a camera battery. A radiograph reveals the battery to be in the stomach. Appropriate management would include:
    A. Daily abdominal radiograph to demonstrate progression.
    B. Flexible endoscopy.
    C. Rigid endoscopy.
    D. Administration of cathartics and metoclopramide.
    E. Administration of ipecac syrup.

17. A 2-year-old boy ingested a lithium camera battery. On the battery's removal from the esophagus via endoscopy, the mucosa was noted to be focally burned and damaged. Appropriate management would include:
    A. Administration of steroids.
    B. Close observation to rule out perforation.
    C. Nonionic radiopaque contrast study (i.e., Gastrografin).
    D. Barium swallow.
    E. Administration of antibiotics.

18. All of the following are complications of having ingested a button battery *except:*
    A. Tracheoesophageal fistula.
    B. Erosion into the aorta.
    C. Heavy metal poisoning.
    D. Death.
    E. Obstruction at the pylorus.

19. A 20-month-old boy is playing with his marbles while waiting in the ED. Suddenly he chokes, turns blue and limp, and is noted to be bradycardic. The most appropriate initial management is:
    A. Cycles of five back blows and five chest thrusts.
    B. Repeated subdiaphragmatic abdominal thrusts.
    C. Blind finger sweep.
    D. Endotracheal intubation.
    E. Oxygen.

20. After unsuccessful attempts at endotracheal intubation of the patient in question 19, he is noted to be apneic and pulseless. The most appropriate next step in management is:
    A. Nasotracheal intubation.
    B. Nasopharyngeal airway.
    C. Surgical cricothyrotomy.
    D. Needle cricothyrotomy.
    E. Tracheotomy.

21. An 8-month-old boy is brought to the pediatric ED with coughing and gagging. He has stridor and is cyanotic and unable to cry. Before he began coughing, his 5-year-old sister had been playing with him. The most correct initial management is:
    A. Cycles of five back blows and five chest thrusts.
    B. Repeated subdiaphragmatic abdominal thrusts.
    C. Blind finger sweep.
    D. Endotracheal intubation.
    E. Oxygen.

22. Resuscitative maneuvers for the patient described in question 21 fail to produce foreign body expulsion. Upon direct laryngoscopy there is visualization of a plastic cap in the hypopharynx. The most appropriate next step in management is:
    A. Back blows and chest thrusts.
    B. Subdiaphragmatic abdominal thrusts.
    C. Removal with finger sweep.
    D. Endotracheal intubation.
    E. Removal with Magill forceps.

23. Which of the following regarding aspiration of foreign body into the tracheobronchial tree is true?
    A. It occurs equally in males and females.
    B. It occurs mostly in children less than 1 year of age.
    C. Less than 50% of children with foreign body aspiration have a suggestive history.
    D. Ninety percent of airway foreign bodies lodge in the mainstem bronchi.
    E. Fifty percent of airway foreign bodies are radiopaque.

24. Characteristics of foreign body aspiration into the tracheobronchial tree include which of the following?
    A. Nonorganic materials are the most commonly aspirated foreign body.
    B. Slightly more than half of all bronchial foreign bodies are found on the left side.
    C. Children with incomplete dentition are at greater risk for aspiration of solid foods.
    D. Tracheal or laryngeal foreign bodies are associated with a lower morbidity and mortality.
    E. In most cases patients have coughing, wheezing, and a decrease in or absence of breath sounds.

25. A 2-year-old child aspirated a piece of hot dog. Which of the following statements regarding patients with foreign body aspiration is true?
    A. Radiologic studies are diagnostic.
    B. Physical findings include stridor and retractions.
    C. In more than half of children with foreign body aspiration the condition is diagnosed in the first 24 hours.
    D. More than half of children with foreign body aspiration have the triad of coughing, wheezing, and decrease in or absence of breath sounds.
    E. More than half of all children may be asymptomatic when they come to the ED.

26. A 2-year-old girl was eating snack foods when she suddenly began coughing and gagging. In the pediatric ED she is crying and wants to drink from her bottle. Appropriate *initial* radiologic studies for the evaluation of foreign body aspiration include all of the following *except:*
    A. Posteroanterior (PA) and lateral views of the chest and neck.
    B. CT scan of the chest.
    C. Lateral decubitus views.
    D. Assisted expiratory film.
27. Which of the following radiologic findings is *not* compatible with foreign body aspiration?
    A. Normal (PA) chest radiograph.
    B. Unilateral atelectasis.
    C. Unilateral hyperinflation.
    D. Increased anteroposterior (AP) diameter.
    E. Pulmonary infiltrates.

28. Removal of a bronchial foreign body is best accomplished by:
    A. Rigid bronchoscopy.
    B. Balloon catheter technique.
    C. Flexible fiberoptic bronchoscopy.
    D. Open thoracotomy.
    E. Chest percussion and postural drainage.
29. Which of the following statements regarding aspiration hazards is incorrect?
    A. Food and objects with rounded edges pose an increased threat.
    B. Balloons are responsible for the majority of toy-related choking deaths.
    C. Children who lack back molars are at the greatest risk for solid food aspiration.
    D. The Consumer Product Safety Commission requires that toys with small parts carry a specific choking-hazard warning for children under 5 years of age.
    E. Three fourths of deaths from foreign body aspiration occur in the first 3 years of life.

ANSWERS [See Barkin et al: Chapter 26.]

1. The answer is **D,** pages 372 and 373.
   AP and lateral soft tissue neck or chest films are diagnostic in the case of radiopaque esophageal foreign bodies. Radiographs in two planes are always required to confirm the location of a foreign body.
2. The answer is **A,** page 372.
   Flat circular objects, such as coins or buttons, in the esophagus tend to lodge in the coronal plane on AP or PA radiographs, whereas those in the trachea are oriented in the sagittal plane. Since the object is radiopaque and easily visualized on plain films, further radiologic studies, such as a barium swallow or CT scan, are not necessary.
3. The answer is **D,** pages 372 to 374.
   Smooth-edged round esophageal foreign bodies spontaneously pass into the stomach in 16% to 76% of patients during observation. There is a very low incidence of complications associated with impaction in the esophagus in the first 12 hours. It is both safe and cost effective to observe asymptomatic children before attempting removal in this setting. Glucagon has been used to promote passage of food boluses lodged in the distal esophagus into the stomach in adults. It is rarely applicable to the pediatric patient. The Heimlich procedure is reserved for airway obstruction. Discharge to home is not indicated for any esophageal foreign body.

4. The answer is **E,** pages 373 and 374.
   All retained esophageal foreign bodies must be removed, particularly those in the upper third of the esophagus, because of the risk for aspiration and perforation. Endoscopy is the procedure of choice for removal of esophageal foreign bodies, since it enables direct visualization of mucosal injury, as well as safe removal of the foreign body. Esophageal bougienage is a risky procedure and not recommended. Balloon catheter removal is performed in an outpatient setting with its advantage being the avoidance of general anesthesia.
5. The answer is **B,** pages 371 and 372.
   Unfortunately, diagnosis of foreign body ingestion is often difficult, since less than half of these patients have a history of a witnessed event. Because the posterior wall of the trachea is compressible, acute symptoms may be of airway compromise, such as gagging, choking, coughing, or stridor. These airway-related symptoms should not eliminate the possibility of a retained foreign body in the esophagus. Foreign body ingestion is seen in females and males equally. Food impaction is rarely seen in young children, except in those who have undergone an esophageal surgical procedure.
6. The answer is **A,** pages 371 and 372.
   Foreign body ingestion must be considered in children who have any GI or respiratory complaints. The majority of ingestions occur in young children, ages 6 months to 6 years. A history of a specific event is seen in only half of these children. Children may be asymptomatic, but symptoms referred either to the GI tract or to the airway are often seen.

7. The answer is **A,** page 372.

   Objects tend to lodge in the esophagus at one of three anatomic sites of narrowing: the cricopharyngeus muscle, the level of the aortic arch, and the gastroesophageal junction. The majority of impacted foreign bodies are found at the level of the cricopharyngeus.

8. The answer is **D,** pages 376, 378, and 379.

   In the face of a strong history and clinical examination suggestive of aspiration, observation, further radiologic evaluation, and medical management are unnecessary. Airway foreign body removal is best achieved by rigid bronchoscopy under general anesthesia. Peanuts are the most common offending agent. Rapid diagnosis and retrieval are essential, since peanut oil may cause an inflammatory reaction and dislodgment of the peanut may result in further obstruction with rapid clinical deterioration. Flexible fiberoptic bronchoscopy is useful when the diagnosis is in question. However, its use for removal of the object is discouraged.

9. The answer is **B,** page 372.

   Nonradiopaque objects may be diagnosed by xeroradiography, CT scan, or contrast studies when history or examination is suggestive of a retained esophageal foreign body. Endoscopy is preferable when plain films are nondiagnostic, allowing for examination of multiple foreign bodies, evaluation of esophageal damage, and definitive therapy. Balloon catheter removal is not indicated for nonradiopaque, sharp-edged objects.

10. The answer is **D,** pages 371 and 375.

    Coins are the most common nonfood ingestant. Small toy parts, buttons, pins, and batteries are also commonly described. The incidence of GI foreign bodies is equal in males and females. Children often are asymptomatic with intestinal foreign bodies. Smooth esophageal foreign bodies often pass spontaneously into the stomach. Perforation is rare.

11. The answer is **B,** page 374.

    Balloon catheter removal of an esophageal foreign body is safe and efficacious for an object that is:
    • A single piece
    • Smooth
    • Radiopaque
    • Located in the esophagus
    • Lodged for less than 72 hours
    • Causing incomplete obstruction
    For a child who:
    • Is cooperative and unsedated
    • Has no signs or symptoms of airway compromise
    • Has no history of prior esophageal disease or surgery
    • Is being treated by a skilled and experienced technician

12. The answer is **C,** page 375.

    Regarding intestinal foreign bodies, it is estimated that 80% to 90% will pass uneventfully through the GI tract. The incidence of perforation is less than 1%. A conservative approach of outpatient observation is appropriate for most asymptomatic children. Cathartics and stool softeners have no proven benefit. If the foreign body is not identified in the stool, repeat radiographs at 2 weeks may be obtained. Parents should be advised to return for symptoms or signs of obstruction or perforation such as abdominal pain, vomiting, fever, or bloody stool.

13. The answer is **B,** page 375.

    Complications of foreign body in the intestinal tract are rare. They include perforation, obstruction, and GI hemorrhage, the latter two being rare in children. The most common sites for perforation are sites of anatomic narrowing, including the pylorus, duodenum, duodenojejunal flexure, ileocecal valve, or appendix. The ileocecal valve is the most frequent site. Long, pointed, slender objects such as sewing needles or bones have a greater risk of perforation, while large blunt objects may become impacted and cause mucosal ulceration.

14. The answer is **E,** page 372.

    Major complications usually occur more than 24 hours after impaction. The nature of such complications depends on the site of esophageal perforation. Complications are not asymptomatic.

15. The answer is **D,** page 375.

    Observation and discharge are not options with button batteries in the esophagus. Immediate removal of a button battery retained in the esophagus is required, since esophageal burns as early as 4 hours after ingestion have been documented. Removal is best done endoscopically with direct visualization. Blind removal with a tube or catheter is not recommended, since it has a greater potential for iatrogenic perforation and precludes assessment of mucosal damage.

16. The answer is **A,** pages 375 and 376.

    There is little risk of complications from button batteries once they have passed into the stomach. In a large series, more than 95% passed through the GI tract spontaneously, with a transit time of less than 96 hours in most cases; most patients remained asymptomatic. High failure rate of attempts at retrieval from the stomach or beyond, anesthetic risk, and lack of significant injury from the battery ingestion militate against removal once the battery is past the esophagus. Daily radiographs are recommended to demonstrate progression from the stomach. If a battery remains in the stomach for several days, it may become embedded in the gastric wall. Therefore it is advisable to remove it if no progress is made after 3 to 7 days. Removal is also indicated if signs of peritonitis develop. Once past the pylorus, the majority of batteries pass through the GI tract without problems. Ipecac is contraindicated; it is ineffective in expelling batteries from the stomach and duodenum and could lead to lodgment in the esophagus. The data are insufficient to support the use of cathartics and metoclopramide.

17. The answer is **B,** page 375.

Impacted esophageal batteries can cause burns within 4 hours of ingestion, and perforation has been reported. Steroids and antibiotics are indicated only in the management of circumferential burns and have no role in the treatment of focal esophageal mucosal burns from button battery ingestion. Because of potential for perforation and possible need for surgical repair, barium swallow is not recommended. Nonionic radiopaque contrast medium, because it is water soluble, is the diagnostic study of choice. However, because of the risk of aspiration, the most appropriate management is close observation and surgical consultation.

18. The answer is **E,** page 375.

Complications from an esophageal burn include perforation with possible tracheoesophageal fistula formation, erosion into the aorta, mediastinitis, and death. Esophageal burns predispose to stricture formation. Heavy metal poisoning (from mercury-containing batteries) has been described. Since button batteries are so small, obstruction is not much of a concern.

19. The answer is **B,** page 378.

Treatment for an apneic and unconscious child older than 1 year of age with complete airway obstruction is subdiaphragmatic abdominal thrusts. A series of five back blows and chest thrusts is recommended for children younger than 1 year of age. Blind finger sweep is never indicated in children, and endotracheal intubation is used only if initial airway maneuvers are unsuccessful. Oxygen does not alleviate the airway obstruction.

20. The answer is **D,** page 378.

Needle cricothyrotomy is indicated in pediatric complete airway obstruction that has been resistant to abdominal thrusts. Emergency surgical tracheotomy or cricothyrotomy is contraindicated in young children, since these techniques have high morbidity in the emergency setting. The nasopharyngeal airway maintains airway patency only through the nasopharynx.

21. The answer is **A,** page 378.

Treatment for an apneic and unconscious child less than 1 year old with complete airway obstruction is a series of five back blows and chest thrusts. Subdiaphragmatic abdominal thrusts in children younger than 1 have the potential risk of injury to the abdominal viscera.

22. The answer is **E,** page 378.

If initial obstructed airway maneuvers fail to produce foreign body expulsion, direct laryngoscopy may permit visualization of the upper airway. Removal with Magill forceps is indicated if a foreign body is seen in the upper airway. Removal with finger sweep should not be attempted if Magill forceps are available. Endotracheal intubation may dislodge the object into a mainstem bronchus, thereby converting a complete obstruction to a partial obstruction; this should be done only if removal with Magill forceps is unsuccessful.

23. The answer is **D,** page 376.

Approximately 75% of cases of foreign body aspiration occur in children less than 3 years of age. The male/female ratio is approximately 2:1. Most airway foreign bodies lodge in a mainstem bronchus. Tracheal or laryngeal foreign bodies account for only 3% to 11% but are associated with a greater morbidity and mortality. Organic debris is the most common offending agent. In contrast to esophageal foreign bodies, airway foreign bodies are rarely radiopaque. Between 50% and 90% of children with foreign body aspiration have a suggestive history, most commonly of an acute episode of paroxysmal cough.

24. The answer is **C,** page 376.

Lack of an efficient grinding surface before eruption of the back molars, presence of small food and nonfood objects in the house, and the natural curiosity of the toddler explain the high propensity for choking in those younger than 3 years old. Organic debris, particularly peanuts, is the most commonly aspirated material. Slightly less than half of all bronchial foreign bodies are left-sided. Tracheal or laryngeal foreign bodies are associated with a higher morbidity and mortality than foreign bodies in the mainstem bronchi. The classic triad of acute onset of wheezing, coughing, and absent or diminished breath sounds is present in only about 40% of cases.

25. The answer is **B,** page 376.

Radiologic studies are often normal or nondiagnostic for airway foreign body. Only half of aspirations in children are diagnosed correctly in the first 24 hours after an aspiration event, and there may be delays in diagnosis of weeks to years. One fourth of children may be asymptomatic when they come to the ED, and up to 39% may have no supportive physical findings. The classic triad of coughing, wheezing, and decreased or absent breath sounds is present in about 40% of cases.

26. The answer is **B,** page 377.

Initial radiologic evaluation involves PA and lateral views of the chest and neck. Although plain films may be interpreted as normal, differential inflation of the affected lung, the most common abnormality identified, may be documented by fluoroscopy, lateral decubitus views, or an assisted expiratory film. Although CT scan, xeroradiography, and ultrasonography have been advocated for foreign body imaging, their utility has not been demonstrated.

27. The answer is **D,** page 377.

Although the chest radiograph may appear normal in foreign body aspiration, in some cases it offers clues to the presence of the foreign body. Unilateral hyperinflation from a ball-valve effect, resorption atelectasis distal to the location of complete bronchial obstruction, or persistent pulmonary infiltrates are the most common abnormal chest radiograph findings.

28. The answer is **A,** page 378.

   Fiberoptic flexible bronchoscopy may be used to visualize a foreign body if the diagnosis is in question, but removal through a rigid scope is advocated, since the patient can be ventilated through the rigid bronchoscope during the episode.

29. The answer is **D,** page 376.

   Hot dogs, grapes, and other small, rounded, pliable foods and objects pose a significant aspiration risk for infants and toddlers. The CPSC does not require that toys with "small parts" carry an aspiration warning label, only that they be labeled "Not for children under 3 years."

Musculoskeletal and Soft Tissue Injuries

Tom Kwiatkowski

See Barkin et al: Chapters 27 to 32.

1. When the hand and wrist are being splinted, which of the following best describes the position of function or "hooded cobra" position?
   A. The wrist is in 20 to 30 degrees of flexion, the metacarpophalangeal (MCP) joints are flexed 60 to 70 degrees, and the interphalangeal (IP) joints are flexed 10 to 20 degrees.
   B. Wrist is neutral, MCP joints are flexed 20 to 30 degrees, and IP joints are flexed 10 to 20 degrees.
   C. Wrist is neutral, MCP joints are flexed 60 to 70 degrees, and IP joints are flexed 10 to 20 degrees.
   D. Wrist is in 20 to 30 degrees of flexion, MCP joints are flexed 20 to 30 degrees, and IP joints are flexed 10 to 20 degrees.
   E. Wrist is in 20 to 30 degrees of flexion, MCP joints are flexed 20 to 30 degrees, and IP joints are flexed 60 to 70 degrees.

2. A 16-year-old boy was involved in a fight at school and is brought to the ED by his father. On examination he has tenderness over the fifth metacarpal of his left hand. X-ray reveals a nondisplaced fracture of the neck of the fifth metacarpal. The best approach to this patient would be:
   A. Arrange an immediate orthopedic referral for fixation and admission.
   B. Place the injured hand in a thumb spica splint or cast with outpatient referral to orthopedics.
   C. Place the injured extremity in a sling, since the fracture is nondisplaced, with outpatient referral to orthopedics.
   D. Place the injured hand in an ulnar gutter splint with outpatient orthopedic referral.
   E. Arrange an immediate orthopedic referral for closed reduction and long-arm cast application.

3. Which of the following best describes a Salter-Harris type II fracture?
   A. The fracture is transverse through the physeal-metaphyseal interface (epiphyseal plate) with extension into the metaphysis.
   B. The fracture is transverse through the physeal-metaphyseal interface (epiphyseal plate) with extension through the epiphyseal ossification center and the articular cartilage.
   C. The fracture line extends from the articular surface to the metaphyseal cortex, traversing the epiphysis, physis, and metaphyseal bone.
   D. It is a compression fracture through the epiphyseal plate with microvascular compromise.
   E. It is a fracture through the epiphyseal plate, with no extension into the diaphyseal or epiphyseal bone.

4. A 10-year-old girl was at gym class and injured her wrist doing a cartwheel. She is brought by her mother to the ED several hours later because of continued wrist pain. On examination she has point tenderness over the dorsal surface of the distal radius. A slight amount of soft tissue swelling is also noted. X-rays are unremarkable. The best treatment for this patient is:
   A. Since there is no fracture on x-ray, the child should be instructed to refrain from gym classes until the pain resolves and use Tylenol if necessary.
   B. Arrange an immediate orthopedic referral for circular cast application.
   C. Place the injured extremity in a sling and tell the mother to follow up with orthopedics if the pain does not resolve in 1 week.
   D. Place the injured extremity in a thumb spica splint and provide outpatient orthopedic referral.
   E. Place the injured extremity in a volar forearm splint that extends to the distal palmar crease, with outpatient orthopedic referral.

5. Which of the following statements is true regarding bony dislocations in children?
   A. Dislocations are common in children because of bone immaturity and ligament laxity.
   B. Dislocations are less common than in adults, since ligaments and their attachments are the most stable elements of joints in children.
   C. Dislocations are common in children, since most dislocations result from childhood sports injuries.
   D. Dislocations are less common than in adults because the periosteum in children is much stronger than the ligaments surrounding a joint.
   E. Dislocations are common in children, in contrast to adults, in whom avulsion injuries are much more common.

6. The best position of the wrist for examining the scaphoid (navicular) bone is:
   A. Flex the wrist approximately 30 degrees with mild ulnar deviation.
   B. Extend the wrist approximately 30 degrees with mild ulnar deviation.
   C. Extend the wrist approximately 30 degrees with mild radial deviation.
   D. Flex the wrist approximately 30 degrees with mild radial deviation.
   E. Keep the wrist in a neutral position with mild radial deviation.

7. The most common carpal bone fracture in children is:
   A. Boxer's fracture.
   B. Mallet fracture.
   C. Scaphoid fracture.
   D. Fracture of radial styloid process.
   E. Gamekeeper's thumb.

8. The best location on the hand to test for pure median nerve sensation is:
   A. The palmar surface of the tip of the ring finger.
   B. The web space between the thumb and index finger.
   C. The dorsal surface of the tip of the index finger.
   D. The palmar surface of the base of the ring finger.
   E. The palmar surface of the tip of the index finger.

9. A 10-year-old child sustained a laceration to the distal palmar surface of the index finger. Gross sensation is intact. When testing for two-point discrimination, neuronal integrity is confirmed when the child can distinguish which of the following distances?
   A. 15 mm or less.
   B. 5 mm or less.
   C. 1 cm or less.
   D. 8 mm or less.
   E. 12 mm or less.

10. Which of the following is true regarding extension of the MCP joints of the fingers?
    A. The muscles involved are supplied by the median nerve.
    B. This action is performed by the intrinsic muscles of the hand.
    C. This action is best tested with the fingers in extension at the proximal interphalangeal (PIP) joint.
    D. This action is maintained even with the loss of wrist extension.
    E. This action is best tested with the fingers in flexion at the PIP joint.

11. Flexion at the PIP joint of the finger is primarily a function of:
    A. The flexor digitorum superficialis.
    B. The ulnar nerve.
    C. The interossei.
    D. The flexor digitorum profundus.
    E. The lumbricals.

12. Following an injury to the wrist and hand, a 12-year-old child has difficulty with finger adduction. Finger adduction is a function of:
    A. The median nerve.
    B. The palmar interossei.
    C. The radial nerve.
    D. The lumbricals.
    E. The dorsal interossei.

13. A 15-year-old boy was working with his father cutting glass and sustained a laceration to the palmar surface of his index finger. On examination he is unable to flex this finger at the distal interphalangeal joint (DIP). This represents an injury to:
    A. Radial nerve.
    B. Palmar interosseous.
    C. Flexor digitorum profundus.
    D. Flexor digitorum superficialis.
    E. Lumbrical.

14. A 15-year-old boy fell while jogging at school. He is brought to the ED because of wrist pain. On examination he has pain in the anatomic snuffbox, and an x-ray reveals a nondisplaced fracture of the scaphoid. Appropriate management includes:
    A. Placing the forearm in a sling, with outpatient orthopedic referral.
    B. Immediate orthopedic consultation for internal fixation, since a high incidence of nonunion exists with these fractures.
    C. Placing the patient in a volar splint for orthopedic follow-up.
    D. Placing the patient in a thumb spica splint or cast, with close orthopedic follow-up.
    E. Placing the hand in a bulky dressing to minimize movement, with outpatient orthopedic referral.

15. Which of the following statements is true regarding carpometacarpal (CMC) joint dislocations in children?
    A. Flexion of the involved digit is usually normal.
    B. They are difficult to diagnose clinically, since swelling, tenderness, and joint deformity are uncommon.
    C. They most commonly involve the thumb.
    D. Closed reduction is difficult and should be avoided.
    E. They most commonly involve the fifth finger.

16. A 16-year-old girl fell while skiing during a school trip. After returning home she is brought to the ED by her mother because of left thumb pain. Her mother tells you that the physician at the ski lodge examined her and made the diagnosis of "gamekeeper's thumb." Her x-ray is seen in Fig. 24-1. Which of the following is true regarding this condition?
    A. Tenderness and swelling are noted over the radial aspect of the MCP joint of the thumb.
    B. The injury is caused by hyperextension of the CMC joint of the thumb.
    C. Ulnar deviation of the thumb exacerbates the pain.
    D. The injury results in instability of the radial collateral ligament of the thumb.
    E. Radial deviation of the thumb exacerbates the pain.

17. A 14-year-old girl comes to the ED after an injury to her right index finger, resulting in a boutonniere deformity. Which of the following statements is true regarding this condition?
    A. The DIP joint is held in flexion while the PIP joint is held in extension.
    B. The dorsal DIP joint has overlying tenderness and swelling.
    C. The MCP joint is held in extension while the DIP is held in flexion.
    D. Surgical repair of the tendon is required, since these injuries do not respond to conservative management.
    E. The dorsal PIP joint has overlying tenderness and swelling.

18. A 5-week-old infant is brought to the ED by his mother after she noticed a "bulge" on the right side of the chest near the shoulder. Physical examination reveals a bony prominence on the clavicle. An x-ray reveals callus formation surrounding a clavicular fracture. At this point you should:
    A. Obtain urgent orthopedic evaluation for stabilization and management.
    B. Reassure the parent that this injury probably occurred during birth and will resolve spontaneously over the next several months.
    C. Place the infant in a figure-of-8 splint for 3 to 4 weeks.
    D. Consider the diagnosis of child abuse, since this a rare injury in this age group.
    E. Place the infant in an arm sling for 2 to 3 weeks.

19. Which of the following statements is true regarding clavicular fractures in childhood?
    A. The clavicle is the most frequently fractured bone in children.
    B. They are associated with high-energy trauma, such as motor vehicle accidents or falls of more than 5 feet.
    C. Fractures are most common at the junction of the medial and middle thirds of the clavicle.
    D. They are a common manifestation of child abuse.
    E. Fractured clavicles usually bow posteriorly, making the affected clavicle less prominent on inspection.

20. A 15-year-old boy sustains an injury to his right shoulder during football practice. Examination in the ED reveals tenderness over the distal clavicle and pain with abduction. X-ray of the right shoulder is negative. At this point you would:
    A. Place the patient in a figure-of-8 splint for a presumed occult clavicular fracture.
    B. Request urgent orthopedic consultation.
    C. Obtain a posteroanterior (PA) view of the chest.
    D. Discharge the patient on analgesics and assure him that he has only a shoulder sprain.
    E. Assume the patient has a shoulder dislocation and place the patient in a long-arm splint.

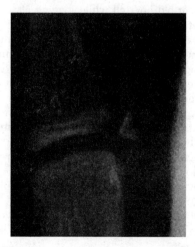

FIG. 24-1 Gamekeeper's thumb. (From Ogden JA: *Skeletal injury in the child*, ed 2, Philadelphia, 1990, WB Saunders.)

21. While practicing on the parallel bars during gymnastics, a 15-year-old girl suddenly has acute right shoulder pain. On examination in the ED the patient cannot abduct or externally rotate her arm. There is also prominence of the acromion. Which of the following statements is true regarding this patient?
    A. Vascular injuries are common with this disorder.
    B. Decreased sensation over the lateral portion of the shoulder and upper arm may be associated findings.
    C. This is a true orthopedic emergency.
    D. X-rays are not helpful in making the diagnosis.
    E. Once the diagnosis is confirmed, the patient will require general anesthesia and operative repair.

22. Which of the following statements is true regarding shoulder dislocations in children?
    A. This disorder is common in young children because of ligament laxity.
    B. Posterior dislocations are much more common than in adults.
    C. Recurrences are rare.
    D. The mechanism of injury is abduction and extension of the shoulder.
    E. The patient is at increased risk for dislocations in the uninvolved shoulder.

23. A 17-year-old boy complains of left shoulder pain after lifting a 100-lb bag of gravel at work. On examination he has pain with abduction and external rotation. However, passive range of motion of the shoulder is normal. Which of the following statements is true regarding this injury?
    A. Treatment usually involves immobilization in a sling and analgesia, followed by passive range of motion exercises.
    B. Plain x-rays confirm the diagnosis in more than 75% of cases.
    C. Urgent referral to orthopedics is necessary to prevent long-term complications.
    D. Steroid injection in the ED is indicated and will markedly reduce the pain.
    E. The patient needs an arthrogram to decide whether early surgical intervention is indicated.

24. A 13-year-old girl fell backward while playing volleyball at school. In the ED she has significant tenderness and mild swelling over the proximal humerus. She is reluctant to move her arm because of the pain. Anteroposterior (AP) x-ray of the affected shoulder is negative for shoulder dislocation or clavicular fracture. At this point you should:
    A. Obtain a lateral view of the affected shoulder.
    B. Examine the patient more thoroughly with passive range of motion of the shoulder for better localization of the injury.
    C. Place the patient in a sling, with orthopedic follow-up if the pain does not resolve.
    D. Admit the patient for an arthrogram or magnetic resonance imaging (MRI).
    E. Place the patient in a figure-of-8 sling for a presumed occult clavicular fracture.

25. Which of the following statements is true regarding humeral shaft fractures in children?
    A. These fractures are common because of bone immaturity.
    B. The distal third is the most common location for fractures.
    C. Anesthesia in the web space between the first and second metacarpals suggests neuronal injury.
    D. Child abuse frequently results in transverse fractures.
    E. Admission to the hospital for observation is necessary to monitor blood loss, which is often significant.

26. The most common elbow fracture in pediatric patients is:
    A. Supracondylar fracture of humerus.
    B. Radial head fracture.
    C. Lateral condyle of distal humerus.
    D. Medial epicondyle of humerus.
    E. Olecranon fracture of ulna.

27. An 8-year-old boy fell while playing soccer. He comes to the ED 2 hours later complaining of pain in the elbow. On examination there is tenderness and swelling over the distal humerus and marked pain with flexion of the elbow. At this point you should:
    A. Splint the elbow in flexion to stabilize the fracture and prevent further injury.
    B. Obtain x-rays of the elbow and humeral shaft.
    C. Evaluate distal neurovascular function.
    D. Evaluate the fracture site for deformity and, if present, obtain immediate orthopedic consultation.
    E. Establish intravenous (IV) access and administer Valium 0.1 ml/kg to minimize muscle spasm and vascular compromise.

28. Which of the following is an early sign of vascular compromise in a patient with a supracondylar fracture of the humerus?
    A. Absent radial pulse.
    B. Absent ulnar pulse.
    C. Forearm pain exacerbated by passive extension of the fingers.
    D. Forearm pain exacerbated by passive flexion of the fingers.
    E. Decreased grip strength.

29. A 15-year-old boy struck his elbow on the ground while in-line skating. He was brought to the ED 3 hours later by his father for evaluation. On examination he has a 5-cm abrasion over the lateral aspect of the elbow. He has full range of motion at the elbow joint and minimal tenderness. You obtain an x-ray that demonstrates a small anterior fat pad sign and no evidence of fracture. What most likely describes this patient?
    A. The patient most likely has a radial head fracture.
    B. The patient has evidence of a joint effusion.
    C. The patient does not show clinical or radiologic evidence of a fracture.
    D. The patient will require a circular cast to immobilize his fracture.
    E. Arthrocentesis should be performed as the next step in evaluation of this patient.

30. Which of the following statements is true regarding elbow dislocations in children?
    A. They are rare because of the ligamentous support and osseous stability of this joint.
    B. Volkmann's contracture is seen with the same frequency as with supracondylar fractures.
    C. Spontaneous reduction is rare because of the rapid development of muscle spasm.
    D. Closed reduction should be avoided because of frequent neurovascular injury.
    E. They are most common in children less than 3 years of age.

31. A 3-year-old child is brought to the ED because of refusal to lift his right arm. His mother states that after his father picked him up briskly by his hands, he began complaining of pain in his arm. On examination the child refuses to lift his right arm and holds it partially flexed, pronated, and close to his body. Physical examination is unremarkable except for the child's refusal to lift his arm. Which of the following is true regarding the patient's diagnosis?
    A. X-rays should be obtained before reduction to rule out an associated fracture.
    B. Orthopedic consultation should be obtained in the ED.
    C. Following reduction, the patient should be placed in a sling and swathe for 5 to 7 days to prevent recurrent dislocation.
    D. The social worker should be notified regarding the possibility of child abuse.
    E. Reduction should be attempted without x-rays and if it is successful, the child can be discharged from the ED without x-rays or immobilization.

32. Which of the following best describes the components of a Monteggia's fracture?
    A. Fracture of the distal ulna associated with anterior dislocation of the radial head.
    B. Fracture of the proximal ulna associated with a radial head fracture.
    C. Fracture of the proximal ulna associated with anterior dislocation of the radial head.
    D. Fracture of the proximal ulna associated with posterior dislocation of the radial head.
    E. Fracture of the distal ulna associated with a fracture of the radial head.

33. Which of the following statements is true regarding pelvic fractures in young children in contrast with pelvic fractures in adults?
    A. A single break in the pelvic ring occurs more commonly because of the mobility of the sacroiliac joint and symphysis pubis.
    B. A single break in the pelvic ring occurs less commonly because of the relatively increased strength of the ligamentous structures of the sacroiliac joint and symphysis pubis.
    C. Massive hemorrhage is more common because of the increased vascularity of immature bone.
    D. Rectal examinations should not be performed because of the high incidence of rectal injuries.
    E. Pubic fractures are common even with relatively trivial injuries in children less than 5 years of age because of bone immaturity.

34. Which of the following statements is true regarding hip fractures in children?
    A. They are common in children, especially those younger than 1 year of age.
    B. The femoral neck of a child is strong, and high-velocity forces (e.g., motor vehicle accident) are required to break it.
    C. The femoral neck of a child is relatively weak, and simple injuries (e.g., fall off a bicycle) can result in a fracture.
    D. They are difficult to diagnose on routine x-rays. A tomogram or MRI is usually necessary to confirm the diagnosis.
    E. Avascular necrosis of the femoral head is uncommon because of its rich blood supply, especially in children younger than 10 years of age.

35. A 12-year-old boy is involved in a multivehicle accident. He was not wearing a seatbelt, and his right knee was thrust against the dashboard of the car. He comes to the ED with his right leg internally rotated, adducted, flexed, and shortened. Which of the following statements is true regarding his diagnosis?
    A. He most likely has a fracture of the femoral neck of his right femur.
    B. He most likely has an anterior dislocation of the right hip.
    C. Sciatic nerve injuries are commonly associated with this diagnosis, occurring in more than 50% of cases.
    D. X-rays may reveal associated fractures, especially of the posterior wall of the acetabulum.
    E. This injury is uncommon in children younger than 5 years of age.

36. A 5-year-old child is sent to the ED by his pediatrician to rule out Legg-Calvé-Perthes disease. Which of the following statements is true regarding this condition?
    A. It is rare after 6 years of age.
    B. It is a congenital process unrelated to injury.
    C. Pain is present with active range of motion of the involved joint, with few to no findings on passive range of motion.
    D. Management includes minimal weight bearing with the involved extremity maintained in adduction.
    E. These patients often have knee pain.

37. A 14-year-old boy comes to the ED with right knee pain. The onset of pain has been gradual over the previous month. The patient is afebrile and has no systemic complaints. X-ray of the knee is unremarkable. At this point, you should:
    A. Refer the patient to orthopedics for consideration of a bone scan to rule out Legg-Calvé-Perthes disease.
    B. Immobilize the knee in a compression dressing together with no weight bearing for 1 week for a presumed ligamentous injury.
    C. Obtain a complete blood count (CBC) and sedimentation rate.
    D. Obtain AP and frog leg films of the right hip.
    E. Obtain lumbosacral and sacroiliac joint films.

38. A 3-year-old boy is brought to the ED because of inability to bear weight on his right leg. His mother states that according to the baby-sitter, he fell to the floor while climbing out of his crib. X-rays reveal a spiral fracture of the femoral shaft. Which of the following statements is true regarding this injury?
    A. A fall from a crib does not explain this injury.
    B. This fracture can result from indirect rotational forces consistent with this child's mechanism of injury.
    C. Significant swelling is usually present on physical examination.
    D. This fracture is pathognomonic of child abuse.
    E. Significant blood loss is common.

39. Which of the following statements is true regarding ligamentous injuries to the knee in childhood?
    A. A significant ligamentous injury is uncommon in a child with open physes.
    B. The anterior cruciate ligament is most commonly involved.
    C. The medial collateral ligament is most commonly involved.
    D. The majority of tense acute hemarthroses are caused by posterior cruciate ligament damage.
    E. Surgical correction is necessary more commonly than in adults for third-degree sprains.

40. A 13-year-old boy comes to the ED complaining of right knee pain. The patient states that he was running and stopped suddenly when an automobile crossed his path unexpectedly. He states that he heard a "pop" in his knee when he stopped. Within 1 hour, his knee became swollen. On physical examination the patient has a tense right knee effusion with limited and painful range of motion. The most likely diagnosis is:
    A. Posterior cruciate ligament tear.
    B. Anterior cruciate ligament tear.
    C. Medial meniscus injury.
    D. Lateral meniscus injury.
    E. Medial collateral ligament tear.

41. 41. Which of the following best describes Osgood-Schlatter disease?
    A. Avascular necrosis of the femoral head.
    B. Avulsion of the tibial spine associated with chronic anterior cruciate ligament stress.
    C. Partial avulsion and separation of the tibial tubercle.
    D. Necrosis and softening of the overlying cartilage of the proximal tibia.
    E. Avulsion of the tibial tubercle.

42. A 16-year-old boy fell after tripping on a curb while running. He comes to the ED complaining of left ankle pain. On examination there is swelling and tenderness over the lateral aspect of the ankle joint, although range of motion is intact. X-rays are negative for fracture. The most likely cause of this injury is:
    A. Tear of the posterior talofibular ligament.
    B. Tear of the deltoid ligament.
    C. Tear of the anterior tibiofibular ligament.
    D. Tear of the anterior talofibular ligament.
    E. Tear of the posterior tibiofibular ligament.

43. Which of the following statements is true regarding the talar tilt test?
    A. It is intended to evaluate the integrity of the anterior talofibular ligament and the calcaneofibular ligament.
    B. The foot is everted to determine the degree of talar tilt.
    C. A 20-degree difference between the affected side and contralateral side is considered significant.
    D. It is intended to evaluate the integrity of the deltoid ligament.
    E. It is associated with many false positive findings during the acute period.

44. Which of the following statements is true regarding ankle fractures in children?
    A. The distal fibular physis is one of the weakest components of the ankle joint and is more likely to be disrupted than the adjoining ligaments.
    B. Fractures through the distal tibial physis are common.
    C. Isolated fractures through the physis of the distal fibula are common.
    D. Growth disturbances are common with Salter type I and II injuries.
    E. Salter type III fractures have the poorest prognosis for normal growth of affected bone.

45. The most commonly fractured tarsal bone in children is the:
    A. Talus.
    B. Cuneiform.
    C. Cuboid.
    D. Navicular.
    E. Calcaneus.

46. An 8-year-old boy comes to the ED complaining of foot pain. According to his mother, he sustained a puncture wound to the sole of his foot from a piece of glass 2 days ago, while at camp. He was barefoot when the injury occurred. On examination the wound is warm and tender, with an early developing cellulitis. The most likely causative organism is:
    A. *Staphylococcus epidermidis.*
    B. *Streptococcus pyogenes.*
    C. *Pseudomonas.*
    D. *Staphylococcus aureus.*
    E. *Pasteurella.*

47. A 10-year-old girl comes to the ED with difficulty walking. On examination there is pain and swelling on the plantar aspect of the left foot over the first MCP joint. Her father states that approximately 5 days ago, she stepped on a nail while on vacation. Which of the following statements is true regarding this injury?
    A. This patient most likely has a streptococcal infection.
    B. With deep space infections, systemic findings (e.g., fever, increased white blood cells) are usually present.
    C. Deep space infections are usually caused by *Pseudomonas.*
    D. Deep space infections are usually caused by *S. aureus.*
    E. Deep space infections are uncommon at the MCP joints.

48. A 17-year-old boy comes to the ED after sustaining a puncture wound to his left foot. On examination a puncture wound is noted on the plantar surface of the foot just distal to the first MCP joint. The wound is cleaned, and there is no obvious foreign body. The patient states that he received his childhood immunizations but has not been to a doctor since he was 10 years old. Which of the following options is appropriate regarding tetanus prophylaxis?
    A. Tetanus and diphtheria (Td) toxoid 0.5 ml and 250 units tetanus immune globulin (TIG).
    B. Td toxoid 0.5 ml and 500 units TIG.
    C. TIG 250 units.
    D. Td toxoid 0.5 ml.
    E. No tetanus prophylaxis is indicated.

49. A 13-year-old girl comes to the ED with a jagged wound on the plantar surface of her left foot. Before irrigation and debridement, you decide to perform a posterior tibial nerve block. The best method for performing this block is:
    A. Inject lidocaine with epinephrine medial to the posterior tibial artery pulse inferior to the medial malleolus.
    B. Inject lidocaine without epinephrine lateral to the posterior tibial artery pulse at the level of the proximal half of the medial malleolus.
    C. Inject lidocaine with epinephrine lateral to the posterior tibial artery pulse at the level of the proximal half of the medial malleolus.
    D. Inject lidocaine without epinephrine medial to the posterior tibial artery pulse at the level of the proximal half of the medial malleolus.
    E. Inject lidocaine with epinephrine medial to the posterior tibial artery pulse at the level of the proximal half of the medial malleolus.

50. A 5-year-old boy weighing approximately 20 kg sustained several lacerations to his hand and fingers with broken glass. The maximum volume of 1% lidocaine without epinephrine you can use for infiltration of his wounds is:
    A. 5 ml.
    B. 8 ml.
    C. 10 ml.
    D. 12 ml.
    E. 14 ml.

51. The sensory distribution of the radial nerve usually includes:
    A. Entire dorsal surface of hand except tip of thumb.
    B. Dorsal surface of index, middle, and ring fingers.
    C. Dorsal surface of thumb, index, and middle fingers.
    D. Dorsal surface of forearm and hand to DIP joint.
    E. Dorsal surface of hand to PIP joint.

52. A 13-year-old boy injured his right index finger while playing football. The distal phalanx is held in flexion, and he is unable to extend the DIP joint. X-ray reveals no fracture. Appropriate management for this injury is:
    A. An ulnar gutter splint.
    B. Splinting the DIP joint in mild hyperextension.
    C. Splinting the DIP joint in mild flexion.
    D. Buddy taping the index and middle fingers.
    E. Orthopedic consultation for operative repair.

53. While playing football, a 15-year-old injures his right ring finger. On examination he is unable to flex the DIP joint, which is swollen and tender. X-ray is unremarkable. The best treatment for this patient is:
    A. Referral for surgical repair of flexor digitorum profundus tendon.
    B. Splinting the DIP joint in extension.
    C. Splinting the DIP joint in flexion.
    D. Volar splint in position of function until swelling and pain subside.
    E. Radial gutter splint.

54. A 10-year-old girl is brought to the ED after injuring the distal tip of her finger in a car door. Which of the following management options is appropriate?
    A. Recent data suggest that a partially avulsed nail does not have to be removed when associated with a tuft fracture unless there is a large subungual hematoma.
    B. Subungual hematomas do not have to be drained unless they exceed 50% of the nailbed surface.
    C. Tuft fractures in young children, unlike in adults, are often complex and require orthopedic referral.
    D. Nailbed lacerations are best repaired with 6-0 nylon, which can be left in place for 10 days.
    E. Recent data suggest that an intact nail does not have to be removed when there is no associated fracture, even with a large subungual hematoma.

55. An 8-year-old boy cut his hand with a piece of glass. Examination reveals a laceration on the flexor surface of the middle finger over the proximal phalanx. An arterial pumper was present and responded to elevation and pressure. Motor function is intact. Which additional injury is most likely present?
    A. Laceration of a palmar interossei.
    B. Laceration of the digital nerve.
    C. Laceration of the lumbrical.
    D. Laceration of the flexor digitorum profundus.
    E. Laceration of the flexor digitorum superficialis.

56. A 7-year-old boy comes into the ED with an amputation injury to his right index finger incurred in a lawnmower accident. Management recommendations include:
   A. Wrap the amputated part in dry gauze, seal in a plastic bag, and place in ice water.
   B. If more than 4 hours has elapsed since the injury, reimplantation is not an option for a finger because of its limited vascularity.
   C. Reimplantation of single digits as in this case is not indicated.
   D. Distal amputations not involving bone are best treated with skin grafting.
   E. If a single digit is involved, successful reimplantation of cooled tissue can occur up to 24 hours after amputation.

57. A 14-year-old skier is brought to the ED after prolonged exposure to the elements after a fall. Both feet are cold and appear frostbitten. The appropriate rewarming technique is:
   A. Rapid rewarming with warm water ($40°$ to $42°$ C) for 20 to 30 minutes continuously.
   B. Slow rewarming with warm water ($40°$ to $42°$ C) applied for 5-minute intervals separated by rest periods of 5 to 10 minutes.
   C. Slow rewarming with elevation and passive warming techniques (e.g., wrapping with blankets).
   D. Slow rewarming with water at room temperature ($20°$ to $25°$ C) for 45 to 60 minutes.
   E. Rapid rewarming with water at room temperature ($20°$ to $25°$ C) together with vigorous massage.

58. A 15-year-old boy comes to the ED complaining of pain in his right middle finger. He thinks he injured it last week when he climbed over a barbed wire fence. On examination the volar aspect of the distal phalanx is red, swollen, indurated, and painful. Correct management options include:
   A. If no fluctuance is present, begin warm soaks, elevation, and oral antibiotics.
   B. A longitudinal incision is the preferred technique for drainage.
   C. A horizontal incision is the preferred technique for drainage.
   D. With good surgical drainage, antibiotics are unnecessary.
   E. Needle drainage, followed by warm soaks and broad-spectrum antibiotics, has been shown to be equally effective to more aggressive measures.

59. A medical student requests your assistance to examine a child who he thinks has a scapular fracture. Which of the following is true regarding this injury?
   A. Fractures are common in young children because of the superficial location of this bone.
   B. In contrast to older children and adults, relatively minor trauma can fracture the scapula in a young child.
   C. Fractures are usually displaced because of numerous muscle insertions.
   D. Most fractures are associated with shoulder dislocation.
   E. Isolated fractures are treated with a sling and swathe for 3 to 4 weeks.

60. Dislocation of the shoulder may be associated with:
   A. Fracture of the greater tuberosity of the humerus.
   B. Injury of the brachial artery.
   C. Fracture of the lesser tuberosity of the humerus.
   D. Fracture of the coracoid process.
   E. Injury to the radial nerve.

61. The muscular components of the rotator cuff include:
   A. Supraspinatus, infraspinatus, teres major.
   B. Subscapularis, infraspinatus, deltoid.
   C. Supraspinatus, infraspinatus, teres minor.
   D. Subscapularis, infraspinatus, teres major.
   E. Supraspinatus, infraspinatus, deltoid.

62. The vast majority of supracondylar fractures are secondary to this mechanism of injury:
   A. Hyperextension.
   B. Abduction.
   C. Hyperflexion.
   D. Distraction.
   E. Supination.

63. Volkmann's contracture is caused by injury to the:
   A. Median nerve.
   B. Radial nerve.
   C. Axillary artery.
   D. Ulnar nerve.
   E. Brachial artery.

64. When splinting a child with a suspected supracondylar fracture, particular attention must be paid to the following:
   A. Excessive extension must be avoided.
   B. Excessive flexion must be avoided.
   C. The degree of flexion and extension are not as important as keeping the forearm in a supinated position.
   D. The degrees of flexion and extension are not as important as keeping the forearm in a pronated position.
   E. The splint should be wrapped as firmly as possible to limit edema formation and the likelihood of neurovascular compromise.

65. A 10-year-old boy fell on a partially flexed outstretched hand while running. He comes to the ED in significant pain with swelling around the elbow. Physical examination is significant for shortening of the forearm and protrusion of the olecranon posteriorly. Neurovascular status is intact. The most likely diagnosis is:
   A. Anterior dislocation of the elbow.
   B. Displaced supracondylar fracture.
   C. Posterior dislocation of the elbow.
   D. Monteggia's fracture.
   E. Anterior dislocation of the humerus.

66. The correct technique for reduction of radial head subluxation (nursemaid's elbow) is:
    A. Flexion of the elbow followed by rapid supination and extension.
    B. Flexion of the elbow followed by rapid pronation and extension.
    C. Extension of the elbow followed by rapid supination and flexion.
    D. Extension of the elbow followed by rapid pronation and flexion.
    E. Pronation is the most important maneuver; the amount of elbow flexion or extension is probably not important.

67. Which of the following statements is true regarding forearm fractures in children?
    A. Single forearm fractures commonly occur because of ligament laxity.
    B. Compartment syndromes and ischemia seldom occur.
    C. Injuries to the median, ulnar, or radial nerves are common and require urgent referral and follow-up.
    D. Longitudinal bone growth disturbances occur most commonly with fractures involving the proximal growth plates.
    E. Greenstick fractures are best treated with splinting and early mobilization.

68. A 10-year-old girl is brought to the ED after falling off a 10-foot ladder onto a concrete surface. After initial stabilization, she is noted to have pain in her right hip, which is flexed, externally rotated, and shortened. Which of the following statements is true regarding this injury?
    A. The majority are secondary to transepiphyseal injuries.
    B. These injuries do not typically affect growth potential.
    C. Transcervical (neck) fractures are far more common than transepiphyseal fractures.
    D. Avascular necrosis is unusual in nondisplaced fractures.

69. A referring pediatrician wants you to evaluate a child to rule out toxic synovitis. Which of the following is true regarding this condition?
    A. It is uncommon below 3 years of age.
    B. About 25% of cases are secondary to bacterial infection.
    C. *S. aureus* is the most common organism isolated.
    D. The peak incidence is at 2 years of age.
    E. The patient usually has significant pain on abduction and external rotation of the hip.

70. A 14-year-old boy comes to the ED with knee pain following a soccer injury. You perform the McMurray test and note a click when moving the leg into external rotation. The patient most likely has an injury to:
    A. Medial meniscus.
    B. Medial collateral ligament.
    C. Anterior cruciate ligament.
    D. Lateral meniscus.
    E. Posterior cruciate ligament.

71. Which of the following statements is true regarding patellar dislocations?
    A. In adolescents, it is much more common in girls than boys.
    B. Most patients do not have a hemarthrosis.
    C. Reduction is best accomplished with the hip and knee in full extension.
    D. Dislocations of the patella almost always occur medially.
    E. After reduction, the knee is immobilized in 30 degrees of flexion.

72. A 14-year-old girl injured her ankle while playing basketball. On examination there is significant tenderness and swelling medially. Which of the following statements is true regarding this injury?
    A. The mechanism of injury was inversion of the ankle.
    B. This is the most common type of ankle sprain in adolescents.
    C. The talar tilt test will most likely be positive.
    D. The calcaneofibular ligament is most likely involved.
    E. This usually is a more serious injury than a lateral ankle injury.

73. Which of the following statements is true regarding hair removal before laceration repair?
    A. Leaving hair in contact with a wound significantly increases infection rate.
    B. Shaving is the preferred method of hair removal.
    C. Hair is best removed with scissors.
    D. Depilatories are associated with higher wound infection rates.
    E. If hair is not removed for cosmetic reasons, the sutures should be removed within 5 days.

74. Which of the following statements is true regarding laceration repair?
    A. Wound antiseptics containing detergent are preferred to clean open wounds.
    B. Most wounds can be adequately cleaned with normal saline alone.
    C. Povidone-iodine solution has been shown to have deleterious effects on wound healing.
    D. Vicryl and Dexon are associated with higher wound infection rates than plain gut or chromic sutures.
    E. Facial lacerations should be repaired with layered closures whenever possible.

75. The most common pathogen causing osteomyelitis of the foot following a puncture wound is:
    A. *Pseudomonas.*
    B. *S. aureus.*
    C. *Streptococcus.*
    D. *Salmonella*
    E. *S. epidermidis.*

ANSWERS   [See Barkin et al: Chapters 27-32.]

1. The answer is **C,** page 387.
   When splinting the wrist and hand, placing the hand in the correct position of function is important to minimize joint stiffness following removal of the splint.

2. The answer is **D,** pages 387 and 394 to 395.
   The patient has a boxer's fracture, a common injury. Since the fracture is nondisplaced, no reduction is necessary and an ulnar gutter splint, with outpatient orthopedic referral, is the appropriate treatment.

3. The answer is **A,** pages 382 to 384.
   A Salter-Harris type II fracture is the most common type of fracture seen in children that involves the growth plate and is treated with reduction and immobilization. (See Fig. 24-2.)

4. The answer is **E,** pages 382 to 389.
   The patient clinically has a Salter-Harris type I fracture of the distal radius. These fractures are difficult to diagnose radiographically if there is no displacement. In this example, there is no displacement, and reduction is not necessary. Treatment is immobilization, usually for 3 to 4 weeks, with outpatient orthopedic follow-up.

5. The answer is **B,** page 381.
   Ligaments around major joints in children are much stronger and more resistant to tensile forces than the adjacent epiphyseal plate. Therefore dislocations are uncommon in children, and epiphyseal displacements or apophyseal avulsions are seen much more frequently.

6. The answer is **B,** pages 391 to 394.
   Extending the wrist with mild ulnar deviation allows the scaphoid to slip out from beneath the styloid process of the radius, making it easily palpable in the anatomic snuffbox.

7. The answer is **C,** page 394.
   As in adults, the scaphoid is the most commonly fractured carpal bone in children. It is the largest bone in the proximal row of carpals and forms the floor of the anatomic snuffbox.

8. The answer is **E,** page 392.
   The median nerve consistently supplies sensation to the palmar surface of the index finger and frequently supplies the distal dorsal surface of the index finger as well. (See Figs. 24-3 and 24-4 on page 130.)

9. The answer is **D,** page 392.
   Two-point discrimination is important to perform in order to pick up subtle neuronal injuries that are not apparent on gross sensory testing (e.g., pin prick, light touch).

10. The answer is **E,** pages 392 and 393.
    This maneuver establishes intactness of the radial nerve at the level of the digits and should always be performed to establish distal motor radial nerve integrity. This test should be performed with the PIP joints in *flexion* to prevent compensatory assistance from the intrinsic muscles of the hand.

11. The answer is **A,** page 393.
    The flexor digitorum superficialis is the primary flexor of the finger's PIP joint and is supplied by the median nerve.

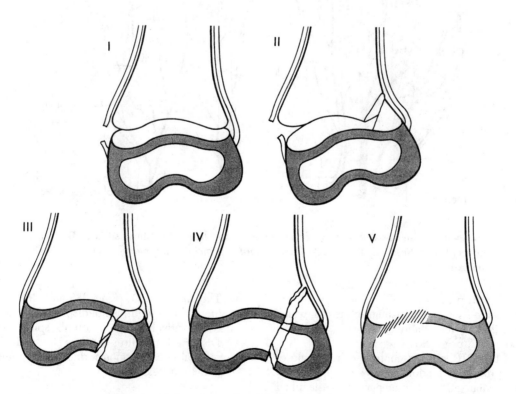

FIG. 24-2   Salter-Harris classification of epiphyseal fractures.

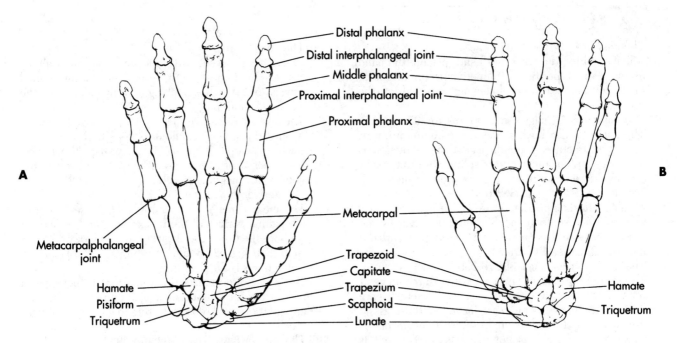

FIG. 24-3   Bones of the right hand. **A,** Palmar surface. **B,** Dorsal surface. (From Fess EE, Philips CA: *Hand splinting, principles and methods,* ed 2, St Louis, 1987, Mosby.)

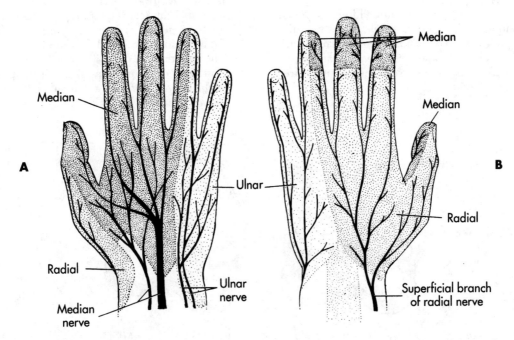

FIG. 24-4   Cutaneous distribution of the nerves of the hand. **A,** Palmar surface. **B,** Dorsal surface. (From Fess EE, Philips CA: *Hand splinting, principles and methods,* ed 2, St Louis, 1987, Mosby.)

12. The answer is **B,** page 393.
    The ulnar nerve supplies the palmar interossei, which are responsible for finger adduction.

13. The answer is **C,** page 393.
    Flexion of the DIP joints is controlled by the flexor digitorum profundus tendons. They are supplied by both the median nerve (lateral part) and the ulnar nerve (medial part).

14. The answer is **D,** pages 388 and 394.
    Since this fracture is nondisplaced, it can be managed conservatively with a thumb spica splint or cast. Displaced fractures require immediate orthopedic referral because open reduction and internal fixation may be necessary.

15. The answer is **C**, page 396.

CMC joint dislocations usually are dorsal dislocations involving the thumb. Closed reduction is usually accomplished easily, followed by the application of a thumb spica cast. *Unstable* injuries usually require internal fixation to prevent long-term complications.

16. The answer is **E**, page 397.

Gamekeeper's thumb is a hyperextension injury of the MCP joint of the thumb resulting in instability of the ulnar collateral ligament. Radial deviation of the thumb exacerbates the pain. Treatment involves the application of a thumb spica splint or cast with orthopedic follow-up.

17. The answer is **E**, page 398.

The boutonniere deformity is secondary to a disruption of the central slip of the extensor tendon at the PIP joint with concomitant volar subluxation of the lateral bands of the tendon. The DIP joint is held in extension while the PIP is held in flexion. Management is conservative, such as splinting of the involved finger with outpatient orthopedic follow-up.

18. The answer is **B**, pages 403 and 404.

Clavicular fractures are common birth injuries, most frequent with vaginal breech deliveries. Rarely, such injuries require a sling for comfort shortly after birth, but once callus formation has occurred, no further treatment is necessary.

19. The answer is **A**, pages 403 and 404.

The clavicle is the most frequently fractured bone in childhood, usually associated with birth injuries or *low*-energy trauma. The clavicle usually fractures at the junction of the middle and lateral thirds of the bone, causing it to bow *anteriorly* and making the fractured side more prominent on physical examination.

20. The answer is **C**, page 405.

The patient most likely has an acromioclavicular sprain. A posteroanterior (PA) chest film will allow comparison of the space between clavicle and acromion on the affected and nonaffected sides. If the x-ray is normal, it can be repeated with the patient holding a weight to enhance the sensitivity of making the diagnosis. For first- and second-degree injuries, when acromioclavicular separation is less than 1 cm, the patient should be treated with a sling and swathe, with orthopedic follow-up. (See Fig. 24-5.)

21. The answer is **B**, pages 405 to 407.

This patient has an anterior shoulder dislocation, a common orthopedic injury. The axillary nerve may be involved, resulting in decreased sensation over the deltoid. Vascular injuries are uncommon. Most anterior shoulder dislocations can be easily reduced in the ED by a variety of techniques. Following reduction the patient should be placed in a sling and swathe, with orthopedic follow-up.

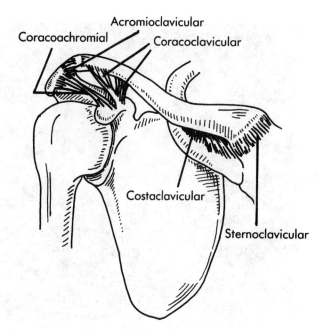

FIG. 24-5 Ligaments of the acromioclavicular joint. (From Jackimczyk KC, Goy W: *Musculoskeletal trauma.* In Rosen P, Doris PE, Barkin RM, et al: *Diagnostic radiology in emergency medicine,* St Louis, 1992, Mosby.)

22. The answer is **D**, pages 405 to 407.

Anterior shoulder dislocations are secondary to indirect trauma to the arm, causing abduction and extension of the shoulder and disrupting the joint capsule. This injury is more common in adolescents and adults than young children, and 95% are *anterior* dislocations. Recurrences are not uncommon. However, there is no increased risk in the uninvolved extremity. (See Fig. 24-6 on page 132.)

23. The answer is **A**, page 407.

The patient has a rotator cuff injury, which initially is treated conservatively with sling immobilization. X-rays are rarely helpful in making the diagnosis. There is no indication for steroid injection in the ED, and an arthrogram should be considered only if the patient has severe and persistent weakness.

24. The answer is **A**, pages 407 and 408.

The mechanism of injury in this patient suggests a proximal humeral fracture. It may be difficult to diagnose on x-ray examination, and both AP and lateral views of the shoulder must be obtained. Passive range of motion should be avoided, since this will only worsen the pain and can cause axillary nerve damage. These injuries are usually treated conservatively with a sling and swathe, unless there is significant separation, angulation, or malrotation of the epiphyseal fragment.

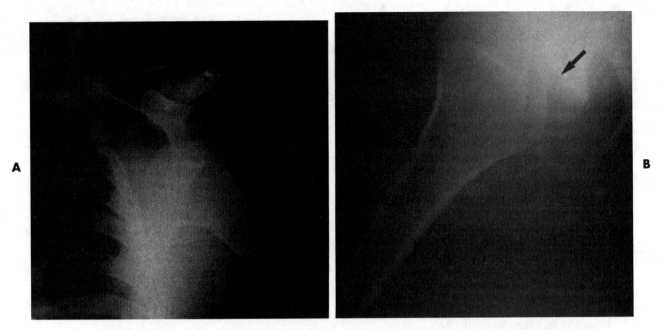

FIG. 24-6   Anterior dislocation of the shoulder becomes more common in adolescence. **A,** Anteroposterior view. **B,** Axillary view demonstrates displacement of the humeral head from the glenoid. Note the humeral head is anterior to the anterior rim of the glenoid fossa. (From Jackimczyk KC, Goy W: *Musculoskeletal trauma.* In Rosen P, Doris PE, Barkin RM, et al: *Diagnostic radiology in emergency medicine,* St Louis, 1992, Mosby.)

25. The answer is **C,** pages 408 and 409.
    Humeral shaft fractures are uncommon in children because the proximal and distal cartilaginous structures are more likely to fail. The middle third is the most common location of fractures, and radial nerve injuries are associated with anesthesia of the dorsum of the hand and weakness of wrist and finger extensors. Child abuse usually results in spiral fractures. Uncomplicated fractures are treated with immobilization (sling and swathe or long arm splint) with close outpatient orthopedic follow-up.

26. The answer is **A,** page 409.
    Supracondylar fractures are the most frequent elbow fracture in children, peaking between the ages of 3 and 10. These fractures have the potential for serious neurovascular compromise and require prompt and appropriate evaluation and management. (See Fig. 24-7 on page 133.)

27. The answer is **C,** pages 409 to 411.
    Supracondylar fractures of the humerus can become orthopedic emergencies because of vascular compromise. This requires immediate evaluation of distal neurovascular function to determine the need for immediate orthopedic consultation. Following this evaluation, the elbow should be splinted in *extension,* and x-rays and orthopedic consultation obtained. If not treated appropriately, these fractures can cause a compartment syndrome, resulting in muscle necrosis and subsequent fibrosis with a permanent disability known as Volkmann's contracture.

28. The answer is **C,** pages 409 to 411.
    With supracondylar fractures, forearm pain is suggestive of increased pressure within the volar fascial compartment of the forearm. Exacerbation of this pain by passive extension of the fingers is a useful finding of early vascular compromise. Loss of distal pulses is a late finding as are distal sensory and motor neurologic abnormalities.

29. The answer is **C,** pages 409 to 411.
    A small anterior fat pad sign is frequently seen in normal individuals. This patient has full range of motion at the elbow with minimal tenderness. There is no evidence of a fracture on x-ray and no *posterior* fat pad sign, which should always raise the suspicion of a fracture. There is no clinical or x-ray evidence of a joint effusion, and there is no indication to perform arthrocentesis.

30. The answer is **B,** pages 413 and 414.
    Volkmann's contracture and neurovascular compromise are seen commonly in children with elbow dislocations or supracondylar fractures. The elbow has little osseous stability in children, and it is frequently dislocated, particularly from age 8 years through adolescence. Spontaneous reductions are common, and x-rays may reveal only an associated fracture or effusion. Closed reduction should be performed on an urgent or emergency basis depending on the presence of neurovascular compromise.

31. The answer is **E,** pages 414 and 415.
    "Nursemaid's elbow" or radial head subluxation is common in children between the ages of 6 months and 5 years. X-rays are not helpful in making the diagnosis, and return to normal function following reduction rules out associated injuries.

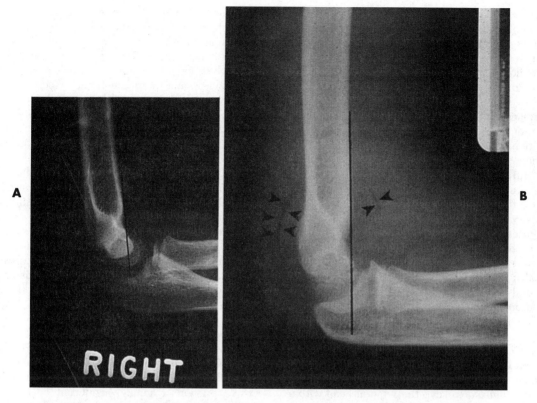

FIG. 24-7 **A,** Normal lateral radiograph of the elbow. The anterior fat pad is visible adjacent to the humerus, and the posterior fat pad is not seen. **B,** Greenstick supracondylar fracture. The posterior fat pad is visible, and the anterior fat pad is displaced anteriorly. Posterior angulation of the distal humerus causes the anterior humeral line to intersect the capitellum in its anterior portion.

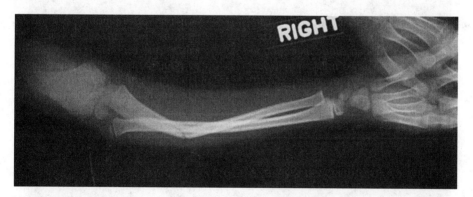

FIG. 24-8 Monteggia's fracture-dislocation. Isolated fracture of the ulna is uncommon. Dislocation of the radial head must be suspected. (From Jackimczyk KC, Goy W: *Musculoskeletal trauma.* In Rosen P, Doris PE, Barkin RM, et al: *Diagnostic radiology in emergency medicine,* St Louis, 1992, Mosby.)

32. The answer is **C,** pages 416 and 417.
A Monteggia's fracture includes a proximal ulnar fracture associated with anterior dislocation of the radial head. There may also be associated wrist injuries. All children with ulnar fractures must have x-rays of both the wrist and elbow to rule out associated injuries, since an isolated fracture of the ulna is uncommon. (See Fig. 24-8.)

33. The answer is **A,** pages 421 and 422.
Isolated fractures of the pelvic ring occur more commonly in children because of the mobility of the sacroiliac joint and symphysis pubis. Massive hemorrhage is less common in pediatric pelvic fractures. The rectal examination is helpful in the clinical diagnosis of sacral and coccygeal injuries and should be performed with pelvic injuries. Pubic fractures typically result from high-velocity trauma and are not seen with trivial injuries.

34. The answer is **B,** page 422.

    The femoral neck of a child is strong. In contrast to adults, a *high-velocity* force, such as a motor vehicle accident, is required to fracture it. Hip fractures are rare in children. Routine AP and lateral films should be adequate to identify most injuries. Avascular necrosis of the femoral head is common, especially with displaced fractures.

35. The answer is **D,** page 423.

    This patient has a classic case of a posterior hip dislocation. Dislocations are frequently associated with fractures, especially of the posterior wall of the acetabulum. In contrast, a hip fracture typically involves a hip in *external* rotation and *abduction*. Sciatic nerve injuries do occur, but in 10% or less of such injuries. This injury is more common in children younger than 5 years of age because of ligament laxity.

36. The answer is **E,** page 423.

    Legg-Calvé-Perthes disease is avascular necrosis of the femoral head. It usually occurs in children 5 to 9 years old and is more common in boys. The disease may follow injury to the hip. The knee is a common site for referred pain. On examination there is pain with *passive* range of motion and limited hip movement, particularly internal rotation and abduction. Management includes minimal weight bearing with the femur *abducted* to keep the femoral head within the acetabulum. (See Fig. 24-9.)

37. The answer is **D,** pages 423 and 424.

    Referred pain to the knee is common with hip problems in children. Slipped capital femoral epiphysis is common in boys 12 to 15 years old and may include knee pain. Symptoms may be acute or gradual in onset, and there may be no associated injury. Both hips may also be affected. Legg-Calvé-Perthes disease is uncommon at this age and also would require x-rays of the hip for evaluation.

38. The answer is **B,** pages 424 to 425 and 605 to 606.

    Indirect rotational force is frequently responsible for spiral femoral fractures in young children. The child typically catches his foot (e.g., between the bars of a crib) and then falls, resulting in a twisting motion of the femur. Spiral fractures typically have minimal swelling and deformity and are not suspected until the child refuses to bear weight. Significant blood loss is unusual. Epiphyseal-metaphyseal fractures are virtually pathognomonic of child abuse. This fracture may also occur with child abuse, and this should be considered when the mechanism of injury cannot explain the fracture.

39. The answer is **C,** pages 426 and 427.

    The most common ligamentous injury of the knee in childhood involves the medial collateral ligament, and it frequently occurs during contact sports. In contrast to previous teaching, significant ligamentous injury can occur in a child with open physes. Most tense acute hemarthroses (approximately 85%) are caused by anterior cruciate ligament injuries. Surgical correction is rarely necessary, even for third-degree sprains.

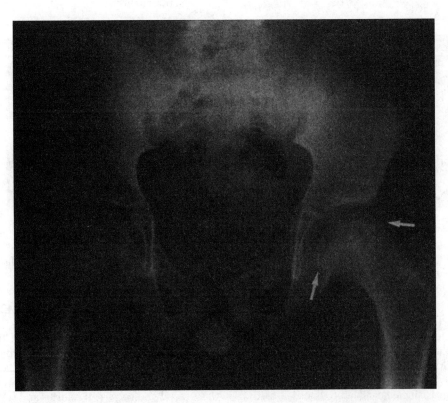

FIG. 24-9   Legg-Calvé-Perthes disease, anteroposterior view. Involved femoral head is flattened and mottled *(arrows).* (From Jackimczyk KC, Goy W: *Musculoskeletal trauma.* In Rosen P, Doris PE, Barkin RM, et al: *Diagnostic radiology in emergency medicine,* St Louis, 1992, Mosby.)

40. The answer is **B,** pages 426 and 427.

Anterior cruciate ligament (ACL) injury is usually secondary to forcible hyperextension or sudden deceleration with the foot flexed, causing abduction and external rotation of the leg. A loud pop is frequently heard, and 85% of acute tense hemarthroses are secondary to ACL tears.

41. The answer is **C,** page 427.

Osgood-Schlatter disease is generally seen in early adolescence in active children 11 to 15 years of age. It results from repetitive microscopic injury that produces inflammation of the apophysis of the tibial tubercle and *partial* avulsion and separation of the tibial tubercle. *Complete* avulsion of the tibial tubercle results from forceful contraction of the quadriceps muscle (as in jumping), which has an increased incidence in association with Osgood-Schlatter disease. It is important to distinguish between the two because complete disruption of the tibial tubercle may require open reduction and pinning.

42. The answer is **D,** pages 429 to 432.

The ligament most commonly injured with inversion stress is the anterior talofibular ligament. Of lateral ligament sprains, 65% are restricted to the anterior talofibular ligament and 20% have concomitant calcaneofibular ligament tears. The posterior talofibular ligament is the strongest of the lateral ligaments and is injured only in severe sprains. (See Fig. 24-10.)

43. The answer is **A,** pages 430 and 431.

The talar tilt test evaluates the integrity of the anterior talofibular ligament and the calcaneofibular ligament. The examiner stabilizes the patient's leg and firmly *inverts* the foot to determine the degree of talar tilt. A 10-degree difference between the affected and contralateral side is considered significant. During the acute period, there may be *false negative* findings caused by muscle spasm and swelling. (See Fig. 24-11 on page 136.)

44. The answer is **B,** pages 432 and 433.

Fractures of the distal tibial physis are most common, comprising nearly 10% of all physeal injuries. It is also one of the weakest components of the ankle joint. Isolated fractures through the physis of the distal fibula are uncommon. Growth disturbances rarely occur with Salter I and II injuries; *Salter V* fractures have the worst prognosis.

45. The answer is **E,** pages 433 and 434.

Although relatively uncommon, fractures of the calcaneus are the most frequent tarsal injuries in children. Children younger than 3 years old may fracture the calcaneus with relatively minor trauma. Most are secondary to a fall from a height, and there may be associated spinal injuries. (See Fig. 24-12 on page 136.)

46. The answer is **D,** pages 434 to 436.

S. aureus is the causative agent in the majority of cases. *Pseudomonas* rarely causes cellulitis after a puncture wound and is more commonly associated with deep space infections such as osteomyelitis and septic arthritis.

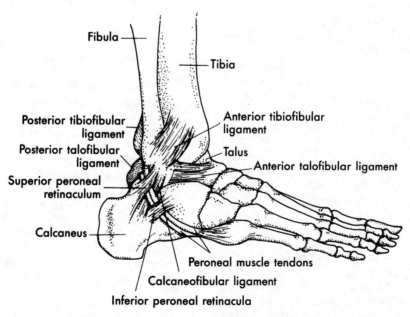

FIG. 24-10 Lateral view of the ankle showing the lateral ligaments (anterior talofibular, calcaneofibular, posterior talofibular), as well as the anterior and posterior tibiofibular ligaments, which contribute to the tibiofibular syndesmosis. (From Hergenroeder AC: *Am J Dis Child* 144:809, 1990.)

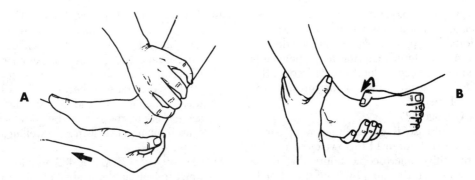

FIG. 24-11 Tests for joint stability. **A,** The anterior drawer test. **B,** The talar tilt test. (From Hergenroeder AC: *Am J Dis Child* 144:809, 1990.)

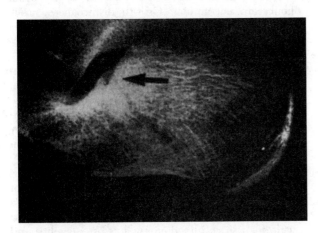

FIG. 24-12 Intraarticular fracture of the calcaneus. (From Ogden JA: *Skeletal injury in the child,* ed 2, Philadelphia, 1990, WB Saunders.)

47. The answer is **C,** pages 434 to 436.
Deep space infections are usually caused by *Pseudomonas* and generally come several days after injury. Typically there are few systemic signs of infection. Puncture wounds near the metatarsophalangeal joint may penetrate more deeply because of the weight-bearing nature of this area.

48. The answer is **D,** pages 434 to 436 and 953 to 954.
A puncture wound is considered to be prone to tetanus. Since this patient received his initial childhood immunizations, tetanus immune globulin is not indicated. However, since his last booster was longer than 5 years ago, a Td booster is indicated.

49. The answer is **B,** pages 454 and 455.
The posterior tibial nerve runs lateral and posterior to the posterior tibial artery. Solutions containing epinephrine should *not* be used for this block.

50. The answer is **B,** page 444.
The maximum dose of lidocaine without epinephrine that should be used for infiltration is 4 mg/kg. For a 20-kg child the total dose would be 80 mg or 8 ml of a 1% lidocaine solution (10 mg/ml).

51. The answer is **C,** page 392.
The superficial branch of the radial nerve supplies the dorsal surfaces of the thumb, index, and middle fingers at least as far as their distal IP joints, and also innervates the whole dorsum of the hand lying on the radial side of the third metacarpal. (See question 4, Fig. 24-4 on page 130.)

52. The answer is **B,** page 397.
This patient has a mallet finger caused by injury of the extensor tendon at its attachment to the DIP joint. In the absence of a significant fracture, splinting the DIP joint in mild hyperextension with a dorsal or ventral splint is adequate.

53. The answer is **A,** page 398.
The patient most likely has a "jersey finger," which is an avulsion of the flexor digitorum profundus tendon. It is most frequently seen in contact sports when one player's finger catches on another's shirt or jersey. This injury requires surgical referral and repair.

54. The answer is **E,** page 399.
Nailbed lacerations often complicate distal tuft crush injuries and usually need to be repaired. However, recent data suggest that if the nail and its borders are intact and there is no associated fracture, the nail does not have to be removed to search for a nailbed laceration regardless of the size of the subungual hematoma. Nailbed lacerations are repaired with *absorbable* sutures. Subungual hematomas should always be drained. Tuft fractures are common in children, and as in adults, typically require only conservative treatment.

55. The answer is **B,** page 398.
If the digital artery has been injured (identified by pulsating blood flow), it should be assumed that the nerve is also injured because the nerve lies superficial to the artery. The artery should never be clamped, since the nerve may become damaged. In children the digital nerve should be repaired as far as the DIP joint, and the results are usually excellent.

56. The answer is **E,** pages 399 to 400.
    Since fingers contain essentially no muscle tissue, successful reimplantation of *cooled* tissue can occur up to 24 hours after amputation. Amputated parts are wrapped in sterile gauze that has been *soaked* in an isotonic solution before being sealed in a plastic bag and placed in ice water. Reimplantation of single digits is indicated especially for the index finger. Distal *soft tissue* amputations heal well by *secondary intention* after good cleaning and debridement.

57. The answer is **A,** page 400.
    Frostbitten areas need to be *rapidly* rewarmed, preferably with *warm* water (40° to 42° C).

58. The answer is **B,** pages 400 and 401.
    A felon must be treated aggressively with surgical drainage and antibiotics even if fluctuance is not present. Longitudinal incisions are advocated to avoid iatrogenic complications (e.g., neurovascular compromise and scarring).

59. The answer is **E,** page 405.
    Scapular fractures are rare in children and usually associated with high-energy trauma or crushing injuries. Most fractures are not displaced and occur along the lateral border involving the acromion, coracoid, or glenoid.

60. The answer is **A,** pages 405 and 406.
    In addition to fracture of the greater tuberosity, shoulder dislocations may be associated with injuries to the glenoid capsule—a Hill-Sachs compression fracture of the posterior humeral head, and damage of the *axillary* artery and nerve.

61. The answer is **C,** page 407.
    In addition to the supraspinatus, infraspinatus, and teres minor, the subscapularis is included by many authors as part of the rotator cuff or "SITS" muscle group.

62. The answer is **A,** page 409.
    The vast majority (more than 90%) of supracondylar fractures result from hyperextension such as a fall on an outstretched hand with the elbow locked in extension.

63. The answer is **E,** page 409.
    The most feared complication of supracondylar fractures, Volkmann's contracture, is secondary to entrapment or injury to the brachial artery, resulting in ischemia and subsequent necrosis of muscles of the forearm.

64. The answer is **B,** pages 409 to 411.
    Immobilization is important with supracondylar fractures to prevent secondary injury to soft tissues, nerves, and vessels. However, excessive flexion of the elbow can compromise perfusion, and the arm should be secured with no more than 20 to 30 degrees of flexion. The splint should not be applied tightly, to allow frequent and accurate assessment of neurovascular function.

65. The answer is **C,** pages 413 and 414. Elbow dislocations in children are posterior. In contrast to a supracondylar fracture, which may seem similar, there is shortening of the forearm and posterior prominence of the olecranon.

66. The answer is **C,** pages 414 and 415.

67. The answer is **B,** pages 419 and 420.
    Forearm fractures are common in childhood, second only to fractures of the clavicle. Complications including compartment syndrome and nerve injuries are uncommon. Isolated fractures rarely occur, and there is usually a subtle greenstick or plastic deformation fracture of the other bone or an associated dislocation. Therefore always include the wrist and elbow in radiographs. Greenstick fractures require overcorrection or completion of the fracture to prevent subsequent angulation.

68. The answer is **C,** pages 421 to 423.
    Most hip fractures in children are either transcervical (femoral neck) or cervicotrochanteric. Transepiphyseal injuries are rare. Injuries can significantly affect growth potential of the femur. Avascular necrosis occurs in displaced *and* nondisplaced fractures.

69. The answer is **D,** pages 423, 1025, and 1032.
    Toxic synovitis is a benign cause of hip pain in children, thought to be secondary to nonspecific inflammation and hypertrophy of the synovial membrane. It is seen in children until skeletal maturity, 1½ to 7 years of age, with a peak incidence at 2 years of age. The child usually has a limp with minimal or no pain on abduction and external rotation of the hip. It is a diagnosis of exclusion once more serious causes (e.g., septic arthritis, osteomyelitis) have been ruled out.

70. The answer is **A,** pages 426 and 427.
    Injury to the menisci occurs when a twisting motion is applied to the knee when it is flexed. The McMurray test duplicates this motion. A clicking noise on external rotation indicates a tear of the medial meniscus, and on internal rotation, injury to the lateral meniscus.

71. The answer is **A,** page 427.
    Patellar dislocation is common in adolescent girls, probably for anatomic reasons. It is the second most common cause of acute hemarthrosis (anterior cruciate ligament tears are first). Reduction is performed by relaxing the quadriceps by *flexing* the hip and extending the knee (straight leg raise) with gentle pressure on the patella. Dislocations are almost always lateral, and following reduction, the knee is immobilized in extension.

72. The answer is **E,** pages 429 to 432.
    Medial injuries to the ankle involve the *deltoid* ligament and follow an eversion stress. They are far less common than inversion injuries, which involve the lateral ligaments. The talar tilt test assesses the integrity of the lateral ligaments. Greater force is required to injure the deltoid ligament. Therefore these injuries are usually more serious than inversion injuries.

73. The answer is **C,** pages 443 and 444.
    In most wounds, including the scalp, hair removal is not necessary and does not increase infection rate. Shaving should be avoided because this has been shown to increase infection rate. Depilatories are good agents for hair removal and are associated with a much lower infection rate than shaving.

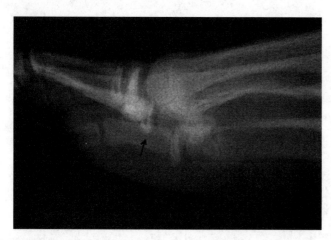

FIG. 24-13   Radiograph showing periosteal new bone in a case of osteomyelitis of the foot following a puncture wound. Cultures in this case were positive for *Pseudomonas aeruginosa*.

74. The answer is **E,** pages 440 and 446.
    Layered closures on the face improve cosmetic outcome and should be used whenever possible. Normal saline is an excellent irrigating solution but has no antibacterial activity. Wound antiseptics should *not* contain detergents because these have been associated with tissue necrosis. *Povidone-iodine solution* is an excellent antiseptic with relatively few toxic effects. Some authorities recommend diluting 10% povidone-iodine solution to a 1% solution before irrigating. Plain gut and chromic sutures are associated with higher infection rates than Vicryl or Dexon absorbable sutures.

75. The answer is **A,** page 455.
    P. aeruginosa frequently colonizes tennis shoes, which may contribute to its frequency as a cause of osteomyelitis following a deep puncture wound of the foot. Cellulitis is a much more common complication of puncture wounds. *S. aureus* is the usual pathogen. (See Fig. 24-13.)

Animal and Human Bites

Cathy Schwartz

See Barkin et al: Chapter 33.

1. A mother notices bite marks on her 3-year-old son's right hand. The nanny is not sure how the wound occurred but thinks either the 5-year-old sister or the 2-year-old brother may have done it. The family has no pets. The distance between the center of the canine teeth on the bite wound is 4 cm. The biter is most likely:
   A. A neighbor's dog
   B. The younger brother.
   C. The older sister.
   D. The nanny or other adult.
   E. A mouse.

2. A 2-year-old girl is bitten on the arm by a squirrel in the park. Which of the following therapeutic options is most appropriate?
   A. Suture the wound.
   B. Culture the wound and wait for culture results before starting antibiotics.
   C. Treat with oral penicillin only.
   D. Initiate rabies treatment.
   E. Irrigate the wound with 100 ml of normal saline.

3. A 10-year-old boy comes in with a small cat bite. He is allergic to penicillin. The best choice for a prophylactic antibiotic in this patient is:
   A. No antibiotic, since it is a very small wound.
   B. Amoxicillin–clavulanic acid after penicillin desensitization.
   C. Erythromycin.
   D. Trimethoprim-sulfamethoxazole.
   E. Tetracycline.

4. Which of the following animals should be killed and have its brain examined for rabies after it bites a person?
   A. A ferret.
   B. A dog.
   C. A hamster.
   D. A gerbil.
   E. A rat.

5. A 12-year-old boy has a painful hand and a laceration over the fifth metacarpophalangeal joint after a fight at school. Which of the following statements regarding this injury is true?
   A. The children involved must be tested for HIV.
   B. The hand should be x-rayed.
   C. The wound should be sutured.
   D. An appropriate antibiotic would cover *Pasteurella multocida*.
   E. The patient must receive a tetanus booster.

6. Which of the following is the most appropriate treatment for a dog bite in the periorbital region?
   A. The patient should be referred to an ophthalmologist.
   B. The wound should be irrigated with antibiotics.
   C. Prophylactic antibiotics need not be prescribed.
   D. Intravenous (IV) antibiotics should be administered to prevent meningitis that may result from the ensuing periorbital cellulitis.

7. Which of the following statements concerning dog bites is true?
   A. The infection rate is 30%.
   B. The bite should never be sutured.
   C. Prophylactic antibiotics will prevent infection and are recommended for all dog bites.
   D. The most common infecting organisms are *P. multocida* and *Staphylococcus aureus*.
   E. Dog bites occur mainly on the extremities in children.

8. Which of the following is true about cat bites and scratches?
   A. Boys are bitten twice as often as girls.
   B. About 10% of cat bites and scratches become infected.
   C. Almost 90% of cat wounds near the eye are associated with corneal abrasions.
   D. Irrigation of cat bites with a syringe and needle effectively prevents infection from occurring.
   E. Cats transmit rabies more often than dogs in the United States.

1. The answer is **D,** page 460.

The suspicion of child abuse should be considered in any child with a human bite. Bruise marks left from the bite can be measured to determine whether a young child or an older person caused the bite. The distance between the center of the canine teeth (the third tooth on either side separated by four central incisors) should be measured in centimeters. If the distance is greater than 3 cm, the biter has permanent teeth. If the distance is less than 3 cm, the biter has primary teeth. Bite mark evidence has been admitted in courts of law.

2. The answer is **E,** page 461.

Thorough cleaning is the most important factor in reducing infections of bite wounds. Oral penicillin is not the antibiotic of choice for bite wounds. Other antibiotics such as amoxicillin-clavulanate should be considered. Squirrels are not known to transmit rabies in the United States. Primary suturing of animal bites is generally not recommended.

3. The answer is **D,** page 462.

Patients with cat bites should be treated with an antibiotic because of the difficulty in cleaning puncture wounds and the high rate of associated infections. An appropriate antibiotic should cover *P. multocida;* erythromycin does not. In a patient not allergic to penicillin, amoxicillin-clavulanate would be an excellent choice.

4. The answer is **A,** page 462.

Rabid pet ferrets have been reported in the United States, but no rabies vaccine is available for ferrets. Because the natural history of rabies in ferrets is unknown, quarantine is not thought to be reliable, and it is recommended that the animal be sacrificed and the brain examined. Rabbits and rodents (rats, mice, gerbils, hamsters, and squirrels) are not known to transmit rabies in the United States. A dog can be observed for 10 days to see if it exhibits any signs of rabies.

5. The answer is **B,** pages 460 to 462.

The fifth metacarpal bone is often fractured in fistfights. Although HIV has been isolated in human saliva, this route is considered to be low risk by the Centers for Disease Control and Prevention. In general, bites should be left open, especially in wounds at high risk for infection. A serious infection in closed-fist injuries may occur when bacteria are introduced into the joint space on an extensor tendon by an incisor puncture. Appropriate antibiotics should cover *S. aureus, Streptococcus,* and anaerobes. A tetanus booster is usually not needed in school age children from the United States, since schools require immunizations be up to date.

6. The answer is **A,** page 462.

Bites in the periorbital area that may involve ocular structures should be referred to an ophthalmologist. The eye should be evaluated for repair of the lacrimal gland and treatment of corneal abrasions. Studies involving the irrigation of bite wounds with antibiotics or IV administration of prophylactic antibiotics are inconclusive. Good wound cleaning and debridement are the most important factors for reducing infection.

7. The answer is **D,** pages 460 to 462.

Dog bites have a low infection rate (2% to 5%) despite the crushing nature of the injury. Primary repair may be attempted in an area in which unsightly scarring might result. This should be tried only in bites that occurred a few hours before the patient came into the ED and after thorough cleaning. Deep puncture wounds that are difficult to clean should never be closed. The head and neck are involved in 58% of dog bites in children.

8. The answer is **E,** pages 459 to 462.

Cats transmit rabies more frequently than dogs. Even a cat scratch contaminated with saliva can cause transmission. Wounds caused by cats occur more often in girls. Approximately 40% of cat bites become infected despite initial cleaning. This happens because cat bites tend to be small but potentially deep puncture wounds. Corneal abrasions are associated with 40% of cat wounds near the eye.

26

Venomous Animal Bites and Stings

Stuart M. Caplen

See Barkin et al: Chapter 34.

1. Which of the following is true regarding snakebites?
   A. Between October and May is when 90% of envenomations occur.
   B. Snakebites most commonly occur on the feet and toes.
   C. Children are the most common victims of snakebite.
   D. Elapidae (coral snakes) are found in Arizona and the southern Gulf States.
   E. Snakebites are frequently fatal.

2. Which is true regarding identification of snakes?
   A. Crotalidae (pit vipers) have round pupils.
   B. Coral snakes all have yellow rings next to red rings.
   C. Pit vipers have a round head.
   D. Coral snakes have vertical elliptical pupils.
   E. *Agkistrodon* (copperheads and water moccasins) have terminal rattles on their tails.

3. A 6-year-old boy has been bitten by a rattlesnake. Which one of the following statements regarding this problem is *true?*
   A. The snakebite should be packed in ice to decrease venom toxicity.
   B. An arterial tourniquet is recommended.
   C. Excessive activity of the victim may increase venom toxicity.
   D. Symptoms may not occur for up to 6 hours.
   E. Coma and seizures are common within the first hour after a bite.

4. A 3-year-old girl is bitten by a pit viper on the right leg. There is some local swelling and severe pain. A lymphatic constriction band has been placed on the extremity. Treatment of this patient would include which one of the following?
   A. Perform a prophylactic fasciotomy.
   B. Administer ultrapurified antivenin to prevent serum sickness.
   C. Administer 15 vials of antivenin.
   D. Administer an antivenin skin test. A positive test is an absolute contraindication to administering antivenin to the patient.
   E. Administer a larger dose of antivenin than you would give an adult.

5. Which one of the following statements regarding pit viper therapy is *true?*
   A. Hyperbaric oxygen is considered definitive therapy.
   B. Corticosteroids have been shown to decrease damage from snake venom and should be given routinely.
   C. Direct current electric shocks have decreased tissue damage from snake venom experimentally.
   D. Colloids are superior to crystalloids in the treatment of venom shock.
   E. Incision of the bite and suction of serum are effective for removing venom up to 2 hours after the bite.

6. Which of the following is true regarding pit viper bites?
   A. All patients should receive antivenin.
   B. Serum sickness is uncommon after antivenin treatment.
   C. Respiratory muscle paralysis is common after envenomation.
   D. In 20% of snakebites there is no envenomation.
   E. Acetaminophen will potentiate the venom.

7. Which of the following statements regarding coral snake envenomation is *true?*
   A. Local edema and swelling are characteristic.
   B. Antivenin should be given for all suspected envenomations.
   C. Coagulation and bleeding problems are characteristic of severe envenomation.
   D. Incision and suction have proved to be helpful.

8. A 2-year-old boy is stung by a scorpion. There is mild central nervous system stimulation. Proper management of this condition includes which one of the following?
   A. Warm compresses.
   B. Meperidine for pain.
   C. Naloxone as a direct antagonist.
   D. Phenobarbital.
   E. Diazepam.

9. A 10-year-old boy with a *Latrodectus* (black widow spider) bite on the left hand is complaining of severe stomach pain. Which of the following statements regarding his diagnosis and treatment is *true?*
   A. There is a specific monoclonal antibody test that can confirm the diagnosis of black widow spider envenomation.
   B. Antivenin should be given routinely to all children younger than 12.
   C. Diazepam can be given intravenously for muscle contractions.
   D. Ulceration at the site of the bite is common.
   E. Human antivenin is available and should be used in this case.
10. A *Loxosceles reclusa* (brown recluse spider) bite:
   A. Causes severe pain at the time of the bite.
   B. Produces a diffuse macular rash 12 to 18 hours after it happens.
   C. Produces only local skin symptoms.
   D. Produces a vesicle surrounded by an ischemic ring.
   E. Is commonly found in the northeastern United States.
11. A 7-year-old boy in St. Louis, who was crawling in a closet, is bitten by a brown recluse spider on the right thigh. Treatment would include:
   A. Dapsone.
   B. Hydrocortisone.
   C. Prophylactic antibiotics.
   D. Heparin.
   E. Urokinase.
12. Which of the following is true regarding centipedes and millipedes?
   A. Both have one pair of legs per body segment.
   B. Millipede bites typically result in lymphangitis.
   C. Centipede bites can be treated with antivenin.
   D. Millipede toxin causes a contact dermatitis.
   E. Millipede bites are treated with intradermal calcium gluconate.

13. A 2-year-old girl is seen after being stung by a Portuguese man-of-war. The tentacles are still attached to the skin. The correct method of removal is to:
   A. Wash with sterile water.
   B. Wash with sodium bicarbonate.
   C. Wash with vinegar.
   D. Wash with soap and water.
   E. Wash with milk.
14. A 10-year-old boy steps on a stingray and has a barb in his right foot. Management of this problem would include:
   A. Injecting sodium bicarbonate around the wound.
   B. Immersing the limb in hot water.
   C. Delaying removal of the barb until 48 hours after the injury.
   D. Soaking the wound in calcium gluconate.
15. Which of the following is true with respect to marine envenomations?
   A. Initial treatment for sea urchin envenomation is to put ice packs on the affected area.
   B. Granulomas are common after a sea urchin envenomation.
   C. Catfish and lionfish envenomate by specialized fangs in front of their mouths.
   D. Sea urchin envenomation is mostly local with necrosis common.
   E. Lionfish envenomations are painless with severe systemic toxicity.

ANSWERS [See Barkin et al: Chapter 34.]

1. The answer is **D,** page 465.
   Because snakes hibernate during the winter, 90% of snake envenomations occur between April and October; 80% of snakebites occur on the hands and fingers, 15% on the ankles and feet. Young men ages 18 to 28 account for 50% of all snakebites, frequently in association with alcohol intoxication. There are an estimated 45,000 snakebites per year in the United States, 12,000 to 15,000 being by venomous snakes. There have been only 1 to 2 deaths annually from snakebites since 1990. Coral snakes are found only in Arizona and the southern Gulf States.

2. The answer is **B,** page 465.
   Pit vipers have vertical elliptical pupils. They also have a triangular head with a pit located between the eye and nostril, as well as terminal rattles. Copperheads and water moccasins do not have rattles on their tail. Coral snakes have round pupils. They have a black snout and yellow rings alternating with red ones ("Red next to yellow kills a fellow").

3. The answer is **C**, pages 466 and 467.

Ice is contraindicated for snakebites as it may increase tissue damage. Arterial tourniquets are also contraindicated. A lymphatic constriction band that allows one finger to be inserted underneath the band may be used. The most effective method of reducing venom spread is to use an elastic wrap while immobilizing the extremity. In 25% of snakebite victims, there is no venom released. Symptoms of envenomation are primarily localized; pain, swelling, and hemorrhagic blisters are common. If the victim has no symptoms after 30 minutes, there probably has been no envenomation. Excessive activity of the victim increases the toxicity of the venom.

4. The answer is **E**, pages 467 and 468.

In snakebites, treatment fasciotomy is rarely needed because tissue necrosis is due to the direct action of the venom and not due to increased pressure. If significant tissue swelling is noted, compartmental pressures should be measured. Use of antivenin may prevent the need for fasciotomy. There is no ultrapurified pit viper antivenin. The antivenin used in the United States is made from horse serum and has a large number of foreign proteins. Serum sickness frequently occurs 7 to 14 days after administration of the antivenin. Serum sickness develops in 100% of the patients who receive more than 7 vials. It is usually not life-threatening and can be treated with prednisone. A positive skin test is not an absolute contraindication to antivenin administration, but if antivenin is given, it should be in an intensive care unit (ICU) setting with consultation of someone who has experience in treating snakebites. The patient should be pretreated with cimetidine and diphenhydramine. Epinephrine should be nearby or administered as a slow infusion if anaphylaxis occurs. The number of vials of antivenin administered initially is dependent on the symptoms:

No symptoms	No antivenin
Local symptoms only	5 vials
Multiple bites or mild systemic symptoms	10 vials
Severe systemic symptoms or severe local symptoms	15 vials

Children weighing less than 25 kg require 50% more antivenin as an initial dose because of a higher dose/body weight of venom.

5. The answer is **D**, page 468.

In animal models, colloids such as albumin were superior to crystalloids in the treatment of venom shock. Corticosteroids have not been found to be definitive therapy. Incision and suction are useful only up to 30 minutes after the bite, and their use has caused morbidity in the past. Direct current shock therapy has not been shown to be effective.

6. The answer is **D**, pages 466 to 468.

In approximately 20% of snakebites there is no envenomation. With pit snake envenomation, except with the Mojave rattlesnake, local signs of venom toxicity such as pain and swelling will start to be present by 30 minutes after the bite. Thus, with one exception, if there are no local symptoms by the time the patient arrives in the ED, there is probably no envenomation. However, the patient should still be observed for several hours. It is recommended that prophylactic antivenin be given to all patients bitten by the Mojave rattlesnake, since there may be no local symptoms and its effects are mainly neurotoxic.

Serum sickness is seen in 100% of patients who receive more than 7 vials of antivenin, since it is made of horse serum. Purer monoclonal antibody–specific antivenin is under investigation and when available may decrease the incidence of posttreatment serum sickness.

Pit viper venom does not cause respiratory paralysis, and acetaminophen does not potentiate venom.

7. The answer is **B**, pages 467 to 468.

Coral snake envenomation is mainly neurotoxic. Local reactions at the bite are minimal. Symptoms include vomiting, weakness, seizures, and bulbar and respiratory paralysis. It is recommended that 6 to 10 vials be given for all coral snake bites because of an estimated 10% to 20% fatality rate if untreated.

8. The answer is **D**, page 470.

Scorpion stings by the *Centruroides sculpturatus* usually cause pain and local hyperesthesia. In severe cases, tachycardia, sweating, central nervous system stimulation with hyperactivity, and seizures can occur.

Dysrhythmias may also occur. Management of scorpion stings includes cold compresses, which may be enough with analgesics. Phenobarbital is considered the drug of choice to treat seizures and central nervous system stimulation. Other drugs such as narcotic analgesics can potentiate the venom. Propranolol can be used to treat tachyarrhythmias. An antivenin is available in Arizona from goat serum for severely envenomated children.

9. The answer is **C**, page 469.

Black widow spiders are about 1.5 cm in diameter with a red hourglass in the venomous female's ventral abdomen. Venom proteins cause acetylcholine release, leading to painful muscle contractions. Norepinephrine release causes hypertension. Children under 6 years of age can be more severely envenomated because of increased venom dose for size. Symptoms include headaches, eyelid edema, nausea, vomiting, increased salivation, and perspiration. The most pathognomonic feature is painful muscle contractions of the abdomen and thorax. Treatment includes using intravenous (IV) diazepam for muscle cramps. Antivenin should routinely be used for children under 6. The antivenin is made from horse serum, and a skin test should be performed before use. Laboratory tests are not helpful in the diagnosis.

10. The answer is **D,** pages 469 and 470.

The brown recluse spider is 9 to 12 cm in diameter with a violin-shaped marking on the cephalothorax. The bite causes little or no pain initially. A vesicle may develop, surrounded by an ischemic ring of extravasated blood (target legion). Pain develops several hours after envenomation. The central part of the lesion becomes necrotic. This is thought to be because of activation of complement and migration of leukocytes to the arteriole endothelium, which causes thrombosis and infarction of tissue. Systemic symptoms may include nausea, vomiting, malaise, fever, and chills. Disseminated intravascular coagulation may occur, as well as intravascular hemolysis. The most common area in which these bites occur is the midwestern United States, although they can occur anywhere.

11. The answer is **A,** page 470.

The necrosis from the brown recluse bite can be severe and extensive. Skin grafting may be necessary. Dapsone, by inhibiting leukocyte migration, may decrease the area of infarction and should be given for the first 5 days. Antibiotics are indicated for secondary infection. Experimental rabbit antivenin is being studied, and it may be effective if administered within 48 hours.

12. The answer is **D,** pages 470 and 471.

Centipedes are elongated and flat with each segment having one pair of legs. Centipedes can bite. The toxin causes burning, localized swelling, and erythema with lymphadenitis and regional lymphadenopathy. Systemic symptoms include nausea, dizziness, and fever. The local inflammation usually disappears in 4 to 6 hours, although edema and tenderness may last or recur up to 3 weeks. Treatment consists of pain relief, wound cleaning, and tetanus prophylaxis. Antihistamines or corticosteroids may be effective for severe local symptoms. No antivenin exists.

Millipedes are elongated and cylindrical with two pairs of legs per segment. Glands on the side of the body excrete a defensive toxin. The toxin causes a contact dermatitis, which may blister and exfoliate. "Mahogany" skin discolorations in the shape of a curled up millipede have been confused with signs of child abuse. If the toxin gets in the eye, severe pain, lacrimation, and blepharospasm occur, followed by conjunctivitis, periorbital edema, and possible corneal ulceration.

Treatment is to irrigate copiously with water or saline to remove the toxin. After that, the wound should be treated like a second-degree burn. Eye injuries need ophthalmologic consultation.

13. The answer is **C,** page 471.

Coelenterata include jellyfish, anemones, and corals. The nematocyst is a venom-producing apparatus. The stings usually produce paresthesias and burning, linear wheals. Severe envenomation can cause headaches, vertigo, seizures, coma, nausea, vomiting, and bronchospasm. Field management includes bathing the site with seawater. Fresh water causes the nematocysts to fire and is contraindicated. Vinegar (3% to 5% acetic acid) will inactivate the nematocysts in most species. It should be applied for 30 minutes, and then the area can be washed clean. Topical steroids and Burow's solution may help relieve local discomfort. Tetanus prophylaxis should be given if needed.

14. The answer is **B,** pages 472 and 473.

Hot water immersion (45° to 50° C) for 1 to 1½ hours will inactivate the venom. After immersion the barb should be removed as completely as possible. Prophylactic antibiotics may be useful. Symptoms include severe pain, edema and hemorrhage, muscle cramps, nausea, vomiting, diarrhea, diaphoresis, cardiac arrhythmias, and hypertension. Warm water immersion will also inactivate the venom of the lionfish, stonefish, and scorpionfish.

15. The answer is **B,** pages 472 and 473.

A sea urchin of the phylum Echinodermata usually envenomates when a victim steps on it. The urchin leaves toxic spines in the victim's skin and soft tissue. Initial treatment for this type of envenomation is hot water immersion. The initial reaction is a severe burning followed by swelling and redness. In severe poisoning, symptoms may include weakness, syncope, paresthesias of the face, and muscle paralysis, especially of the facial muscles. The patient may go on to suffer respiratory arrest. Spines that can be easily removed should be. Antibiotics are indicated if infection develops. Granulomas may form that require excision.

Catfish and lionfish envenomate with dorsal and pectoral spines. Scorpaenidae (lionfish, stonefish, sculpin, and scorpion fish) are found in the coastal waters of Florida, California, and Hawaii and in the Gulf of Mexico. The lionfish, a popular aquarium fish, accounts for the majority of reported stings. In Scorpaenidae envenomations the wound immediately becomes ischemic and cyanotic with intense pain. Edema, paresthesias, and tissue necrosis may develop. Systemic symptoms include seizures, tremors, muscle weakness, delirium, dysrhythmias, hypotension or hypertension, and myocardial ischemia with congestive heart failure. Granulomas occur frequently.

Treatment includes hot water immersion to inactivate the venom and relieve pain, and careful wound care. An antivenin is available for the stonefish in Australia.

Catfish envenomations are mild but similar to stingray envenomations. Treatment consists of hot water immersion and exploration of the wound for foreign bodies.

27

Drowning and Near Drowning

Christopher Shields

See Barkin et al: Chapter 35.

1. Which one of the following statements concerning the diving reflex in drowning is *true?*
   A. Shunts the blood from the core to the periphery.
   B. Induces hypothermia.
   C. Occurs in the majority of cold water immersions.
   D. Probably has little influence on outcome.
   E. Causes dysrhythmias.

2. Which one of the following statements concerning drowning is correct?
   A. About 40% occur in freshwater.
   B. Chlorinated water has a worse prognosis than freshwater.
   C. Saltwater increases the need for mechanical ventilation.
   D. Hypoxemia rather than water type dictates therapy.
   E. Most cases involve aspiration of large amounts of fluid.

3. All of the following are considered risk factors for drowning *except:*
   A. Seizure disorder.
   B. Asthma.
   C. Alcohol and drug abuse.
   D. Head trauma.
   E. Spinal trauma.

4. Which of the following is a *true* statement concerning the initial chest x-ray in a drowning case?
   A. Fluffy infiltrates indicate poor ultimate prognosis.
   B. Normal chest x-ray is a definite indication of no pulmonary damage.
   C. Clavicle and rib fractures are indications of trauma.
   D. Signs of foreign body aspiration are frequently seen.
   E. Spontaneous pneumothorax is frequently encountered.

5. Prehospital treatment of drowning victims in cardiac arrest includes all of the following *except:*
   A. Cervical spine precautions.
   B. Chest compressions.
   C. Heimlich maneuver.
   D. Early intubation.
   E. Intravenous (IV) access.

6. A 6-year-old boy is brought to the hospital after a near drowning at the ocean and is found to be hypotensive. Which of the following statements is *true?*
   A. Saline and Ringer's lactate solutions are contraindicated in saltwater drowning.
   B. Fluid boluses are given in 10 ml/kg aliquots.
   C. Fluid status should be monitored immediately by a central venous catheter.
   D. The patient's hypotensive state may indicate associated trauma.

7. Which one of the following is the best immediate treatment in drowning?
   A. Oral β-agonist for bronchospasm.
   B. Hyperbaric oxygen.
   C. Steroids.
   D. Inhaled racemic epinephrine.
   E. Continuous positive airway pressure (CPAP) for worsening hypoxemia.

8. A 7-year-old boy is seen in the ED following a near drowning. On physical examination he is found to have tachypnea, tachycardia, and mild expiratory wheezing. The initial chest radiograph is negative. The most appropriate disposition will be:
   A. Discharge if symptoms resolve within 6 hours.
   B. Admit to general pediatric floor if initial chest x-ray is negative.
   C. Discharge on oral steroids if symptoms resolve within 6 hours.
   D. Observe for 12 hours in the pediatric ED.
   E. Admit to pediatric intensive care unit (ICU).

9. Which of the following factors is associated with a poor outcome in drowning cases?
   A. Return of spontaneous cardiac rhythm following cardiopulmonary resuscitation (CPR).
   B. Submersion longer than 9 minutes.
   C. CPR for less than 5 minutes.
   D. Low blood glucose level.
   E. Spontaneous respirations after CPR.

10. Which one of the following statements concerning increased intracranial pressure in drowning victims is correct?
    A. A ventriculostomy should be inserted while the patient is in the ED.
    B. It is treated with corticosteroids and induced hypothermia.
    C. It is treated with elevation of the head of the bed to 30 degrees.
    D. It is treated by maintaining the $Paco_2$ at 40 mm Hg.
    E. It is treated with restricted glucose-containing fluids.

ANSWERS [See Barkin et al: Chapter 35.]

1. The answer is **D,** page 475.
   The diving reflex is thought to have beneficial effects in a few selected submersion victims. However, it is probably not active in children and has little influence on outcome. The reflex is stimulated by cold water immersion but does not itself cause hypothermia. It does cause a shift of blood preferentially to the heart and brain and results in bradycardia.

2. The answer is **D,** page 475.
   The mechanism of pulmonary injury may vary slightly between saltwater and freshwater drowning. Therapy is dictated by hypoxemia. More than 90% of drownings occur in freshwater, even in areas with saltwater beaches. Chlorinated water does not change the prognosis. Most cases involve only a small amount of aspirated fluid.

3. The answer is **B,** page 476.
   Patients with a seizure disorder have a fourfold to fivefold greater risk of drowning, even with therapeutic levels of anticonvulsants. Alcohol and drug abuse are risk factors for drowning and diving accidents, especially in adolescent boys. Spinal injury and head trauma are associated with submersion injuries.

4. The answer is **C,** pages 476 and 477.
   The chest x-ray may show signs of associated trauma. The fluffy infiltrates may not be seen on the initial film and are not correlated with hypoxemia or outcome. The initial chest x-ray may be normal, but this does not eliminate the possibility of pulmonary damage. The signs of foreign body aspiration and spontaneous pneumothorax may be seen occasionally.

5. The answer is **C,** page 477.
   CPR must be performed on all drowning victims in cardiac arrest. Cervical spine precautions are necessary when trauma is a possibility. The use of early intubation to ensure ventilation and further airway protection is important. IV or intraosseous access is necessary for fluid and epinephrine administration. The Heimlich maneuver is not routinely recommended in submersion cases, but the airway is handled in a manner similar to that in other unresponsive patients.

6. The answer is **D,** page 478.
   Hypotension is treated with normal saline or Ringer's lactate, regardless of the water type in which the drowning occurs. The patient should be treated initially with repeated IV boluses of 20 ml/kg. If hypotension persists, the fluid status should be monitored via a central venous catheter. Other causes of hypotension are *associated trauma* with blood loss, cervical spine injury, ischemic cardiomyopathy, vascular shunting, and hypothermia.

7. The answer is **E,** pages 477 and 478.
   Persistent hypoxemia should be treated with CPAP on self-ventilating patients and positive end-expiratory pressure (PEEP) on patients requiring mechanical ventilation. Hyperbaric oxygen is used to treat patients with carbon monoxide poisoning or scuba diving injuries. Antibiotics and corticosteroids have not been shown to be effective in treating aspiration pneumonitis.

8. The answer is **E,** page 479.
   Patients with hypoxemia or symptoms such as tachypnea, wheezing, rales, or confusion should be admitted to the pediatric ICU for monitoring. Initial radiographs in these patients may be negative even though respiratory failure may subsequently develop.

9. The answer is **B,** page 479.
   Factors associated with a poor outcome following ischemic injury are: submersion greater than 9 minutes, CPR for more than 25 minutes, an elevated blood sugar level, and the lack of spontaneous respiration after CPR.

10. The answer is **C,** pages 478 and 479.
    Increased intracranial pressure is not usually seen for several hours after a drowning. Treatment with corticosteroids, barbiturates, and induced hypothermia is controversial. The head of the bed should be elevated 30 degrees, and the $Paco_2$ maintained at 25 to 30 mm Hg. Fluids should be administered judiciously. Glucose-containing fluids should be avoided in the initial resuscitation because of poor outcome.

28

Electrical and Lightning Injuries

Steve Gottesfeld

See Barkin et al: Chapter 36.

---

1. Which of the following is the correct order for *increasing* resistance?
   A. Nerves, blood vessels, muscle, skin, bone.
   B. Bone, skin, blood vessels, muscle, nerves.
   C. Nerves, blood vessels, muscle, bone, skin.
   D. Blood vessels, nerves, muscle, bone, skin.
   E. Blood vessels, nerves, skin, bone, muscle.

2. Initial management of a 6-year-old boy who has sustained a high-voltage electrical burn to the chest should include which one of the following?
   A. Chest computed tomographic (CT) scan to rule out esophageal injury.
   B. Exploration of the wound with deep debridement.
   C. Intravenous (IV) fluid administration based on the surface area of the wound.
   D. Attention to the cervical spine if a history of loss of consciousness is present.

3. A child sustains an electrical injury to his hand. Which of the following statements regarding skin resistance is true?
   A. A newborn's skin is relatively thick and has high resistance.
   B. Callused adult skin has low resistance.
   C. The resistance of hands decreases with perspiration.
   D. The presence of an entrance or exit wound is unrelated to skin resistance.
   E. A child who is electrocuted in a bathtub will have multiple skin wounds as a result of high resistance.

4. A 2-year-old boy has bitten an electrical cord and has burned his lips. Which of the following is most correct?
   A. The child should be watched for delayed bleeding.
   B. Late complications are extremely uncommon.
   C. The child will have severe pain.
   D. The wound should be excised and sutured to prevent complications.
   E. The patient should be admitted, since severe complications can occur immediately.

5. An awake 2-year-old boy is taken by his parents to the ED after sticking his finger in an electrical wall outlet. Which of the following is the most appropriate next step?
   A. Insert two large-bore IV lines.
   B. Insert a Foley catheter to monitor urinary output.
   C. Administer tetanus prophylaxis.
   D. Place the child on a cardiac monitor.
   E. Examine the child's fingers to determine if he actually received an electrical injury.

6. Which of the following statements regarding pulmonary complications of electrical injures is *true?*
   A. Respiratory arrest can outlast cardiac arrest.
   B. Pulmonary emboli frequently form.
   C. Respiratory arrest is caused by massive diaphragmatic thermal damage.
   D. The duration of apnea is unrelated to survival.
   E. Massive pulmonary hemorrhage leads to hypoxia.

7. Which of the following statements regarding lightning injuries is *true?*
   A. Few lightning strikes go unreported.
   B. There is a 70% to 80% mortality rate.
   C. Less than 5% sustain permanent sequelae.
   D. Lightning is alternating current.
   E. Each year approximately 100 fatalities occur in the United States.

8. Which of the following electrical pathways carries the greatest risk of death?
   A. Foot to foot.
   B. Hand to foot.
   C. Mouth to foot.
   D. Mouth to hand.
   E. Hand to hand.

9. Which of the following lightning strikes carries the highest mortality rate?
   A. Flashover.
   B. Side flash.
   C. Glancing strike.
   D. Direct strike.
   E. Strike potential.

10. Which of the following is true regarding cardiac complications from electrical injuries?
    A. Asystole is the most common cause of cardiac arrest in alternating current injuries.
    B. The majority of nonfatal rhythm disturbances occur immediately and resolve spontaneously.
    C. Ventricular fibrillation is the most common cause of cardiac arrest in lighting injuries.
    D. Creatinine phosphokinase (CPK)-MB isoenzymes are of no value in the evaluation and management.
    E. Dysrhythmias should not be treated because they are likely to resolve spontaneously.

ANSWERS   [See Barkin et al: Chapter 36.]

1. The answer is **A,** page 482.
Joule's law states that increased resistance to the passage of a current generates greater heat. This heat may then cause thermal injury to tissues. Body tissues vary in their electrical resistance capacity in the following order from lesser to greater: nerves, blood vessels, muscle, skin, tendon, fat, bone.

2. The answer is **D,** page 486.
Initial management of a high-voltage electrical injury should include immediate attention (as in all emergencies) to the airway with cervical spine control, breathing, and circulation. Electrically injured patients can have both medical and traumatic injuries, and therefore cervical spine immobilization and evaluation are critical.

Patients with signs suggestive of transfer of current through the thorax should have a 12-lead electrocardiogram (ECG), chest x-ray, and serial CPK-MB measurements. Fluid administration is not based on surface area of the wound as in thermal wounds but should be based on maintenance of adequate urinary output (1 ml/kg). In general, thoracic wounds should not be probed or explored.

3. The answer is **C,** page 483.
Normal palms have approximately 40,000 ohms of resistance, which may drop to 300 to 1000 ohms when moisture, such as perspiration, is present. Callused adult skin has high resistance (100,000 ohms). The appearance of entrance and exit wounds is related to resistance. Dry (high-resistance) skin in contact with an electrical current has a well-demarcated area of whitish yellow ischemia and necrosis. This is in contrast to a child electrocuted in a bathtub filled with water, where there may be no skin wounds because of the large area of contact and low skin resistance.

4. The answer is **A,** page 485.
An oral burn of the commissure of the lip is commonly complicated by delayed bleeding from the labial artery as healing progresses and the eschar sloughs off. This phenomenon occurs approximately 5 to 14 days after the injury. The parents should be educated at discharge about this potential problem and instructed how to control the bleeding temporarily. Late complications of mouth electrical injuries include microstomia, speech problems, labial adhesions, ankyloglossia, and deterioration of dentition. These wounds are often relatively painless.

5. The answer is **D,** page 486.
Initial stabilization of an electrically injured patient involves the maintenance of "airway, breathing, and circulation." Cardiac monitoring is indicated early in the resuscitation and evaluation. Examination of the fingers is part of the secondary survey and may be misleading because the absence of a skin wound does not give much information about the severity of the underlying tissue damage. Fluid loss from electrical injuries is difficult to assess. Therefore following adequate urinary output is the most reliable method.

6. The answer is **A,** page 485.
The most important pulmonary complication is respiratory arrest. Respiratory center paralysis can outlast cardiac arrest following electrical injuries. The duration of apnea is a critical factor in survival and therefore must be aggressively treated even in the patient who appears clinically dead. Respiratory center paralysis or forced tetanic contractions of the muscles of respiration are the causes of respiratory arrest in an electrocuted patient.

7. The answer is **E,** page 482.
Lightning is extremely high-voltage direct current that kills approximately 100 people annually in the United States. Most strikes, however, go unreported. Nevertheless, two thirds of lightning strike victims suffer some degree of permanent sequelae. Most victims of lightning strikes are outdoors participating in recreational activities such as hiking, camping, and golf. Surprisingly, 70% to 80% of victims survive.

8. The answer is **E,** page 483.
   Once an electrical current penetrates the skin, it tends to flow directly from the contact point to the ground. Because internal body tissues have relatively uniform resistance, the current tends to travel directly without deflection. The hand to hand pathway carries the greatest mortality rate (more than 60%) because of transection of the spinal cord from C4 to C8.
9. The answer is **D,** page 483.
   Lightning current may contact a victim several ways. Direct strike is the most serious type, since the major pathway of current flow is through the victim. Strike potential refers to a current that hits the ground, enters the victim's leg, and exits through the other leg. Flashover phenomenon occurs when lightning energy flows outside the body of the victim, usually facilitated by wet clothes.
10. The answer is **B,** page 485.
    Cardiac complications occur in between 5% and 54% of electrical exposures. Most nonfatal rhythm disturbances occur immediately and resolve spontaneously, but their appearance may be delayed up to 12 hours in electrical injuries and up to 2 weeks in lightning injuries. The massive direct current exposure of a lightning strike causes a total depolarization of the heart, resulting in asystole. Ventricular fibrillation is more commonly seen in alternating current injuries. CPK-MB isoenzymes may be helpful in evaluating the electrically injured patient, since myocardial damage and infarction have been reported.

CHAPTER

29

Thermal Injury

Jeffrey Schor

> See Barkin et al: Chapter 37.

1. A 2-year-old girl is seen in the ED with a sharply demarcated partial-thickness burn covering 50% of her chest. There are also isolated erythematous areas scattered around her trunk, left arm, and left leg. The most likely etiology for this injury is:
   A. A scald burn from hot liquid.
   B. A flame burn from ignition of her clothing.
   C. A contact burn from lying on a radiator.
   D. A flash burn from an exploding firecracker.
   E. An electrical burn from grabbing an exposed wire.

2. A 12-year-old boy is brought to the ED with burns covering all of the anterior trunk, his entire left arm, and his left anterior thigh. The total body surface area (TBSA) affected in this patient is approximately:
   A. 5% to 9%.
   B. 10% to 14%.
   C. 15% to 20%.
   D. 21% to 25%.
   E. 26% to 30%.

3. Significant increases in overall mortality and morbidity occur with burns covering a TBSA of greater than:
   A. 20%.
   B. 30%.
   C. 40%.
   D. 50%.
   E. 60%.

4. A 4-year-old boy is taken to the ED after being removed from a house fire. On evaluation, he is awake and alert but covered with soot. According to the Emergency Medical Service (EMS) workers who brought him in, he has sustained burns on his arms and face. You examine the burns on his right arm and note that the arm's appearance is mottled with areas of waxy white skin. The burns on his face are red and moist with blisters. His facial burns appear to be causing him the most distress. The TBSA affected by burns is estimated at 12%. In assessing the depth of the burn, the burn on the arm is most likely a:
   A. First-degree burn.
   B. Superficial partial-thickness burn.
   C. Deep partial-thickness burn.
   D. Full-thickness burn.
   E. Third-degree burn.

5. The patient described in question 4 is at *highest* risk of:
   A. Significant fluid deficits.
   B. Significant muscle breakdown leading to myoglobinuria.
   C. Significant infection.
   D. Significant pulmonary injury.
   E. Significant facial scarring.

6. A 2-year-old girl is brought to the local ED with burns covering 18% of her body. They are mostly second-degree burns. The appropriate management of this patient would be:
   A. Intravenous (IV) hydration with normal saline, stabilization, and transfer to a regional burn center.
   B. Silver sulfadiazine (Silvadene) cream, debridement, and discharge with follow-up.
   C. Silver sulfadiazine (Silvadene) cream, debridement, and hospitalization with oral hydration.
   D. IV hydration, hospitalization, and prophylactic antibiotics.
   E. IV hydration via central lumen catheter, pain medication, and admission.

7. A 16-year-old girl sustains a minor second-degree burn to her hand. Her last tetanus immunization was at 10 years of age. All of the following are appropriate in the management of this patient except:
   A. Placing of burn under cool water.
   B. Cleansing of wound with soap and water.
   C. Applying bland ointment and nonstick gauze to wound and wrapping it with gauze.
   D. Having patient perform active range of motion exercises.
   E. Administering tetanus prophylaxis.

ANSWERS   [See Barkin et al: Chapter 37.]

1. The answer is **A,** page 489.

   Scald burns result from contact with a hot liquid or gas. They are most commonly seen in children younger than 3 years of age, are usually sharply demarcated, and often result in second- and third-degree burns. There are often isolated areas of burns scattered in the direction of the splash.

   Flame burns result from direct ignition of clothing or skin. They are most commonly seen in children older than 2 years of age who play with matches, open fires, or flammable material.

   Contact burns occur in children who come in contact with a hot object. These burns usually have a well-demarcated border, with either partial- or full-thickness injury.

   Flash burns are often caused by explosions and result in a uniform, partial-thickness burn.

   Electrical burns occur as a result of electric current passing through the skin and tissue structures of the body, usually an extremity.

2. The answer is **D,** pages 490 and 491.

   The "rule of nines" is a reasonably accurate way to estimate total body surface area (TBSA) in patients older than 9 years of age. This rule states that each lower extremity is counted as 18% of TBSA (9% anterior and 9% posterior), the anterior trunk as 18%, the posterior trunk as 18%, and each upper extremity and the head as 9%. The remaining 1% is allocated to the perineum. For younger children, however, the Lund and Browder chart should be used to correct for the smaller surface area of the lower extremities (see Fig. 37-1, page 490 in Barkin et al). The burn percentage for the patient in this question includes: 9% for the anterior chest, 9% for the entire left arm, and 4.5% for the anterior left thigh. So the patient has a 22.5% TBSA burn.

3. The answer is **B,** page 491.

   Most fatal injuries occur in children sustaining a greater than 60% TBSA burn. A minor burn is considered less than 10% TBSA, moderate burns are 10% to 20% in children, and major burns are greater than 20% TBSA in children. Significant increases in overall mortality and morbidity occur with greater than 30% TBSA burns.

4. The answer is **C,** pages 490 and 491.

   First-degree burns usually result from brief contact with scalding fluids and sunburns. They result in local tissue destruction, pain, and redness, but no blister formation.

   Second-degree burns are divided into superficial and deep partial-thickness burns. Superficial partial-thickness injuries appear moist and red, blister, and are painful. The facial burn on this patient is an example of a superficial partial-thickness burn.

   Deep partial-thickness burns involve the entire epidermis and dermis. These injuries have a mottled appearance with areas of waxy white injury. The surface of the burn is dry and anesthetic.

   Third-degree, or full-thickness burns, involve destruction of the epidermal, dermal, and subcutaneous layers, leaving a dry, leathery appearance. The wounds appear white, red, or black and may or may not have blisters. Thrombosed blood vessels may be visible.

5. The answer is **D,** pages 491 and 492.

   House fires cause 75% of all fire-related deaths, with most patients dying of smoke inhalation as opposed to complications of burns. The patient described in question 4, who is covered with soot, obviously has been exposed to smoke. Smoke inhalation can result in significant pulmonary injury. Direct inhalation of toxic particles or heat from the smoke may produce upper or lower airway complications. Carbon monoxide poisoning is also a risk.

   Although the burn on the patient's arm may ultimately require some excision and grafting, he probably will not suffer any other major complications from a 12% TBSA burn. Fluid deficits and muscle breakdown usually occur with burns of greater than 30% TBSA. Infection is possible but not as high a risk in this patient as smoke inhalation. Finally a superficial partial-thickness burn such as the patient has on his face is unlikely to scar.

TABLE 29-1 Tetanus Prophylaxis in Routine Wound Management

History of tetanus immunizations	Clean minor wound		All other wounds*	
	Td†	**TIG**	**Td**	**TIG**
Unknown or less than 3 doses	Yes	No	Yes	Yes
3 or more doses‡	No§	No	No‖	No

From *MMWR* 39(3):37-41, 1990; Committee on Infectious Diseases: *AAP* 409-414, 1994.

*Such as, but not limited to, wounds contaminated with dirt, feces, soil, and saliva; puncture wounds; avulsions; and wounds resulting from missiles, crushing, burns, and frostbite.

†For children younger than 7 years of age give DTP (or DT if pertussis is contraindicated).

‡If only 3 doses of *fluid* toxoid have been received, a fourth dose of absorbed toxoid should be given.

§Yes, if more than 10 years since the last dose.

‖Yes, if more than 5 years since the last dose.

6. The answer is **A,** pages 492 to 494.

The severity of burns is determined by the depth of the burn, TBSA, location of the injury, age and health of the patient, and associated injuries. These will be the first pieces of information required of the emergency physician in the transfer of a patient to a burn center.

Major burns have partial-thickness involvement of 15% to 20% in children. Full-thickness burns of greater than 10% are also considered in this category as are burns of the hands, face, eyes, ears, feet, or perineum. Any child with these findings should be admitted to a pediatric burn center.

Children with greater than 15% TBSA burns will need IV hydration while urine output is monitored over several days. Those with greater than 40% TBSA burns usually need a central line. Potassium chloride should be avoided in the ED as children tend to have high initial potassium levels because of massive red blood cell breakdown. Children should also not receive anything by mouth because an ileus may develop, leading to the possibility of vomiting and subsequent aspiration.

Antibiotics should not be administered prophylactically but rather for specific signs and symptoms of infection after appropriate cultures.

Pain medication should be used once vital signs are normalized.

7. The answer is **E,** pages 494 and 953 to 954.

Tetanus prophylaxis should be administered according to Table 29-1.

CHAPTER

30

Heat Injury

Jeffrey Schor

See Barkin et al: Chapter 38.

1. The greatest amount of heat loss from the body occurs through:
   A. Conduction.
   B. Convection.
   C. Radiation.
   D. Evaporation.
2. As the temperature rises because of increased environmental heat, the body:
   A. Increases the metabolic rate by increasing thyroxin release.
   B. Releases endogenous pyrogens, which results in resetting the hypothalamic thermostat.
   C. Dilates cutaneous blood vessels by inhibiting sympathetic centers in the posterior.
   D. Decreases sweating initially.
   E. Decreases the heart rate to preserve normal cardiac output.
3. A 6-year-old boy who comes to the ED has a maculopapular, erythematous rash with scattered vesicles over part of his trunk and back. The rash is intensely itchy. No other areas are affected. He is otherwise healthy with no previous underlying problems. He frequently plays outdoors because it is summer, but his mother makes sure he is always wearing clothes. The most appropriate treatment for this rash is:
   A. Light, loose clothing and a cool environment.
   B. Frequent use of talcum powder.
   C. Topical antibiotics with an antistaphylococcal component.
   D. Oral acyclovir.
   E. Topical steroids.
4. A 16-year-old boy is in the finals of the U.S. National Tennis Tournament, which is being held in Miami. After 3 hours of play the boy suddenly drops to the ground holding his left leg. Although vigorous massage is attempted, he is forced to quit the match because of leg cramps. The most likely etiology for his cramps is:
   A. Poor conditioning.
   B. A black widow spider bite.
   C. Fluid replacement with sports fluid only.
   D. Fluid replacement with water only.
   E. Not enough bananas.
5. Which of the following is often associated with heat exhaustion?
   A. Altered mental status.
   B. Temperature elevation, typically greater than 40° C (104° F).
   C. Rhabdomyolysis.
   D. Absent sweating.
   E. Nausea, vomiting, and irritability.
6. Heatstroke is characterized by:
   A. A core temperature greater than 40.6° C (105° F).
   B. Profuse sweating.
   C. Hypoventilation and bradycardia.
   D. Normal mental status.
   E. Normal electrolyte values.
7. Early in the first heat wave of the summer, a 15-year-old girl is brought into the ED after fainting at an outdoor rock concert. She is awake and alert on arrival, has a temperature of 37.3° C, and has a heart rate (HR) of 92 beats per minute. She is mildly orthostatic. She is otherwise healthy with no previous medical history. The best course of action would be to:
   A. Secure a large-bore intravenous (IV) line with rapid normal saline infusion.
   B. Obtain a nonurgent computed tomographic (CT) scan.
   C. Have the patient rest and offer her fluids.
   D. Obtain serum electrolytes to determine management strategy.
   E. Perform a serum toxicologic screen.

8. On a hot August Sunday, a 12-year-old boy is brought into the ED after collapsing at a soccer game. He had otherwise been healthy and had been playing well. On arrival his core temperature is 41.1° C (106° F), and his skin is dry. He is also incoherent. Which of the following statements regarding management of this patient is true?
   A. Cool water immersion is contraindicated because it may precipitate cardiac arrhythmias.
   B. Shivering should not be suppressed because it is a protective mechanism that helps control temperature.
   C. IV fluids should be infused slowly because these patients are often in renal failure.
   D. Lukewarm water should be sprayed on the patient while air is blown over him until his core temperature is less than 39° C (102° F).
   E. Ice packs should be placed in the groin, axilla, and neck area because that is the most rapid way of cooling the patient.

9. Of the following, the most appropriate preventive measure against heat illness is:
   A. Salt tablets.
   B. Fluid loading before activity.
   C. Replenishment of fluids with high-glucose solutions.
   D. Constant sipping of fluids to quench thirst.
   E. Use of heavy clothing to cause sweating.

10. At the end of a warm summer day, a 15-year-old boy comes to the ED with a complaint of swollen hands and feet. He is awake and alert. His temperature and blood pressure are normal. The hands are non-erythematous and do not hurt; they are edematous but nonpitting. The rest of the examination is normal. The most appropriate management of this child should include:
    A. Fluid restriction.
    B. A salt-free diet.
    C. A short course of diuretics.
    D. Warm compresses.
    E. A cool environment.

ANSWERS   [See Barkin et al: Chapter 38.]

1. The answer is **C**, page 496.
   The greatest amount of heat loss from the body occurs through radiation, accounting for about 60% of the total loss. The effective heat loss from evaporation is approximately 25% and is due mainly to sweating.

2. The answer is **C**, pages 496 and 497.
   With increased heat, the hypothalamus lowers the core temperature by three mechanisms:
   - Dilatation of cutaneous blood vessels by inhibition of sympathetic centers in the posterior hypothalamus that cause vasoconstriction.
   - Stimulation of sweating by transmission down the autonomic pathways and through the sympathetic outflow tract to the sweat glands.
   - Inhibition of heat production from shivering and chemical thermogenesis including decreased discharge of thyrotropin-releasing hormone.

   When the core temperature equals or exceeds 40° C (104° F), there is maximal peripheral vasodilation. Sequestration of large volumes of blood with a reduction in effective circulating volume often takes place. This leads to an increase in heart rate and contractility to maintain cardiac output in the face of this low total peripheral resistance. During fever (such as that caused by infection) endogenous pyrogens stimulate prostaglandins, which resets the hypothalamic thermostat. This would be a maladaptive response to high external temperatures as an additional heat load on a higher than normal set point could predispose to extremely high temperatures.

3. The answer is **A**, page 497.
   The description of the rash and its temporal association is characteristic of prickly heat. Prickly heat is an acute inflammatory skin eruption caused by a blockage of sweat glands. It typically occurs in hot, humid weather and is generally found on clothed areas of the body. The affected area frequently is devoid of sweat.
   A child with prickly heat should wear light, loose clothing. Maintaining a cool environment is the ideal way to avoid the rash and is helpful in relieving it. Cool baths often help relieve the itching. Topical agents, such as talcum, other powders, and antibiotics should be avoided. If the rash becomes diffuse and pustular, systemic antibiotics should be considered.

4. The answer is **D**, page 498.
   Heat cramps can be seen in both unconditioned and highly trained athletes. These cramps are normally found in the muscle groups actually used while working, although any muscle may be affected. Typically they occur after individuals sweat profusely and relieve their thirst with hypotonic solutions. Although the exact etiology is unknown, salt depletion is believed to play a large role. Differential diagnoses include a black widow spider bite and hypokalemia, but these are rare, and usually there is something in the patient's history to suggest those possibilities. Management includes removal from the hot environment where the cramping occurred and replacement of fluids with a salt-containing solution (one teaspoon of salt in 500 ml of water over 1 to 2 hours).

5. The answer is **E,** page 498.

Heat exhaustion is a mild form of heat illness and the most common heat-related illness seen in athletes. Typical causes include exposure to high temperatures, excessive sweating, and inadequate replenishment of water and salt. It can be differentiated from heatstroke mainly by lower core temperatures (almost always lower than 40° C) and normal mental functioning. Thirst, headache, nausea, vomiting, and irritability are common. Management includes removal from heat, rehydration, and rest.

6. The answer is **A,** pages 498 and 499.

Heatstroke is a medical emergency characterized by a temperature greater than 40.6° C, neurologic dysfunction, and anhidrosis. Hyperventilation and tachycardia are universal, and severe electrolyte abnormalities are common.

Heatstroke occurs when the body is unable to dissipate heat, causing loss of temperature control. As a result there is a rapid rise in core temperature, which is injurious to cells and organs throughout the body.

7. The answer is **C,** page 497.

Heat syncope is often seen during the early phase of heat acclimatization. It is associated with orthostatic hypotension and mild dehydration and is caused by vasodilation of cutaneous blood vessels with shunting of the blood to peripheral tissues. Prolonged standing or vigorous activity can worsen this generally self-limited condition. Placing the patient in a supine position is helpful. Oral rehydration is usually sufficient.

8. The answer is **D,** pages 498 and 499.

Heatstroke is a medical emergency. After the airway is secured, rapid cooling of the patient should be performed. Although ice packs cool a patient, the most rapid method is to use a fine spray of water with air currents to dry. Cool water immersion may be used but is often impractical. Shivering often occurs but is not advantageous, since it raises body temperature and can be controlled with IV diazepam 0.2 to 0.3 mg/kg.

Complications of heatstroke include seizures, rhabdomyolysis, hepatic damage, renal failure, and disseminated intravascular coagulation (DIC). Rapid central nervous system collapse is also a danger.

9. The answer is **B,** page 499.

Adequate fluid preloading (300 to 500 ml of fluid) and periodic drinking (150 ml for a 40-kg child every 15 minutes while exercising) should be mandatory during hot weather. Quenching thirst alone does not ensure sufficient fluid replenishment.

Salt replacement with salt tablets is unnecessary. The average American diet has enough sodium to offset deficits in most situations. Use of high-osmolar solutions can cause gastric distension and delay gastric emptying. Light clothing is preferred in hot weather because it allows for better dissipation of heat.

10. The answer is **E,** page 497.

Heat edema is dependent swelling of the hands and feet that often occurs at the onset of hot weather. It is self-limited and spontaneously resolves after the patient is in a cool environment for a period of time. Aldosterone, salt, and water retention are thought to contribute to this condition but play no role in management.

Accidental Hypothermia and Frostbite

Anne F. Brayer

See Barkin et al: Chapter 39.

1. A 2-year-old girl and her 30-year-old mother are brought to the ED after spending the night on a boat stranded in a lake. The lowest temperature overnight was 40° F (4° C). Compared with her mother, the child is likely to be:
   A. Less hypothermic because of her increased ability to shiver.
   B. Less hypothermic because of her surface area to body mass ratio.
   C. More hypothermic because of her surface area to body mass ratio.
   D. More hypothermic because of her increased ability to shiver.
   E. More hypothermic because her mother was protected by having had alcohol.

2. A child is standing on icy cold but dry pavement in bare feet. Heat loss from his feet into the pavement is largely due to:
   A. Conduction.
   B. Radiation.
   C. Evaporation.
   D. Transpiration.
   E. Convection.

3. A 5-year-old patient who had been lost for several hours in the woods on a winter day is brought to the ED. He is somewhat confused, not shivering, and his extremities are slightly stiff. His vital signs are normal, and he has dilated and reactive pupils. Assuming no injury or ingestion has occurred, his core temperature is most likely to be:
   A. 37° C (98.6° F).
   B. 35° C (95° F).
   C. 32° C (89° F).
   D. 28° C (82° F).
   E. 20° C (68° F).

4. The J wave, or Osborne wave, seen on the electrocardiogram (ECG) of hypothermic patients is:
   A. A negative deflection between the P and Q waves.
   B. A negative deflection between the R and T waves.
   C. A negative deflection after the T wave.
   D. A positive deflection between the P and Q waves.
   E. A positive deflection between the R and T waves.

5. The paramedics call on the medic control line to say they are at the scene of a motor vehicle crash that was undiscovered for many hours. They have a young child who was ejected into a snow bank, has no vital signs, and is asystolic on the monitor. The most appropriate prehospital management would be:
   A. Defibrillation followed by intubation and transport.
   B. Initiation of breathing control through bag-valve-mask (BVM) ventilation followed by intubation, cardiopulmonary resuscitation (CPR), and transport.
   C. Initiation of CPR and insertion of an intravenous (IV) catheter for administration of warmed fluids.
   D. Intubation and defibrillation followed by CPR.
   E. No resuscitative efforts because the patient is dead.

6. A 4-year-old patient with a tympanic temperature of 35° C (95° F) is being transported by prehospital personnel. She is wet, shivering, and alert. Prehospital management most appropriately would include:
   A. Giving warmed, humidified oxygen and inserting a Foley catheter, irrigating the catheter with warmed fluids.
   B. Inserting a Foley catheter and nasogastric tube and irrigating both with warmed fluids.
   C. Inserting an IV catheter and administering bretylium to prevent ventricular fibrillation.
   D. Removing wet clothing, wrapping child in warmed blankets, and administering warmed, humidified oxygen.
   E. Transporting as is to begin active core rewarming in the ED.

7. A patient with severe hypothermia (core temperature below 30° C) is noted by the paramedics to have ventricular fibrillation and no respiratory effort. The most appropriate treatment would be:
   A. Insertion of IV catheter and administration of lidocaine.
   B. Insertion of IV catheter and administration of bretylium.
   C. Initiation of CPR and administration of bretylium before intubation.
   D. Intubation, CPR, and consideration of defibrillation with 1 watt-sec/kg.
   E. Intubation, CPR, and administration of IV epinephrine.

8. A 15-year-old patient who has spent the night outdoors in winter after running away from home is brought to the ED. He has a core temperature of 32° C (89° F). Management should include:
   A. Diuresis with furosemide because of likely congestive heart failure.
   B. Administration of maintenance IV fluids.
   C. Administration of isotonic fluids to correct intravascular volume depletion.
   D. Administration of IV bicarbonate to correct likely metabolic acidosis.
   E. Fluid restriction to prevent pulmonary edema.

9. A child is being treated for ventricular fibrillation secondary to severe hypothermia. The rewarming technique most likely to be effective is:
   A. Rewarming hemodialysis.
   B. Gastric lavage with warmed fluids.
   C. Peritoneal lavage with warmed fluids.
   D. Giving of warmed, humidified oxygen.
   E. External rewarming with heated blankets.

10. Attempts to resuscitate a child who has apnea and asystole have been unsuccessful despite successful core warming to 32° C (89° C). This outcome can be predicted by:
    A. The initial core temperature of 28° C (82° F).
    B. The rapid onset (over 2 hours) of hypothermia.
    C. The initial arterial pH of 7.20.
    D. The initial serum potassium of 12 mEq/L.
    E. The initial presence of ventricular fibrillation.

11. A 6-year-old child is going outdoors to go sledding on a winter day when the ambient temperature is -4° C (25° F) and a 15-mph wind is blowing. Her parents are attempting to dress her to prevent hypothermia. They should:
    A. Dress her for warmer weather, since she is likely to be active.
    B. Make sure to take advantage of the wind to allow drying.
    C. Dress her in close-fitting garments to hold the heat close to her skin.
    D. Pay special attention to the legs, since most heat loss comes from there.
    E. Dress her in layers to allow air trapping and pay special attention to hands, feet, and face, which are more susceptible to freezing.

12. The 6-year-old girl described in question 11 spends 2 hours sledding. She negates her parents' efforts when she removes a mitten to pull the sled more easily. When she returns home, her fourth and fifth fingers on that hand are cold, pink, and painful. Capillary refill time is 2 seconds. When her parents warm the hand, it remains pink, and the pain gradually resolves. She has likely suffered:
    A. Hypothermia.
    B. Frostnip.
    C. Superficial frostbite.
    D. Deeper frostbite.
    E. Freezing-refreezing injury.

13. A 2-year-old child was taken on a winter hike by his parents and rode in a backpack on his father's back. Unbeknownst to his parents, he lost the boot on his right foot during the trip. When the family returns home, the boy's toes on that foot are white and waxy. He does not complain of pain until his parents place the foot in warm water. It then becomes swollen and red, and he is screaming in pain. He likely is suffering from:
    A. Hypothermia.
    B. Frostnip.
    C. Superficial frostbite.
    D. Deep frostbite.
    E. Freezing-refreezing injury.

14. At this point the parents of the child described in question 13 should:
    A. Immerse his foot in cold water until the pain resolves.
    B. Pack his foot in snow to recool it and go to the nearest ED.
    C. Rub his foot vigorously and leave it open to room temperature to allow slow rewarming.
    D. Warm his foot over dry heat such as a heat register.
    E. Place his foot in warm water and go to the nearest ED.

15. A 14-year-old boy is brought to the ED for evaluation of possible frostbite to his foot. After rapid warming in 40° C (105° F) water for an hour, he is found to have hemorrhagic blisters and a blackish coating on his toes. The best management at this point would be:
    A. Debridement of the blisters and coating, and replacement of the foot in the water for another hour.
    B. Initiation of anticoagulation.
    C. Administration of tetanus prophylaxis and dressing of wound to prevent infection and further trauma.
    D. Immediate referral for surgical debridement and possible amputation to prevent gangrene.
    E. Debridement of blisters and discharge of patient taking oral analgesics.

ANSWERS   [See Barkin et al: Chapter 39.]

1. The answer is **C**, page 500.
   Young children have a larger surface area to body mass ratio, making them more susceptible to hypothermia. Other things that may make them more susceptible include minimal subcutaneous fat, thinner skin with increased permeability, delayed shivering, and developmental immaturity leading to a delayed behavioral response to cold. Alcohol causes vasodilatation and increased susceptibility to hypothermia.

2. The answer is **A**, page 501.
   Radiation refers to heat transfer by electromagnetic waves. Conduction is the transfer of heat from one form of matter to another such as from the child's feet to the pavement. Convection refers to heat being lost from matter to moving matter, and evaporation to heat being transferred as matter changes form. Transpiration refers to vapor loss from plant material.

3. The answer is **C**, page 502.
   The symptoms and signs are consistent with moderate hypothermia. With mild hypothermia, shivering is usually present. With severe hypothermia, changes in vital signs are nearly always present because the patient rapidly progresses to stupor and coma. Pupils often are not reactive (Fig. 31-1).

4. The answer is **E**, page 504.
   The J wave (Osborne wave) is pathognomonic of hypothermia and has been found in both adult and pediatric patients. It is a positive deflection on the RT segment and is usually seen when the core temperature nears 30° C (86° F) (Fig. 31-2).

5. The answer is **B**, pages 504 and 505.
   This patient very likely is hypothermic. The apparent absence of vital signs is not uncommon in patients with severe hypothermia. Unless obvious injuries incompatible with life exist, resuscitation should be initiated and the patient should be transported without delay. Defibrillation is not indicated for asystole and is likely to be ineffective in a severely hypothermic patient anyway. Warming in the field also is contraindicated for patients with severe hypothermia, since it is difficult to monitor, is likely to delay transport, and can lead to metabolic disturbances, complicating resuscitation.

6. The answer is **D**, pages 504 and 505.
   Patients with mild hypothermia who are alert and shivering do not require internal core rewarming. They are not at risk for ventricular arrhythmias. These patients do benefit from efforts to prevent further heat loss such as removal of wet clothing and drying of skin and hair.

7. The answer is **D**, page 505.
   Treatment of patients with severe hypothermia includes intubation and CPR. Recent evidence suggests that intubation does not trigger fibrillation in hypothermic adults, and this patient already has fibrillation anyway. Resuscitative drugs are unlikely to be effective in patients with core temperatures less than 30° C and can complicate hospital management, since they pool in the body.

8. The answer is **C**, pages 502 and 503.
   This patient probably has suffered slow onset of hypothermia and is likely to have significant intravascular volume loss. The initial treatment of metabolic acidosis, if it exists, would be isotonic fluid resuscitation rather than bicarbonate infusion. Pulmonary edema is not a likely consequence of hypothermia.

9. The answer is **A**, page 506.
   External rewarming alone is unlikely to be effective in a patient with severe hypothermia, especially with a collapse rhythm. Although various internal core-rewarming techniques have been shown to be effective in some cases, extracorporeal techniques including bypass and hemodialysis are the most effective.

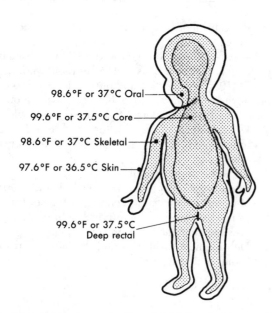

98.6°F or 37°C Oral
99.6°F or 37.5°C Core
98.6°F or 37°C Skeletal
97.6°F or 36.5°C Skin
99.6°F or 37.5°C Deep rectal

FIG. 31-1   Temperature profile of child in normal homeothermic state. (Adapted from Pozos RS, Born DO, editors: *Hypothermia: causes, effects, prevention,* Piscataway, NJ, 1982, New Century Publishing.)

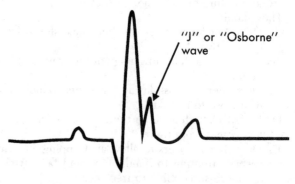

"J" or "Osborne" wave

FIG. 31-2   Electrocardiogram demonstrating appearance of J or Osborne wave.

10. The answer is **D,** page 506.

Survival has been shown to be unlikely in victims of hypothermia with serum potassium level of greater than 10 mEq/L. Patients with rapid onset of hypothermia do better overall than those with slow onset, assuming there are not other complications (such as near drowning). Many patients with initial core temperatures of 28° C (82° F) survive. Although ventricular fibrillation and low serum pH are associated with hypothermia, they have not been shown to be accurate predictors of survival.

11. The answer is **E,** pages 506 and 507.

Dressing for cold weather involves protection from heat loss by protecting body from contact with wind and water (or snow). Dressing in loose clothing allows more air trapping, which acts as an insulator. Dressing in layers also accomplishes this and allows for adjustments to changes in environment and activity level. Hand, feet, and face are particularly susceptible to freezing and should be especially protected.

12. The answer is **B,** page 507.

Frostnip is an early stage of freezing injury characterized by an intense cold feeling, pain, and eventually numbness. Total loss of sensation does not occur. Capillary refill time often is normal. The skin remains erythematous on rewarming. Frostbite is characterized by loss of sensation, pallor, and little or no capillary refill. Pain occurs on rewarming.

13. The answer is **C,** page 507.

See answer to question 12. Superficial frostbite typically becomes painful on rewarming as reperfusion occurs. On rewarming deeper frostbite often remains gray and without signs of perfusion and may remain nonpainful.

14. The answer is **E,** pages 507 and 508.

Rapid rewarming of frostbite in water heated to 38° to 43° C (100° to 110° F) appears to give the best result. Slow rewarming is less effective and can result in further tissue damage. Recooling and especially refreezing can result in a particularly poor outcome and should be prevented at all costs.

15. The answer is **C,** pages 507 and 508.

The patient has frostbite with potential deep tissue damage. After rewarming, frostbitten patients should be managed similar to patients with burns. Tetanus prophylaxis is indicated. Dressing the affected part to prevent further trauma and infection is important. Fluid management and analgesia often are necessary. Anticoagulation has not been shown to be effective. Amputation surgery should be delayed until clear demarcation of nonviable tissue has occurred.

CHAPTER 32

High-Altitude Illness and Dysbarism

Jeffrey Schor

See Barkin et al: Chapter 40.

1. Altitude-related illness first becomes symptomatic above which altitude?
   A. 8000 feet.
   B. 12,000 feet.
   C. 16,000 feet.
   D. 20,000 feet.
   E. 24,000 feet.

2. The most important factor affecting the incidence of altitude-related illnesses is:
   A. Age.
   B. Sex.
   C. Prior conditioning.
   D. Rate of ascent.
   E. Altitude.

3. Pathophysiologic changes that occur during ascent to high altitudes include all of the following *except:*
   A. Increase in minute ventilation.
   B. Increase in 2,3-diphosphoglycerate (DPG).
   C. Decrease in plasma volume by 10% to 20%.
   D. Impaired functioning of the adenosine triphosphate (ATP)-dependent sodium pump.
   E. Decrease in heart rate.

4. A 17-year-old boy with a history of mild acute mountain sickness (AMS) asks for advice before going on a camping trip in the Rockies. Along with your general tips, you offer him:
   A. Acetazolamide to be taken before the trip.
   B. Acetazolamide to be taken before the trip and for the first few days of ascent.
   C. Acetazolamide to be taken if symptoms occur.
   D. An intramuscular shot of dexamethasone before the trip.
   E. A warning not to go because he is predisposed to severe illness.

5. On the third day of a high-altitude ski vacation, an 8-year-old child has respiratory difficulties. Physical examination of the chest reveals bilateral crackles. The most important form of management is:
   A. Oxygen (100%) until symptoms resolve, followed by bed rest.
   B. Furosemide (Lasix) 1 mg/kg orally.
   C. Furosemide (Lasix) 1 mg/kg intravenously.
   D. Immediate descent.
   E. Methylprednisolone (Solu-Medrol) 1 mg/kg intravenously.

6. Which of the following statements regarding high-altitude pulmonary edema (HAPE) is correct?
   A. It is more common in children than adults.
   B. It is usually precipitated by inactivity at higher altitudes.
   C. It is less common in children who have previously lived at high altitudes.
   D. It is often related to the heart.
   E. It occurs within the first 8 to 16 hours of ascent.

7. A 14-year-old girl begins to experience an excruciating headache after hiking for 2 days at 13,000 to 14,000 feet. She is becoming increasingly confused and ataxic. Your management should be to:
   A. Avoid rapid descent because the severe change in barometric pressure may precipitate spontaneous intracranial hemorrhage.
   B. Administer acetazolamide.
   C. Administer dexamethasone.
   D. Administer mannitol.
   E. Avoid intubation because of the risk of increasing intracranial pressure.

8. All of the following are complications of dysbaric diving injuries *except:*
    A. Ruptured tympanic membrane.
    B. Lung rupture.
    C. Air embolism.
    D. Nitrogen narcosis.
    E. Splenic rupture.

9. A 10-year-old boy complains of headache and right leg weakness 8 hours after scuba diving to a depth of 60 feet. The best treatment for this patient is:
    A. Dexamethasone intravenously.
    B. Placement of bilateral chest tubes.
    C. Hyperbaric treatment at 2.8 atmospheres.
    D. Hyperbaric treatment at 6 atmospheres initially, then 2.8 atmospheres.
    E. Mannitol intravenously.

ANSWERS [See Barkin et al: Chapter 40.]

1. The answer is **A,** page 511.
    Altitude-related illness is rare below 8000 feet, the elevation at which arterial oxygen saturation falls below 90% for most individuals. Hypoxia results from decreased partial pressure of oxygen at reduced barometric pressures and is the major physiologic consequence of high-altitude exposure.

2. The answer is **D,** pages 511 and 512.
    High-altitude disorders occur when the rate of onset of altitude stress exceeds the body's ability to adapt. They occur in the young and healthy and are common in well-conditioned athletes. Although altitude affects symptoms, most people become acclimatized if they ascend at a predictable rate. Typically, climbers should allow 1 day to ascend 1000 feet from elevations of 8000 to 10,000 feet and 2 days to ascend 1000 feet at elevations greater than 14,000 feet.

3. The answer is **E,** page 511.
    Stimulation of the aortic and carotid bodies resulting from hypoxia leads to a compensatory increase in minute ventilation. Within 24 hours of ascent, a rise in 2,3-DPG facilitates oxygen delivery to the tissues. Hypoxia also impairs the function of ATP-dependent sodium pump, which causes fluid shifts from the intravascular space into hypoxic cells and the interstitial space.

    A rapid decrease in plasma volume by 10% to 20% occurs within a few hours of ascent to high altitude. Cardiovascular effects include sinus tachycardia, venoconstriction, pulmonary artery vasoconstriction, and decreased cardiac output. Central nervous system (CNS) hypoxia results in cerebral vasodilation, increased cerebral blood flow, and a slight increase in cerebrospinal fluid (CSF) pressure.

4. The answer is **B,** page 512.
    Prophylaxis is recommended for climbers who have experienced prior episodes of AMS or for rescue workers who must make rapid ascents. Acetazolamide has been approved by the Food and Drug Administration for this purpose. It prevents AMS by acting as a diuretic and respiratory stimulant. The medication should be started 24 hours before ascent and continued for 2 to 3 days after attaining high altitude.

    Several studies indicate that dexamethasone may be useful in preventing AMS. However, until more data are available, dexamethasone is still considered primarily an emergency drug for the treatment of high-altitude cerebral edema in conjunction with descent and oxygen.

5. The answer is **D,** page 513.
    High-altitude pulmonary edema (HAPE) is an uncommon but potentially fatal form of high-altitude sickness that affects more than 10% of individuals who go above 14,500 feet. The cornerstones of therapy are immediate descent, rest, and oxygen. At high altitude even small changes in altitude can result in large changes in hemoglobin saturation, and descent should take priority in symptomatic individuals. Although the overall mortality rate is 11%, the mortality rate without descent is 44%. Descent is the definitive treatment, and all other therapies should be regarded as temporizing measures until descent occurs.

    Oxygen administered at 6 to 8 L/min decreases pulmonary artery pressures, heart rate, and respiratory rate and improves hemoglobin oxygen saturation. However, it should never be the sole method of management.

    Diuretics are contraindicated because patients at high altitudes are often hypovolemic. Steroids have not been shown to be of any benefit.

6. The answer is **A,** page 513.
    HAPE is a unique pulmonary edema of noncardiac origin. It occurs more frequently in children, adolescents, and young adults and is often precipitated by exercise at altitude. It has been reported at higher frequencies in children who have lived at high altitudes and subsequently return after a visit to a lower altitude.

    HAPE rarely occurs below 8000 feet but affects more than 10% of individuals who go above 14,500 feet. The onset of HAPE occurs within 24 to 96 hours after arrival at high altitude.

7. The answer is **C,** page 514.
    High-altitude cerebral edema (HACE) is the most severe high-altitude illness. Symptoms include severe incapacitating headache, ataxia, loss of coordination, confusion, diplopia, emotional lability, and hallucinations. This can progress to lethargy, stupor, and coma, followed by death.

    Rapid descent and oxygen administration are the major treatment modalities. Severely affected patients need 30 degree elevation of the head, and intubation with hyperventilation should be considered. Rapid sequence induction should be performed with increased intracranial pressure precautions.

    Dexamethasone (4 mg q6hr IV) may produce dramatic improvement and should be given. Acetazolamide and osmotic diuretics are not effective in the treatment of HACE.

8. The answer is **E,** pages 516 to 519.

Because of unequal pressure on ascent, barotrauma may occur. This can cause hemotympanum or tympanic membrane rupture. Sinusitis may also occur.

Pulmonary overpressurization syndrome occurs when compressed air expands on ascent faster than it can be vented. This can result in pneumothorax, pneumomediastinum, pneumopericardium, subcutaneous emphysema, and air embolism. Air embolism is caused when air enters the circulation via ruptured pulmonary veins. This usually occurs on breath-holding ascent that expands the air and ruptures the lung. Symptoms depend on the particular organ to which the air embolizes.

Nitrogen narcosis (similar to ethanol intoxication) is seen when nitrogen is inhaled at elevated partial pressures. The symptoms include laughter, impaired judgment and memory, and muscle incoordination. Symptoms resolve with ascent. If deep dives are required, helium can be substituted for nitrogen. Splenic rupture is not a symptom of dysbaric diving injury.

9. The answer is **D,** pages 519 and 520.

Decompression sickness, or the bends, is due to liberation of gas bubbles of nitrogen from saturated tissues when pressure is decreased. This usually results from ascending too rapidly and not allowing the nitrogen to wash out of the tissues. Type 1, or mild illness, causes pruritus, lymph node pain, periarticular pain, vertigo, tinnitus, and deafness. It is treated with hyperbaric oxygen at 2.8 atmospheres. Type 2 is more common in children and consists of the spectrum of headaches, seizures, visual impairment, paralysis, dyspnea, respiratory failure, and shock. Initial treatment consists of 100% oxygen, IV crystalloids, and monitoring of urine output. The patient should be placed on the left side with the head bent down to prevent gas embolism to the brain. Definitive treatment is to use a hyperbaric chamber of 6 atmospheres for 30 minutes to reduce the size of the bubbles and then to treat the patient at 2.8 atmospheres. Hyperbaric oxygen improves tissue oxygen and provides a large diffusion gradient to reabsorb the nitrogen bubbles.

Pneumothoraces should be treated only if present. Dexamethasone has been used for neurologic complications, but evidence is lacking for efficacy. Mannitol is not a mainstay of treatment.

Radiation Exposure

Anne F. Brayer

See Barkin et al: Chapter 41.

1. A 2-year-old child is exposed to total body radiation. His prognosis can best be predicted by:
   A. Skin changes at 24 hours.
   B. Degree of vomiting and diarrhea over first few days.
   C. Hematocrit at 48 hours.
   D. Hair loss at 1 week.
   E. Absolute lymphocyte count at 48 hours.

2. X-rays are an example of:
   A. α-Particles.
   B. β-Particles.
   C. β-Decay.
   D. γ-Rays.
   E. Neutrons.

3. A 12-year-old child was found playing near a garbage dump that contained radioactive waste material and was brought to the ED. Initial management should include:
   A. Shielding patient with lead to prevent further contamination.
   B. Fluid resuscitation similar to that for thermal burns.
   C. Internal decontamination to prevent absorption of radioactive material.
   D. Administration of calcium disodium edetate (EDTA).
   E. Washing of skin and shaving of hair to prevent further contamination.

4. A child has been exposed to external radiation contamination. On examination an obvious open fracture of the left ankle is noted. Which of the following is the correct management sequence?
   A. Removal of clothing, copious irrigation and covering of wound, washing of the rest of the body, and surgical debridement as soon as possible.
   B. Removal of clothing, washing of body progressing from head to foot, and cleansing and covering of wound.
   C. Internal decontamination followed by external washing and nonsurgical treatment of fracture.
   D. Removal of clothing, copious irrigation and covering of wound, washing of the rest of the body, and delay of surgery for at least 24 hours.
   E. Immediate covering of wound, then casting, internal gastrointestinal (GI) decontamination, and washing of rest of the body.

5. A patient who has had 24 hours of nausea and vomiting, followed by thrombocytopenia, granulocytopenia, and lymphopenia, at 48 hours has most likely received a whole body irradiation dose of:
   A. 10 mrem.
   B. 10 rad.
   C. 50 rad.
   D. 200 rad.
   E. 1000 rad.

6. Which of the following statements concerning early central nervous system (CNS) symptoms in a patient with radiation exposure is correct?
   A. Symptoms are common and should resolve within 24 hours.
   B. Symptoms are variable and difficult to interpret.
   C. Symptoms usually result from hypoxic injury.
   D. Symptoms usually result from intracranial bleeding.
   E. Symptoms should be interpreted as a sign of high-dose radiation exposure.

7. You order a chest radiograph on a 2-year-old child. Her parents question the amount of radiation exposure. You would be correct in telling them that the exposure:
   A. Is about twice the annual natural radiation exposure the child gets.
   B. Is not measurable so they shouldn't concern themselves.
   C. May result in a mild degree of radiation sickness that will likely resolve without treatment.
   D. Is roughly equal to radiation sustained from two coast-to-coast jet flights.
   E. Is less than the exposure she gets from 1 hour of television watching.

8. Ionizing radiation includes:
   A. Neutrons from nuclear reactors, x-rays, and carbon-14.
   B. X-rays, radioisotopes, and microwaves.
   C. Plutonium, radio waves, and tritium.
   D. Microwaves, plutonium, and neutrons from nuclear accelerators.
   E. Solar rays, microwaves, and radio waves.

9. An adolescent ingests a large quantity of tritium as a suicide attempt. Possible useful treatment would include:
   A. Chelation with calcium EDTA.
   B. Administration of Prussian blue.
   C. Dilution with 3 to 4 liters of fluid.
   D. Shampooing and trimming of hair.
   E. Administration of 300 mg of potassium iodide.

10. A 3-year-old accidentally ingests a large amount of radioactive iodide 1 hour before arrival in the ED. Initial treatment should include:
   A. Gastric lavage and administration of activated charcoal.
   B. Gastric lavage followed by administration of potassium iodide.
   C. Administration of syrup of ipecac followed by chelation with calcium EDTA.
   D. Administration of activated charcoal alone.
   E. Administration of activated charcoal followed by chelation with the zinc salt of diethylenetriamine pentaacetic acid (DTPA).

ANSWERS   [See Barkin et al: Chapter 41.]

1. The answer is **E,** page 523.
   Skin changes and hair loss have not been associated with overall prognosis. Although early onset of nausea and vomiting can be indicative that significant exposure has occurred, there is no clear dose-response relationship. The most common hematologic changes include depression of the lymphocyte and platelet counts. The absolute lymphocyte count obtained within 48 hours of exposure has been correlated with ultimate prognosis.

2. The answer is **D,** page 522.
   X-rays are an example of γ-rays, which are pure electromagnetic radiation. α-Particles are positively charged fragments from heavy radioactive elements. β-Particles are electrons emitted by isotopes such as tritium and carbon-14. β-Decay is another example of γ-radiation and results from decay from radioisotopes and radiation produced by linear accelerators. Neutrons are particulate radiation resulting from nuclear reactors, accelerators, and weapons.

3. The answer is **B,** page 524.
   X-ray exposure is an example of irradiation, not contamination. Irradiation victims require fluid resuscitation similar to thermal burn patients. Irradiation does not result in the victim's becoming radioactive, and efforts at decontamination are unnecessary.

4. The answer is **A,** pages 524 and 525.
   Open wounds should be treated first and covered to prevent washing radioactive material into the wound. External decontamination should then proceed with washing of the skin and hair and irrigation of the eyes. When surgery is necessary, it is safest to perform early, before fluid and electrolyte imbalance, coagulation disorders, or infection occurs.

5. The answer is **D,** page 523, Table 41-2, and page 525.
   This person would fall into the survival-possible group. Problems with fluid and electrolyte imbalance, hematologic abnormalities, and infection would be likely complications.

6. The answer is **E,** page 525.
   CNS symptoms are rarely a part of low-level radiation exposure. When CNS symptoms appear early, it can be assumed that the patient has had a very large exposure.

7. The answer is **D,** page 523, Table 41-1.
   Natural radiation exposure is about 100 mrem/person/year. A chest radiograph results in about 10 mrem/film. A coast-to-coast flight results in about 5 mrem exposure. Color television results in only 1 mrem/year under typical conditions. By contrast, measurable laboratory effects of radiation exposure begin at about 10 rad (equal to 10,000 mrem of x-ray exposure). Clinical findings are rare below 50 rad exposure.

8. The answer is **A,** page 522.
   Solar rays, microwaves, and radio waves are examples of nonionizing radiation. Nonionizing radiation produces neither radiation sickness nor contamination. Ionizing radiation results from exposure to α-particles, β-particles, γ-rays, or neutrons. It can cause radiation sickness, contamination, or both, depending on the type of particle or ray involved.

9. The answer is **C,** page 525.
   Dilution can be effective treatment for tritium or technetium-99 exposure by production of diuresis. Chelation is useful for internal contamination with specific heavy metals. Antacids and Prussian blue are used to precipitate other heavy metals. Potassium iodide is used as a blocking agent for radioactive iodide ingestions.

10. The answer is **B,** page 525.
   See answer to question 9. Activated charcoal has not been shown to be effective for heavy metal ingestions.

General Management Principles for Poisoning

Morton Salomon • *Waseem Hafeez*

See Barkin et al: Chapter 42.

1. Which of the following interventions is most important in determining the outcome of patients following an ingestion?
   A. Administration of activated charcoal.
   B. Gastric emptying.
   C. Supportive care.
   D. Hemodialysis.
   E. Administration of an antidote.
2. All of the following statements regarding an *accidental* ingestion compared with a *nonaccidental* ingestion are true except:
   A. The quantity of the ingestion is usually unknown.
   B. The timing of the ingestion is more likely to be known.
   C. The ingestion most often occurs in young children and the elderly.
   D. Outcome of the ingestion generally is more benign.
   E. An accidental ingestion is more likely to involve a single substance.
3. Which of the following statements concerning drug kinetics in an overdose is *correct?*
   A. The kinetics of drug overdose can be predicted by the kinetics of a pharmacologic dose of the drug.
   B. The volume of distribution of a drug is calculated from the tissue concentrations divided by the serum concentration.
   C. Drugs with a large volume of distribution are more easily dialyzable.
   D. Drugs that are protein bound are more easily eliminated from the body.
   E. Drugs with a volume of distribution less than 1L/kg are more amenable to hemodialysis.
4. A 17-year-old girl comes to the ED 1 hour after ingesting 36 g of sustained release–enteric coated aspirin tablets. Which of the following statements concerning this patient's condition is *true?*
   A. It is unlikely that any aspirin remains in the stomach at the time the patient arrives.
   B. Peak serum levels of aspirin will occur at approximately 6 hours.
   C. The pills should be visible on a plain radiograph of the abdomen.
   D. Management should be withheld until a serum drug level confirms the overdose or the patient becomes symptomatic.
   E. Arrangements should be initiated to perform hemoperfusion for the patient.
5. Which of the following household substances, if ingested by a toddler, should cause the most concern?
   A. Silica gel (dehumidifying packets).
   B. Pencil lead.
   C. Eye makeup.
   D. Mercury from a broken thermometer.
   E. A whole cigarette.
6. Which of the following compounds is *least* likely to be adsorbed to activated charcoal?
   A. Syrup of ipecac.
   B. Cyanide.
   C. Polyethylene glycol.
   D. Acetaminophen.
   E. Sorbitol.
7. Which of the following poisons is *correctly* matched with its antidote?
   A. Cyanide/thiosulfate.
   B. Iron/calcium EDTA.
   C. Oleander/pralidoxime.
   D. Isoniazid/thiamine.
   E. β-Blockers/β-agonists.

8. Which one of the following toxins is correctly matched with the most *appropriate* method of *enhanced excretion?*
   A. Phencyclidine/urinary acidification.
   B. Theophylline/multiple-dose activated charcoal (MDAC).
   C. Tricyclic antidepressants/hemoperfusion.
   D. Ethylene glycol/ethanol.
   E. Acetaminophen/*N*-acetylcysteine (NAC).

9. Which of the following toxins is correctly matched with the most *appropriate* method of *enhanced elimination?*
   A. Theophylline/hemodialysis.
   B. Nicotine/urinary alkalinization.
   C. Salicylates/hemoperfusion.
   D. Methanol/hemodialysis.
   E. Phenobarbital/urinary acidification.

10. Whole bowel irrigation would be the most appropriate management strategy in which of the following ingestion scenarios?
    A. An asymptomatic cocaine body packer.
    B. An asymptomatic 3-year-old child who ingested iron 4 hours ago.
    C. An asymptomatic 16-year-old adolescent who ingested 20 sustained-release verapamil tablets 2 hours ago.
    D. Answers A and B are correct.
    E. Answers A and C are correct.

11. Which of the following statements about the use of whole bowel irrigation is *most correct?*
    A. It should always be used in severe iron overdose.
    B. The recommended irrigation rate is 10 ml/kg/hr.
    C. It should never be used with activated charcoal.
    D. Electrolyte disturbances rarely occur.
    E. Antiemetics should be avoided when using polyethylene glycol.

12. A 14-year-old boy is found unconscious in an alley. He is brought to the ED and is noted to be responsive only to pain. Vital signs reveal: blood pressure (BP) 110/70 mm Hg, heart rate (HR) 116 beats per minute, respiratory rate (RR) 12 breaths per minute and shallow, and temperature (T) 96.1° F (35.6° C). His pupils are small, and needle marks ("tracks") are noted on both forearms. The most correct sequence of management strategies for this patient would be:
    A. Intravenous (IV) access, naloxone 0.4 mg IV, 50 ml of dextrose-50, thiamine 100 mg.
    B. Bag-valve-mask (BVM) assisted ventilation with 40% oxygen, IV access, naloxone 2 to 4 mg, 50 ml of dextrose-50.
    C. BVM with 100% oxygen, intubation of the patient's trachea, naloxone 2 to 4 mg, IV access, 50 ml of dextrose-50.
    D. Intubation of the patient's trachea with assisted ventilation, IV access, naloxone 0.4 mg, gastric lavage, 50 ml of dextrose-50.
    E. Intubation of the patient's trachea and assisted ventilation with 100% oxygen, gastric lavage, naloxone 2 to 4 mg, 50 ml of dextrose-50, thiamine 100 mg.

13. Which statement about MDAC is most correct?
    A. It should be used in all overdose situations because it might help and certainly cannot hurt.
    B. It has been shown to enhance the clearance of a small number of toxins.
    C. It has not been shown to cause constipation and bowel obstruction.
    D. It enhances the clearance of theophylline because theophylline undergoes enterohepatic recirculation.
    E. It is important in the management of serious awake cyclic antidepressant overdoses.

14. Which statement best describes the role of cathartics in gastric decontamination?
    A. Sorbitol has been shown to be the most effective cathartic in decreasing gut transit time.
    B. All cathartics have been shown to reduce absorption of toxins.
    C. Cathartics should be given whenever charcoal is administered.
    D. Cathartics work by reducing desorption (unbinding) of the toxin from activated charcoal.
    E. Use of sorbitol has been shown to improve clinical outcome in certain situations.

ANSWERS   [See Barkin et al: Chapter 42.]

1. The answer is **C**, pages 529 to 533.

   In most poisonings, supportive care and attention to advanced life support are critical to the patient's outcome. Gastric emptying, in most situations, has little influence on drug absorption and even less influence on patient outcome. Multiple-dose activated charcoal (MDAC) has been demonstrated to increase the clearance of several drugs, such as phenobarbitol and theophylline, but has had little influence on clinical outcome. The administration of specific antidotes (e.g., N-acetylcysteine [NAC] in acetaminophen poisoning) and the use of hemodialysis (e.g., in salicylate poisoning) can be lifesaving interventions but are applicable only in select situations and not in the majority of overdoses.

2. The answer is **A**, pages 527 and 530.

   Accidental ingestions, which are most common in children younger than 6 and the elderly, are more likely to involve a *known* quantity of a single substance with a better estimate of the timing of the event. Intentional ingestions are more likely to be serious, and the history is less reliable.

3. The answer is **E**, pages 527 and 528.

   A volume of distribution less than 1 L/kg is relatively small, indicating that a large proportion of the absorbed drug remains in the serum and is therefore more amenable to methods that enhance the elimination of drugs. Drugs that are protein bound are difficult to eliminate because they are not amenable to exchange across membranes. During an overdose situation the kinetics that have been predicted for a pharmacologic dose of the drug are no longer applicable. Rates of absorption and elimination change because of the saturation of biologic mechanisms. The volume of distribution of a drug is calculated by dividing the total dose of the drug by the serum concentration.

4. The answer is **C**, pages 528 to 531 and 560.

   Enteric-coated tablets are often visible on plain x-ray films, especially enteric-coated salicylate tablets. Salicylate induces pyloric spasm and forms concretions that adhere to the gastric mucosa, thereby making it probable that some aspirin remains in the stomach. Although the Done nomogram uses 6 hours for the peak level in salicylate overdoses, this is an overdose of enteric-coated tablets, and the nomogram is therefore unreliable because it is unlikely that the peak level will be achieved in 6 hours. Because this is a potentially serious overdose, management should begin as soon as possible pending the results of the drug level. The definitive treatment of choice for salicylate poisoning is hemodialysis, not hemoperfusion. Arrangements need not be instituted until the levels are obtained from this patient because it is early in the poisoning and hemodialysis might not be necessary.

5. The answer is **E**, box on page 528.

   A whole cigarette can produce symptomatic nicotine poisoning in a small child. Pencil lead, of course, is not really lead but carbon. Silica gel and eye makeup are nontoxic. The amount of mercury ingested from a broken thermometer would also be nontoxic, especially because its absorption would be minimal.

6. The answer is **B**, page 531.

   Cyanide is a small molecule and thus does not readily adsorb to activated charcoal. Although syrup of ipecac, sorbitol, and polyethylene glycol are used in conjunction with activated charcoal as part of gastrointestinal decontamination regimens, they all adsorb to activated charcoal. Acetaminophen, a complex molecule, is readily adsorbed by activated charcoal.

7. The answer is **A**, page 533, Table 42-1.

   Thiosulfate is the third component of the cyanide antidote kit along with amyl nitrite and sodium nitrite. Iron is chelated by deferoxamine. Oleander is a naturally occurring cardiac glycoside and should be treated with digoxin immune fragments of antibodies (Digibind). Pyridoxine (vitamin B_6) is the antidote for a symptomatic isoniazid overdose. β-Blocker toxicity is not effectively reversed by β-agonists and is usually treated with glucagon.

8. The answer is **B**, pages 532 and 533.

   The clearance of theophylline in serum is enhanced by MDAC via gastrointestinal dialysis. Phencyclidine (PCP), as a weak base, can have its excretion enhanced by urinary acidification, but this can also cause precipitation of myoglobin in the renal tubules and therefore is no longer recommended. Tricyclic antidepressants have a large volume of distribution, are also largely protein bound, and thus are not significantly extracted by hemoperfusion. Ethanol is used as an antidote in the treatment of ethylene glycol poisoning but acts by slowing the conversion of ethylene glycol to its toxic metabolite, oxalic acid, and plays no role in enhancing elimination of the compound. Similarly N-acetylcysteine prevents the formation of toxic metabolites in the liver in an acetaminophen overdose and makes no significant contribution to clearance.

9. The answer is **D**, pages 532 and 533.

   The definitive treatment for both methanol and ethylene glycol elimination is hemodialysis after blocking the toxic effect with ethanol. Theophylline can be eliminated by hemodialysis, but hemoperfusion is more effective. Salicylate is effectively eliminated by hemoperfusion, but hemodialysis is equally effective and corrects electrolyte disturbances in the process. Phenobarbital is a weak acid and is treated with *alkalinization*. Nicotine is a weak base and can have its elimination expedited by urinary acidification, but this is not recommended because of the risk of seizures and rhabdomyolysis.

10. The answer is **E**, page 532.

    Both A and C are correct. Whole bowel irrigation (WBI) has been used successfully with body packing and is especially useful for ingestions of sustained-release preparations that happened hours before the patient comes in. WBI has been successfully used with iron ingestion as well because iron does not bind to activated charcoal. However, a young child who is asymptomatic 4 hours after ingesting iron would not need treatment.

11. The answer is **D**, page 532.

    Because WBI uses a balanced electrolyte solution, it is not expected to cause electrolyte imbalances. Although valuable in severe iron overdoses, WBI is contraindicated if the overdose causes gastrointestinal hemorrhage. The recommended rate of irrigation is 500 ml/hr in children and 1 to 2 L/hr in adolescents and adults. Although the solution is expected to bind to activated charcoal, a preliminary single dose of activated charcoal can be given before the initiation of WBI if deemed useful. IV antiemetics are recommended if the patient is vomiting WBI solution.

12. The answer is **C**, page 529.

    The patient in the scenario has compromised vital signs and coma of unknown etiology. The first priority in management of the patient is stabilization of the airway followed by administration of an antidote followed by gastric decontamination efforts. Begin BVM with *100% oxygen* followed by intubation of the patient's trachea to secure the airway. Naloxone can be given via the endotracheal tube. Dextrose should be administered to all coma victims unless an accurate glucose reading in the high normal range can be obtained immediately. Thiamine is rarely necessary in the treatment of adolescents and children in coma.

13. The answer is **B**, page 533.

    MDAC has been clearly demonstrated to enhance the clearance of phenobarbital, theophylline, possibly aspirin, and a few other drugs. Its effect on other toxins has not been studied or demonstrated, and its effect on clinical outcome is even less clear. Repeated doses of charcoal pose the risk of aspiration, especially in unconscious or struggling patients or those with vomiting or seizures. Repeated doses of cathartic, along with the charcoal, may lead to serious electrolyte disturbances. Theophylline does not undergo significant amounts of enterohepatic recirculation. MDAC enhances the clearance of theophylline by gastrointestinal dialysis. In serious cyclic antidepressant overdoses a significant risk of seizure and rapid loss of consciousness makes MDAC therapy hazardous.

14. The answer is **A**, pages 531 and 532.

    Of the cathartics commonly used in overdose management, sorbitol has the greatest impact on gut transit time, followed by magnesium citrate. Research has failed, however, to demonstrate any benefit regarding reduced drug absorption or clinical outcome from the use of cathartics. Cathartics are not needed to prevent constipation or obstruction from charcoal and can cause severe electrolyte disturbances if administered repeatedly with MDAC. Desorption of toxin from activated charcoal is best prevented by large doses of charcoal.

35

Specific Toxins

Morton Salomon • *Waseem Hafeez*

See Barkin et al: Chapter 43.

1. An 18-year-old girl is brought to the ED in active seizure. After learning that she was pregnant, she ingested an unknown quantity of isoniazid tablets. The first step in the management of this patient is to:
   A. Stabilize airway and provide 100% oxygen.
   B. Establish intravenous (IV) access and administer anticonvulsant.
   C. Administer activated charcoal via nasogastric tube.
   D. Avoid giving activated charcoal because the patient is pregnant.
   E. Perform gastric lavage.

2. Which of the statements regarding emesis induced by syrup of ipecac is true?
   A. It may be used in children older than 1 month of age.
   B. It can be used safely with any ingestion.
   C. If successful, activated charcoal should not be needed.
   D. It is more useful when applied at home than when administered in the ED.
   E. The standard dose is 1 ml/kg to a maximum of 60 ml.

3. A 17-year-old girl comes to the ED with a history of nausea, vomiting, diaphoresis, and pallor. On questioning she admits to taking 25 "extra strength" acetaminophen tablets about 8 hours ago. Initial management should be to:
   A. Obtain an acetaminophen level and await results.
   B. Administer activated charcoal followed by *N*-acetylcysteine (NAC) 2 hours later.
   C. Administer NAC 70 mg/kg intravenously.
   D. Start forced diuresis.
   E. Administer NAC 140 mg/kg orally.

4. To obtain the greatest effectiveness, NAC should be administered within how many hours following the ingestion of acetaminophen?
   A. 72 hours.
   B. 48 hours.
   C. 24 hours.
   D. 16 hours.
   E. 8 hours.

5. A patient vomits a dose of NAC within 1 hour of administration. All of the following statements regarding this problem are correct except:
   A. Wait 4 hours for next dose.
   B. Repeat the same dose.
   C. Use an antiemetic before NAC administration.
   D. Use a nasogastric tube or duodenal tube to administer NAC by continuous infusion.
   E. Mix with fruit juice or soda and let the patient drink it through a straw.

6. The major route of metabolism of acetaminophen in a 4-year-old child is:
   A. The kidney.
   B. Cytochrome P-450 pathway.
   C. Glucuronidation.
   D. Sulfation.
   E. Demethylation.

7. A 19-year-old pregnant patient is seen in the ED with a 4-hour acetaminophen level that is greater than 250 µg/ml. The correct management approach would be to:
   A. Avoid NAC because it is a known teratogen.
   B. Avoid NAC because it does not prevent fetal hepatotoxicity.
   C. Proceed with gastric emptying only.
   D. Use activated charcoal alone.
   E. Use the same dosage and route of administration as in any acetaminophen ingestion.

8. Which statement is *true* regarding liver toxicity from acetaminophen overdose?
   A. It is likely because acetaminophen plasma half-life is approximately 2 to 3 hours.
   B. It usually is clinically evident 12 to 24 hours after ingestion.
   C. For a given toxic plasma level, children have a higher incidence of hepatic aminotransferase elevation than adults have.
   D. Hepatic toxicity results from *N*-Acetyl-p-benzoquinoneimine (NAPQI).
   E. Diet, nutritional status, and age are not related to liver toxicity.

9. A patient has a 4-hour acetaminophen level of 150 μg/ml. After an oral dose of NAC of 140 mg/kg the next acetaminophen level is below the toxic zone. You would now:
   A. Discontinue NAC therapy and observe for 24 hours.
   B. Continue NAC 140 mg/kg every 4 hours for 17 doses.
   C. Continue NAC 70 mg/kg every 4 hours for 17 doses.
   D. Discontinue NAC therapy and repeat acetaminophen level every 4 hours and restart therapy only if level reaches hepatic toxic zone.
   E. Discontinue therapy, discharge home, and monitor daily for renal, hepatic, and coagulation function tests.

10. A mother brings in her 1-year-old after accidentally spilling a bottle of rubbing alcohol over his face while giving him an alcohol sponge bath for fever. The child is drowsy, and the pupils are midpoint and reactive. Blood alcohol and isopropanol levels are pending. Which statement regarding this scenario is correct?
    A. Isopropanol is oxidized to oxalic acid by alcohol dehydrogenase.
    B. Isopropanol is less toxic than ethanol at equivalent blood levels.
    C. Emesis with syrup of ipecac is recommended.
    D. High serum ketone levels with little or no acidosis is characteristic of isopropanol exposure.
    E. Hemodialysis is not effective.

11. A 20-year-old suicidal man comes to the ED saying he ingested something. He is inebriated but responds to commands. He complains of nausea, abdominal cramps, and blurry vision. Visual examination shows fixed, dilated pupils with retinal hyperemia. The signs and symptoms are most consistent with ingestion of which of the following?
    A. Ethanol.
    B. Ethylene glycol.
    C. Methanol.
    D. Paraldehyde.
    E. Isopropanol.

12. The arterial blood gas measurement for the patient described in question 11 shows: pH 7.15, $Paco_2$ 25 mm Hg, Pao_2 94 mm Hg. Serum chemistries are: Na 142 mEq/L, K 3.5 mEq/L, Cl 100 mEq/L, HCO_3 10 mEq/L, glucose 90 mg/dl, BUN 18 mg/dl, Cr 0.8 mg/dl. Which of the following best describes the patient's acid-base status?
    A. Respiratory acidosis.
    B. Combined metabolic with respiratory acidosis.
    C. Metabolic acidosis with decreased anion gap.
    D. Metabolic acidosis with increased anion gap.
    E. Metabolic acidosis with normal anion gap.

13. Which of the following ingestions could be seen with an increased anion gap?
    A. Acetaminophen.
    B. Isopropanol.
    C. Ethylene glycol.
    D. Ethylene dibromide.
    E. Methane.

14. The major toxic effects of methanol ingestion are due to the accumulation of which metabolite?
    A. Glycoaldehyde.
    B. Glycolic acid.
    C. Formic acid.
    D. Glyoxylate
    E. Oxylate.

15. Following a methanol ingestion, the goal of inhibiting alcohol dehydrogenase is best achieved by maintaining the serum ethanol concentration between:
    A. 5 and 20 mg/dl.
    B. 20 and 50 mg/dl.
    C. 50 and 100 mg/dl.
    D. 100 and 200 mg/dl.
    E. 200 and 300 mg/dl.

16. Hemodialysis is indicated for any patient with a peak methanol level greater than:
    A. 10 mg/dl.
    B. 20 mg/dl.
    C. 50 mg/dl.
    D. 100 mg/dl.
    E. 150 mg/dl.

17. A 19-year-old brought in by Emergency Medical Service (EMS) is stuporous but responds to commands. He acts intoxicated but has no odor of alcohol on his breath. He has nystagmus, but his pupils are equal and reactive, and funduscopy examination is normal. He was given 2 mg naloxone, 100 mg thiamine, and 100 ml 50% dextrose by EMS during transport to the ED with no change in the patient's clinical status. Which of the following urinary findings would suggest a potential toxin?
    A. Gross hematuria.
    B. Proteinuria.
    C. Granular cast.
    D. Calcium oxalate crystals.
    E. Urinary ketones.

18. Ethylene glycol poisoning is characterized by all of the following *except*:
    A. Metabolic acidosis.
    B. Increased anion gap.
    C. Hypocalcemia.
    D. Hypomagnesemia.
    E. Hypokalemia.

19. A 15-year-old girl comes to the ED with a history of ingesting a bottle of diphenhydramine (Benadryl) tablets. Which one of the following signs and symptoms would be expected on examining the patient?
    A. Sweating, lacrimation, salivation, miosis, and blurred vision.
    B. Lethargy, slow respirations, hypotension, and miosis.
    C. Agitation, tachycardia, sweating, and mydriasis.
    D. Flushed face, agitation, dry mucous membrane, and dilated pupils.
    E. Headache, tachycardia, tachypnea, cherry red mucous membrane, and dim vision.

20. A 6-month-old baby was accidentally given 50 mg of diphenhydramine (Benadryl) 2 hours before coming to the ED. The patient is flushed, tachycardic, and agitated. Which statement regarding antihistamine overdose is most accurate?
    A. Gastrointestinal (GI) decontamination will not be useful beyond 1 hour of ingestion.
    B. Seizures generally are resistant to diazepam.
    C. Anticholinergic effects are a result of decreased production of acetylcholine.
    D. Dialysis should be considered.
    E. Drug elimination occurs through hepatic metabolism and urinary excretion.

21. A 5-year-old patient with a history of a seizure disorder controlled with carbamazepine (Tegretol) comes to the ED with nausea, vomiting, and ataxia. All of the following statements are true for carbamazepine (CBZ) toxicity *except:*
    A. Its complications mimic those of both phenytoin and tricyclic antidepressants (TCAs).
    B. Clinical presentations are unpredictable because GI motility and absorption is delayed.
    C. The half-life is longer after chronic use than after a single ingestion.
    D. No minimal lethal dose is known.
    E. A common complication of it is seizures.

22. A 2-year-old is brought to the ED by his mother, who says her son may have ingested a few CBZ (Tegretol) chewable tablets used by his sibling. Which of the following clinical findings would best support the possibility of an ingestion?
    A. Vomiting.
    B. Confusion and excitation.
    C. Tachycardia.
    D. Hyperreflexia.
    E. Nystagmus.

23. A grandmother brings in a 15-month-old infant who may have swallowed one clonidine tablet (0.1 mg) about 30 minutes ago. The child is sitting quietly on her lap with heart rate (HR) 80 beats per minute, blood pressure (BP) 130/80 mm Hg, and respiratory rate (RR) 20 breaths per minute. Which of the following would be the most appropriate management of this patient?
    A. The patient can be discharged after initial assessment.
    B. Look for other ingestants because hypertension is unlikely with a clonidine overdose.
    C. Naloxone 0.1 mg/kg IV bolus should be given because the patient is bradycardic.
    D. Emesis should be immediately attempted with syrup of ipecac.
    E. Only supportive care and monitoring are needed because most patients recover in 12 to 24 hours.

24. A 2-year-old who swallowed digoxin tablets is found to have bradycardia. An electrocardiogram (ECG) shows ventricular bigeminy. Which of the following is true?
    A. ECG findings of T wave depression and scooped ST segments correlate with significant digoxin toxicity.
    B. Digoxin immune FAB (Digibind) is indicated for life-threatening dysrhythmias.
    C. There is a wide margin between therapeutic and toxic doses.
    D. Hyperkalemia is not affected by digoxin immune FAB (Digibind) therapy.
    E. Forced alkaline diuresis may increase renal excretion.

25. Which statement regarding caustic injury to the esophagus is *correct?*
    A. Acid burns are usually deeper than alkali burns in the esophagus and thus cause greater long-term complications.
    B. If there are no oropharyngeal lesions, esophagoscopy is not required because esophageal burns are unlikely.
    C. Patients who ingest caustics appear to have an increased risk of esophageal carcinoma.
    D. Only 50% of all stricture formation results within 2 months of ingestion.
    E. About 10% of first-degree burns result in esophageal strictures.

26. A frantic mother calls you saying her 2-year-old child just swallowed some household bleach. She gave him milk, which he drank without any drooling or vomiting. Which of the following is the most appropriate action to take?
    A. Tell the mother to give her son syrup of ipecac immediately.
    B. Tell the mother to bring her son to the ED for endoscopy to rule out esophageal burns.
    C. Reassure the mother that it is a mild irritant and that her son will do fine as he has been drinking without problems.
    D. Warn the mother that because household bleach is an alkali, it can cause esophageal strictures even if oral lesions are not seen.
    E. Tell the mother to give her son antacid to buffer the effect of the bleach.

27. A 16-year-old girl comes to the ED in status epilepticus. Her ECG shows a widened QRS complex (more than 0.12 sec). All of the following ingestions can cause the above *except:*
    A. Propoxyphene.
    B. Quinidine.
    C. Phenothiazine.
    D. Amphetamine.
    E. Imipramine.

28. A 17-year-old distraught girl walks into the ED saying she ingested a handful of nortriptyline pills after an argument with her boyfriend. She is alert, with BP 120/70 mm Hg and HR 120 beats per minute, and the lead II on the ECG reveals a QRS with a duration of 0.12 sec. The most appropriate immediate management should be:
    A. Emesis with syrup of ipecac.
    B. Activated charcoal with cathartic.
    C. Sodium bicarbonate 1 to 2 mEq/kg slow IV push.
    D. Phenytoin 10 to 20 mg/kg slow IV over 20 minutes.
    E. Physostigmine 0.5 mg IV over 1 minute.

29. All of the following statements regarding TCA overdosage are true except:
    A. The quinidine-like effects on the myocardium occur before neurologic symptoms.
    B. Limb-lead QRS duration is helpful in choosing patients at risk for ventricular dysrhythmias or seizures.
    C. Patients with a Glasgow Coma Scale (GCS) score less than 8 are at a greater risk for complications than those with prolonged QRS greater than 0.1 sec.
    D. TCA levels, if immediately available, correlate with the ECG findings.
    E. Hypotension unresponsive to fluid therapy should be treated with norepinephrine.

30. Asymptomatic patients with a history of TCA ingestion or suspected overdose must be observed and monitored for *at least* how many hours after ingestion before discharge?
    A. 2 hours.
    B. 6 hours.
    C. 12 hours.
    D. 24 hours.
    E. 48 hours.

31. Which statement most accurately describes the effects of insecticides?
    A. Carbamates create an irreversible bond with cholinesterase.
    B. Organophosphates stimulate the release of excessive amounts of acetylcholine at the synaptic junction.
    C. Insecticide poisoning can be confirmed by a rise in cholinesterase level in the blood.
    D. Humans have no biotransformation mechanism for metabolizing (detoxifying) insecticides.
    E. Organophosphates inhibit the degradation of acetylcholine.

32. Which statement most accurately characterizes the difference between organophosphate and carbamate insecticides?
    A. Carbamate exposure is more common than organophosphate exposure.
    B. Carbamate poisoning is usually of shorter duration.
    C. Pralidoxime must be started sooner to be effective in carbamate poisoning.
    D. Only organophosphates are absorbed through the skin.
    E. Both answers B and C are correct.

33. Which of the following statements concerning cholinergic poisoning treatment is most correct?
    A. Pralidoxime is used to prevent irreversible deactivation of cholinesterase.
    B. Atropine restores the biologic activity of cholinesterase.
    C. The dose of atropine should not exceed 2 mg.
    D. Pralidoxime is more useful as a treatment for carbamate exposure than for organophosphate exposure.
    E. Bronchorrhea must be treated by loop diuretics because atropine is ineffective for this symptom.

34. Which of the following statements concerning the use of laboratory tests in iron ingestion is *most* accurate?
    A. If the total iron-binding capacity (TIBC) is elevated, chelation should be instituted.
    B. A negative deferoxamine challenge indicates that there is unbound iron in the serum.
    C. A serum iron level greater than 300 μg/dl is considered to be an indication for starting chelation.
    D. An elevated white blood cell count (WBC), low serum glucose level, and an anion gap metabolic acidosis suggest iron toxicity.
    E. Both answers A and C are correct.

35. A 22-month-old, 15-kg girl is found with an empty bottle of chewable vitamin tablets (15 mg of elemental iron per tablet). Although originally 100 tablets were in the bottle, the mother believes that at least 75 tablets had been consumed before the ingestion. Five tablets are found on the floor in the house. The child is asymptomatic when she comes to the ED 90 minutes after the ingestion. Which of the following is the next most appropriate action?
    A. Administer an immediate dose of activated charcoal and observe for 6 hours.
    B. Obtain a serum iron level, complete blood count, serum electrolytes, and liver function studies and observe the patient for 6 hours in the ED.
    C. Obtain an abdominal radiograph, and if no iron tablets are seen, discharge the child.
    D. Administer syrup of ipecac and observe for 6 hours in the ED.
    E. Administer a deferoxamine challenge of 50 mg/kg intramuscularly.

36. A 16-year-old, 50-kg girl in her third trimester of pregnancy comes to the ED with vomiting, bloody diarrhea, and lethargy. Her pulse (P) is 120 beats per minute and her BP 85/50 mm Hg. Her family fears she might have ingested an entire bottle of prenatal vitamins (65 mg of elemental iron per tablet, 100 tablets in the bottle). Which of the following would be the best therapeutic approach in this patient?
    A. Administer IV fluids and begin a deferoxamine infusion at 15 mg/kg/hr.
    B. Administer deferoxamine 90 mg/kg intramuscularly immediately to support the possibility of an ingestion.
    C. Administer syrup of ipecac.
    D. Administer whole bowel irrigation to decontaminate the gut while initiating oral deferoxamine therapy.
    E. Avoid chelation therapy because deferoxamine is toxic to the fetus. Begin hemodialysis instead.

37. Which of the following statements regarding naloxone (Narcan) is most correct?
    A. It can be administered intravenously, intramuscularly, and endotracheally, but *not* intraosseously.
    B. It is often effective in reversing miosis associated with barbiturate overdose.
    C. It can reverse the respiratory depression of a clonidine overdose.
    D. It is effective with natural and semisynthetic opioids and is ineffective with synthetic opioids.
    E. It has agonist as well as antagonist effects at higher doses.

38. A 3-year-old is found on the bathroom floor with several medication bottles scattered about. The child is responsive only to pain with 3-mm pupils, HR 76 beats per minute, BP 78/44 mm Hg. These symptoms are consistent with toxicity from all of the following drugs *except:*
    A. Difenoxin (Lomotil).
    B. Ethanol.
    C. Chloral hydrate.
    D. Physostigmine.
    E. Clonidine.

Questions 39 through 42 apply to the following case scenario:

A 14-year-old boy comes in 3 hours after ingestion of salicylate. The maximal amount ingested is 35 g of salicylate. He is complaining of tinnitus, nausea, and vomiting. At the time he arrives in the ED his vital signs are BP 108/68 mm Hg, P 124 beats per minute, and RR 26 breaths per minute. An arterial blood gas reveals a pH of 7.44, and his serum salicylate level is 44 mg/dl.

39. Which of the following would *not* be expected in this patient?
    A. Normal anion gap metabolic acidosis.
    B. Elevation of prothrombin time (PT).
    C. Lactic acidosis.
    D. Hypoglycemia.
    E. Decreased serum ionized calcium.

40. Which of the following statements concerning the patient described is *most* accurate?
    A. Activated charcoal is unlikely to be of value in this patient's management because of the length of time since ingestion.
    B. The patient should not receive IV dextrose and $NaHCO_3$ concomitantly because of the risk of cerebral edema.
    C. Alkalinization of the urine is unnecessary in this case because the salicylate level places the patient in a "mild" category.
    D. Effective alkalinization of the urine will require adequate replacement of potassium.
    E. $NaHCO_3$ therapy should be avoided because the patient's serum is already alkaline.

41. Which of the following statements concerning the patient described is correct?
    A. Hemodialysis and hemoperfusion would be about equally effective in removing salicylate from this patient.
    B. The serum salicylate level indicates that dialysis will not be needed.
    C. An acute ingestion of salicylates is more likely to require dialysis than a chronic ingestion.
    D. Hypothermia, seizures, and renal failure are indications for dialysis.
    E. If pulmonary edema develops, dialysis should be avoided.

42. The patient is given 2 mEq/kg of sodium bicarbonate, and an infusion of 1 mEq/kg HCO_3 is initiated. An hour later his urine pH is measured at 7.0. What strategy regarding urine alkalinization would be *most* appropriate at this time?
    A. Maintain current management as long as urine pH stays at 7.0 or higher.
    B. Check serum potassium and replenish potassium if needed.
    C. Check serum pH and increase bicarbonate drip only if patient is now acidotic.
    D. Maintain the same rate of bicarbonate administration, double the rate of fluid administration.
    E. Do not be concerned about urine alkalinization at this point in this patient's management.

In questions 43 through 48 choose the drug from the list below that is *most* likely to cause the effect or symptom described: (Each drug can be used once, more than once, or not at all.)
    A. Barbiturates.
    B. Benzodiazepines.
    C. Opioids.
    D. Ethanol.
    E. Phenothiazines.
    F. Salicylates.

43. Miosis _____
44. Potentiates γ-aminobutyric acid (GABA) effect _____
45. Quinidine-like effects on ECG _____
46. Isoelectric electroencephalogram (EEG) _____
47. Positive ferric chloride test of the urine _____
48. Anticholinergic symptom complex _____

49. Which of the following modalities is *least* likely to enhance the clearance of phenobarbital in an overdosed patient?
    A. Repeat dosage of activated charcoal.
    B. Fluid diuresis.
    C. Administration of furosemide.
    D. Acidification of the urine.
    E. Peritoneal dialysis.

50. Which constellation of findings would *not* be expected in a barbiturate overdose?
    A. Slurred speech/adult respiratory distress syndrome (ARDS).
    B. Miosis/acute tubular necrosis (ATN).
    C. Mydriasis/prolonged QTc interval.
    D. Cutaneous bullae/cerebral edema.
    E. Hypothermia/hypercapnia.

51. All of the following may suggest a phenothiazine overdose *except:*
    A. Phenistix test of the urine.
    B. ECG.
    C. Elevated anion gap.
    D. Abdominal radiograph.
    E. Therapeutic trial of diphenhydramine.

52. Which one of the following is not seen with a phenothiazine overdose?
    A. Flushed warm skin, dry mouth, and mydriasis.
    B. Torticollis, opisthotonos, and tongue spasm.
    C. Hyperthermia, skeletal muscle activity, and renal failure.
    D. Prolongation of the QT interval, flattened T waves, and U waves on an ECG.
    E. Miosis, hypotension, and cutaneous bulla.

53. All of the following are associated with maternal cocaine abuse *except:*
    A. Placenta previa.
    B. Prolonged withdrawal syndrome.
    C. Spontaneous abortion.
    D. Limb defects.
    E. Postmaturity syndrome.

54. Which statement about the pharmacokinetics of cocaine is most accurate?
    A. The half-life of crack (free-base cocaine) is approximately 60 to 90 minutes.
    B. Cocecognine, its principal metabolite, is found in the urine up to 12 hours after use.
    C. It is absorbed significantly only through the lungs.
    D. It is metabolized mainly in the plasma.
    E. Less than 1 mg/kg is nontoxic.

55. Which of the following is *least* likely to be associated with intranasal cocaine abuse?
    A. Status epilepticus.
    B. Noncardiogenic pulmonary edema.
    C. Bowel infarction.
    D. Aortic dissection.
    E. Subarachnoid hemorrhage.

56. Which of the following strategies is most appropriate for the treatment of phencyclidine (PCP) intoxication?
    A. Multiple-dose activated charcoal (MDAC) to elimination.
    B. Acidification of the urine to enhance elimination.
    C. Haloperidol to control agitation.
    D. Propranolol for the management of hypertension.
    E. IV hydration to prevent renal failure.

57. Which diagnostic test would be *least* useful in the management of an amphetamine overdose?
    A. Serum potassium.
    B. Creatine kinase.
    C. Urine myoglobin.
    D. Serum drug level.
    E. ECG.

58. All of the following may be seen in a patient following a theophylline ingestion *except:*
    A. Hypokalemia.
    B. Hypophosphatemia.
    C. Hypomagnesemia.
    D. Hypoglycemia.
    E. Metabolic acidosis.

59. The fact that theophylline clearance is enhanced by MDAC is best supported by which of the following statements?
    A. It undergoes significant hepatic excretion.
    B. It is largely (more than 90%) protein bound.
    C. It has a relatively low volume of distribution.
    D. It assumes an ionized form in the serum.
    E. It undergoes gastric resecretion.

60. Which statement concerning the management of theophylline toxicity is *correct?*
    A. Propranolol may be effective in the treatment of hypotension.
    B. Activated charcoal has no role in the treatment of IV aminophylline toxicity.
    C. Whole bowel irrigation enhances clearance of theophylline from the serum.
    D. Cimetidine can be used to control theophylline-induced hyperemesis because it decreases theophylline levels.
    E. Hemoperfusion and hemodialysis are equally effective in removing theophylline.

ANSWERS [See Barkin et al: Chapter 43.]

1. The answer is **A,** page 535.
   The principles of management in all toxicology cases involve supportive care. Initial stabilization and attention to the ABCs (airway, breathing, circulation) should be the first priority. Activated charcoal is not contraindicated in pregnancy. The antidote for isoniazid-induced seizures is pyridoxine.

2. The answer is **D,** page 535.
   Syrup of ipecac now is generally reserved for home use after minor pediatric ingestions and rarely used in ED settings. Ipecac is not recommended in children younger than 12 months of age. The dose is 15 ml for children younger than 12 years of age and 30 ml for older children. It is not used in patients who are comatose, lack a gag reflex, or have ingested a caustic substance.

3. The answer is **E,** pages 538 and 539.
   N-Acetylcysteine (NAC) is the drug of choice for acetaminophen ingestion. The patient in the scenario has taken 25 extra strength acetaminophen tablets (500 mg), which equals 12.5 g, and is in phase I (1½ to 24 hours) of acetaminophen poisoning. Liver damage may occur in adults who ingest 7.5 g or 140 mg/kg. Although an acetaminophen level should be measured, NAC therapy should be initiated immediately because 8 hours already has elapsed, and that is the time in which NAC may be expected to maximally prevent hepatotoxicity. The dose of NAC is 140 mg/kg followed by 70 mg/kg for 17 more doses. Activated charcoal may bind NAC and reduce its effectiveness. Therefore a 2-hour interval between these two therapies is theoretically desirable, although probably unnecessary. However, NAC takes priority here and should not be delayed. Forced diuresis is ineffective because only 5% of the drug and its toxic metabolite are excreted in the urine.

4. The answer is **E,** page 538.
   If the acetaminophen level drawn 4 hours after the ingestion is in the hepatotoxic range on the Rumack-Matthew nomogram, treatment with NAC should be initiated immediately. It is 100% effective if used within 8 hours, 8% to 33% within 8 to 16 hours, and 4% to 50% within 6 to 24 hours after ingestion.

5. The answer is **A,** page 539.
   If the patient in the scenario vomits NAC within 1 hour, the same dose should be repeated. NAC (Mucomyst) tastes foul, smells like rotten eggs, and irritates the stomach. To reduce the likelihood of vomiting, dilute to a 5% solution (1:1 of 10% or 1:3 of 20% solution of Mucomyst) with chilled juice or a sweet soda drink. Covering it and having the patient drink through a straw, pretreating with metoclopramide IV, and administrating it through a nasogastric tube radiologically placed in the duodenum have all been successful. Waiting 4 hours would not prevent vomiting and is harmful because NAC's effectiveness is reduced.

6. The answer is **D,** page 536.
   More than 90% of the acetaminophen dose is conjugated by the liver to sulfate (52%) and gluconate (42%) metabolites. Less than 5% is excreted unchanged in the urine and 4% to 5% is metabolized via the hepatic cytochrome P-450 mixed function oxidase system to an active intermediate metabolite N-acetyl-p-benzoquinoneimine (NAPQI). Demethylation is not known to be a metabolic pathway of acetaminophen.

7. The answer is **E,** page 539.
   Current data suggest that use of NAC protects both the mother and fetus, since fetal hepatotoxicity is possible with an overdose. NAC does not appear to be teratogenic. The current consensus is to treat pregnant women with the same protocol as any acetaminophen ingestion, since the risk of not treating exceeds the potential risk of NAC to the fetus.

8. The answer is **D,** pages 536 and 537.
   Liver toxicity results when NAPQI, a reactive intermediary, is formed by cytochrome P-450 activity. Glutathione conjugates NAPQI to nontoxic conjugates. In an overdose glutathione becomes depleted, and NAPQI binds covalently with the hepatocyte to produce centrilobular hepatic necrosis. The normal half-life for acetaminophen is 2 to 3 hours. In patients with intoxication the plasma half-life increases. A plasma half-life over 4 hours suggests liver toxicity and over 12 hours suggests the possibility of hepatic coma. Hepatic enzymes increase in the second stage of acetaminophen overdose (24 to 48 hours), and progressive hepatic encephalopathy develops in the final hepatic stage (3 to 4 days). Children seem to have a lower incidence of clinical toxicity, which may be related to the fact that children younger than 12 years primarily use the sulfate pathway of conjugation. Diet, nutritional status, and age all affect cytochrome P-450 activity, which regulates the amount of NAPQI formed.

9. The answer is **C,** page 539.
   Once an acetaminophen level is found to be in the hepatic toxic zone, the full NAC course of 18 doses over 72 hours is to be administered. Only if the exact time of ingestion is determined to be different from what was originally thought and the level found to be under the toxic range can the NAC treatment be discontinued. If the time of ingestion is not known and the acetaminophen level is more than 10 μg/ml (level drawn at least 4 hours after ingestion), the fully recommended course of therapy should be given.

10. The answer is **D,** pages 541 and 542.

Isopropyl alcohol exists as a 70% solution in rubbing alcohol, and toxicity may occur easily as it is absorbed through the skin, by inhalation, or by ingestion. Isopropanol is oxidized to acetone by alcohol dehydrogenase. Serum acetone levels continue to rise as isopropyl alcohol levels fall, resulting in high serum ketones without acidosis. Death has been reported with isopropanol levels as low as 150 mg/dl in adults, but similar ethanol levels would not be expected to be lethal. Isopropyl alcohol is readily absorbed from the gastrointestinal (GI) tract, 80% within 30 minutes, resulting in rapid central nervous system (CNS) depression. Thus, induction of emesis with ipecac is hazardous. Although forced diuresis is ineffective, hemodialysis has been used in patients with levels greater than 150 mg/dl with severe symptoms. One word of caution, a complete physical and neurologic examination is essential to rule out physical abuse because it may be manifested in many different ways.

11. The answer is **C,** page 542.

GI tract findings (nausea, vomiting, abdominal cramps, GI bleeding, pancreatitis), eye findings (blurring of vision similar to "stepping into a snowstorm"), and severe metabolic acidosis with an elevated anion gap are classic signs and symptoms of methanol ingestion. The pupils are dilated with sluggish or absent reaction to light and accommodation with hyperemia of the optic disc, resulting in temporary or permanent blindness. The ocular toxicity correlates directly with the severity of metabolic acidosis, and delay in management may result in permanent blindness.

12. The answer is **D,** page 539.

The patient in the scenario has a metabolic acidosis with an elevated anion gap of 35.5. Metabolic acidosis may be associated with a normal or an increased anion gap. Anion gap can be calculated by subtracting the measured anions from the measured cations:

$$[(Na^+ + K^+) - (Cl^- + HCO_3^-)]$$

The gap is normally 12 to 16 mEq/L. Organic acids that are unmeasured anions contribute to the elevated gap.

13. The answer is **C,** page 539.

The etiologies of metabolic acidosis with elevated anion gap can be recalled with the mnemonic MUD-PILES: **M**ethanol, **U**remia, **D**iabetic ketoacidosis, **P**araldehyde, **I**ron, **I**soniazid, or **I**nhalants, **L**actic acidosis, **E**thylene glycol or chronic **E**thanol abuse, and **S**alicylates or **S**olvents. In acetaminophen poisoning metabolic acidosis is uncommon. Isopropyl alcohol ingestion results in high serum ketones with little or no acidosis. Methane (natural gas) is a simple asphyxiant and is biologically inactive but may cause hypoxemia. Ethylene dibromide is a fumigant pesticide that may lead to intractable metabolic acidosis with *decreased* anion gap.

14. The answer is **C,** page 542.

Methanol is oxidized by alcohol dehydrogenase (a rate-limiting enzyme) to formaldehyde, which in turn is converted to formic acid by aldehyde dehydrogenase. Formaldehyde is 30 times more toxic and formic acid 6 times more toxic than methanol. These metabolites are responsible for metabolic acidosis with increased anion gap, and ocular toxicity. Glycoaldehyde, glycolate, glycoxalate, and oxalic acid are all hepatic metabolites of ethylene glycol.

15. The answer is **D,** page 543.

Symptoms of methanol poisoning may be delayed 12 to 24 hours because of slow accumulation of the toxic metabolites. This lack of symptoms may lead to a false sense of security and management delay. In any suspected case of methanol (or ethylene glycol) intoxication, aggressive management with ethanol infusion is essential, even before the blood level is available, to prevent death. Ethanol has a ninefold to twentyfold greater affinity for alcohol dehydrogenase than methanol, and at levels of 100 to 150 mg/dl the formation of formic acid is fully inhibited. A loading dose of 0.8 g/kg of 100% ethanol is given either orally as a 20% to 30% solution via nasogastric tube or intravenously as a 5% to 10% solution in D5W. A maintenance dose of about 130 mg/kg/hr is used until the methanol level is below 20 mg/dl with no more acidosis. Frequent monitoring of ethanol level and blood glucose should be done. Ethanol levels greater than 200 mg/dl will prevent metabolism of methanol but will result in significant toxicity as well.

16. The answer is **C,** page 543.

Hemodialysis is indicated if the peak methanol level is greater than 50 mg/dl or if renal failure, visual impairment, or intractable metabolic acidosis develops. During hemodialysis the ethanol infusion should be doubled to maintain a blood level of 200 to 300 mg/dl, since ethanol also will be dialyzed. Since formic acid is further metabolized to CO_2 and H_2O by a folate-dependent pathway, some authorities advocate the use of IV folate.

17. The answer is **D,** pages 543 and 544.

Ethylene glycol is oxidized by alcohol dehydrogenase to oxalate, which is highly toxic. Patients usually have CNS depression, appear intoxicated without alcohol on the breath, and have profound metabolic acidosis with an increased anion gap. Urinalysis may reveal massive calcium oxalate crystals if a significant amount of metabolism already has occurred. Other *nonspecific* urinary findings include microscopic hematuria and proteinuria, which precede renal failure.

18. The answer is **E,** pages 543 and 544.

Metabolic acidosis with increased anion gap is suggestive of methanol and ethylene glycol ingestion. Ethylene glycol toxicity results from its metabolite oxalate, which chelates calcium ion to form insoluble calcium oxalate crystals and results in hypocalcemia. Hypomagnesemia usually occurs with hypocalcemia. However, *hyperkalemia* results from muscle necrosis, the development of acute tubular necrosis and renal failure, and metabolic acidosis.

19. The answer is **D**, page 545.
    Benadryl (diphenhydramine) is an anticholinergic agent. This toxidrome is easily remembered by: "Hot as a hare, Blind as a bat, Dry as a bone, Red as a beet, and Mad as a hatter." The other answers represent other toxidromes:
    A = anticholinesterase or cholinergic agents, as in organophosphates.
    B = narcotic overdose.
    C = sympathomimetic agents such as amphetamines, cocaine, and aminophylline.
    E = carbon monoxide toxicity.

20. The answer is **E**, pages 545 and 546.
    Drug elimination occurs through hepatic metabolism and urinary excretion of metabolites. Delayed GI decontamination may be helpful, since gastric emptying can be delayed by 12 hours or more. Anticholinergic effects result from competitive inhibition of muscarinic receptors in the autonomic nervous system and neuromuscular junctions of skeletal muscles. Antihistamines are not dialyzable.

21. The answer is **C**, page 546.
    The half-life of CBZ after a single dose is 20 to 65 hours; after chronic use it is 8 to 19 hours. Oral absorption occurs over 4 to 36 hours as GI motility is delayed. Since serum levels do not correlate with symptoms, no minimal toxic dose is known. CBZ is structurally related to both phenytoin and tricyclic antidepressants (TCAs) and it shares their toxicity. Seizures and status epilepticus are common complications.

22. The answer is **E**, page 546.
    Dizziness, ataxia, and nystagmus with deviating pupils are the classic triad seen in CBZ toxicity. Although vomiting, confusion and excitement, tachycardia, and hyperreflexia are all possible signs of toxicity, they are nonspecific.

23. The answer is **E**, pages 547 and 548.
    All children who are symptomatic after clonidine ingestion require admission, monitoring, and supportive care because symptoms may persist for up to 24 hours. Although the toxic dose of clonidine is not known, significant toxicity has resulted with as little as 0.1 mg 30 minutes after ingestion. Since it rapidly causes lethargy and respiratory depression, which is characterized by periodic gasping or sighing and agonal respiration, emesis with syrup of ipecac is contraindicated. The central effects of clonidine predominate and cause tachycardia and hypotension, but initially there may be peripheral α_2 stimulation and reduced uptake of epinephrine, resulting in benign, transient paradoxic hypertension. Aggressive therapy of this hypertension may result in profound hypotension. Naloxone reverses the CNS opiate effects of clonidine and may improve lethargy and reduce respiratory depression but is less effective against tachycardia and hypotension.

24. The answer is **B**, pages 548.
    Digoxin immune FAB (Digibind) is indicated for use in treating life-threatening digoxin-induced dysrhythmias and for hyperkalemia. The ECG findings of T wave depression and scooped ST segments are known as *digitalis effect* but do not indicate toxicity. Alkaline diuresis is not useful in digitalis elimination.

25. The answer is **C**, pages 548 and 549.
    Drain pipe cleaners usually contain sodium hydroxide as their principal component. Patients who ingest caustics have an increased risk of developing esophageal carcinoma. In the esophagus, acid burns usually cause a superficial coagulation necrosis with eschar formation of the mucosa, which limits penetration of the injury. However, bases cause liquefaction necrosis of the fat and protein involving the mucosa, submucosa, and muscle and penetrate deeply, causing the potential for greater tissue damage. Oropharyngeal lesions do not predict esophageal burns as only a third of patients with oral lesions develop esophageal burns, and about 10% to 15% of those with esophageal burns have no oral lesions. First-degree burns do not develop strictures; 15% to 30% of second-degree burns do; and almost 100% of third-degree burns do.

26. The answer is **C**, page 549.
    Household bleach usually contains chlorine or sodium hypochlorite, which is a mild irritant and usually causes no tissue destruction. Syrup of ipecac is not indicated, nor is esophagoscopy, since bleach is a mild alkali and not a caustic substance. Immediate dilution with water or milk is all that is required. Antacid buffer is ineffective and may be harmful. The use of weak acid to neutralize the alkali is absolutely contraindicated as the chemical reaction releases heat and gas that may cause additional tissue damage.

27. The answer is **D**, page 551.
    β-Blockers, propoxyphene, quinidine, phenothiazines, and cyclic antidepressants all cause seizures, slow cardiac conduction, and widen the QRS complex. Amphetamine and other sympathomimetics may cause seizures and ventricular dysrhythmias without prolongation of the QRS complex.

28. The answer is **C**, pages 551 and 552.
    Alkalinization is the first priority for the patient in the scenario with a widened QRS complex greater than 100 ms. Alkalinization can be achieved by the use of sodium bicarbonate to maintain the blood pH between 7.45 and 7.55. This serves to increase the binding of the free drug, which is responsible for the toxic effects. Emesis with syrup of ipecac is to be avoided because of the potential for seizures and hypotension. Activated charcoal with a cathartic may be helpful because the anticholinergic effects delay GI motility and gastric emptying. Lavage may be attempted if the ingestion was not too long ago. The use of phenytoin and physostigmine in TCA overdose is controversial.

29. The answer is **D**, pages 550 to 552.

TCA levels do not correlate with ECG findings. Limb-lead QRS duration less than 0.1 sec may be helpful because these patients are at negligible risk for seizures or ventricular dysrhythmias. One study that compared GCS score of less than 8 and QRS greater than 0.1 sec showed a greater risk of complications from the low GCS. Since hypotension is a result of excessive blockade of norepinephrine reuptake at the postganglionic synapse and results in norepinephrine depletion, norepinephrine should be used if IV fluids and Trendelenburg positioning are unsuccessful.

30. The answer is **B**, page 552.

Patients with a history of TCA ingestion or suspected TCA overdose should be monitored and observed in the ED with frequent 12-lead ECGs for at least 6 hours.

31. The answer is **E**, pages 552 and 553.

Organophosphates exert their effect by interfering with the enzyme cholinesterase, which degrades acetylcholine at the synaptic junction. They do not influence the release of acetylcholine but rather cause its accumulation by preventing degradation. Insecticide poisoning causes cholinesterase levels to *fall,* and this test can be used to confirm the clinical impression of insecticide poisoning. Humans are, in fact, able to detoxify organophosphates by conjugation in the liver. Carbamates form a *reversible* bond with cholinesterase. In contrast, organophosphates *irreversibly* bind to cholinesterase via phosphorylation.

32. The answer is **B**, pages 552 and 553.

Carbamate toxicity generally is of shorter duration (8 to 24 hours) and creates fewer CNS symptoms. Both carbamate and organophosphates are readily absorbed through the skin. Use of organophosphates is more prevalent. Therefore organophosphate poisoning is more common. Although some studies indicate a valuable role for pralidoxime in carbamate poisoning, pralidoxime is not as essential here because the bond to cholinesterase is reversible without pralidoxime.

33. The answer is **A**, page 554.

Pralidoxime reactivates cholinesterase by competing for the phosphate moiety of the organophosphate compound, thus releasing it from the cholinesterase enzyme. Atropine counteracts the effects of acetylcholine excess but has no effect on the biological activity of cholinesterase. There is no maximum dose of atropine in insecticide poisoning. Rather, the dose must be titrated to the patient's clinical response. As discussed above, pralidoxime generally is used for organophosphate poisoning and not carbamate exposure. Loop diuretics such as furosemide should be avoided in insecticide poisoning because they exacerbate already excessive urinary output. Bronchorrhea generally is controlled with ventilation and atropine.

34. The answer is **C**, pages 555 and 556.

Iron levels greater than 300 µg/dl are widely accepted as an indication for chelation therapy. Total iron-binding capacity (TIBC) can be falsely elevated by a high serum iron level and therefore is not considered a reliable guide in determining the need for chelation. A negative deferoxamine challenge test indicates that all the iron in the serum is bound to protein. An elevated WBC and increased anion gap acidosis along with an *elevated* serum glucose (greater than 150 mg/dl) suggest iron toxicity when serum levels are not available.

35. The answer is **B**, page 556.

A quick calculation indicates that the child in this scenario ingested approximately 20 mg of elemental iron per kilogram. This is the lower range at which toxicity can occur. However, this child is currently asymptomatic. Because we cannot base our management approach on history alone, it is best to observe the child in the ED for symptoms while we wait for laboratory tests. Iron does not bind to activated charcoal, and its administration will not be helpful. An abdominal radiograph is useful when it is positive, but a negative radiograph is more commonly seen with chewable tablet ingestions. The use of ipecac is questionable in this case because it is already 90 minutes after ingestion. A deferoxamine challenge test would be overly aggressive in this asymptomatic child with an estimated ingestion of 20 mg/kg.

36. The answer is **A**, page 556.

The patient in the scenario is hypotensive as a result of the toxic effects of iron in the GI tract. Fluid resuscitation is the first priority in management followed by administration of a specific antidote. It is safer to give 15 mg/kg/hr of deferoxamine than a single dose of 90 mg/kg in this patient because deferoxamine may further reduce blood pressure. Ipecac is contraindicated in all lethargic patients. In this case whole bowel irrigation might exacerbate intravascular fluid depletion and would be difficult to perform if the patient is unable to cooperate. However, whole bowel irrigation may often be the best method of iron decontamination. Although the safety of deferoxamine in pregnancy is not completely established, growing experience with its use in this situation is reassuring. Deferoxamine has been found to be less toxic to the fetus than an iron overdose. Hemodialysis is only indicated as an adjuvant to chelation therapy in patients with renal failure. Hemodialysis removes chelated iron but not free iron.

37. The answer is **C**, page 559.

Naloxone has been shown to be an effective antidote in narcotic and clonidine overdoses, although its effect with clonidine is less consistent. Naloxone can be safely administered via all routes, including intraosseous infusion. It is effective against all forms of opioids, including synthetic ones, but has no effect on barbiturate reversal. Naloxone is a pure antagonist with no agonist effects.

38. The answer is **A,** page 558.

Difenoxin (Lomotil), a combination of diphenoxylate and atropine, often shows anticholinergic symptoms such as delirium, tachycardia, and mydriasis. Ethanol (typically causes mydriasis, but in 35% of children in deep coma, miosis can be seen), chloral hydrate, and other sedative hypnotics can cause miosis and cardiovascular depression. Clonidine occupies opiate receptors, mimicking their effects. Physostigmine, a cholinergic agent, also can cause miosis and bradycardia.

39. The answer is **A,** page 560.

Salicylates are a common cause of increased anion gap metabolic acidosis (MUDPILES). Salicylate overdose may cause hepatotoxicity, which affects the production of vitamin K–dependent clotting factors and elevates the prothrombin time and the bleeding time. Through its inhibition of the Krebs cycle, salicylate poisoning may cause a buildup of lactic acid, as well as other organic acids. Hyperglycemia occurs initially because of a decreased use of glucose via the Krebs cycle but is often followed by hypoglycemia. Salicylate toxicity stimulates excessive losses of water, sodium, and potassium through the urine.

40. The answer is **D,** page 561.

Replacing potassium losses and maintaining a normal serum potassium is the key to successful alkalinization of the urine. The kidneys will continue to reabsorb bicarbonate and add hydrogen ion to the urine if potassium replacement is not instituted. Even though the patient in the scenario comes in 3 hours after ingestion, charcoal can be of value because salicylates empty slowly from the stomach. Multiple-dose activated charcoal (MDAC) may also enhance clearance. Glucose is an essential component of therapy because patients with salicylate overdose are prone to hypoglycemia. It is unlikely that the patient in the scenario is an example of a mild overdose. At 3 hours his level does not yet reflect maximum absorption. As this is a potentially serious overdose, alkalinization should be aggressively pursued. Alkalinization of both the serum and urine should be attempted. Serum pH can be increased to 7.55 if therapeutically necessary. However, the patient should be monitored for electrolyte disturbances and arrhythmias.

41. The answer is **A,** page 561.

Hemodialysis and hemoperfusion are equivalent in removing salicylate, although hemodialysis is preferred because it also allows for the correction of metabolic abnormalities. This is a potentially serious overdose (maximum total dose 35 g), and the 3-hour level does not reflect true toxicity expected in this case. The Done nomogram is not accurate until 6 hours after ingestion. It also cannot be used for enteric-coated aspirin ingestions, chronic ingestions, or ingestions that take place over a number of hours. Chronic salicylate overdosage is generally more toxic than acute salicylate overdose, and the patient may require dialysis at a lower serum salicylate level. Although seizures and renal failure are indications for hemodialysis, hypothermia is not expected to occur. *Hyperthermia* can occur in salicylate poisoning and usually occurs in patients with the most severe toxicity. Noncardiogenic pulmonary edema would be another indication for hemodialysis because alkaline diuresis is untenable.

42. The answer is **B,** page 561.

Maximal elimination through alkalinization requires a urine pH of 7.5 to 8.0. Alkalinization cannot be accomplished if the serum K^+ is low because the renal tubules will exchange H^+ for K^+ to conserve potassium. Therefore the serum K^+ should be maintained above 4.0. Alkalinization of the serum is as important as that of the urine. Once the patient becomes acidotic, salicylate will enter tissue rapidly, and increased toxicity will ensue. Fluid diuresis per se is not an effective approach to enhanced elimination, although large fluid losses are expected from salicylate toxicity. Alkalinization is definitely indicated in this patient, since he is symptomatic, and his salicylate level is 44 at only 3 hours.

43. The answer is **C,** page 558.

Opioids most consistently cause miosis, although barbiturates, ethanol, cholinergics, and phenothiazines can cause miosis as well, but not as frequently.

44. The answer is **B,** page 563.

Benzodiazepines exert their effect by increasing the GABA effect at the postsynaptic inhibitory neuronal junction.

45. The answer is **E,** page 563.

Phenothiazines have a membrane-depressing effect similar to those of TCAs. These effects, which include prolongation of the QT interval, are rarely life threatening in phenothiazine overdose.

46. The answer is **A,** page 562.

Barbiturate coma may lead to an isoelectric EEG.

47. The answer is **E or F,** page 560.

Salicylates and phenothiazines can cause a color change when ferric chloride is added to the urine. They also cause a positive Phenistix test of the urine.

48. The answer is **E,** pages 563 and 564.

Phenothiazines have varying anticholinergic properties, which is why they are sometimes used as decongestant medications.

49. The answer is **D,** pages 562 and 563.

Phenobarbital, a weak acid, can have its excretion enhanced fivefold to tenfold by *alkalinization* of the urine. This property is not shared by shorter acting barbiturates, which have a more alkaline pKa. MDAC has been shown to decrease the half-life and increase the clearance of phenobarbital. Forced fluid diuresis and furosemide also may have a similar effect. Peritoneal dialysis, hemodialysis, and hemoperfusion have been shown to speed clearance of barbiturates from the body, especially long- and intermediate-acting barbiturates. Hemoperfusion is the method of choice.

50. The answer is **C,** page 562.

Prolonged QTc is not likely to be associated with a barbiturate overdose. Mydriasis is seen 69% of the time in barbiturate poisoning. Slurred speech occurs early in barbiturate exposure, imitating alcohol intoxication. Adult respiratory distress syndrome (ARDS), acute tubular necrosis (ATN), and cerebral edema are all sequelae of anoxic damage from a severe overdose. Barbiturates also can cause blisters indirectly in dependent areas of the skin, as well as miosis. Hypothermia and hypercapnia are the results of coma and respiratory depression.

51. The answer is **C,** pages 563 and 564.

Phenothiazines are not among the drugs known to cause an increased anion gap metabolic acidosis (MUDPILES). Phenothiazines are detectable by both ferric chloride and Phenistix tests performed on the urine. Many phenothiazines cause quinidine-like effects on ECG, particularly prolongation of the QT interval. Phenothiazines are often radiopaque (CHIPS). Dystonic reactions caused by phenothiazines are reversible with diphenhydramine. This response can be considered a diagnostic confirmation.

52. The answer is **E,** page 563.

Although phenothiazines can cause miosis, especially in children, the triad of miosis, hypotension, and cutaneous bullae suggests barbiturate poisoning. Warm skin, dry mouth, mydriasis, and other anticholinergic symptoms are seen with phenothiazines. Dystonic reactions can occur with phenothiazines even in therapeutic levels. They also may occur with a single therapeutic dose, chronic usage, or acute overdose. Hyperthermia and muscle overactivity may lead to rhabdomyolysis and renal failure and are seen in neuroleptic malignant syndrome. Mild quinidine-like effects on the ECG are seen with various phenothiazine overdoses.

53. The answer is **A,** page 564.

Spontaneous abortion along with abruptio placentae (not placenta previa), prematurity (not postmaturity), and intrauterine growth retardation has been associated with prenatal use of cocaine by the mother. Cocaine causes a mild and short-lived withdrawal syndrome in newborns.

54. The answer is **D,** page 564.

Cocaine is rapidly metabolized in the plasma by cholinesterase. Although the half-life of standard cocaine is 60 to 90 minutes, that of the free-base is only a few minutes. Benzoylecgonine is the principal metabolite and it persists in the urine up to 72 hours. Cocaine is absorbed through the GI tract and mucous membranes as well as the lungs. Although toxic reactions usually occur at doses greater than 1 mg/kg, individual reactions to cocaine are idiosyncratic, and there is no absolutely safe dose.

55. The answer is **B,** page 564.

Noncardiogenic pulmonary edema is reported with salicylate and narcotic overdoses but not with cocaine. Pulmonary edema occurring in association with cocaine usage is most likely to occur on a cardiogenic basis. Cocaine is one of the few drugs that cause status epilepticus (as opposed to isolated seizures) in an overdose. Bowel infarction, aortic dissection, and subarachnoid hemorrhage are complications associated with the vasoconstricting properties of cocaine.

56. The answer is **E,** page 566.

Since agitation associated with muscle overactivity and hyperthermia can lead to rhabdomyolysis in phencyclidine (PCP) poisoning, vigorous hydration is recommended to prevent myoglobin precipitation in the renal tubules. MDAC might enhance clearance of the drug, but the risk of aspiration outweighs the benefit in extremely agitated patients. Acidification of the urine will enhance elimination of this weak base, but it is unsafe to attempt in the presence of myoglobinuria. Since haloperidol may lower the seizure threshold, benzodiazepines are a safer choice to control agitation. PCP exerts its effect as an α-agonist, and therefore the use of propranolol (pure β-blocker) may cause unopposed α-effects and lead to an increased blood pressure.

57. The answer is **D,** page 567.

Although amphetamines are readily identified on drug screens of the urine, a specific serum level is of little value in patient management. Obtaining a serum potassium level would alert you to hypokalemia; an increase in creatine kinase (CPK) would indicate muscle breakdown; a urine myoglobin would alert you to the possibility of renal failure; and an ECG would demonstrate ischemia or dysrhythmias.

58. The answer is **D,** page 568.

Theophylline overdose, like most sympathomimetic drugs, will cause hyperglycemia in the initial phases of an acute overdose. Acute theophylline ingestion is associated with many metabolic disturbances, including low serum potassium, phosphorus, and magnesium levels. Metabolic acidosis may be seen in severe overdoses. Chronic overdoses are more likely to cause hyperkalemia and hypocalcemia.

59. The answer is **C**, pages 568 and 569.

Because theophylline has a relatively low volume of distribution (0.5 L/kg), it largely remains in the serum and is therefore available for removal by GI dialysis with MDAC. The fact that theophylline remains only partially protein bound and does not assume an ionized form makes it more amenable to diffusion across the gut lumen. Gastric resecretion occurs primarily with small molecules such as lithium.

60. The answer is **A**, page 569.

Hypotension occurs late in theophylline overdoses and results from β_2-induced vasodilation. Therefore the use of small doses of propranolol can counteract this β_2 toxicity. However, it should not be used in patients with a history of asthma. MDAC has been shown to remove theophylline from the serum by "GI dialysis," irrespective of the route of administration. Whole bowel irrigation can be very effective in sustained-release theophylline overdoses but acts by reducing absorption rather than enhancing clearance. Cimetidine should be avoided in theophylline overdoses because it inhibits theophylline metabolism. Ranitidine is a better choice for controlling hyperemesis. Hemoperfusion is the most effective method of extracorporeal theophylline removal.

Inhalation Injuries

Waseem Hafeez • Morton Salomon

See Barkin et al: Chapter 44.

1. All of the following statements concerning pneumonia resulting from smoke inhalation are *true except:*
   A. Pneumonia may develop days after the initial injury.
   B. Pneumonia carries a high mortality rate.
   C. Prophylactic antibiotics are associated with a reduced incidence of pneumonia.
   D. Infecting organisms include *Staphylococcus aureus.*
   E. Bronchoscopy is more effective in diagnosing pneumonia than a xenon lung scan.

2. The most common inhalation injuries in the pediatric population are caused by:
   A. Hydrocarbon aspiration.
   B. Smoke from a house fire.
   C. Bleach.
   D. Methane (natural gas).
   E. Inhaled organophosphates (insecticide).

In questions 3 to 7 match each inhalant with its most common mechanism of injury:
   A. Displacement of oxygen (O_2).
   B. Binding to hemoglobin.
   C. Cellular anoxia.
   D. Respiratory irritant.
   E. Mechanical obstruction of bronchioles.

3. Chlorine _____
4. Methane _____
5. Baby powder _____
6. Hydrogen cyanide _____
7. Carbon monoxide _____

8. Emergency Medical Service (EMS) workers bring in an 8-year-old from a burning building where he was found to be lethargic. He was given 100% O_2 using a nonrebreather mask and intravenous (IV) fluids. On arrival in the ED he is awake but complains of tightness around the forehead with severe headache, nausea, and poor vision. His physical examination reveals tachycardia, tachypnea, and reactive pupils with bilateral retinal hemorrhages. The patient's hemoglobin level is 12 g/dl, and an arterial blood gas (ABG) drawn while breathing room air reveals pH 7.32, $Paco_2$ 38 mm Hg, Pao_2 68 mm Hg, and carboxyhemoglobin (COHb) level of 30%. Appropriate management includes which of the following?
   A. Decrease to 50% the O_2 by face mask.
   B. Immediately arrange for transfer for hyperbaric O_2 (HBO) therapy.
   C. Intubate the patient's trachea and institute mechanical ventilation.
   D. Transfuse packed red blood cells to increase the O_2-carrying capacity of the blood.
   E. Correct the metabolic acidosis by administering sodium bicarbonate.

9. Which of the following is the most important physical characteristic in determining the aspiration potential of a hydrocarbon?
   A. Volatility.
   B. Surface tension.
   C. Viscosity.
   D. Solubility.
   E. pH of the vehicle.

10. A 3-year-old is rescued from a smoke-filled room and brought immediately to the ED with tachypnea. Which of the following tests is *most* likely to give the most information regarding the initial management of this patient?
   A. Chest radiograph.
   B. Pulse oximetry.
   C. COHb level.
   D. Blood cyanide level.
   E. Electrocardiogram (ECG).

11. Which of the following is most often indicated during the initial resuscitation in severely compromised smoke inhalation victims?
   A. Antibiotics.
   B. Corticosteroids.
   C. Positive end expiratory pressure (PEEP).
   D. D5W 0.45 normal saline.
   E. All of the above.

12. All of the following patients are candidates for HBO therapy after carbon monoxide (CO) exposure *except:*
   A. Patients with CO level greater than 25%.
   B. Patients with recurrent neurologic or cardiovascular symptoms up to 3 weeks after initial O_2 therapy.
   C. Patients with neurologic or cardiovascular symptoms not resolving after 6 hours of 100% O_2.
   D. All pregnant patients.
   E. Patients with neuropsychiatric symptoms.

13. A patient found stuporous at the scene of a house fire is brought to the ED, receiving 100% O_2 by face mask on the way. Vital signs, mental status, and physical examination are now normal. You should:
   A. Admit for HBO therapy.
   B. Discharge home, since the patient is fine.
   C. Place on nonrebreather mask for 2 hours, then discharge home.
   D. Check COHb level and discharge home if normal.
   E. Observe for 6 hours, then discharge home if 6-hour x-ray film of chest is normal.

14. A 2-year-old boy is brought in by his mother with complaints that the child swallowed kerosene stored in a beverage bottle. The patient coughed initially but has not vomited. He is alert and comfortable. His vital signs are respiratory rate (RR) 28 breaths per minute and heart rate (HR) 110 beats per minute. Pulse oximeter readings are 96% while breathing room air. The next most appropriate step is:
   A. Institute early gastric emptying.
   B. Administer activated charcoal.
   C. Administer corticosteroids to reduce the inflammatory response.
   D. Administer systemic antibiotics to prevent complications of hydrocarbon aspiration.
   E. Observe the patient for 6 to 8 hours in the ED and discharge home if the chest radiograph is negative.

15. All of the following statements are true concerning smoke inhalation *except:*
   A. Extensive thermal injuries cause more deaths than toxic gas inhalation.
   B. Adding moisture to the air increases injury and probability of death.
   C. The most common fatal gas from smoke inhalation is CO.
   D. Acrolein vapor can cause severe ocular irritation and pulmonary edema.
   E. Fire victims who die immediately do so from asphyxiation.

16. The O_2-hemoglobin dissociation curve is shifted toward the left in all of the following conditions *except:*
   A. Carboxyhemoglobinemia.
   B. Acidosis.
   C. Hypothermia.
   D. Fetal hemoglobin.
   E. Cyanide poisoning.

17. A patient who is brought into the ED from a burning apartment has irritability, tachypnea, and tachycardia. Which of the following is *least* likely to be affected by CO poisoning?
   A. Serum pH.
   B. Serum lactate level.
   C. Pulse oximetry readings.
   D. ECG.
   E. $Paco_2$.

18. All of the following statements concerning inhalational injury to the airways are *true except:*
   A. Bronchospasm occurs between 1 and 6 hours following the exposure.
   B. Pulmonary edema is a common early finding.
   C. Bronchopneumonia can occur more than 60 hours after exposure.
   D. Smoke destroys alveolar epithelial type II cells.
   E. Pulmonary capillary hyperpermeability may be secondary to inhaled carbon dioxide.

ANSWERS [See Barkin et al: Chapter 44.]

1. The answer is **C**, page 584.
   Prophylactic antibiotic use has not been shown to be beneficial in the reduction of incidence of pneumonia. Bronchopneumonia usually develops more than 60 hours after the burn, and chest radiographic abnormalities lag behind the physical findings by 12 to 24 hours. In the first week the primary organism is usually penicillin-resistant *S. aureus,* while later in the course, *Pseudomonas* and gram-negative organisms become more common. Xenon lung scans do not add to the information obtained by clinical assessment or bronchoscopy.

2. The answer is **B**, page 578.
   Children are rarely involved in occupational chemical exposures. The most common exposure is from house fires in which burns, carbon monoxide (CO), and cyanide all contribute to injury. The other sources are common but less frequent.

3. **D**
4. **A**
5. **E**
6. **C**
7. **B**
   Chlorine is a respiratory irritant that causes membrane damage and inflammation of the upper respiratory tract. Methane gas is nonirritating but causes displacement of oxygen (O_2) from the airways, thus resulting in asphyxiation. Baby powder can obstruct small bronchioles and alveoli because of its small particle size (less than 5 mm). Particles larger than 10 mm can obstruct medium and large airways. Hydrogen cyanide causes cellular anoxia while CO binds avidly to hemoglobin with an affinity of 230 to 270 times that of O_2. (See page 580 in Barkin et al.)

8. The answer is **B**, pages 589 and 590.
   The patient has signs and symptoms that correlate with a COHb level greater than 25%. This is the level at which most authorities would recommend the use of hyperbaric O_2 (HBO) therapy. Oxygen at 100% delivered by a nonrebreather mask at 2 atm reduces the half-life of COHb from 4 to 6 hours to approximately 60 minutes, while HBO at 3 atm reduces the half-life to 20 to 30 minutes.

9. The answer is **C**, pages 590 and 591.
   Viscosity is defined as the resistance to flow over a surface and is measured as Saybolt universal seconds (SUS). Agents with SUS less than 60 have a very high potential for aspiration. This is because the substance can reach the tracheobronchial tree and subsequently result in toxicity.

10. The answer is **C**, page 584.
    Arterial blood gas changes demonstrating hypoxemia, hypercarbia, and metabolic acidosis are all early findings. Chest radiograph is usually normal initially while pulse oximetry overestimates the true O_2 saturation in the presence of COHb. ECG changes are mostly seen in adults, and blood cyanide levels are rarely useful because the turnaround time is too slow to be of any therapeutic value. Arterial blood gas results do not reflect the level of CO exposure.

11. The answer is **C**, pages 585 and 586.
    Positive end-expiratory pressure (PEEP) as an early intervention is useful in hypoxemia and respiratory insufficiency. Corticosteroids increase mortality from sepsis, delay wound healing, and may produce fluid and electrolyte problems. Prophylactic antibiotics have been associated with a higher rate of pulmonary infections. Ringer's lactate solution is recommended for initial resuscitation.

12. The answer is **D**, page 589.
    Pregnant patients with COHb levels greater than 15% or with fetal distress evident on fetal monitoring are candidates for HBO. Other indications include coma and other neurologic signs and cardiovascular involvement, as well as the conditions mentioned in the question.

13. The answer is **A**, page 590.
    Admission criteria include: (a) history—if patient was stuporous or unconscious at the scene, or if initial vital signs were abnormal, (b) physical—mental status changes, vital sign changes, and (c) laboratory—COHb level of more than 15% to 20%, metabolic acidosis, or elevated lactate regardless of symptoms.

14. The answer is **E**, pages 590 to 593.
    Kerosene has a low viscosity and high potential for aspiration pneumonia but has little if any systemic toxicity unless ingested in massive quantities. If the child remains asymptomatic at 6 to 8 hours, obtain a radiograph and send him home. About 92% of the patients in whom pneumonia eventually will develop have a positive radiograph within 8 hours. One study suggests that radiographs are necessary in asymptomatic patients. Since children ingest only a small amount and kerosene does not cause systemic effects, gastric emptying is not recommended. Similarly, the use of activated charcoal is not recommended unless other toxic substances are concomitantly ingested. Prophylactic antibiotics to prevent pneumonia have not been found to be beneficial. The use of corticosteroids in aspiration pneumonia has been associated with increased morbidity.

15. The answer is **A**, pages 579 to 581.
    Although thermal injuries to the skin, especially on the face, neck, and chest, can result in severe upper airway edema and airway obstruction, the majority of deaths in burn victims result from smoke inhalation and toxic gases that cause pulmonary injury. The upper airway, including the nasal turbinates, has excellent heat-reducing properties. Dry air of temperatures greater than 150° C has little effect on the lower airway. Adding moisture to the air (steam inhalation) gives it 4000 times the heat capacity, resulting in pulmonary edema, pneumonitis, and coagulation necrosis of the lower airway. CO has been reported as the single leading cause of death by poisoning in the United States. Acrolein vapor, resulting from combustion of wood and cotton, causes severe ocular irritation and is a major contributor to pulmonary injury in smoke inhalation. It may cause pulmonary edema at concentrations of 10 ppm within seconds.

16. The answer is **B**, page 586.
    Acidosis shifts the O_2-hemoglobin dissociation curve to the right. All the other conditions cause leftward shift of the curve and change the shape of the curve from sigmoid to hyperbolic. As a result the O_2 is tightly bound to hemoglobin and is released to the tissues at a much lower tissue O_2 tension, resulting in severe hypoxemia.

17. The answer is **C,** pages 588 and 589.

Pulse oximetry evaluates O_2 saturation by sampling two wavelengths of light. This measurement may overestimate the true oxyhemoglobin saturation in the presence of elevated COHb levels. In canine studies, even with COHb levels of 50%, the pulse oximeter recorded saturations of 95%. Hypoxia and inhibition of cellular energy cause metabolic and lactic acidosis. Respiratory acidosis is common in smoke inhalation because of respiratory insufficiency. Cardiotoxicity results from hypoxemia and may lead to a diminished cardiac output, hypotension, myocardial ischemia with ST segment changes, intraventricular conduction blocks, and arrhythmias. These changes most commonly affect the elderly, but an ECG is recommended as a part of the assessment in any child over 12 years of age. In younger children the most common finding is a sinus tachycardia.

18. The answer is **E,** pages 579 to 582.

Carbon dioxide is a simple asphyxiant and causes hypoxemia; it does not have a direct toxic effect on the lungs. Capillary hyperpermeability results from systemic toxins inhaled during smoke inhalation that cause vascular injury and increase in bronchial blood flow with the formation of exudates and interstitial edema. Smoke destroys alveolar type I and II cells, which affects ventilation-perfusion balance.

Abuse and Neglect

Jill C. Glick

See Barkin et al: Chapter 45.

1. All of the following are historical clues or "red flags" that should raise concern that an injury was more likely *intentional except:*
   A. Delay in seeking medical care.
   B. Discrepancies in the history of the injury between caretakers.
   C. Inconsistencies between the injury and the explanation of the injury.
   D. Explanation of the injury that is consistent with the child's developmental capabilities.
   E. History of recurrent injuries.

2. Which of the following statements concerning physical abuse is correct?
   A. A decrease in the number of child abuse reports occurred in the early 1990s because of prevention programs.
   B. Girls and boys are physically abused with equal frequency.
   C. The highest frequency of physical abuse occurs in children 4 to 6 years old.
   D. Each year, 2.5% of the children in the United States are abused.
   E. The abuser is a noncaretaker in 60% of the cases.

3. A 7-month-old boy is brought to the ED by his mother for treatment of burns on his feet. The mother describes the infant being in a bath seat in the sink when the infant turned on the hot water and sustained a partial-thickness burn to both feet. The next appropriate step in your management for this child is:
   A. Corroborate the history by talking with another caretaker.
   B. Call the regional welfare agency and do not inform the mother of the report.
   C. Admit the child for a child protective services investigation.
   D. Treat the burns and arrange outpatient follow-up with the burn service.
   E. Educate the mother about safety and prevention.

4. Which of the following is a true statement regarding child maltreatment?
   A. Child abuse is the leading cause of death in the first year of life following the neonatal period.
   B. An organic etiology for failure to thrive (FTT) is diagnosed in 75% of cases.
   C. Sexual abuse occurs more often in lower economic groups.
   D. Victims of fatal child abuse infrequently have been reported to welfare agencies before their deaths.
   E. Once investigated, 80% of child abuse reports to welfare agencies are substantiated.

5. Which of the following statements regarding the findings from the medical evaluation for sexual abuse is true?
   A. Condyloma acuminatum and herpes simplex are diagnostic of sexual abuse in all age groups.
   B. Nonperinatally acquired gonorrhea is diagnostic of sexual abuse in children.
   C. Evaluation of a vaginal discharge in a prepubertal child must be reported to a welfare agency pending antigen testing for *Chlamydia*.
   D. The best marker of sexual abuse is the size of the hymenal opening.
   E. Sexual abuse that happened more than 72 hours ago requires emergency evaluation.

In questions 6 through 9 choose the best answer from the list below:
   A. Head magnetic resonance imaging (MRI).
   B. Head computed tomographic (CT) scan.
   C. Ophthalmologic examination.
   D. Bone scan.
   E. Skeletal survey.
   F. Single-view "babygram."

6. First-line imaging to evaluate for presence of intracranial bleeding. _____

7. More sensitive radiographic study to define shearing injuries to the brain. _____

8. Radiographic screening indicated in children younger than 1 year old with evidence of medical neglect. _____

9. Radiographic study most specific to diagnose metaphyseal injuries. _____

10. A 2-year-old boy with cerebral palsy and developmental delay is seen in the ED because of inconsolable crying for the past 8 hours. According to the caretaker the child has had a low-grade fever and fell out of his bed last night. The child's vital signs are within normal limits, and he is crying. The left humerus is swollen and deformed. The x-ray films of the humerus show a spiral fracture. The caretaker consistently reports that the child fell out of his bed onto a wooden floor the night before the visit. The examination shows no other cutaneous lesions. The appropriate management of this child is to:
   A. Contact the regional child protective agency if the skeletal survey exhibits other injuries.
   B. Perform a head CT and ophthalmologic examination and see if the findings are consistent with shaken infant syndrome.
   C. Contact the regional child protective agency only if the orthopedic surgeon suspects child abuse.
   D. Treat the fracture, contact the regional child protective agency, and discharge the child with orthopedic follow-up.
   E. Admit the patient, obtain a skeletal survey, and contact the regional child protective agency.

11. A 6-month-old full-term infant is brought to the ED by the mother because of fever, refusal to eat, vomiting, and lethargy. On examination the child weighs 5 kg and is afebrile with a heart rate (HR) of 80 beats per minute, blood pressure (BP) of 75/40 mm Hg, and shallow respirations. She has no skin rashes or markings. Her fontanelle is full, left pupil is 2 mm and reactive, and right pupil is sluggish at 4 mm. No retinal hemorrhages are apparent on your examination. The Glasgow Coma Scale score is 7. Your immediate plan for this child is to:
   A. Arrange for a head CT.
   B. Empirically treat for meningitis and rehydrate.
   C. Empirically administer dextrose and naloxone (Narcan).
   D. Intubate and treat for signs of increased intracranial pressure.

12. A 5-year-old girl is brought to the ED by police for evaluation for sexual abuse. The patient's kindergarten teacher called the police because the child told the teacher that her father had touched her vagina and it hurt her. The appropriate management at this time would be to:
   A. Contact the regional child protective agency and arrange for a follow-up examination with the child's pediatrician.
   B. Interview and examine the child and her father simultaneously.
   C. Not obtain cultures for Chlamydia and gonorrhea because the history does not include vaginal intercourse.
   D. Obtain specimens for culture from the vagina, rectum, and oropharynx because of the patient's age and lack of verbal abilities and empirically treat her for sexually transmitted diseases.
   E. Interview and examine the child, perform cultures of the three orifices, and determine home disposition with the regional child protective agency.

13. Which of the following are pathognomonic findings for child abuse?
   A. Vaginal discharge in a prepubertal female.
   B. Venereal warts in the perirectal area in a 2-year-old boy.
   C. Hymenal ring with a diameter of 7 mm in a 6-year-old.
   D. A positive Chlamydia antigen test from the vagina of a 2-year-old.
   E. Positive gonorrhea culture from the vagina of a 2-year-old whose mother had gonorrhea during pregnancy.

14. Which physical finding is pathognomonic for child maltreatment?
   A. Spiral fractures of extremities in toddlers.
   B. Fifth percentile for weight of a 1-month-old who was born prematurely at 34 weeks.
   C. Metaphyseal fractures in an 18-month-old.
   D. Posterior rib fractures in a 6-month-old.

15. A 3-year-old boy has a high fever and signs of compensated shock. He has a medical history of severe, recurrent abdominal pain, fevers, and polymicrobial sepsis. He was a full-term baby and followed an uncomplicated course until the age of 18 months when fevers and chronic diarrhea began. His mother is a respiratory therapist in your hospital and is an excellent medical historian. She is frustrated that a diagnosis for her child's condition has not been made and has seen many subspecialists for medical evaluation. A true statement regarding this medical entity is:
   A. This form of child abuse usually affects adolescent females.
   B. The mortality rate is close to 10%.
   C. The patient can be discharged to his primary caretakers if they receive adequate counseling.
   D. The siblings are not at risk for similar symptoms.
   E. The long-term morbidity associated with this syndrome is minor.

16. A 3-year-old boy in cardiopulmonary arrest is brought to the ED. The mother called 911 after finding her child in her bed not breathing. He has a history of asthma and developmental delay. The child this evening had bilious vomiting and a low-grade fever after returning from his dad's home, according to his mother. He became tired, and the mother put him into her bed. He fell asleep easily, but she found him unresponsive when she checked him. During the resuscitation you find that he is anemic. Which of the following is a true statement?
    A. The majority of abdominal injuries caused by child abuse are due to penetrating injuries.
    B. Because of the mechanism of injury, the mortality rate is low for this type of physical abuse.
    C. Abdominal abuse injuries include contusions, lacerations, and ruptures of abdominal structures.
    D. Blunt abdominal injuries are part of the shaken infant syndrome.
    E. Thoracic injuries caused by child abuse are more common than abdominal injuries.

17. A 6-month-old who was born prematurely is being evaluated for fever and cough. A chest x-ray film reveals two healed posterior rib fractures. The child received mechanical ventilation for 1 week and currently is not receiving any medications. The child is with her grandmother, and the mother is attending school. The grandmother denies history of trauma. Which one of the following statements is correct?
    A. Rib fractures are common in neonates admitted to an intensive care unit (ICU).
    B. Vigorous chest physiotherapy is associated with rib fractures.
    C. Rib fractures are associated with difficult deliveries.
    D. Rib fractures prompt suspicion of child abuse and warrant further investigation.
    E. Anterior and lateral fractures often are more associated with child abuse.

18. Which of the following is a true statement regarding cutaneous lesions resulting from child abuse?
    A. Burns are the most common cutaneous manifestation of child abuse.
    B. The sequence of color change in bruises that are healing is time dependent.
    C. Linear contusions are more common in unintentional injuries than in intentional injuries.
    D. The location of bruises as an indication of child abuse is not as reliable in older children.
    E. Human bite marks are more likely to leave puncture wounds than bites of carnivores.

19. A 2-month-old boy is brought to the ED by his teenage mother because his left knee is swollen. She noted that his knee appeared mildly swollen this morning and has progressively become worse through the day. The child has become fussy and is refusing to eat. The mother reports that the child fell out of her arms yesterday while they were lying on a couch, and he fell onto a carpeted floor. The child is crying and has stable vital signs except for a 38.5° C rectal temperature. His left knee is swollen and warm to touch. Which of the following is a true statement?
    A. A skeletal survey is indicated.
    B. A report for medical neglect must be filed with the regional child protective agency.
    C. Metaphyseal fractures are best diagnosed by bone scan.
    D. An emergency CT scan is warranted because of the association of skeletal trauma with shaken infant syndrome.
    E. Evaluation for an infectious etiology is warranted.

20. A 2½-year-old comes to the ED with burns to his perineum, lower back, and thighs with sparing of the buttocks. He has healed cutaneous markings consistent with "loop marks" on his back. Which one of the following statements is correct?
    A. Each state has its own legal requirements for health care workers regarding reporting child abuse cases.
    B. The physician should not inform the caretaker of the report to the regional welfare agency.
    C. The health care worker must consult a child protective service team to diagnose child abuse before reporting a suspected child abuse.
    D. The physician is protected against legal action for reporting a child abuse case by the good faith reporting laws.
    E. By law social workers are the only health care workers who must file the reports with state welfare agencies.

ANSWERS [See Barkin et al: Chapter 45.]

1. The answer is **D**, pages 600 and 601.

When eliciting a history about a child who has sustained an injury, focus on the following key points to help differentiate between an inflicted and a noninflicted injury: (a) a history of delay of seeking care, (b) the given mechanism for the injury not fitting with the physical findings, (c) the child's developmental ability being inconsistent with the history given for the injury, (d) inconsistencies between caretakers' histories of the injury, (e) history of recurrent injuries, (f) claims that the injury was self-inflicted, or (g) comments such as "the child bruised easily." These elevate the suspicion that the injuries were in fact inflicted.

2. The answer is **D**, pages 599 and 600.

Caregivers must recognize that child maltreatment continues to be on the increase with 30,000 cases reported in the mid-1970s compared with nearly 3.5 million reports made yearly to child welfare groups currently. Boys are more frequently abused than girls, and the majority of children abused are younger than 4 years old. The abuser is a caretaker in 90% of the cases. The multiple risk factors for physical abuse include characteristics of the child such as prematurity and mental retardation; characteristics of the abusive caretaker such as young age, being unmarried, and being a substance abuser; and characteristics of the abusive family such as social isolation and poverty. The interaction of these risk factors leads to child maltreatment. However, it is essential to understand that sexual abuse has different risk factors that are epidemiologically and psychosocially distinct from the risk factors for physical abuse.

3. The answer is **C**, page 601.

Given the patient's age, it is unlikely that the infant could turn on the water and sustain a burn to his feet. It is crucial to determine if the history and the injury sustained are compatible. Because of the location of the burn to the extremities and the age of the child the case must be reported. The safety of the child is paramount, and admission may be warranted for both medical and psychosocial reasons.

4. The answer is **A**, pages 599 and 604.

Child abuse is the most frequent cause of death in infants outside the neonatal period. Most children with failure to thrive (**FTT**) have an environmental or nonorganic reason for their FTT. Sexual abuse occurs equally among different economic groups and does not have a propensity to occur in the lower socioeconomic groups. Welfare agencies are able to substantiate about 30% of hotline reports.

5. The answer is **B**, pages 609 to 612.

The physician must acknowledge that the diagnosis of sexual abuse is usually based on the history with the possibility of supportive physical findings. The absence of physical findings rarely confirms the absence of sexual abuse. All children who come to the ED for evaluation for sexual abuse within 72 hours of the assault must be evaluated and treated as a medical emergency. Certain laboratory results are diagnostic of sexual abuse, such as a positive culture for gonorrhea outside of the prenatal period. Evidence of condyloma acuminatum, *Chlamydia, Trichomonas vaginalis,* and herpes simplex is cause for suspicion but cannot be considered proof of sexual abuse. Primary syphilis in infants younger than 4 months old or secondary syphilis in those older than 1 also is suggestive of sexual abuse. Much attention is focused on the morphology and size of the hymen in the diagnosis of sexual abuse. Although a hymenal opening greater than 5 mm in the horizontal plane has been described as consistent with abuse, size is affected by examination technique. Therefore a complete description of the hymenal tissue, particularly signs of scarring, tears, or paucity of hymenal tissue, should be documented and considered consistent with the diagnosis of sexual abuse.

6. The answer is **B**, pages 606 and 607.
7. The answer is **A**, pages 606 and 607.
8. The answer is **E**, pages 606 and 607.
9. The answer is **E**, pages 606 and 607.

A noncontrast head computed tomographic (CT) scan is the diagnostic study of choice to evaluate for intracranial bleeding. Magnetic resonance imaging (MRI) has some advantages over CT in visualizing shearing injuries and can also provide information regarding the existence of multiple subdural hematomas and timing of the bleeding. All children younger than 1 who the physician suspects have been abused or neglected should have a skeletal survey. Children younger than 5 who possibly have been abused physically also should have skeletal surveys for screening purposes. A "babygram" is not a suitable substitute for a skeletal survey. Metaphyseal injuries are pathognomonic for physical abuse and are best diagnosed by plain radiographs compared with bone scans.

10. The answer is **E,** page 606.

Spiral fractures are worrisome in nonambulating children, and a spiral fracture of the humerus in a young child is especially suspect, indicating a rotational force to cause the injury. Developmentally delayed children are at more risk to be abused, and a delay in seeking care is of concern in this case. The child should have been in pain and requiring medical attention the night before, when the injury happened. The child's injury should be treated, and because of the suspicion of physical abuse the child should be admitted for safety concerns and the regional welfare agency promptly contacted. The parents or caretaker should be informed of the report. The diagnosis of abuse should be made after a thorough psychosocial assessment has been made. The primary physician can corroborate with the orthopedic subspecialist, but it is the role of the admitting physician along with the primary attending physician to make the diagnosis of child abuse and convey this diagnosis to the welfare agency.

11. The answer is **D,** pages 604 to 606.

The physical examination of this child indicates that the child is in shock and requires aggressive stabilization. Even though retinal hemorrhages are not apparent on the initial examination, this does not exclude the diagnosis of abusive head trauma. Abusive head trauma is the leading cause of death from child abuse. In this case the child is a victim of shaken infant syndrome, and immediate management would consist of intubation; management of the child's airway, breathing, and circulation; and treatment of increased intracranial pressure. Also, the child's weight is far below the fifth percentile for weight, which must be addressed by the evaluating team.

12. The answer is **E,** pages 610 and 611.

Determining when the abusive act(s) occurred will be difficult because of the age of the child. The evaluation most likely will cause significant parental anxiety and thus needs to be performed in the ED. The child deserves a thorough history and physical examination for documentation. Because of this child's lack of verbal skills or fear to disclose the complete history, cultures for gonorrhea and *Chlamydia* should be obtained from all three orifices. Because of the low probability of this child's having a sexually transmitted disease, it is reasonable to withhold treatment pending cultures. A history should be obtained in a nonthreatening way without any promises or assurances, and the caretakers should be interviewed separately. The ultimate goal is to prevent child abuse from recurring, hence the need to determine the safest disposition for the child where more abuse will not occur.

13. The answer is **E,** pages 611 and 612.

A positive vaginal culture for gonorrhea after the neonatal period is pathognomonic for sexual abuse. Although a discharge suggests the possibility of sexual abuse, it deserves thorough evaluation, which includes diagnoses outside of the realm of abuse. Condylomata acuminata (venereal warts) have a long incubation period and could be consistent with abuse or be perinatally acquired. Much discussion has been focused on the dimension of the hymenal ring as evidence of child sexual abuse, but hymenal findings must be interpreted with caution and compared with the given history. Hymenal size depends on many factors, including examination technique, which is important. Scarring, tearing, and loss or absence of tissue are considered consistent with, but not proof of, sexual abuse. Accurate descriptions including the morphology and dimensions of the hymenal opening are extremely important. *Chlamydia* antigen tests are considered unreliable, and therefore only culture should be used.

14. The answer is **C,** pages 605 and 606.

Epiphyseal-metaphyseal fractures are virtually pathognomonic for abuse. They result from shearing forces when an extremity is pulled or twisted. Spiral fractures prompt suspicion of abuse in the nonambulating child, yet they are not pathognomonic in the ambulating child and warrant investigation. Although a child's being in less than the fifth percentile is a concern, the calculation for a child who was born prematurely must be corrected for growth delay. Hence a child at the fifth percentile cannot be labeled an FTT child unless the calculation has been corrected for gestational age. Posterior rib fractures are a reason to suspect abuse, but they can also result from noninflicted injuries, and the history must be searched regarding an explanation for these findings.

15. The answer is **B,** pages 607 and 608.

Munchausen syndrome by proxy is a form of child abuse in which a caretaker simulates or produces illness in a child. It has a mortality rate of close to 10%. Boys and girls are equally affected, with a mean age of 15 months for the syndrome's onset. The forms of Munchausen syndrome by proxy are protean, including reports of bleeding, seizures, apnea, and fevers. The caretakers usually are knowledgeable medically and thrive in the medical setting. The siblings are also at risk for involvement and require evaluation and treatment. Because of the high mortality and morbidity of this syndrome, children must be placed in a safe environment once the diagnosis is suspected.

16. The answer is **C,** page 605.

Although abdominal trauma resulting from child abuse is infrequent, it has a high mortality related to both the severity of the injury and the delay in seeking care. The majority of abdominal injuries are caused by blunt trauma, and the wide range of injuries includes lacerations, contusions, and ruptures of abdominal organs, vasculature, and mesentery. Shaken infant syndrome refers to babies who sustain intracranial bleeding manifested classically by subdural hematomas, often with associated physical findings of bruising or fractures where the baby was grasped. Abdominal trauma should always be considered in children who have unexplained shock or peritonitis, especially if associated with anemia. Thoracic injuries caused by abuse are less frequently reported than abusive abdominal trauma.

17. The answer is **D,** page 606.

Rib fractures are uncommon in childhood and should alert the physician to evaluate for child abuse. Signs of healing rib fractures in varying ages are indicative of abuse if there is no bone disease. Rib fractures are rare in neonatal intensive care graduates because posterior rib fractures are not associated with vigorous chest physiotherapy or cardiopulmonary resuscitation. Posterior rib fractures are the rib fractures most commonly associated with child abuse.

18. The answer is **B,** pages 602 to 604.

The sequence of color change in healing bruises is time dependent (see Table 45-1, page 602 in Barkin et al). Bruises are the cutaneous lesions most commonly associated with child abuse, and the suspicion of inflicted injuries is elevated for all ages of children when bruises are seen on the inner thighs, inner arms, and thorax, likewise with multiple bruises in the penis, scrotum, buttocks, and face. Nature does not leave injuries with well-demarcated lines that indicate the use of an implement to bruise or burn. Human bites leave an ovoid pattern and do not cause puncture wounds as carnivores' bites frequently do.

19. The answer is **E,** pages 605 and 606.

This is a good case for a workup of infection, either a joint or bone infection. Although the mother has risk factors as a ward of the state and a teenager, the case calls for an ED evaluation for infection. A bone survey is not warranted to evaluate for prior abuse, and metaphyseal fractures are diagnosed by skeletal radiograph. A head CT scan is not warranted for this baby with stable vital signs and a focus for infection.

20. The answer is **D,** page 613.

All 50 states have the same mandatory reporting laws for child abuse. Physicians are highly encouraged to inform families of the decision to file a report with a child protective services agency, although doing so is not required by law in all states,. If a caretaker attempts to remove a child for whom there are concerns of abuse, the physician must consider taking protective custody to ensure that a complete workup is performed and the child is not returned to a potentially harmful environment. Health care workers and other mandated reporters are not required to contact a child protective service team before reporting cases. Mandated reporters are protected from legal action as good faith reporters even in cases in which abuse is not proved. Failure to report child abuse can result in legal action. Physicians should be competent in filing a child abuse report with the county or state child protective agency. It is not a law that a social worker is the only capable person to file a child abuse report.

Allergic and Immunologic Disorders

Won Baik-Han • Arabella C. Stock

See Barkin et al: Chapter 46.

1. A 15-year-old girl with a history of migraine headaches controlled with propranolol is seen in the ED with sudden onset of palpitations, pruritus, generalized hives, and difficulty in breathing after eating shellfish. The diagnosis of anaphylactic reaction is made, and the patient receives three subcutaneous (SQ) doses of epinephrine 1:1000 0.01 ml/kg with no response. The next drug of choice should be:
   A. Intravenous (IV) aminophylline.
   B. Diphenhydramine.
   C. Nebulized atropine sulfate.
   D. IV cimetidine.
   E. Nebulized albuterol.

2. Which of the following is associated with polyarticular juvenile rheumatoid arthritis (JRA) with rheumatoid factor negative?
   A. Common small joint involvement.
   B. Significant improvement with therapy.
   C. Onset in late childhood or adolescence.
   D. Associated vasculitis.
   E. Tendency to affect younger males.

3. A 10-year-old girl is brought to the ED after the gradual onset of swelling of the upper extremities associated with cramping abdominal pain and vomiting following an episode of strenuous exercise. She has no associated urticaria, pruritus, or difficulty in breathing. The most likely diagnosis is:
   A. Systemic mastocytosis.
   B. Hereditary angioneurotic edema.
   C. Cold urticaria.
   D. Anaphylaxis.
   E. Vasovagal reaction.

4. A 7-year-old boy is seen in the ED with complaints of malaise, generalized urticarial rash, painful swelling of knees and elbows, low-grade fever, and tender lymphadenopathy that developed progressively over the past 3 days. His medical history includes an episode of otitis media, for which he was treated with cefaclor, 2 weeks before the onset of the new symptoms. All of the following diagnoses should be included in the differential diagnosis of the patient *except:*
   A. Acute rheumatic fever.
   B. Infectious hepatitis.
   C. Rubella.
   D. Collagen vascular disease.
   E. Anaphylactoid reaction.

5. Which of the following laboratory findings *will not* be associated with the patient's condition described in question 4?
   A. Elevated sedimentation rate.
   B. Hyaline casts.
   C. Decreased complement levels.
   D. Microscopic hematuria.
   E. Elevated blood urea nitrogen level.

6. A 10-year-old child with a known case of type I pauciarticular JRA comes to the ED with fever, pain in the right knee, rash, and red, painful eyes for 3 months. The temperature (T) is 39.2° C, respiratory rate (RR) 26 breaths per minute, heart rate (HR) 90 beats per minute, and blood pressure (BP) 90/70 mm Hg. The most likely diagnosis is:
   A. Conjunctivitis.
   B. Uveitis.
   C. Kawasaki disease.
   D. Optic neuritis.
   E. Acute glaucoma.

7. What is the most important therapeutic option for the patient described in the previous question?
   A. Systemic corticosteroids.
   B. Acetylsalicylic acid.
   C. Nonsteroidal antiinflammatory agents.
   D. Topical steroids.
   E. Immunosuppressive agents.

8. A 12-year-old child comes to the ED with a 13-week history of persistent fever, pain in the left knee, and acute onset of chest pain and dyspnea. The child looks ill. Which of the following is the most likely complication of this child's condition?
   A. Cerebral abscess.
   B. Hydrops of the gallbladder.
   C. Pulmonary embolus.
   D. Pericarditis.
   E. Acute renal failure.

9. A 5-year-old is seen in the ED for the sudden onset of wheezing, erythema, generalized pruritic urticaria, and chest tightness. The airway is stabilized, and oxygen, epinephrine, and IV diphenhydramine are administered. The patient's respiratory status improves, but his urticaria persists. Which of the following should be given as the next step in the management of this patient?
   A. IV cimetidine.
   B. Another dose of diphenhydramine.
   C. IV epinephrine at 0.1 mg/kg/min.
   D. IV dopamine at 0.1 mg/kg/min.
   E. IV methylprednisolone 10 mg/kg.

10. A 16-year-old boy requires a radiologic study with IV contrast. The patient's medical history includes severe pruritus and wheezing after exposure to shellfish. Which of the following should be considered in the management of this patient?
    A. Use of an ionic dye.
    B. Pretreatment with IV steroids and diphenhydramine.
    C. Pretreatment with diphenhydramine only.
    D. Pretreatment with IV steroids.

11. A 6-year-old child is seen in the ED for the acute onset of pruritic hives that developed after he played with cats. His vital signs are stable, and he is not in respiratory distress. The best therapeutic option for this patient would be:
    A. Corticosteroids.
    B. Epinephrine 0.2 ml (1:1,000) SQ.
    C. Atropine.
    D. Diphenhydramine.
    E. Ice packs.

12. A 7-year-old boy with a history of chronic asthma is seen in the ED with complaints of coughing and wheezing. He is treated with continuous nebulized albuterol and IV steroids. After 2 hours of therapy, the patient becomes anxious, with deep retractions and wheezing. The oxygen saturation is 91%. An arterial blood gas study is performed and shows pH 7.24, $Paco_2$ 55 mm Hg, Pao_2 65 mm Hg. The next step in the management of this patient is:
    A. Increase the dose of nebulized albuterol.
    B. Obtain a radiograph of the chest.
    C. Administer IV aminophylline.
    D. Intubate and start mechanical ventilation.
    E. Administer IV terbutaline.

13. A 13-year-old boy is seen in the ED for the acute onset of shortness of breath and difficulty talking. He was stung on the forearm 20 minutes ago by a bee. He also has diffuse urticaria and periorbital edema. The best therapeutic option is:
    A. Administer albuterol by nebulization.
    B. Administer epinephrine SQ.
    C. Initiate IV therapy with 0.45% normal saline.
    D. Apply tourniquet above the forearm.
    E. Sedate the patient and intubate the trachea.

14. An 8-year-old boy is seen in the ED with diffuse pruritic skin lesions on his face, upper chest, and all extremities. He has had the papulovesicular eczematous lesions for 48 hours. He has no angioedema, urticaria, or wheezing. The patient was camping with his family 1 week ago. What is the best therapeutic option in this patient?
    A. Diphenhydramine.
    B. Topical corticosteroid.
    C. Oral cimetidine.
    D. Epinephrine SQ.
    E. Systemic corticosteroid.

15. A previously well 9-year-old girl has a history of generalized headache, lethargy, and vomiting for 1 week. She has been treated with oral antibiotics for sinusitis for the past 2 weeks. She has a history of chronic allergic rhinitis. Examination of the patient shows blurred optic disc margins without any abnormal physical or neurologic signs. The next step in the management of this patient is:
    A. X-ray film of the sinus.
    B. Cerebral angiography.
    C. Computed tomographic (CT) scan of the head with contrast medium.
    D. Electroencephalography.

ANSWERS   [See Barkin et al: Chapter 46.]

---

1. The answer is **C**, page 622.
   β-Blockers are infrequently used in children and adolescents. Their presence, however, may counteract the effectiveness of epinephrine, making an anaphylactic reaction more severe, prolonged, and refractory to treatment. Agents to consider in the treatment of patients receiving β-blockers are nebulized atropine sulfate or glucagon because of its positive inotropic and chronotropic effects.

2. The answer is **B**, page 624.
   Polyarticular juvenile rheumatoid arthritis (JRA) with rheumatoid factor negative typically affects younger girls, involves fewer joints with less systemic involvement, generally tends to improve with therapy, and rarely involves the small joints of the hands and feet. Systemic manifestations may accompany the disease but are not as acute or persistent as those in systemic onset JRA.

3. The answer is **B,** page 621.

Hereditary angioneurotic edema caused by C_1 esterase inhibitor deficiency is episodic, localized, and nonpitting. The edema results from vasodilatory effects of kinin on the capillary venules. Swelling of the affected parts develops slower than in anaphylactic reaction, without urticaria, itching, discoloration, or redness. Swelling of the intestinal wall may lead to intensely cramping abdominal pain associated at times with vomiting and diarrhea. This entity may occur at sites of trauma, after vigorous exercise, or with menses or emotional stress.

4. The answer is **B,** page 629.

Serum sickness is a systemic type III hypersensitivity reaction that usually follows the administration of foreign proteins or chemicals. It is characterized by fever, skin rash, arthritis, and lymphadenopathy. Erythema multiforme, Stevens-Johnson syndrome, toxic shock syndrome, anaphylaxis or anaphylactoid reactions, JRA, septic arthritis, viral illness, collagen vascular disorders, and acute rheumatic fever should be considered in the differential diagnosis of serum sickness.

5. The answer is **E,** page 629.

Laboratory tests are of limited usefulness in serum sickness. However, the sedimentation rate may be elevated at times, complement levels may be decreased, leukocytosis or leukopenia may be seen, and eosinophilia may or may not be present. Urinalysis may reveal hyaline casts, slight proteinuria, and microscopic hematuria. Electrolyte levels usually are normal.

6. The answer is **B,** page 626.

The findings are consistent with the diagnosis of uveitis or iridocyclitis. Occasionally uveitis in older boys causes a red, painful eye with or without visual disturbances.

7. The answer is **D,** page 628.

Patients with uveitis should be treated with topical steroid therapy. Systemic steroids are seldom used. They are indicated for patients with severe refractory disease, patients with life-threatening complications such as pericarditis, or patients in whom topical steroid therapy has failed.

8. The answer is **D,** pages 625 and 626.

The patient in this scenario has findings consistent with JRA with pericarditis. Symptoms of pericardial involvement include chest pain, tachycardia, and dyspnea. Pericarditis may be the initial symptom or may occur at any time during the course of the disease.

9. The answer is **A,** page 622.

Cimetidine, an H_2-blocker, has been found to be useful in cases of refractory anaphylaxis. Administer in IV doses of 5 to 10 mg/kg every 6 hours.

10. The answer is **B,** page 623.

If the radiologic procedure is required on an emergency basis, consider using a nonionic dye or select another procedure without the use of contrast. Pretreatment with steroids and diphenhydramine would be indicated for the patient described in the scenario.

11. The answer is **D,** page 622.

Acute urticaria caused by exposure to an allergen can occur without evidence of cardiovascular collapse or upper airway obstruction. If the vital signs are stable, the patient should be treated with diphenhydramine 1 to 2 mg/kg IV or intramuscularly with subsequent administration every 4 to 6 hours orally to treat urticaria.

12. The answer is **E,** page 1085.

The patient in the scenario has clinical findings of respiratory distress. He has been treated with the appropriate asthma medications for an acutely ill patient. However, he has not responded well and discloses signs of severe acidosis. IV terbutaline is a good treatment because of its selective β-agonist properties. If this treatment does not produce improvement, intubation and mechanical ventilation should be considered. Other treatment modalities before intubation include magnesium sulfate and ipratropium bromide.

13. The answer is **B,** page 622.

The patient in the scenario has findings consistent with acute anaphylaxis caused by bee sting. Symptoms of anaphylaxis include urticaria, angioedema, coughing, wheezing, laryngeal edema, abdominal discomfort, and syncope. Circulatory collapse, including hypotension and tachycardia, may also occur. The immediate management is epinephrine 1:1000 subcutaneously 0.01 ml/kg (maximum 0.3 ml).

14. The answer is **E,** page 683.

The treatment for this patient is a systemic steroid because multiple sites are involved. Mild cases may be treated with topical steroids, antihistamines, or cool compresses. The patient in this scenario displays a type IV delayed cell-mediated reaction caused by sensitized T-lymphocytes with a specific receptor site for a certain antigen. Subsequent exposure to the antigen results in proliferation of these cells and the recruitment of other cytotoxic cells. Examples of this reaction are contact dermatitis, poison ivy, and tuberculin skin test.

15. The answer is **C,** page 748.

The patient in the scenario displays a history and symptoms of cerebral abscess. The complications of sinusitis include otitis media, nasal polyposis, hearing loss, orofacial deformities, mastoiditis, alveolar hypoventilation, and intracranial abscess.

39

Cardiovascular Disorders

Peter H. Lee • David E. Bank • Arthur Klein

See Barkin et al: Chapter 47.

1. A 15-year-old girl is seen in the ED with a 1-month history of chest pain that does not radiate. Meals do not exacerbate the pain, but movement does. Physical examination shows a swollen, tender costochondral junction without erythema. Pain is reproducible on palpation of the sternum. The rest of the physical examination is normal. What is the next step in the workup for this patient?
   A. Obtain an electrocardiogram (ECG).
   B. Obtain serum cardiac enzyme measurements.
   C. Obtain an echocardiogram.
   D. No workup is necessary.
   E. Aspirate material from the patient's sternum for cell count, Gram's stain, and culture.
2. Which infectious agent is responsible for pleurodynia (i.e., Bornholm disease or "the devil's grip")?
   A. Respiratory syncytial virus.
   B. Epstein-Barr virus.
   C. Coxsackievirus type B.
   D. Human immunodeficiency virus.
   E. *Streptococcus pneumoniae.*
3. A 6-year-old Asian boy comes to the ED with a 3-week history of afebrile illness consisting of prolonged irritability, fever, conjunctivitis, lymphadenopathy, and erythroderma. The patient experienced an episode of sudden, severe chest pain approximately 45 minutes before arrival. The patient's ECG is shown in Fig. 39-1 on page 196. Which is the most likely diagnosis in this patient?
   A. Pericarditis.
   B. Myocardial infarction.
   C. Pericardial effusion.
   D. Prolonged QTc interval.
   E. Torsades de pointes.

4. A 14-year-old obese girl complains of shortness of breath and chest pain on deep inspiration for 5 days. She was discharged from the hospital 10 days ago after an open femur fracture reduction. Medical history is negative for asthma. She takes oral contraceptives. She does not appear toxic. Her pulse (P) is 120 beats per minute, blood pressure (BP) 110/60 mm Hg, respiratory rate (RR) 24 breaths per minute, and oxygen (O_2) saturation 94% on room air, and she is afebrile. Her physical examination shows bibasilar wheezing. Chest radiographs are negative. What is the next step in managing this patient?
   A. Admit the patient and arrange for a ventilation-perfusion scan.
   B. Administer three sequential albuterol nebulizer treatments.
   C. Administer oral prednisone.
   D. Administer intravenous (IV) methylprednisolone.
   E. Empirically treat with antibiotics for a presumed pneumonia.
5. Which of the following heart sounds in children is most suggestive of organic pathology?
   A. Vibratory, systolic murmur.
   B. Diastolic murmur.
   C. Associated split S2 (physiologic) heart sound, not fixed.
   D. Murmur disappearing when supine.
   E. Murmur disappearing when standing.
6. *True or False:* The ECG is the gold standard to exclude structural cardiac disease in children.
   A. True.
   B. False.
7. In a neonate, what would be the most appropriate initial test to help distinguish between persistent pulmonary hypertension and cyanotic congenital heart disease?
   A. Arterial blood gas (ABG).
   B. ABG and chemistry panel.
   C. Hyperoxic test.
   D. Chest radiograph.
   E. Echocardiogram.

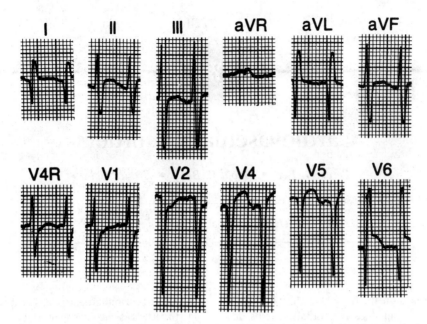

FIG. 39-1   (From Park MK: *How to read pediatric ECGs*, St Louis, 1992, Mosby.)

8. A 2-day-old infant, discharged from the hospital in the morning, is brought into the ED by his parents because he "turned blue." Compared with their firstborn, this baby was noted to be less active and had difficulty feeding while in the hospital. On physical examination the infant is mildly tachypneic and tachycardic, afebrile, with a BP of 70/40 mm Hg. O_2 saturation is 78% on room air. Breath sounds are coarse. No murmurs, rubs, or gallops are noted. What is the most likely diagnosis?
   A. Tetralogy of Fallot.
   B. Transposition of the great arteries.
   C. Patent ductus arteriosus.
   D. Ebstein's anomaly of the tricuspid valve.
   E. Total anomalous pulmonary venous return (obstructed).

9. What is the best immediate step in management of the patient described in question 8?
   A. IV administration of furosemide.
   B. Immediate operative repair.
   C. Indomethacin therapy.
   D. Prostaglandin therapy.
   E. Dopamine infusion.

10. An 18-year-old man comes to the ED complaining of palpitations and diaphoresis. He appears uncomfortable. Medical history is significant only for a "heart problem" when he was younger. Heart rate (HR) is 220 beats per minute, BP is 100/55 mm Hg, and O_2 saturation is 97% on room air. Physical examination reveals a midline sternotomy scar and an irregular rhythm with no murmurs, rubs, or gallops. Lung examination is normal. ECG is consistent with atrial fibrillation. What was his most likely preoperative diagnosis?
   A. Transposition of the great arteries.
   B. Tetralogy of Fallot.
   C. Tricuspid atresia.
   D. Aortic stenosis.
   E. Pulmonary atresia.

11. Which of the following is the most common congenital heart defect seen in children?
   A. Bicuspid aortic valve.
   B. Ventricular septal defect.
   C. Atrial septal defect.
   D. Tetralogy of Fallot.
   E. Coarctation of the aorta.

12. Patients with which of the following congenital heart defects do *not* require antibiotic prophylaxis for bacterial endocarditis?
   A. Ventricular septal defect.
   B. Tetralogy of Fallot.
   C. Atrial septal defect.
   D. Mitral valve prolapse.
   E. Bicuspid aortic valve.

13. What are the *two* determinants of cardiac output?
   A. Heart rate.
   B. Central venous pressure.
   C. Stroke volume.
   D. Systemic vascular resistance.
   E. Blood pressure.

14. Which of the following increases the risk of developing digoxin toxicity?
   A. Hypokalemia.
   B. Hyponatremia.
   C. Hypocalcemia.
   D. Hyperthyroidism.
   E. Sympatholytic drugs.

15. Which of the following is the single most important laboratory test in the diagnosis of infective endocarditis?
   A. White blood cell count.
   B. Blood culture.
   C. Serum complement level.
   D. Serum C-reactive protein level.
   E. Erythrocyte sedimentation rate.

16. For patients with congenital heart disease, which of the following procedures requires antibiotic prophylaxis?
    A. Incision and drainage of infected tissue.
    B. Shedding of primary teeth.
    C. Cardiac catheterization.
    D. Endoscopy with gastrointestinal (GI) biopsy.
    E. Tympanostomy tube insertion.
17. Which of the following bacterial infections has a high occurrence of associated myocarditis?
    A. *Streptococcus pyogenes.*
    B. *Neisseria meningitidis.*
    C. *Corynebacterium diphtheriae.*
    D. *Chlamydia psittaci.*
    E. *Staphylococcus aureus.*

18. A 16-year-old girl with diagnosed systemic lupus erythematosus comes into the ED with a 3-day history of low-grade fevers and cough. She was brought into the ED today by her mother because of difficulty breathing. Additionally she complains of mild chest pain that is relieved by sitting up. Vital signs are HR 120 beats per minute, RR 22 breaths per minute, T 38.8° C, BP 130/60 mm Hg, and O_2 saturation of 99% on room air. Physical examination reveals mild hepatomegaly and jugular venous distension. The heart sounds are distant. No murmurs are detected. The lung fields are clear to auscultation. What is the most likely diagnosis?
    A. Pneumonia.
    B. Pleural abscess.
    C. Pleuritis.
    D. Pericarditis.
    E. Pneumothorax.
19. What specific dermatologic process can be seen in patients with acute rheumatic fever?
    A. Erythema toxicum.
    B. Erythema marginatum.
    C. Erythema nodosum.
    D. Erythema multiforme.
    E. Erythema infectiosum.

ANSWERS   [See Barkin et al: Chapter 47.]

---

1. The answer is **D**, page 631.
   The patient described exhibits signs and symptoms consistent with a diagnosis of costochondritis, or Tietze's syndrome. This entity is typically seen in adolescents and young adults, particularly females. It is of unknown etiology, causing a nonsuppurative inflammation of the costochondral junction. Although usually self-limiting, it can last for several months. The diagnosis can be based on the physical examination. Nonsteroidal antiinflammatory medication and rest are the treatments of choice.
2. The answer is **C**, page 632.
   One of several enteroviruses, coxsackievirus type B infections are associated with pleurodynia (i.e., costalgia). None of the other infectious agents listed is known to cause this entity. Interestingly, coxsackievirus types B1-B5 also have been associated with myopericarditis.
3. The answer is **B**, page 632.
   The ECG shows the classic signs of myocardial infarction (MI): inverted T waves, ST segment elevations, and Q waves. Several keys in this clinical scenario were presented in the patient's medical history. Patients with untreated Kawasaki disease have a 15% to 25% chance of coronary aneurysms. These aneurysms in turn can lead to MIs, sudden death, and chronic coronary artery insufficiency (Table 39-1 on page 198).

4. The answer is **A**, pages 666 to 668 and 1112 to 1115.
   The diagnosis of pulmonary embolism (PE) in children can be difficult. The reason for this is the low overall incidence in children, with a corresponding low level of suspicion on the physician's part. Autopsy reports of the incidence of PE in children have varied, from 0.5% to 3.7%. This number is likely to increase as more children need deep central lines for chronic medical illnesses. Risk factors for PE include IV drug abuse, oral contraceptive use, protracted immobilization, and previous orthopedic surgeries (see Table 47-16, page 667 in Barkin et al for other risk factors). Radiographic evidence, such as Hampton hump, and ECG evidence, such as an S1 Q3 T3 pattern, right bundle branch block, and right axis deviation, are seldom seen in pulmonary emboli. Although a negative trial of β-agonists would not likely harm the patient, appropriate suspicion, workup, and treatment (heparinization, thrombolytics) are acceptable.
5. The answer is **B**, page 634.
   A diastolic murmur is most worrisome. None of the other choices uniformly denotes significant disease or increased risk thereof. Any diastolic murmur deserves follow-up with a cardiologist (see Table 47-3, page 634 in Barkin et al).
6. The answer is **B, false,** pages 634 and 635.
   Although ECG examinations can be helpful as an initial screening tool, the definitive diagnostic tool remains the echocardiogram.

TABLE 39-1   Causes of Myocardial Infarction in Children

Category	Specific condition
Congenital cardiac disease	Stenosis or atresia of any of the valves, supravalvular aortic stenosis, atrioventricular canal, truncus arteriosus, patent ductus arteriosus, transposition of the great vessels, tetralogy of Fallot, coarctation of the aorta
Coronary artery anomalies	Anomalous origin of coronary arteries, single right or left coronary artery, aneurysm of the coronary arteries (Kawasaki disease)
Primary endocardial or myocardial disease	Endocardial fibroelastosis, cardiomyopathy
Collagen disorders	Rheumatic fever, systemic lupus erythematosus, Kawasaki disease, rheumatoid arthritis
Hematologic/oncologic	Polycythemia, hemoglobinopathy (S-C, SS, H types), anemia, leukemia
Neuromuscular disease	Friedreich's ataxia, muscular dystrophy
Primary cardiac tumors	Myxoma, rhabdomyosarcoma, teratoma, fibroma, lipoma, hamartoma
Miscellaneous	Cocaine use

Adapted from Perry LW: *Contemp Pediatr* 27(Nov-Dec):1985.

7. The answer is **C**, page 635.
   Administration of 100% O_2 *usually* will demonstrate improvement over the Pao_2 documented at a lower FIo_2 in neonates with persistent pulmonary hypertension but not cyanotic heart disease.

8. The answer is **B**, pages 636 to 639.
   Transposition classically appears during the first week of life. Other causes of cyanotic heart disease include tetralogy of Fallot, tricuspid atresia, severe pulmonic stenosis, total anomalous pulmonary venous return, and Ebstein's anomaly. The absence of a murmur is characteristic of transposition.

9. The answer is **D**, pages 637 to 639.
   In addition to O_2 therapy, prostaglandin therapy could be lifesaving for this patient. It should precede emergency surgical repair. Ductal-dependent lesions such as transposition can be "temporized" by prostaglandin therapy (i.e., PGE_1), usually in consultation with a cardiologist.

10. The answer is **A**, page 637.
    After atrial repair for a transposition, atrial dysrhythmias and conduction disturbances can appear. Atrial dysrhythmias are rarely seen as sequelae of the correction of the other congenital heart lesions. Ventricular dysrhythmias can be seen at times in patients with surgically repaired tetralogy of Fallot.

11. The answer is **B**, page 639.
    Ventricular septal defects account for approximately 20% to 40% of the cases of congenital heart disease in children.

12. The answer is **C**, page 657.
    Children with an isolated secundum atrial septal defect have a negligible risk of bacterial endocarditis as compared with the general population. Antibiotic prophylaxis is indicated in all of the remaining choices. See page 657 in Barkin et al for recommendations for patients with heart defects requiring prophylaxis.

13. The answers are **A and C**, pages 644 and 645.

    Cardiac output = heart rate × stroke volume

14. The answer is **A**, page 649.
    Hypokalemia, hypercalcemia, hypoxemia, alkalosis, sympathomimetic drugs, and myocardial ischemia can all *increase the sensitivity* of the myocardium to digoxin. Additionally, decreased renal excretion, hypothyroidism, high doses, and drug interactions can predispose a patient to digoxin toxicity caused by high serum levels.

15. The answer is **B**, page 655.
    The blood culture remains the critical diagnostic test in making the diagnosis of infective endocarditis. One report states that the first two blood cultures will be positive more than 90% of the time. Other studies suggest that the sensitivity may approach 100% with three blood cultures being drawn. Therefore examining three blood cultures in the first 24 hours is recommended. Of practical note, the volume of blood for culture should be equal to about 10% of the culture fluid medium. The other tests mentioned can be significant in acute inflammation (nonspecific) or valuable in monitoring the progression of infective endocarditis. They are not as helpful diagnostically.

16. The answer is **A**, page 657.
    Of the choices given, only the incision and drainage of infected tissue is a procedure that should warrant antibiotic prophylaxis. All of the other choices do not need antibiotic prophylaxis, as per the guidelines of the American Heart Association (see table "Prophylaxis Recommendations," page 657 in Barkin et al).

17. The answer is **C**, page 659.
    Although seen less commonly in recent times, myocarditis occurs in up to 25% of diphtheria cases and is the most frequent cause of death from that disease. Usually bacterial myocarditis is a component of serious bacterial multisystem infection. Remember, *viruses* cause most cases of infectious myocarditis.

18. The answer is **D,** pages 661 to 664.

Numerous infectious and noninfectious causes of pericarditis exist. The exact incidence of pericarditis is unknown. Collagen vascular diseases in general can lead to this morbid condition. The child in this question is a classic example. Often the patient with pericarditis also has a component of myocarditis. Congestive heart failure, shock, dysrhythmias, and death are among the potential complications. Although pneumonia, pleural abscess, and pleuritis can all result in fever and cough, the rest of her symptoms and physical examination should lead you to the diagnosis of pericarditis. A person with a pneumothorax usually would have a more acute presentation.

19. The answer is **B,** page 665.

Erythema marginatum is the only choice that is specific for rheumatic fever (RF). Other major criteria (Jones criteria, see table on page 665 in Barkin et al) include carditis, polyarthritis, chorea (Sydenham's), and subcutaneous nodules. Minor manifestations may include arthralgias, fever, elevated erythrocyte sedimentation rate, and a prolonged PR interval (ECG). Documentation of a prior streptococcal infection is of course also imperative for diagnosis.

Dermatology

J.S. Supure

See Barkin et al: Chapter 48.

1. A 15-month-old infant is brought to the ED with a 3-day history of high fever (104° F). The mother states that the fever resolved today with the appearance of a pinkish maculopapular rash mainly over the trunk. Physical examination reveals a well-looking child with minimal periorbital puffiness. Which one of the following is the most likely cause of this patient's illness?
   A. Erythema infectiosum (fifth disease).
   B. Scarlet fever.
   C. Kawasaki disease.
   D. Human herpes virus 6 (roseola).
   E. Pityriasis rosea.
2. Which one of the following is a *true* statement about scarlet fever?
   A. It is commonly associated with pharyngitis, although it can develop with impetigo.
   B. The risk of a complication such as rheumatic fever is greater than that of the risk from strep throat without the rash.
   C. To control the spread of the disease, children should not return to school until 3 days after starting antibiotics.
   D. The presence of Koplik's spots is diagnostic.
   E. It should be reported to local public health authorities to initiate epidemic control measures.
3. Which of the following is true about rubeola (measles)?
   A. The rash first appears on the soles of the feet and spreads to the head.
   B. Impetigo is the most common complication.
   C. Koplik's spots are not seen.
   D. The patient is most contagious during the prodromal period.
   E. The measles virus belongs to the *Parvovirus* genus.

4. Which one of the following is a *true* statement regarding herpes zoster?
   A. A susceptible person does not contract varicella if exposed to someone with zoster.
   B. The herpes virus cannot be cultured from skin lesions.
   C. Trigeminal nerve dermatome is commonly involved.
   D. Varicella-zoster virus persists in the latent form in spinal nerve sensoryroot ganglia.
   E. Children with active zoster lesions need not be isolated.
5. Which of the following statements is *true* regarding tinea corporis?
   A. This infection is commonly seen in cold climates.
   B. Topical treatment is usually effective.
   C. Itching is not a common problem.
   D. Regional lymph nodes are enlarged.
   E. Wood's lamp examination is helpful for diagnosis.
6. Which one of the following statements is *true* regarding oral candidiasis?
   A. White curds are seen and can be wiped off the mucous membrane easily.
   B. A clear relationship exists between antibiotic use and thrush.
   C. Thrush causes painful inflammation of the tongue.
   D. Thrush is commonly seen in newborns.
   E. Nystatin suspension should be used before feedings to wash off the white spots.
7. The diagnostic findings of tinea capitis include all of the following *except*:
   A. The hair stubs produce the "black dot," which is a common appearance.
   B. Kerion formation develops in about one third of tinea capitis cases.
   C. Generalized scaly papules result from systemic sensitization to fungal products.
   D. Most cases in the United States are caused by *Trichophyton tonsurans*.
   E. *Microsporum audouinii* does fluoresce in Wood's lamp examinations.

8. Which one of the following statements regarding Henoch-Schönlein purpura is *true?*
   A. Renal involvement is severe and complete.
   B. Arthritis occurs in 100% of cases.
   C. The skin rash is distributed asymmetrically.
   D. It may include marked swelling and bruising of the scrotum.
   E. The disease has a seasonal incidence that peaks in the summer.

9. Which one of the following statements regarding perianal streptococcal infection is *false?*
   A. The lesion is superficial rather than cellulitic.
   B. Well-marginated red rings of irritated skin extend evenly from the anus.
   C. No induration and regional lymphadenopathy appear.
   D. The diagnosis is made by obtaining a culture that is positive for group A β-hemolytic streptococcal infection (GABHS).
   E. Oral sulfonamide drugs are the treatment of choice for this illness.

10. A mother brings in her 3-year old child, who has an itching skin rash of 3 weeks' duration on her palms and soles. "Her 12-year-old brother has itchy bumps in the web spaces of his fingers," Mom says. Which is the most likely diagnosis?
    A. Atopic dermatitis.
    B. Insect bites.
    C. Varicella.
    D. Scabies.
    E. Herpes zoster.

11. Which of the following statements regarding acute urticaria is true?
    A. Urticarial lesions involve only the palms and soles.
    B. Laboratory tests are routinely useful in evaluation of etiology.
    C. Individual lesions may last for a few minutes or several hours.
    D. Topical steroids and topical antihistamines are always useful.
    E. Lesions are not itchy.

12. Which of the following statements regarding warts is *true?*
    A. The greatest incidence occurs in infants.
    B. Transmission is through direct contact and auto-inoculation.
    C. The incubation period is short.
    D. Cellular immunity plays no role in resolution of the warts.
    E. Warts are intradermal tumors caused by bacteria.

ANSWERS [See Barkin et al: Chapter 48.]

1. The answer is **D,** page 696.
   The most recognized feature of the illness is the sudden onset of high fever in a well-looking child. Some clinicians describe mild conjunctivitis and peri-orbital cellulitis. Febrile seizures sometimes occur with this illness. Because of the young age of the child with high fever, diagnostic tests may be necessary to eliminate a possible serious treatable illness. The nonspecific illness lasts 3 to 4 days. Then as the child becomes afebrile, the rash develops.

2. The answer is **A,** pages 694 and 695.
   Scarlet fever is commonly associated with group A β-hemolytic *Streptococcus* (GABHS) pharyngitis, although it can also develop with impetigo or cellulitis. The risk of complications such as rheumatic fever is no greater than the risk from strep throat without the rash. To control spread of the disease, children should not return to school until 24 hours after starting antibiotics (Fig. 40-1 on page 202).

3. The answer is **D,** page 693.
   The patient is most contagious during the prodromal period. The exanthem classically begins behind the ears at the hairline and spreads from the head to the feet. Otitis media is the most common complication of measles. Koplik's spots (if present) are diagnostic of measles. The measles virus belongs to the paramyxo-virus group.

4. The answer is **D,** page 692.
   Varicella-zoster virus can persist in its latent form in spinal nerve root ganglia and erupt many years after the original infection. Herpes virus can be cultured from the lesion, and varicella can develop in a susceptible person who has been exposed to someone with zoster. Thoracic nerve dermatomes are most commonly involved. Children with zoster should be isolated.

5. The answer is **B,** page 687.
   Topical treatment is usually effective, so cultures are unneeded unless the patient does not respond to therapy. Regional lymph nodes are not usually enlarged unless impetigo complicates the situation. A Wood's lamp examination is not helpful. Infection is most commonly seen in warm climates. Itching is a common problem.

6. The answer is **C,** page 689.
   Thrush causes painful inflammation of the tongue, palate, and buccal mucosa. The white curds cannot be wiped off the mucous membrane (as opposed to curds of milk). There is not a clear relationship between antibiotic use and thrush. It is rarely seen in new-borns. Nystatin suspension should be used after feedings so that it sits in the mouth for as long as possible.

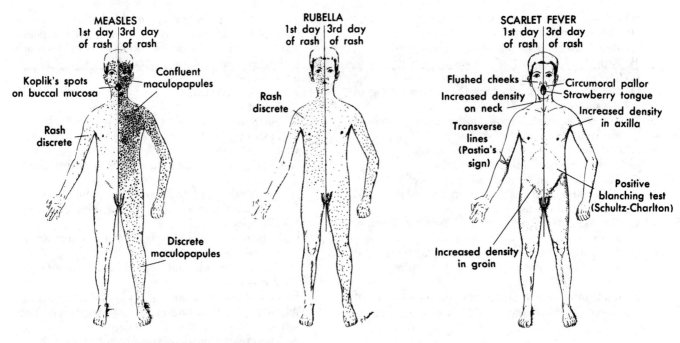

FIG. 40-1 Schematic drawings illustrating differences in appearance, distribution, and progression of rashes of measles, rubella, and scarlet fever. (From Krugman S et al: *Infectious diseases of children*, ed 9, St Louis, 1992, Mosby.)

7. The answer is **A,** page 686.
   The most obvious pattern is characterized by round or oval areas of alopecia that on close inspection show stubby remains of hairs that have broken off. The hair stubs provide the "black dot" appearance. Although this pattern of infection is easy to recognize, it is seen only in 5% of cases. All of the other statements are true.

8. The answer is **D,** page 689.
   The patient may have marked swelling and bruising of the scrotum along with the rash. The skin rash is distributed symmetrically. Arthritis is usually transient and occurs in two thirds of the cases. Renal involvement is usually mild. The disease has a seasonal incidence that peaks in winter.

9. The answer is **E,** page 681.
   Treatment with oral penicillin cures most cases. The infection is superficial with the appearance of a well-marginated, erythematous ring with no induration and no lymphadenopathy. The diagnosis is made by obtaining a culture that is positive for GABHS.

10. The answer is **D,** page 700.
    In older children and adults, scabies papules are found most often on the hands and wrists with typical burrows in the web spaces of fingers. Infants and young children frequently have vesicles on their palms and soles. Severe itching is the most common complaint.

11. The answer is **C,** page 704.
    Urticarial lesions occur on all parts of the body and characteristically have raised erythematous borders and blanched centers. The itchy individual lesions may last for a few minutes or several hours. No routine laboratory tests are used in the evaluation of acute urticaria. Topical steroids and topical antihistamines are not useful in controlling urticaria.

12. The answer is **B,** page 704.
    Transmission through direct contact causes many warts to develop in patterns, which suggests that autoinoculation occurs. The incubation is long and variable. The greatest incidence occurs in children 10 to 19 years of age. Cellular immunity appears to play an important role in resolution of warts.

Ear, Nose, and Throat

Arabella C. Stock

See Barkin et al: Chapter 49.

1. A 4-year-old was taken to the ED after he was found next to a spilled bottle of drain cleaner. He is agitated and drooling and has dysphonia. The next step in the management of this child is:
   A. Administer intravenous (IV) fluids.
   B. Perform immediate endoscopy.
   C. Administer barium swallow.
   D. Obtain a radiograph of the upper airway.

2. A 15-year-old boy with sudden onset of severe right ear pain and inability to close the ipsilateral eye completely says that a few weeks ago he had flu symptoms, sore throat, and a vesicular eruption on the pinna of the right ear. The next step in the management of this patient is:
   A. Administer β-lactamase oral antibiotics.
   B. Use conservative pain control and reassurance.
   C. Start treatment with acyclovir.
   D. Start treatment with prednisone.
   E. Administer broad-spectrum IV antibiotics.

3. A 13-year-old boy comes to the ED with profuse epistaxis on the left side that could not be controlled with digital pressure. In the attempt to identify the bleeding point for cauterization with silver nitrate, a gray mass is noted in the nostril. All of the following may be appropriate *except:*
   A. Packing with topical thrombin.
   B. Topical application of phenylephrine (Neo-Synephrine) 0.5%.
   C. Anterior nasal packing.
   D. Silver nitrate cauterization.
   E. Topical application of cocaine 4%.

4. A 4-year-old boy is seen in the ED with epistaxis on the right side. The bleeding site is visualized, and cauterization is performed until complete hemostasis is achieved. The boy returns to the ED 2 weeks later with respiratory "whistling," which the mother says appeared a few days after the epistaxis episode. The most likely cause of this child's symptoms is:
   A. Foreign body in the nostril.
   B. Sarcoidosis.
   C. Nasal septal perforation.
   D. Allergic rhinitis.
   E. Previously undiagnosed syphilis.

5. A 5-year old-child is seen for sudden hearing loss, facial weakness, headache, and unsteady gait. The most likely cause of these symptoms is:
   A. Late onset of congenital cytomegalovirus.
   B. Ménière's syndrome.
   C. Salicylate ingestion.
   D. Meningitis.
   E. Acoustic neuroma.

6. The most common cause of congenital deafness discovered during childhood is:
   A. Genetic factors.
   B. Intrauterine infections.
   C. Ototoxic drug ingestion during pregnancy.
   D. Birth trauma.
   E. Maternal preeclampsia.

7. A 7-year-old child is brought to the ED after he had a syncopal episode. On arrival in the ED he is awake and alert but is noted to have significant hearing deficit. Which of the following findings may be associated with this child's condition?
   A. Cardiomegaly on the chest radiograph.
   B. Δ-Wave on the electrocardiogram (ECG).
   C. Supraventricular tachycardia on the rhythm strip.
   D. Prolonged QT interval.
   E. Inverted T-waves in the precordial leads.

8. A 2-year-old child comes to the ED with a 1-month history of intermittent low-grade fever and persistent purulent nasal discharge, which does not respond to conservative management with acetaminophen and decongestants. The most likely diagnosis is:
   A. Streptococcosis.
   B. Chlamydial pneumonia.
   C. Allergic rhinitis.
   D. Cribriform plate fracture.
   E. Foreign body.

For questions 9 to 13, match the appropriate diagnosis with the clinical presentation. Each answer may be used once, more than once, or not at all.
   A. Rhabdomyosarcoma.
   B. Congenital epulis.
   C. Odontoma.
   D. Epstein's pearls.
   E. Torus.

9. A 4-day-old infant is seen for multiple small, white lesions on the palate. _____

10. A 15-year-old boy is seen for a slow-growing, firm mass in the midline of the hard palate. _____
    _____

11. A 5-year-old comes to the ED with a history of difficulty in swallowing and an ulcerated mass in the nasopharynx. _____

12. A radiograph shows a radiopaque lesion in the molar region of the mandible, which was taken to exclude a fracture in a 16-year-old who was assaulted with a baseball bat. _____

13. A 5-month-old girl seen in the ED for a 5-mm, round, mucosa-covered, pink mass located on the upper gingiva. _____

14. A 5-year-old child comes to the ED with a 2-day history of fever (39° to 40° C), malaise, headache, and purulent ear discharge. He was seen 3 weeks before this episode and was found to have otitis media, for which he received a 10-day course of amoxicillin. Physical examination disclosed a unilaterally enlarged lymph node, otorrhea, and "sagging" of the posterior external auditory canal with outward protrusion of the pinna. Which of the following tests is most sensitive in establishing the diagnosis?
    A. Blood cultures.
    B. Tympanic cavity aspiration.
    C. Computed tomography (CT) scan of the temporal bone.
    D. Sedimentation rate.
    E. Plain radiographs of the mastoid.

15. The appropriate test is performed for the patient in question 14, and it demonstrates a subperiosteal abscess. The next step in the management of this patient is:
    A. Analgesic therapy with codeine.
    B. Treatment with IV ampicillin 75 mg/kg/day.
    C. Bone scan for confirmation of the above finding.
    D. Prompt otolaryngology consultation for immediate surgery.
    E. Treatment with neomycin otic solution.

16. A 16-year-old diabetic boy known to have been dependent on insulin since he was 6 years old comes in with a severe earache, exacerbated by jaw movement. The patient has had similar episodes of less severity for the past 3 weeks, for which he was treated with topical corticosporin. Physical examination reveals a purulent, thick exudate and swelling of the external ear canal. The most likely organism involved in this patient's condition is:
    A. *Neisseria* species.
    B. *Streptococcus pyogenes*.
    C. *Staphylococcus aureus*.
    D. Herpes simplex virus.
    E. *Pseudomonas aeruginosa*.

17. Which of the following is the most appropriate therapy for the patient described in question 16?
    A. Neosporin-dexamethasone topical spray.
    B. Reassurance and pain management.
    C. Hospitalization and IV antibiotic therapy.
    D. Polymyxin B otic solution.
    E. Acetic acid otic solution.

18. A 5-year-old child fell 5 feet to the ground, landing on his head. He had no loss of consciousness and did not cry. Since the fall, he has had a persistent runny nose. Which of the following tests will be helpful in establishing this child's diagnosis?
    A. Nasal fluid analysis for cell count.
    B. Nasal fluid analysis for sodium.
    C. Nasal fluid analysis for glucose.
    D. Nasal fluid analysis for osmolarity.
    E. Gram's stain of the nasal fluid.

For questions 19 to 22, match the appropriate radiographic views with the corresponding sinus studied. Each answer may be used once, more than once, or not at all.
   A. Sphenoidal sinus.
   B. Frontal and ethmoidal sinuses.
   C. Maxillary sinuses.

19. Waters' (occipitomental). _____

20. Submentovertex. _____

21. Caldwell (anteroposterior). _____

22. Lateral. _____

23. A 16-year-old comes to the ED with a 1-day history of fever, chills, neck stiffness, torticollis, and a tender, indurated swelling around the parotid area. A week ago he was found to have peritonsillar abscess, for which he received a needle aspiration and was discharged from the ED on oral antibiotics. The most likely diagnosis in this patient is:
    A. Pharyngitis with a new organism.
    B. Peripharyngeal extension.
    C. Nonresolved peritonsillar abscess.
    D. Secondary lymphadenitis.
    E. Peritonsillar cellulitis.

24. A 3-year-old child is seen for sudden onset of high fever (40° C), labored breathing, and refusal to eat. The mother states that the child has been sick at home for the past 4 days with sore throat and low-grade fever. The parents have been giving him acetaminophen and decongestants. On examination he appears ill, holds his neck in hyperextended position, and has audible stridor. Which of the following findings on a soft lateral neck tissue radiograph will be consistent with this child's condition?
    A. A prevertebral space less than 40% of the anteroposterior diameter.
    B. A prevertebral space of 7 mm at C3-4.
    C. A prevertebral space of 5 mm at C2.
    D. A prevertebral space of 5 mm at C3-4.
    E. A prevertebral space of 6 mm at C2.

25. All of the following are possible complications of the child described in question 24 *except:*
    A. Empyema.
    B. Hemorrhage.
    C. Peritonsillar abscess.
    D. Airway obstruction.
    E. Pneumonia.

26. A 4-year-old boy comes to the ED with a nontender mass on the anterior border of the sternocleidomastoid muscle. The mass was noted to increase and decrease in size over the past few weeks. The patient's medical history includes tonsillopharyngitis 2 weeks before this new finding. The most likely diagnosis is:
    A. Thyroglossal duct.
    B. Branchial cleft cyst.
    C. Lymphoma of undetermined type.
    D. Tuberculous adenitis.
    E. Esophageal diverticulum.

ANSWERS   [See Barkin et al: Chapter 49.]

1. The answer is **B,** pages 548 to 549 and 710.
   If signs of respiratory compromise are present, no further invasive physical examination should be performed until the airway can be managed. If signs of respiratory compromise are not present, a thorough examination of the aerodigestive anatomy should be undertaken, usually by endoscopy.

2. The answer is **B,** page 712.
   Ramsay Hunt syndrome is an inflammation of the facial nerve resulting from to herpes zoster. Its classic form includes facial paralysis, vesicles on the pinna or the external canal, and associated otalgia, which may be severe and may occur weeks after the resolution of the vesicular eruption. No specific treatment is required except for pain control if severe otalgia is present.

3. The answer is **D,** page 714.
   Angiofibroma, a gray mass in the nose, may appear with epistaxis, although it is rare. Cauterization will worsen the bleeding.

4. The answer is **C,** page 714.
   All of the listed conditions may have respiratory "whistling." Nasal septal perforation has been reported following vigorous application of cautery.

5. The answer is **E,** page 718. All of the above are associated with hearing loss. However, acoustic neuroma can cause acute sensorineural hearing loss. Other cranial nerve involvement may also be present.

6. The answer is **A,** page 719.
   Approximately half of all congenital deafness discovered during childhood is caused by genetic factors. Syndromes associated with hearing loss include Waardenburg's, Turner's, and Treacher Collins to cite a few.

7. The answer is **D,** page 719.
   Jervell and Lange-Nielsen syndrome involves a prolonged QT interval, syncope, and sensorineural hearing loss.

8. The answer is **A,** page 720.
   In children younger than 3 years of age, infection with *Streptococcus pyogenes* causes streptococcosis, a less acute condition characterized by low-grade fever, adenopathy, and rhinitis lasting weeks to months.

All answers for questions 9 to 13 taken from Box 41-1.
9. **D.**
10. **E.**
11. **A.**
12. **C.**
13. **B.**

Box 41-1
Common Masses of the Mouth and Pharynx

A. Oral soft tissues
   1. Benign: hemangioma, lymphangioma, fibrous, epithelial, cystic (ranula, thyroglossal duct, branchial cleft)
   2. Malignant: rhabdomyosarcoma, epidermoid carcinoma
B. Gingiva and jaws
   1. Benign:
      a. Gingiva: congenital epulis, melanotic neuroectodermal tumor, giant cell reparative granuloma, pyogenic granuloma, gingival hypertrophy
      b. Odontogenic: cysts, cementoma, ameloblastoma, central fibroma
      c. Nonodontogenic: hemorrhagic cyst, aneurysmal bone cyst, fibrous dysplasia, cherubism
   2. Malignant: Burkitt's lymphoma, fibrosarcoma, osteogenic sarcoma, Ewing's sarcoma

From Gonzalez C: Tumors of the mouth and pharynx. In Bluestone CD, Stool WC, Scheetz MD, editors: *Pediatric otolaryngology,* Philadelphia, 1990, WB Saunders.

14. The answer is **C**, page 736.

The patient has symptoms and physical findings that correlate with the diagnosis of mastoiditis. A computed tomographic (CT) scan of the temporal bone provides detailed information about the mastoid cavity and is preferred to plain radiographs.

15. The answer is **D**, page 738.

The presence of mastoid osteitis or subperiosteal abscess is an indication for immediate mastoidectomy. Ampicillin is an incorrect choice for an antibiotic. It does not cover staphylococcal species; a broad-spectrum cephalosporin or combination therapy with a penicillinase-resistant penicillin and aminoglycoside are both acceptable until bacterial confirmation is made.

16. The answer is **E**, page 739.

Pseudomonas aeruginosa is usually the etiologic agent in malignant otitis media and typically occurs in patients with diabetes mellitus.

17. The answer is **C**, page 740.

Malignant otitis externa has a high mortality rate. It requires hospitalization, prolonged IV antibiotic therapy, and sometimes surgical debridement.

18. The answer is **C**, page 720.

The history is suggestive of a fracture of the cribriform plate (basilar skull fracture). The detection of cerebral spinal fluid rhinorrhea is important in the diagnosis and is often misinterpreted as allergic or infectious in origin. The basis of a positive test with glucose oxidase–impregnated material is a high glucose level in the nasal discharge, which is consistent with cerebral fluid. The glucose level of nasal discharge can be falsely elevated by the presence of lacrimal secretions or blood. A negative test may be helpful in ruling out cerebral spinal fluid rhinorrhea.

All answers for questions 19-22 taken from Box 41-2.
19. **C.**
20. **A.**
21. **B.**
22. **A.**

Box 41-2

View	Sinus
Occipitomental (Waters')	Maxillary sinuses
Anteroposterior (Caldwell)	Frontal and ethmoidal sinuses
Submentovertex	Sphenoidal sinus
Lateral	Sphenoidal sinus

---

23. The answer is **B**, page 746.

Peritonsillar abscess produces complications that may become evident after the pharyngitis has resolved. Peripharyngeal extension is heralded by spiking fevers, chills, torticollis, and swelling around the parotid area.

24. The answer is **B**, page 747.

The history and physical examination are suggestive of retropharyngeal abscess. A soft tissue lateral neck radiograph in a stable patient demonstrates the retropharyngeal abscess. A normal paravertebral space anterior to C3-4 is 5 mm or less in children and adults or less than 40% of the anteroposterior diameter of the vertebral bodies. The normal prevertebral space anterior to C2 is 7 mm or less.

25. The answer is **C**, page 747.

The most serious complication is airway obstruction. The retropharyngeal abscess may rupture into the mediastinum, lung, and esophagus. Empyema and pneumonia may also occur. The abscess may erode into the blood vessels, resulting in hemorrhage. Peritonsillar abscess is not a complication of retropharyngeal abscess.

26. The answer is **B**, page 722.

Branchial cleft cysts are most commonly seen in children younger than 10 years of age. They typically occur as the persistence of the second branchial groove, located on the anterior border of the sternocleidomastoid muscle (thyroglossal duct has a midline location), and frequently their recognition is precipitated by an infectious process.

Endocrine and Metabolic Disorders

Deborah M. Lopez

See Barkin et al: Chapter 50.

1. All of the following statements concerning failure to thrive (FTT) are *true except:*
   A. FTT is defined as weight between the third and fifth percentiles on a height/weight chart.
   B. FTT is weight 20% or more below ideal weight for height.
   C. FTT may involve a slowing of the velocity of growth.
   D. Poor caloric intake only partially explains FTT.
   E. Nonorganic causes account for 10% of all cases of FTT.

2. A child is seen with normal height and head circumference but abnormal weight gain. Which of the following could *not* explain the failure to gain weight?
   A. Inadequate caloric intake.
   B. Inadequate caloric absorption.
   C. Hyperthyroidism.
   D. Chronic infection.
   E. Intrauterine growth retardation.

3. All of the following clinical findings may be seen in infants with hypoglycemia except:
   A. Vomiting.
   B. Bradycardia.
   C. Tachypnea.
   D. Irritability.
   E. Lethargy.

4. A 4-week-old infant who was normal at birth is seen in the ED with vomiting, diarrhea, jaundice, and failure to thrive (FTT). Physical examination reveals hepatomegaly, ascites, peripheral edema, and possible cataracts. The initial glucose is 20 mg/dl. Which one of the following best accounts for these findings?
   A. Sepsis.
   B. Congenital adrenal hyperplasia.
   C. Galactosemia.
   D. Pyloric stenosis.
   E. Malabsorption syndrome.

5. A 3-week-old boy is seen in the ED with a 3-day history of poor feeding, vomiting, and increased listlessness. Physical examination reveals a moderately dehydrated child. Laboratory values include serum potassium 7.4 mEq/L, sodium 123 mEq/L, and glucose 20 mg/dl. Which of the following best explains these findings?
   A. Sepsis.
   B. Congenital adrenal hyperplasia.
   C. Inborn error of metabolism.
   D. Pyloric stenosis.

6. Which of the following is *not* a characteristic of congenital adrenal hyperplasia?
   A. Hypospadias and impalpable gonads.
   B. Hypokalemia.
   C. Hyponatremia.
   D. Precocious puberty in boys.
   E. Vomiting in the second week of life.

7. Glucocorticoid therapy for a child who has congenital adrenal hyperplasia with cardiovascular collapse is:
   A. No glucocorticoids.
   B. Fludrocortisone 0.1 to 0.2 mg/24 hours.
   C. Hydrocortisone 15 mg/m^2/day orally.
   D. Hydrocortisone 36 to 60 mg/m^2 intravenously (IV).
   E. Cortisone 0.5 to 0.75 mg/kg/day orally.

8. A 30-kg, 6-year-old child is brought in by Emergency Medical Service (EMS) after a motor vehicle accident. The child sustained a severe head injury with a Glasgow Coma Scale (GCS) score of 3. The chest radiograph reveals bilateral neurogenic pulmonary edema. Urine output has increased from 45 ml/hr on arrival to 240 ml/hr a few hours after admission. Which one of the following does *not* support the diagnosis of diabetes insipidus in this child?
   A. Urine osmolality 150 mOsm/L or less.
   B. Serum sodium level 143 mEq/L.
   C. Serum osmolality greater than 290 mOsm/L.
   D. Normal physical examination.

9. Hyponatremia, plasma osmolality 280 mOsm or less, elevated urine specific gravity, and euvolemia are all consistent with the diagnosis of:
   A. Hypovolemic hyponatremia.
   B. Factitious hyponatremia.
   C. Cerebral salt wasting.
   D. Syndrome of inappropriate secretion of antidiuretic hormone (SIADH).
   E. Diabetes insipidus.

10. A 15-year-old boy with Burkitt's lymphoma in remission comes to the ED because he is having seizures. The patient is currently taking antibiotics for pneumonia. His physical examination is nonfocal, and the patient does not appear to be dehydrated. Serum electrolytes reveal a serum sodium level of 112 mEq/L. What is the most appropriate action at this time?
   A. Infusion of hypertonic saline to correct the serum sodium level to 125 mEq/L.
   B. Administration of furosemide at 1 mg/kg.
   C. Fluid restriction to 80% of maintenance fluid.
   D. Immediate correction of serum sodium level to 135 mEq/L.
   E. No therapy indicated at this time.

11. Which of the following is *not* associated with hypoglycemia?
   A. Reye's syndrome.
   B. Sepsis.
   C. Congenital adrenal hyperplasia.
   D. Hypothyroidism.
   E. Phenylketonuria.

12. A 5-kg infant with severe dehydration and delayed capillary refill is seen in the ED. The skin has a "doughy" texture, and the infant appears mildly dehydrated. The initial serum sodium level is 170 mEq/L. Which of the following is the *best* immediate action?
   A. Infusion of hypotonic sodium solution over 24 hours.
   B. Infusion of 10 ml/kg 0.5% of dextrose water.
   C. Administration of 2 mEq/kg of sodium bicarbonate.
   D. Infusion of 20 ml/kg of 0.9% sodium chloride.
   E. Administration of IV antibiotics.

13. The free water deficit in the patient described in question 12 is approximately:
   A. 200 ml.
   B. 400 ml.
   C. 640 ml.
   D. There is no deficit.
   E. Insufficient data to calculate.

14. Which of the following is *incorrect* concerning diabetic ketoacidosis (DKA) in children?
   A. The incidence of DKA has decreased dramatically over the last 20 years.
   B. Ketoacidosis is a rare complication of childhood diabetes.
   C. DKA accounts for about 15% of hospitalizations of diabetic children.
   D. Case fatality rate of childhood diabetes is about 2% to 3%.

15. A 14-year-old child with a history of diabetes mellitus comes to the ED with a 1-day history of vomiting and poor oral intake. Because she was vomiting, she did not take her morning dose of insulin, and her laboratory values include serum sodium 121 mEq/L, serum glucose 1 g/dl, serum potassium 3.4 mEq/L, serum bicarbonate 7.0 mEq/L, and serum pH 6.90. Which one of the following is the best immediate therapeutic intervention?
   A. Administration of potassium chloride bolus of 1 mEq/kg over 1 hour.
   B. Administration of the patient's usual dose of insulin.
   C. IV administration of 0.45% sodium chloride at twice maintenance.
   D. Rapid infusion sodium bicarbonate 2 mEq/kg.
   E. IV administration of 20 ml/kg of 0.9% sodium chloride.

16. The patient described in question 15 begins to complain of a severe headache associated with rapid change in mental status and begins to posture 9 hours after therapy with fluids and an insulin drip at 0.1 unit/kg/hr. Which of the following best explains the patient's change in mental status?
   A. Insulin reaction.
   B. Metabolic acidosis.
   C. Cerebral edema.
   D. Sodium toxicity.
   E. Hypoglycemia.

17. For the patient described in questions 15 and 16, the best immediate course of action would be:
   A. Immediate computed tomographic (CT) scan of the head.
   B. Neurosurgical consult.
   C. Intubation, hyperventilation, and administration of mannitol 1 g/kg.
   D. Administration of dextrose.
   E. Discontinuation of insulin drip.

18. All of the following support the diagnosis of DKA *except:*
   A. Serum glucose greater than 300 mg/dl.
   B. Ketonemia or ketonuria.
   C. Arterial pH less than or equal to 7.30.
   D. Serum bicarbonate level less than or equal to 15 mEq/L.
   E. Elevated serum glucagon levels.

19. Which of the following is *not* a "counterregulatory" hormone to insulin?
   A. Epinephrine.
   B. Glucagon.
   C. Cortisol.
   D. Somatostatin.
   E. Growth hormone.

20. Which of the following statements concerning pheochromocytoma is *incorrect?*
    A. It is a catecholamine-secreting tumor.
    B. It arises from chromaffin cells of the adrenal medulla.
    C. It may be associated with neuroectodermal conditions.
    D. Chromaffin cells of the pheochromocytoma are the source of excess catecholamines.
    E. Hypertension tends to be mild in children.

21. The diagnosis of pheochromocytoma is confirmed by:
    A. Measurement of urinary catecholamines, metanephrines, and vanillylmandelic acid (VMA).
    B. Palpation of an abdominal mass.
    C. CT scan.
    D. Angiography.
    E. Echocardiography.

22. Which of the following statements is *incorrect* concerning hyperthyroidism in children?
    A. It is also known as a diffuse toxic goiter.
    B. It accounts for 10% to 20% of all childhood thyroid disorders.
    C. Males are more often affected than females.
    D. It is an autoimmune thyroid disorder.
    E. The most common clinical presentation is goiter.

23. Which of the following statements concerning neonatal thyrotoxicosis is true?
    A. It results in long-term hyperthyroidism.
    B. Infants are usually born postterm.
    C. It is a contraindication to the use of propranolol.
    D. Usually the anterior fontanelle is widely open.
    E. Heart rate is usually greater than 160 beats per minute.

24. Which of the following statements concerning the treatment of neonatal thyrotoxicosis is true?
    A. Sodium chloride (20 ml/kg of 0.45%) should be infused over 1 hour.
    B. Treatment includes the immediate administration of supersaturated potassium iodide (Lugol's solution).
    C. Propranolol should be administered to ameliorate the cardiovascular symptoms.
    D. Sodium bicarbonate (2 mEq/kg) should be administered over 1 hour.
    E. No therapy is needed.

25. A 10-year-old girl with known Graves' disease comes to the ED with temperature (T) 102° F, heart rate (HR) 150 beats per minute, blood pressure (BP) 148/92 mm Hg, diaphoresis, and decreased capillary refill. Which of the following would *not* be appropriate in her management?
    A. Infusion of 20 ml/kg of Ringer's lactate solution.
    B. IV administration of propranolol at 0.1 mg/kg.
    C. Administration of supersaturated potassium iodide (Lugol's solution).
    D. Treatment with acetaminophen and cooling blankets.

ANSWERS   [See Barkin et al: Chapter 50.]

1. The answer is **E,** pages 755 and 756.
   Failure to thrive (FTT) refers to an infant or child with growth failure. It is defined as weight below the fifth or third percentile on a growth chart or more than 20% below the ideal weight for an infant's height. One of the most important findings is the slowing of the velocity of growth. Nonorganic causes of FTT are common. However, one third to one half of patients with FTT have underlying organic disease.

2. The answer is **E,** page 755.
   Failure to gain weight when the child has normal height and head circumference is due to inadequate caloric intake or absorption, or to organic causes of increased caloric requirements (e.g., hyperthyroidism or chronic infection). Normal head circumference with depressed weight and linear growth are manifestations of intrauterine growth retardation or other types of endocrine disease.

3. The answer is **B,** pages 756 to 758.
   Hypoglycemia is defined in infants and children by a serum glucose level less than 40 mg/dl in a child and less than 30 mg/dl in full-term and preterm neonates. Bradycardia is not seen in hypoglycemia, since the "stress response" elicits an increase in cortisol, growth hormone, and catecholamines; thus tachycardia would be expected.

4. The answer is **C,** pages 757 and 758.
   Glycogen storage diseases usually are accompanied by hepatomegaly and hypoglycemia. Characteristic features vary with type of disease but may include poor feeding, vomiting, diarrhea, growth failure, jaundice, protuberant abdomen, acidemia, hyperlipidemia, hyperuricemia, and bleeding diathesis. Infants with galactosemia experience vomiting, diarrhea, jaundice, and failure to thrive/growth deficiency (FTT/GD) in the first month of life. Hepatomegaly, ascites, peripheral edema, and cataracts may be present.

5. The answer is **B,** pages 758 to 762.

Congenital adrenal hyperplasia is a group of disorders resulting from enzymatic defects in adrenocortical synthesis. Almost all (95%) cases result from 21-hydroxylase deficiency with an incidence of 1 in 10,000 births. Signs of adrenal crisis (insufficiency) include lethargy, vomiting, dehydration, and cardiovascular instability. Common electrolyte abnormalities include hypoglycemia, hyperkalemia, and hyponatremia.

6. The answer is **B,** pages 758 to 762.

Hyponatremia and hyperkalemia may be apparent in classic salt-wasting congenital adrenal hyperplasia because of diminished mineralocorticoid (aldosterone) levels. Hypoglycemia may be present, resulting from low levels of cortisol and complicated by poor feeding or vomiting.

7. The answer is **D,** page 762.

The immediate goal for a child with adrenal crisis is to reverse the hypotension and hypoglycemia. Stress-dose glucocorticoid replacement includes IV administration of hydrocortisone 50 mg/m^2, which is three to five times the physiologic secretion rate. Subsequent maintenance therapy is 12 to 15 mg/m^2/day in two or three divided doses.

8. The answer is **B,** pages 762 to 764.

Diabetes insipidus (DI) is characterized by polyuria with a large urine volume. Laboratory findings include serum osmolality greater than or equal to 290 mOsm/L, serum sodium levels greater than 145 mEq/L, and urine osmolality less than 150 mOsm/L. An assay for antidiuretic hormone (ADH) is not helpful in the acute setting nor is it necessary to make a diagnosis of DI. The physical examination may be normal or reveal signs of dehydration. The serum sodium is greater than or equal to 145 mEq/L in DI.

9. The answer is **D,** pages 763 to 765.

Inappropriate secretion of ADH (SIADH) results in hyponatremia and low serum osmolality. Inappropriate SIADH implies that (a) SIADH is independent from osmoreceptor control, (b) the threshold plasma osmolality is "reset," and ADH is suppressed only at abnormally low osmolality, or (c) there is a "leak" of ADH with hypotonicity and hyponatremia. In summary, the inappropriate presence of ADH results in dilutional hyponatremia, hypotonicity, and urine that is usually hypertonic with euvolemia.

10. The answer is **A,** page 765.

The symptoms of SIADH are not usually severe. Patients with obtundation, coma, or seizures, however, must be managed aggressively. Hypertonic saline (3% saline = 0.513 mEq/ml sodium = 513 mEq/L sodium) is used to correct the sodium to 125 mEq/L. Fluid restriction is the mainstay of therapy, and a trial of furosemide may be helpful after the patient's condition has stabilized. The sodium should not be rapidly corrected above 125 mEq/L, since cerebral edema or central pontine myelinolysis may occur.

11. The answer is **E,** pages 756 to 758.

An optimal blood glucose level is maintained via exogenous substrate supply and appropriate gluconeogenesis and glycogenolysis. Exogenous sources must be present because the body does not tolerate fasting for prolonged periods. Defects in the enzymes necessary for endogenous glucose supply result in less effective glucose homeostasis and leave the child at higher risk for hypoglycemia. Sepsis, Reye's syndrome, hypothyroidism, and poisonings with salicylates, ethanol, and propranolol can cause hypoglycemia. Phenylketonuria is a genetic disorder in which phenylalanine cannot be converted to tyrosine.

12. The answer is **D,** page 763.

The infant has hypernatremic dehydration. The initial resuscitation should focus on restoration of the circulating volume. Hypotonic fluids or free water contributes to cerebral edema and should be avoided.

13. The answer is **C,** page 763.

The free water deficit may be calculated in the following manner:

$$\text{Total body water} = 5 \text{ kg} \times 0.60 = 3 \text{ L}$$

To correct the serum sodium to 140 mEq/L in this 5-kg child with a serum sodium level of 170 mEq/L, the deficit can be calculated as:

$$(170 \text{ mEq/L}/140 \text{ mEq/L}) \times 3 \text{ L} = 3.64 \text{ L}$$

Thus 3.64 L - 3 L = 0.64 L (640 ml) free water deficit

14. The answer is **A,** pages 765 to 768.

Despite advances in the management of insulin-dependent diabetes mellitus (IDDM) in children, the incidence of diabetic ketoacidosis (DKA) has remained essentially unchanged over the last 20 years. DKA is not an uncommon complication, is the most common cause of death, and accounts for 15% of hospitalizations of diabetic children. DKA is a serious and commonly seen illness in the ED.

15. The answer is **E,** pages 765 to 768.

As with any acutely ill child, careful attention is paid to the maintenance of a patent airway. Intravascular volume and tissue perfusion are restored with an isotonic IV solution over the first hour. Fluid and electrolyte deficits are calculated and carefully replaced over 48 hours.

16. The answer is **C,** pages 765 to 768.

Cerebral edema is unpredictable in onset, although it usually occurs 8 to 12 hours after initiation of therapy (recent reports describe its occurrence earlier). Risk factors include rapid rates of fluid infusion and total fluid dose greater than 4 L/m^2/day.

17. The answer is **C,** pages 765 to 768.

As with any brain-injured child, management begins with the ABCs of resuscitation. The child's trachea should be intubated; the child should be hyperventilated and should receive a dose of mannitol at 1 g/kg, which may prove beneficial.

18. The answer is **E**, pages 765 to 769.

DKA accounts for approximately 15% of hospitalizations for diabetes and is the most common cause of death in diabetic children. DKA is classically defined as serum glucose level greater than 300 mg/dl, ketonemia or ketonuria, and a blood pH less than 7.3 or a serum bicarbonate level less than 15 mEq/L. Although serum glucagon levels may be elevated, they are not necessary to make a diagnosis of DKA.

19. The answer is **D**, pages 765 to 769.

Ketoacidosis is generated with insulin deficiency and elevated levels of hormones that oppose the action of insulin ("counterregulatory" hormones). These catabolic hormones are epinephrine, glucagon, cortisol, and growth hormone. These hormones are secreted in response to stress.

20. The answer is **E**, pages 768 and 769.

The clinical manifestations of pheochromocytoma are attributed to sustained or episodic release of catecholamines. The classic triad of headache, palpitations, and diaphoresis is highly sensitive and specific. Hypertension is the most common finding in children and is a sustained reaction rather than episodic or paroxysmal in 90% of cases. Hypertension tends to be more severe in children than in adults and may lead to congestive heart failure.

21. The answer is **A**, pages 768 and 769.

The diagnosis of pheochromocytoma is confirmed by measurement of urinary catecholamines, metanephrines, and vanillylmandelic acid (VMA). One or more of these metabolites is increased in 95% of cases, but urinary metanephrine and plasma catecholamine measurements are the most sensitive indicators of pheochromocytoma. A CT scan or magnetic resonance imaging (MRI) may confirm the location of the tumor.

22. The answer is **C**, pages 769 to 771.

Hyperthyroidism in children is nearly always due to Graves' disease (diffuse toxic goiter) and accounts for 10% to 25% of all childhood thyroid disorders. Girls are much more likely to be affected than boys.

23. The answer is **E**, pages 771 and 772.

Neonatal thyrotoxicosis is a transient hyperthyroidism acquired by transplacental passage of thyroid-stimulating immunoglobulins (TSI) from the mother to the fetus. Affected infants are commonly born before term and may be microcephalic with craniosynostosis. In addition infants are tachycardiac, restless, and hyperthermic and may have respiratory distress.

24. The answer is **C**, page 772.

Treatment of neonatal thyrotoxicosis parallels the treatment of thyroid storm in the child. Propranolol is used to ameliorate the cardiovascular symptoms in a dosage of 1 to 2 mg/kg/24 hr in three divided doses.

25. The answer is **C**, pages 769 to 771.

The patient is having thyroid storm. Thyroid crisis is a life-threatening complication of severe hyperthyroidism, which is usually abrupt in onset. Precipitating factors include infection, trauma, surgery, acute cardiopulmonary disease, and metabolic derangements (DKA and dehydration). Management of these patients includes volume restoration, acetaminophen and cooling blankets for hyperpyrexia, and IV propranolol. Patients should be admitted to a pediatric intensive care unit (PICU) for monitoring. Propylthiouracil (PTU) is used to inhibit thyroid hormone synthesis and peripheral conversion of T_4 to T_3. Iodide solutions are usually begun 1 hour after PTU to avoid causing thyroid storms before the antithyroid effect occurs.

Eye Disorders

Deborah M. Lopez

See Barkin et al: Chapter 51.

1. An adolescent with a minor lid laceration and other facial cuts from a motor vehicle accident is seen in the ED. You note that her left pupil is teardrop-shaped and suspect a corneal laceration. Which of the following would be the most appropriate therapeutic intervention at this time?
   A. Conduct a meticulous examination of the globe.
   B. Immediately patch the eye with a nonpressured protective shield and call the ophthalmologist.
   C. Immediately irrigate the eye with 0.9% normal saline.
   D. Evert the lid for complete examination of the upper lid and palpebral conjunctiva.
   E. Instill fluorescein for evaluation of corneal abrasion.

2. Which of the following statements concerning assessment of visual acuity in children is true?
   A. Fixation in the infant is accomplished by 1 month of age.
   B. Serious ophthalmologic injury with normal acuity is rare.
   C. Subjective testing of vision is possible at 1 year of age.
   D. The adult type of Snellen chart is appropriate for use with children older than 3 years of age.
   E. Using toys to elicit attention is an acceptable screening test of gross visual ability for a 5-year-old.

3. Which of the following statements concerning pediatric ophthalmologic conditions is true?
   A. The most common causes of visual disturbances in children are trauma and infection.
   B. Trauma is rarely seen as a cause of visual disturbance in young infants.
   C. Eye infections such as *Chlamydia* are common from birth through 12 years of age.
   D. A common pediatric ophthalmologic emergency is central retinal artery occlusion.

4. Which of the following is true concerning visual acuity in the preschool population?
   A. An acuity of 20/40 is considered normal for a 3-year-old.
   B. An acuity of 20/30 is considered normal for a 10-year-old.
   C. Normal adult vision of 20/20 is not reached until the adolescent years.
   D. A handheld occluder should be used rather than an eye patch to test each eye's acuity.
   E. A single symbol should be used rather than a full chart of symbols when checking visual acuity.

5. The presence of decreased vision, ophthalmoplegia, and proptosis or pain on eye movement is seen in which one of the following?
   A. Corneal abrasion.
   B. Lens dislocation.
   C. Posterior rupture of globe.
   D. Orbital cellulitis.
   E. Basilar skull fracture.

6. The outcome of which of the following ocular injuries is most critically dependent on the immediate action of the ED physician?
   A. Retinal detachment.
   B. Lid avulsion.
   C. Orbital apex fracture.
   D. Hyphema.
   E. Chemical burn.

7. A 1-month-old is seen with a complaint of head tilt to the right. Pregnancy, labor, and delivery were normal. The child is afebrile and feeds well, and there is no history of trauma. The most appropriate diagnosis would be:
   A. Oculomotor (cranial nerve III) palsy.
   B. Right trochlear nerve (cranial nerve IV) palsy.
   C. Left trochlear nerve (cranial nerve IV) palsy.
   D. Right abducens nerve (cranial nerve VI) palsy.
   E. Left abducens nerve (cranial nerve VI) palsy.

8. Which of the following is true concerning spasmus nutans?
   A. Condition is permanent.
   B. Nystagmus is always unilateral.
   C. It is an inherited form of nystagmus.
   D. The syndrome includes rapid horizontal pendular nystagmus and torticollis.
   E. It usually appears at 5 years of age.
9. A 10-day-old is seen with a mucopurulent discharge from both eyes. The infant is afebrile, and the physical examination is normal. Which of the following statements concerning this infant's problem is true?
   A. The diagnosis of *Chlamydia trachomatis* can be confirmed by demonstrating cytoplasmic inclusions in the discharge material.
   B. *C. trachomatis* is an uncommon cause for this patient's symptoms.
   C. Discharge is the result of silver nitrate administration.
   D. Conjunctival infection by *Neisseria gonorrhoeae* is unlikely because of the age of the patient.
10. Which of the following is the most appropriate management of the patient described in question 9?
    A. If the stain is suggestive of *C. trachomatis*, topical tobramycin should be given for 7 days.
    B. If the stain is suggestive of *C. trachomatis*, oral erythromycin should be given for 14 days.
    C. If the Gram's stain is suggestive of gonococcal conjunctivitis, topical penicillin may be used for 14 days.
    D. If the Gram's stain is suggestive of gonococcal conjunctivitis, intravenous (IV) nafcillin may be used for 14 days.
11. Which of the following is true concerning external hordeolum?
    A. It is a chronic infection of the sebaceous glands lining the lid.
    B. It is a painless lesion causing mainly cosmetic difficulties.
    C. Lesions begin with diffuse eyelid edema and hyperemia, which is painful and localized to the lid margin.
    D. Acute treatments include incision, curettage, and IV antibiotics.
    E. It rarely recurs.

12. Which of the following statements is true concerning ophthalmia neonatorum?
    A. Cause may be related to the use of silver nitrate prophylaxis.
    B. Chemical conjunctivitis occurs in approximately 25% of newborns who receive silver nitrate prophylaxis.
    C. *N. gonorrhoeae* is the infectious agent most commonly causing conjunctivitis.
    D. The potential of long-term complications from untreated *N. gonorrhoeae* infection is minimal.
13. The cardinal signs of a blow-out fracture include each of the following *except*:
    A. Restriction of gaze downward.
    B. Enophthalmos.
    C. Loss of sensation over the malar eminence.
    D. Diplopia.
14. The most common visual sign of retinoblastoma is:
    A. Leukokoria.
    B. Tremulous iris.
    C. Tearing, pain, and photophobia.
    D. Peaked or teardrop pupil.
    E. Periorbital ecchymoses.
15. The most appropriate management for a patient with a painful corneal abrasion is:
    A. Pilocarpine.
    B. Topical ophthalmologic anesthetic agent.
    C. Topical ophthalmologic steroid.
    D. Cycloplegic agent, an antibiotic drop, and a semipressure patch.
    E. No treatment is necessary.
16. All of the following are true concerning orbital cellulitis *except*:
    A. It is characterized by an infection of the orbital tissues posterior to the orbital septum.
    B. It is characterized by periorbital swelling, erythema, proptosis, and ophthalmoplegia or loss of visual acuity.
    C. It is most commonly seen as a complication of sinusitis in children.
    D. The onset of lid edema and erythema is chronic, occurring over 5 to 10 days.
    E. Patients often appear systemically ill.

Match the following findings with the diagnoses listed below. Each answer may be used once:
    A. Curtain moving across visual field.
    B. Tremulous iris.
    C. Peaked or teardrop pupil.
17. Corneal laceration. _____
18. Retinal detachment. _____
19. Lens dislocation. _____

ANSWERS   [See Barkin et al: Chapter 51.]

1. The answer is **B,** page 774.
   If the history or physical examination suggests a penetrating ocular injury or ruptured globe, the eye should be patched immediately with a nonpressured protective shield. No further manipulation or examination should be attempted until an ophthalmologist is present.

2. The answer is **B,** pages 774 and 775.
   Fixation is usually accomplished in children by age 6 months and not at 1 month. Subjective testing of vision is possible at 2 to 3 years of age and not at 1 year. The adult type of Snellen chart is appropriate for children who are 5 to 6 years old (not 3 years old) and who know letters. Using toys to elicit attention is an acceptable screening test of gross visual ability, but not for a 5-year-old.

3. The answer is **A,** pages 774 and 775.
   Trauma and infection are the most common causes of visual disturbance in children. Trauma can be seen easily in young as well as older children. Eye infections such as *Chlamydia* are common from birth through 4 months of age. Although an emergency condition, central retinal artery occlusion is a rare event in the pediatric population.

4. The answer is **A,** page 776.
   The definition of normal visual acuity in the preschool population, when most quantitative testing can be determined, differs by age. An acuity of 20/40 is considered normal for a 3-year-old child, whereas 20/30 is the accepted normal acuity for a 4-year-old child. The normal adult vision of 20/20 is not reached until 5 or 6 years of age. An eye patch should be used rather than a handheld occluder to prevent peeking. Using a full chart of symbols when checking visual acuity will give better results than using a single symbol.

5. The answer is **D,** page 777 and pages 792 to 793.
   Orbital cellulitis is an infection of the orbital tissue posterior to the orbital septum, characterized by periorbital swelling, erythema, and evidence of proptosis, ophthalmoplegia, or loss of visual acuity. In children it is most commonly found as a complication of sinusitis, although it may also be seen following trauma or intraorbital surgery.

6. The answer is **E,** page 774.
   If a history of acid or alkali exposure is obtained, the patient should receive immediate irrigation with saline before further evaluation is attempted.

7. The answer is **C,** page 779.
   Trochlear nerve palsy is more commonly a congenital lesion than an acquired one. When congenital, it presents with head tilt to the side opposite the palsied superior rectus muscle. Signs and symptoms of oculomotor nerve palsies include exotropia and downward deviation of the eye, ptosis, pupillary dilatation and impaired adduction, depression, and elevation. A palsied abducens nerve is usually a nonspecific, nonlocalizing sign of increased intracranial pressure.

8. The answer is **D,** page 780.
   Spasmus nutans is an acquired form of nystagmus presenting in the first year of life with a characteristic triad of rapid, horizontal pendular nystagmus, head nodding, and torticollis. The nystagmus may be variable in different directions of gaze and may be asymmetric or unilateral. The cause is unclear, and the nystagmus usually disappears by age 3.

9. The answer is **A,** pages 785 and 786.
   Chlamydia trachomatis is the most common cause of neonatal conjunctivitis and accounts for 20% to 40% of neonatal conjunctivitis. Chemical conjunctivitis usually is seen in the first 24 to 48 hours of life and not as late as 10 days of life. Conjunctival infection by *Neisseria gonorrhoeae* should be suspected during the first month of life and may have a wide range of symptoms.

10. The answer is **B,** pages 785 and 786.
    Oral erythromycin must be used to eradicate nasopharyngeal carriage (and pneumonia). The treatment of gonococcal conjunctivitis is IV penicillin G (50,000 units/kg/day) or ceftriaxone sodium (50 mg/kg/day) once a day for 7 days in the case of penicillin-resistant gonococci.

11. The answer is **C,** pages 784 and 785.
    An external hordeolum or stye is an acute suppurative infection of the glands of Zeis, which are sebaceous glands attached to the hair follicles. External and internal hordeola are treated with warm compresses several times a day and eyelash scrub with baby shampoo on a washcloth. Both hordeola and chalazia frequently recur. A chalazion is a granulomatous inflammation of a meibomian gland characterized by a firm, nontender nodule in the upper or lower lid. This lesion is usually chronic as opposed to a hordeolum, which is usually an acute inflammatory disorder.

12. The answer is **A,** pages 785 to 787.
    Ophthalmia neonatorum is common during the first month of life. The cause may be infectious or related to silver nitrate prophylaxis. Chemical conjunctivitis occurs in approximately 10% of newborns who receive silver nitrate prophylaxis. The incidence of conjunctival infection with *N. gonorrhoeae* is low, but the potential for destruction and permanent visual disabilities remains high if the diagnosis is delayed.

13. The answer is **A,** page 777.
    A blow-out fracture, resulting from blunt trauma to the orbital rim, most commonly damages the medial wall and orbital floor. Visual impairment, most specifically double vision, may be related to entrapment of the inferior rectus or inferior oblique muscles, causing restriction of upward gaze.

14. The answer is **A,** page 776.
    A white pupillary reflex, leukokoria, is the most common sign of retinoblastoma.

15. The answer is **D**, pages 267 and 778.

If there is a corneal abrasion and if any foreign bodies have been removed, the patient should be treated with a long-acting topical cycloplegic, antibiotic ointment or drops instilled in the eye, and a semipressure patch.

16. The answer is **D**, pages 792 to 793.

Orbital cellulitis is an infection of the orbital tissues posterior to the orbital septum characterized by periorbital swelling, erythema, and evidence of proptosis, ophthalmoplegia, or loss of visual acuity. In children it is most commonly found as a complication of sinusitis. The onset of lid edema and erythema is acute and proceeds rapidly. The patient often appears systemically ill.

17. The answer is **C**, pages 267 and 777.

Corneal lacerations usually result from a sharp object hitting the eye. When considering the diagnosis, carefully assess the pupil for irregularities that may be due to prolapse of the iris (i.e., peaked or teardrop pupil).

18. The answer is **A**, pages 271 and 777.

Retinal tears may lead to detachment, either immediately or months to years later. Patients with retinal detachment may complain of a curtain or cloud of darkness across the visual field. Since the detachment is not limited to any particular part of the retina, the "curtain or cloud" may appear from any direction.

19. The answer is **B**, pages 270 and 777.

Dislocation of the lens occurs when so many of the zonules are broken that the lens falls forward into the anterior chamber or posteriorly into the vitreous cavity. Iridodonesis (trembling iris) may be seen following rapid eye movement if the lens is dislocated. Surgical management of the dislocated lens is urgent.

CHAPTER

44

Gastrointestinal Disorders

Holly M. Bannister

See Barkin et al: Chapter 52.

1. A 16-year-old girl has severe abdominal pain, nausea, and vomiting. On physical examination you note diffuse abdominal, uterine adnexal, and cervical tenderness. The most helpful diagnostic test at this point is:
   A. Serum electrolytes.
   B. Urinalysis and urine culture.
   C. Serum β-human chorionic gonadotropin (HCG).
   D. Flat and upright abdominal radiographs.
   E. Cervical Gram's stain.

2. A 4-year-old child with vomiting and diarrhea that lasted 3 days is brought in 1 week later for irritability, cramping abdominal pain, and recurrence of the diarrhea. The vital signs are temperature (T) 98.8° F, heart rate (HR) 114 beats per minute, respiratory rate (RR) 22 breaths per minute, and blood pressure (BP) 110/68 mm Hg. He is pale, lethargic, and edematous. Your initial diagnostic steps include:
   A. Peripheral blood smear.
   B. Urinalysis.
   C. Measurement of electrolytes, blood urea nitrogen (BUN), creatinine.
   D. Total protein and albumin.
   E. All of the above.

3. An 8-month-old boy is noted by his caretaker to be crying a lot on and off, drawing up his legs, and vomiting over the last day. His last stool this morning was normal. He has no diarrhea or fever. The vital signs are T 97.8° F, HR 136 beats per minute, and RR 28 breaths per minute. He appears extremely irritable. He has a distended abdomen with marked tenderness, an absence of bowel sounds, capillary refill time of 5 seconds, and guaiac-positive stool in the rectum. After you place an intravenous (IV) line and begin hydration, you:
   A. Order abdominal ultrasonography.
   B. Order a barium enema.
   C. Order an air contrast enema.
   D. Request immediate surgical consultation.

4. A 4-year-old boy is brought to the ED because the parents noted brick red stools today. The patient is otherwise well with no constipation, abdominal pain, or fever. His physical examination is normal. The most likely diagnosis is:
   A. Peptic ulcer disease.
   B. Intussusception
   C. Volvulus.
   D. External hemorrhoids.
   E. Meckel's diverticulum.

5. An 8-year-old girl complains of lower abdominal pain and fever. The vital signs are T 101° F, HR 100 beats per minute, RR 24 breaths per minute, BP 106/62 mm Hg. She has mild abdominal tenderness. The remainder of her physical examination is normal. The urinalysis shows 25 to 50 white blood cells (WBCs)/high power field (HPF), 25 to 50 red blood cells (RBCs)/HPF, and 2+ protein. Which one of the following diagnoses is *not* supported by this patient's symptoms?
   A. Henoch-Schönlein purpura (HSP).
   B. Hemolytic uremic syndrome (HUS).
   C. Urinary tract infection.
   D. Acute appendicitis.
   E. Crohn's disease

6. A 3-year-old girl with a runny nose and cough for 3 days complains of fever, abdominal pain, and vomiting for 1 day. The vital signs are HR 132 beats per minute, RR 42 breaths per minute, and T 101.6° F. She is lying in the mother's arms and appears ill. Her physical examination shows voluntary abdominal guarding and right lower quadrant tenderness. Diagnostic workup should include all of the following *except:*
   A. Urinalysis.
   B. Amylase/creatinine clearance ratio.
   C. Complete blood count (CBC).
   D. Abdominal radiograph.
   E. Chest radiograph.

7. The abdominal radiograph of a 3-year-old with abdominal pain demonstrates small radiopaque areas in the right upper quadrant. Which of the following diagnoses is most likely in this patient?
   A. Lead intoxication.
   B. Cholelithiasis.
   C. Appendiceal fecalith.
   D. Meckel's diverticulum fecalith.
   E. All of the above.

8. A 5-year-old girl with large, hard stools every 3 days for 2 weeks now complains of incontinence of stool in school over the past week. The patient has intermittent, severe, cramping abdominal pain with vomiting or fever. Her abdomen is distended, tympanitic, and very tender. Bowel sounds are difficult to hear. Her rectal examination reveals no stool. You:
   A. Suggest increased oral fluids, high-fiber diet.
   B. Give stool softeners.
   C. Administer an enema.
   D. Consult a surgeon.
   E. Follow up in 1 or 2 days if no stool has passed.

9. A 16-year-old girl complains of lower abdominal pain, blood-tinged vaginal discharge, and dysuria. She has lower abdominal, right upper quadrant, uterine adnexal, and cervical tenderness. Which of the following most supports your suspected diagnosis?
   A. Urinalysis.
   B. Abdominal radiographs, flat and upright.
   C. CBC with differential.
   D. Cervical Gram's stain.
   E. Liver function tests.

10. A previously well 6-month-old boy has nonbloody diarrhea, eight stools per day for 2 days, decreased oral intake, and history of lethargy. He is cared for at home, and no family members are ill. In the ED he is alert, and his vital signs are T 100.1° F, HR 150 beats per minute, RR 28 breaths per minute. He has dry mucous membranes and poor skin turgor. His abdominal examination is unremarkable. Microscopic examination of the stool reveals no polymorphonuclear leukocytes. Evaluation of this child should include all of the following *except:*
    A. Serum electrolytes.
    B. BUN/creatinine.
    C. CBC.
    D. Stool culture.
    E. Urinalysis.

11. While in the ED the patient from question 10 has three more episodes of diarrhea and begins to appear toxic. His temperature is now 103° F. Your workup now includes:
    A. Sepsis evaluation with lumbar puncture.
    B. Stool methylene blue stain for lymphocytes.
    C. Stool ova and parasites test.
    D. Abdominal radiographs.
    E. Stool Gram's stain.

12. The first therapeutic maneuver for the patient described in question 10 is:
    A. An attempt at oral hydration with an oral rehydration solution.
    B. IV fluid resuscitation with normal saline (NS) 20 ml/kg.
    C. IV fluid resuscitation with D5⅓ NS at 1½ maintenance.
    D. IV ampicillin.
    E. Oral amoxicillin-clavulanate.

13. A 2-year-old child has a sudden onset of dysphagia. The patient is afebrile and was previously healthy. The most appropriate first therapeutic intervention is:
    A. IV access.
    B. Oral airway placement.
    C. Acetaminophen administered at 10 to 15 mg/kg.
    D. Endotracheal tube placement with sedation.
    E. Allowing the child to assume a position of comfort with 100% oxygen (O_2).

14. For the patient described in question 13, which of the following is the most appropriate first diagnostic step?
    A. Cine-esophagogram.
    B. Computed tomographic (CT) scan of the chest.
    C. Lateral airway radiograph.
    D. Laryngoscopy.
    E. Esophagoscopy.

15. The most likely cause of bright red hematemesis in a 6-year-old girl is:
    A. Esophagitis.
    B. Acute gastritis.
    C. Gastric ulcer.
    D. Duodenal ulcer.
    E. Coagulopathy.

16. The most common cause of lower gastrointestinal (GI) bleeding in a 6-year-old child is:
    A. Meckel's diverticulum.
    B. Henoch-Schönlein purpura.
    C. *Salmonella* enteritis.
    D. Juvenile polyps.
    E. Norwalk virus enteritis.

17. A 3-year-old boy has a rash on his legs, abdominal pain, and bloody diarrhea. Which of the following is the most likely cause of this patient's abdominal pain?
    A. Intussusception.
    B. Rotavirus.
    C. *Shigella.*
    D. *Campylobacter.*
    E. Meckel's diverticulum.

18. A 13-year-old girl complains of abdominal pain for 2 days and of bloody vomitus four times today. The vital signs are T 98.8° F, HR 120 beats per minute, RR 24 breaths per minute, BP 106/58 mm Hg. The remainder of her physical examination reveals minimal, diffuse abdominal tenderness. In the ED you first:
    A. Place an orogastric or nasogastric tube.
    B. Perform an Apt test.
    C. Consult a gastroenterologist for esophagoscopy.
    D. Order a salicylate level.
    E. Obtain a gastric pH.

19. Which of the following is the most appropriate management for the patient described in question 18?
   A. IV vasopressin.
   B. IV cimetidine.
   C. Oral or nasogastric antacids.
   D. Nasogastric lavage with iced saline.
   E. Nasogastric lavage with room temperature saline.

20. A 2-week-old infant is brought to the ED for diaper rash. On physical examination the skin shows only a mild erythematous rash in the diaper area, and you note a smooth, soft, nontender spleen tip palpable 2 cm below the left costal border. The review of systems and of medical and family histories is noncontributory. The infant has been otherwise well. You:
   A. Obtain a CBC.
   B. Order an ultrasound to evaluate liver and spleen size.
   C. Order abdominal radiographs.
   D. Consult a hematologist.
   E. Refer the infant to the regular pediatrician for follow-up.

21. An 18-month-old infant is brought to the ED for evaluation after a fall from the couch onto a coffee table. On examination the child is quiet and pale. The vital signs are T 99° F, HR 142 beats per minute, and RR 28 breaths per minute, and the child is uncooperative for a BP. The physical examination is otherwise normal except for an abdomen with diffuse mild tenderness and hepatosplenomegaly. Which of the following radiologic studies is the most urgent to obtain in this child?
   A. Abdominal radiographs.
   B. Skeletal survey.
   C. Abdominal CT scan.
   D. Abdominal ultrasonogram.

22. Which of the following is the most appropriate first therapeutic intervention for the patient described in question 21?
   A. IV placement and administration of NS.
   B. Placement of a nasogastric tube to low Gomco suction.
   C. O$_2$ 35% by nasal cannula.
   D. IV placement and administration of O-negative packed red blood cells.
   E. IV cefotaxime.

23. A full-term infant who is breastfed is noted to be jaundiced at 16 hours of age. All of the following may explain this clinical finding except:
   A. Sepsis.
   B. Rubella.
   C. Hemolytic disease.
   D. Syphilis.
   E. Physiologic jaundice.

24. A 3-day-old full-term infant was discharged from the hospital at 8 PM with a serum bilirubin level of 7 mg/dl. At 8 AM in your ED his serum bilirubin level is 14.5 mg/dl. According to the mother he has received adequate oral intake. You:
   A. Repeat the serum bilirubin measurement in 6 hours.
   B. Evaluate for sepsis.
   C. Admit for exchange transfusion.
   D. Increase oral feedings.
   E. Begin IV hydration.

25. Risk factors for kernicterus include all of the following except:
   A. Hypoxemia.
   B. Hypercarbia.
   C. Acidosis.
   D. Hyperglycemia.
   E. Hypothermia.

26. The most common cause of unconjugated hyperbilirubinemia in the older child is:
   A. Congenital hemolytic anemia.
   B. Drug ingestion.
   C. Gilbert's disease.
   D. Crigler-Najjar syndrome.
   E. Anorexia nervosa.

27. A 6-week-old boy has been vomiting after every feeding since the age of 1 week. He has no history of fever or change in diet and is otherwise well. The most likely cause of his vomiting is:
   A. Gastroesophageal reflux.
   B. Viral gastroenteritis.
   C. Pyloric stenosis.
   D. Organic acidemia.
   E. Milk allergy.

28. A 7-month-old girl has been vomiting for 2 days. She looks ill and has a distended, tender abdomen with no bowel sounds. You suspect some type of obstruction. Which of the following is the most common cause of obstruction in this age group?
   A. Intussusception.
   B. Volvulus.
   C. Incarcerated inguinal hernia.
   D. Duodenal atresia.
   E. Esophageal foreign body.

29. A 3-year-old boy has mild, intermittent, cramping abdominal pain and bright red blood on the surface of his stool. He has no history of vomiting, diarrhea, or fever. The vital signs are T 98.8° F, P 108 beats per minute, RR 22 breaths per minute. The remainder of his physical examination is normal. The most likely diagnosis is:
   A. Intussusception.
   B. Juvenile polyps.
   C. Salmonella enteritis.
   D. Crohn's disease.
   E. Hemorrhoids.

30. What is the method of choice for diagnosis of the patient described in question 29?
   A. Barium enema.
   B. Upper GI series.
   C. Proctosigmoidoscopy.
   D. Abdominal ultrasound.
   E. Stool culture.

31. The treatment of the patient described in question 29 is:
   A. Soft diet and increased oral liquids.
   B. Stool softeners.
   C. Antibiotics.
   D. Hydrostatic reduction.
   E. Excision.

32. The mother of a 2-year-old boy says she notices something protruding approximately 1 inch from the child's anus during defecation. The boy has no associated pain, and the protrusion disappears after relaxation. All of the following statements are true regarding rectal prolapse *except:*
   A. Rectal prolapse is most common in children older than 3 years of age.
   B. In most cases of rectal prolapse the cause is unknown.
   C. Rectal prolapse is usually painless.
   D. Rectal prolapse may resolve with relaxation.
   E. Pertussis can be a precipitating cause.

33. Which of the following is the best therapeutic option for a patient with rectal prolapse?
   A. Antibiotics.
   B. Stool softeners.
   C. Enzyme replacement therapy.
   D. Peritoneal flap.
   E. Surgical excision.

34. A 16-year-old girl complains of low-grade fever, dyspepsia, abdominal pain, nausea, and vomiting. The vital signs are T 101.2° F, P 110 beats per minute, RR 22 breaths per minute, BP 112/72 mm Hg. Her abdomen is tender in the right upper quadrant with no guarding or rebound. The best procedure to definitively demonstrate this patient's problem is:
   A. Ultrasonography.
   B. Upper GI series.
   C. Serum bilirubin, liver function tests.
   D. Abdominal radiographs.

35. The next day the patient described in question 34 is noted to have shortness of breath with continued abdominal pain, nausea, and vomiting with T 102° F, P 120 beats per minute, RR 28 breaths per minute, BP 118/76 mm Hg, and O$_2$ saturation 98%. The next step is to:
   A. Order liver function tests.
   B. Perform an abdominal ultrasound.
   C. Order cholescintigraphy.
   D. Order abdominal radiographs.
   E. Order chest radiographs.

36. A 3-month-old boy is seen in the ED for fever and irritability that have lasted 1 day. The medical and family histories are negative. The vital signs are T 101° F, P 128 beats per minute, and RR 34 breaths per minute, and the patient is irritable. The liver and spleen are palpable 2 cm below the costal margins. The remainder of the physical examination is unremarkable. The most appropriate next step is:
   A. Abdominal radiographs.
   B. Ultrasound to evaluate liver and spleen size.
   C. A gastroenterology consult.
   D. Sepsis evaluation including lumbar puncture.
   E. Electrocardiogram (ECG).

37. Which of the following is the most common location for GI foreign bodies to lodge?
   A. Ileocecal valve.
   B. Ligament of Treitz.
   C. Pylorus.
   D. Esophagus.
   E. Appendix.

38. A 9-day-old jaundiced boy has a serum bilirubin level of 12 mg/dl. The infant is feeding well with iron-fortified formula and appears well. This patient should be evaluated for:
   A. Congenital hyperthyroidism.
   B. Carotenemia.
   C. Ovalocytosis.
   D. Pyruvate kinase deficiency.
   E. All of the above.

39. A well-appearing 1-year-old is known to have swallowed a button battery. An x-ray film shows the battery in the stomach. The next step in management is:
   A. Whole bowel irrigation.
   B. Administration of steroids and antibiotics for esophageal mucosal burns.
   C. Endoscopic removal.
   D. Allowing the object to pass spontaneously.
   E. Surgical removal.

40. A healthy, full-term 2½-day-old infant has a serum bilirubin of 19 mg/dl. You:
   A. Discharge the baby home with follow-up the next day.
   B. Admit for IV hydration.
   C. Admit for exchange transfusion.
   D. Discharge home with instructions to increase oral hydration and follow up in 12 hours.
   E. Admit for phototherapy.

41. All of the following are true concerning viral gastroenteritis *except:*
   A. Viral diarrhea accounts for 80% of diarrhea in children in the United States.
   B. Carbohydrate malabsorption may occur.
   C. The most common agents are Norwalk virus and rotavirus.
   D. Fat malabsorption may occur.
   E. It commonly causes bloody diarrhea.

42. You have diagnosed acute cholecystitis in a 17-year-old girl who has fever, abdominal pain, and vomiting. The vital signs are T 102° F, P 114 beats per minute, RR 22 breaths per minute, and BP 116/72 mm Hg. She has right upper quadrant tenderness with no guarding or rebound. You now:
    A. Prepare for immediate cholecystectomy.
    B. Prepare for percutaneous lithotripsy.
    C. Discharge home on a bland diet with follow-up in 24 to 48 hours.
    D. Admit for pain control, IV fluids, and antibiotics.
    E. Begin an IV bolus with normal saline 10 ml/kg over 20 minutes.

43. The leading cause of bacterial gastroenteritis in the United States is:
    A. *Campylobacter.*
    B. *Yersinia.*
    C. *Salmonella.*
    D. *Shigella.*
    E. *Escherichia coli.*

44. Which of the following may be a complication of *Salmonella* enteritis?
    A. Meningitis.
    B. Endocarditis.
    C. Urinary tract infection.
    D. Pneumonia.
    E. All of the above.

45. An 18-month-old boy has had a radiopaque foreign body lodged in his midesophagus for approximately 1 week. The best technique for removal is:
    A. Esophagoscopy in the operating room.
    B. Fluoroscopic Foley catheter technique.
    C. Flexible esophagoscopy in the ED.
    D. Allowing the object to pass.
    E. Administration of ipecac.

46. A 3-year-old child who looks well is sent home from day care with diarrhea. You send a stool culture to be analyzed, and it comes back 3 days later positive for *Campylobacter.* On the telephone the father tells you the child is fine with no fever or diarrhea. You advise management of this patient with:
    A. Ampicillin.
    B. Erythromycin.
    C. Trimethoprim-sulfamethoxazole.
    D. Antitoxin.
    E. No medicine. No treatment is necessary.

47. A 4-year-old boy's symptoms include vomiting, drooling, pain on swallowing, and refusal to eat this morning. The mother states that although he seems better this evening, she wants him checked. The vital signs are T 98.8° F, P 116 beats per minute, and RR 24 breaths per minute. In the ED he is playful, smiling, and comfortable in the mother's arms. His physical examination is normal. The most appropriate next step is:
    A. Throat culture.
    B. Posteroanterior (PA) and lateral neck and chest x-ray films.
    C. Indirect laryngoscopy.
    D. Upper GI series.
    E. A consult with a gastroenterologist for upper GI endoscopy.

48. If the workup is normal, the most appropriate next step is:
    A. PA and lateral neck and chest x-ray films.
    B. Throat culture.
    C. Upper GI endoscopy.
    D. Fluoroscopic barium examination of the esophagus.
    E. Indirect laryngoscopy.

49. A 4-year-old child with fever, lethargy, and watery, bloody diarrhea has a seizure in the ED. Which of the following organisms is responsible for this patient's clinical findings?
    A. Rotavirus.
    B. *Campylobacter jejuni.*
    C. *Salmonella enteritidis.*
    D. *Salmonella choleraesuis.*
    E. *Shigella dysenteriae.*

50. The treatment for the patient described in question 49 includes which of the following?
    A. Trimethoprim-sulfamethoxazole.
    B. Penicillin.
    C. Erythromycin.
    D. No antibiotics because the carrier state may be prolonged.
    E. Amoxicillin.

51. A 17-year-old girl comes to the ED to be evaluated because her boyfriend has just been told he has hepatitis B. Her physical examination is normal. Her medications include ibuprofen (Motrin) and birth control pills. After drawing blood for hepatitis studies you:
    A. Send her to her regular doctor for follow-up of her blood work.
    B. Begin hepatitis B vaccine series.
    C. Administer hepatitis B immune globulin and hepatitis B vaccine.
    D. Administer hepatitis B immune globulin 5 ml intramuscularly.
    E. Refer the patient for α-interferon therapy.

52. A 12-year-old boy complains of fever, abdominal pain, weakness, weight loss, and five bloody stools a day. He looks very ill. Vital signs are T 101° F, P 100 beats per minute, RR 20 breaths per minute, and BP 112/62 mm Hg. He has minimal abdominal tenderness. You suspect:
    A. Hirschsprung's disease.
    B. Ulcerative colitis.
    C. Internal hemorrhoids.
    D. Juvenile polyposis.

53. The patient described in question 52 now appears more uncomfortable. His abdomen is distended and tender to palpation. The most appropriate next step is to:
    A. Order a CBC and serum electrolyte measurement.
    B. Order a barium enema.
    C. Order abdominal radiographs.
    D. Consult a gastroenterologist for sigmoidoscopy or colonoscopy.
    E. Administer sulfasalazine and corticosteroids.

54. A 10-year-old girl has nausea, vomiting, and constant, sharp periumbilical pain radiating to the back. Her vital signs are T 99.4° F, P 124 beats per minute, RR 24 breaths per minute, BP 108/62 mm Hg. Her abdomen is distended and tender with voluntary guarding. There are no masses palpable. The most likely diagnosis is:
    A. Hepatitis.
    B. Cholelithiasis.
    C. Pancreatitis.
    D. Renal calculus.
    E. Diabetic ketoacidosis.

55. A 5-year-old child with a history of upper respiratory symptoms 1 week ago now has been vomiting for 3 days. His mother describes him as cranky and drowsy on and off. He has not had abdominal pain, diarrhea, or trauma, and his medical and family histories are negative. Medications include antipyretics. His vital signs are T 98.8° F, P 112 beats per minute, RR 22 breaths per minute, and BP 96/64 mm Hg. He is lethargic with no focal neurologic findings. The skin is clear, and the remainder of the physical examination is normal. You vigorously hydrate the child intravenously and perform a lumbar puncture, which is normal. The child is clinically unchanged. You now:
    A. Perform a toxicology screen (urine and blood).
    B. Order serum amino acids.
    C. Order urine amino acids.
    D. Order a CT scan of the head.
    E. None of the above.

56. The next most appropriate step for the patient described in question 55 is to order which of the following?
    A. Serum ammonia and liver function tests.
    B. Liver biopsy.
    C. Toxicology screen (urine and blood).
    D. CT scan of the head.
    E. None of the above.

57. A 4-week-old girl's vomiting has become progressively worse over the last week, and she has had constipation for 3 days. She has no fever or upper respiratory symptoms. The infant has been feeding well on iron-fortified infant formula. The parents brought her in because the mother noted one episode of blood in the vomit 30 minutes ago. The infant's vital signs are T 99° F, HR 150 beats per minute, and RR 30 breaths per minute. She is alert and feeding vigorously in the mother's arms. You note mild jaundice and the absence of tears. Abdominal examination reveals hyperactive bowel sounds with no distension or tenderness. No masses are palpable, and the remainder of the physical examination is normal. The next most appropriate step is to order:
    A. Urinalysis.
    B. Liver function tests.
    C. Measurements of electrolytes, BUN, glucose.
    D. Abdominal radiographs.
    E. An upper GI series.

58. The next most appropriate step in the evaluation of the patient described in question 57 is to:
    A. Order abdominal radiographs.
    B. Order abdominal ultrasound.
    C. Order an upper GI series.
    D. Consult with a surgeon.
    E. Measure electrolytes, BUN, glucose.

59. A 5-year-old child has a 6-day history of high fever, cervical adenopathy, erythematous lips, conjunctivitis, and erythematous extremities. A potential complication of this disorder is:
    A. Midgut volvulus.
    B. Thrombocytopenia.
    C. Hydrops of the gallbladder.
    D. Retropharyngeal abscess.
    E. Septic arthritis.

ANSWERS   [See Barkin et al: Chapter 52.]

---

1. The answer is **C**, pages 799 and 800.
    Ectopic pregnancy must be considered in every adolescent girl complaining of lower abdominal pain. Abdominal pain is present in 97% of cases. Nausea, vomiting, urinary symptoms, and abnormal vaginal bleeding may be noted. Peritoneal signs may be present in ruptured ectopic pregnancy. The diagnosis is based on a positive pregnancy test and ultrasound. Cervical Gram's stain may be helpful to support a diagnosis of pelvic inflammatory disease (PID), which should also be considered in this patient; however, ruling out ectopic pregnancy is most important.

2. The answer is **E**, page 799.
    This patient with a preceding viral infection has hemolytic uremic syndrome (HUS), which is characterized by a microangiopathic hemolytic anemia, thrombocytopenia, and acute renal failure. Pallor, irritability or lethargy, and weakness develop 5 to 10 days after a viral or bacterial infection. Cramping abdominal pain and diarrhea occur in 25% to 50% of the cases. Renal failure develops over the next 2 weeks. Intussusception, toxic megacolon, and perforation have been associated with HUS. Treatment is peritoneal dialysis and supportive therapy.

3. The answer is **D**, pages 852 to 854.

This 8-month-old boy with intermittent, colicky abdominal pain, vomiting, and blood in the stool must be suspected of having intussusception, which is the telescoping of one segment of the intestine into the lumen of another. Plain abdominal radiographs may be normal early and after 8 to 12 hours may show signs of intestinal obstruction, the soft tissue mass of intussusception, or free air if perforated. With an experienced ultrasonographer, ultrasound may be useful in the diagnosis of intussusception, and there is recent literature to support this. Barium enema is currently the procedure of choice for diagnosis and therapy; however, the patient in the clinical scenario appears ill with marked abdominal tenderness, no bowel sounds, capillary refill time of 5 seconds, and guaiac-positive stools. In a patient with signs of shock and potential perforation and peritonitis immediate surgery is the procedure of choice.

4. The answer is **E**, pages 813 and 854 to 856.

Isolated rectal bleeding is a common sign of Meckel's diverticulum in children under the age of 5 years. The bleeding may appear brick red or like currant jelly when the bleeding is brisk or tarry if the bleeding is minimal. Although classically painless, some children may have abdominal pain and tenderness as well as abdominal distension, hyperactive bowel sounds, and vomiting. Meckel's diverticulum may be a lead point for intussusception; however, patients with intussusception usually complain of intermittent abdominal pain. Although external hemorrhoids may result in rectal bleeding, they are unusual in children and are often associated with constipation, anal pain, and prolapse of the hemorrhoids. Internal hemorrhoids are often seen with portal hypertension. Peptic ulcer disease is more likely to produce dark blood coming from the rectum as a result of upper GI bleeding. Midgut volvulus usually occurs in the neonatal period as abdominal pain, bilious vomiting, and melena.

5. The answer is **E**, page 803.

Urinalysis is essential in the evaluation of a patient complaining of abdominal pain. Hematuria is consistent with urolithiasis and urinary tract infection and when present with proteinuria may be consistent with Henoch-Schönlein purpura (HSP) and HUS. Pyuria can be seen when an inflamed appendix is lying next to a urethra or bladder.

6. The answer is **B**, pages 802 to 803 and 844 to 845.

This patient appears ill with abdominal and respiratory complaints. Laboratory evaluation can provide helpful clues to the diagnosis of abdominal pain. A CBC detects leukocytosis (gastroenteritis, appendicitis) and anemia (blood loss, underlying hematologic abnormality). Urinalysis is helpful to detect urinary tract infection, appendicitis, HSP, HUS, diabetic ketoacidosis (DKA), and porphyria. In a patient in whom intraabdominal pathology is suspected, radiographs should be performed to look for free air, air-fluid levels, obstruction, calcifications, foreign bodies, and masses. When a child is too young or uncomfortable to stand erect, a left lateral decubitus film is a good alternative to an upright film. In a patient with fever, cough, and tachypnea, a chest radiograph is appropriate to rule out pneumonia, which can accompany abdominal pain. Amylase/creatinine clearance ratio may be useful in the diagnosis of acute pancreatitis but would be least helpful in this case of a young child with right lower quadrant pain.

7. The answer is **E**, page 803.

In addition to lead chips, gallstones, and appendiceal or Meckel's fecalith, renal stones may appear as foreign bodies or calcifications on abdominal radiographs. All can be located in the right upper quadrant.

8. The answer is **D**, page 806.

This patient has chronic constipation with intermittent pain; infrequent and large, hard stools; and soiling episodes. Because the abdomen is distended and tympanic, a bowel obstruction is suspected, and surgery staff should be consulted immediately. Fluids, high-fiber diet, stool softeners, and enemas are viable therapies for constipation but not in this patient with signs of possible obstruction.

9. The answer is **D**, page 800.

This patient has PID, which is diagnosed clinically. The diagnosis of gonorrhea is supported by a positive cervical Gram's stain. The most common symptom is lower abdominal pain, but up to 30% of patients have right upper quadrant tenderness. Urinary and GI complaints are heard frequently. The blood-tinged vaginal discharge in this patient makes PID a more likely diagnosis than a urinary tract infection. Liver function tests may be useful in a patient with abdominal pain and right upper quadrant tenderness, but the uterine adnexal and cervical tenderness and bloody vaginal discharge suggest PID.

10. The answer is **D,** page 808.

The patient described in this question is moderately dehydrated as demonstrated by dry mucous membranes, decreased skin turgor, and lethargy. Any patient with moderate to severe dehydration requires electrolytes, BUN, and CBC with differential. Urinalysis is helpful for specific gravity and ketones. A stool culture is particularly helpful in the infant who has bloody diarrhea or polymorphonuclear leukocytes in the stool or who is under 1 year of age with diarrhea and a febrile or toxic appearance. Stool cultures also are useful for the child who has more than 10 stools in 24 hours, is in day care, has a history of travel, is immunosuppressed, or has multiple family members who are ill.

11. The answer is **A,** page 808.

Any child under 2 years of age who appears toxic and has a fever should have a complete evaluation for sepsis. A stool methylene blue stain for polymorphonuclear leukocytes, not lymphocytes, is helpful if a bacterial cause of the diarrhea is suspected. Stool ova and parasites tests and abdominal radiographs may be useful later in the evaluation of this patient.

12. The answer is **B,** page 808.

This patient appears toxic and dehydrated and should receive a 20 ml/kg IV bolus of normal saline. IV antibiotics may be indicated, but ampicillin alone is not adequate. This patient is too ill to receive oral rehydration alone at this time.

13. The answer is **E,** pages 811 and 812.

The child with acute dysphagia most likely has an infectious process or has ingested a foreign body. Maintenance of airway patency is the first goal, and allowing the child to assume a position of comfort with the parent while administering O$_2$ is the simplest way to achieve this. In extreme cases endotracheal intubation may be required.

14. The answer is **C,** page 811.

Lateral airway films may demonstrate obstruction or foreign bodies in the aerodigestive tract and are the simplest and least invasive choice presented. Contrast studies are the procedures of choice for esophageal lesions causing dysphagia. Computed tomography (CT) and magnetic resonance imaging (MRI) also may be useful. Laryngoscopy, bronchoscopy, and esophagoscopy can be diagnostic and therapeutic and should be performed by a subspecialist.

15. The answer is **A,** page 812.

Bright red hematemesis results from bleeding at or above the cardia and indicates little contact with gastric juices. The most common causes in children are varices and esophagitis, although brisk gastric and duodenal bleeding may be bright red. Coffee grounds indicate the action of gastric acid on blood.

16. The answer is **D,** pages 813 and 827.

The most frequent cause of lower GI bleeding in children is juvenile polyps. The peak incidence is age 3 to 7 years. Juvenile polyps result in bright red blood from the rectum, which is intermittent and usually painless. They are nonmalignant, and approximately 75% can be reached by digital examination. These patients should be referred for polyp removal to be certain the lesions are not premalignant. Meckel's diverticulum, HSP, and *Salmonella* are less common causes of lower GI bleeding in children. Viral agents that may be associated with bloody diarrhea include rotavirus and Norwalk virus (Table 44-1).

17. The answer is **A,** pages 813, 853, and 854.

This patient has HSP, which is associated with a characteristic rash on the lower extremities and bloody stools. GI bleeding can result from the generalized vasculitis of HSP or an associated intussusception.

TABLE 44-1   Causes of Upper and Lower Gastrointestinal Bleeding by Age

Age	Upper GI	Lower GI
0-1 month	Idiopathic	Anal fissure
	Gastritis	Upper GI bleeding
	Stress ulcers	Volvulus
	Esophagitis	Necrotizing
	Swallowed maternal	enterocolitis
	blood	Swallowed maternal
	Congenital blood	blood
	dyscrasia	Infectious colitis
	Vascular malfor-	Milk allergy
	mation	Blood dyscrasia
		Duplication
1 month-	Gastritis	Anal fissure
1 year	Esophagitis	Intussusception
	Stress ulcer	Meckel's diverticulum
	Mallory-Weiss tear	Infectious diarrhea
	Vascular	Milk allergy
	malformation	Duplication
	Duplication	Pseudomembranous
		colitis
1-12 years	Esophageal varices	Polyps
	Peptic ulcer disease	Anal fissure
	Stress ulcer	Meckel's diverticulum
	Gastritis	Infectious diarrhea
	Mallory-Weiss tear	HSP
	Foreign body	HUS
	Esophagitis	Intussusception
		Pseudomembranous
		colitis
Adolescent	Esophageal varices	Polyps
	Peptic ulcer disease	Hemorrhoids
	Gastritis	Inflammatory bowel
	Mallory-Weiss tear	disease
	Esophagitis	Infectious diarrhea
	Stress ulcer	

GI, Gastrointestinal; *HSP,* Henoch-Schönlein purpura; *HUS,* hemolytic uremic syndrome.

18. The answer is **A,** pages 814 and 815.
    Aspiration of the stomach via an oral or nasogastric tube should be performed if significant upper GI bleeding is suspected after determining that the bleeding is actually from the GI tract and that the material is actually blood and not other materials that can simulate blood. The screening test specific for gastric contents (e.g., Gastroccult) should be used because an acidic pH can diminish the sensitivity of oxidation/reduction reactions on other screening card tests. The Apt test differentiates swallowed maternal blood in the neonate from neonatal blood. Gastroduodenoscopy identifies the location of bleeding in most cases. A medication history is important because some medications may be associated with gastritis or ulcer formation and upper GI bleeding.

19. The answer is **E,** pages 813 to 815.
    If the gastric contents are positive for blood, a lavage with 10 ml/kg room temperature normal saline should be performed until the active bleeding stops. Iced saline gastric lavage may exacerbate bleeding. Vasopressin, cimetidine, and antacids do have their roles in the treatment of upper GI bleeding but are not the first line of treatment in the patient with an acute upper GI bleed.

20. The answer is **E,** pages 815 to 817.
    Palpation of a 1- to 2-cm spleen tip is normal in the otherwise well infant as long as it is not firm or tender. Life-threatening causes of splenomegaly include hypersplenism (sickle cell), severe hemolytic anemia, trauma, sepsis, and congestive heart failure, which should be ruled out by history and physical examination. Ultrasonography is the best method to evaluate liver and spleen size but is not indicated in this patient at this time.

21. The answer is **C,** page 818.
    A pale tachycardic child with a history of trauma should be evaluated immediately for anemia and possible splenic or hepatic laceration. A hemoglobin hematocrit will define anemia and lead you to the next most urgent diagnostic step, abdominal CT scan. Child abuse must be considered in the differential diagnosis, especially in a patient in whom the mechanism does not appear severe enough to produce such serious intraabdominal injury.

22. The answer is **A,** pages 817 and 818.
    Because you are most concerned about possible hepatic or splenic laceration in this pale, tachycardic patient with a history of trauma and hepatosplenomegaly, an IV should be placed immediately. Normal saline should be administered initially rather than noncrossmatched blood unless the patient is unresponsive to saline or acutely decompensates. Although oxygen would be useful in this patient, nasal cannulas are not tolerated well in this age group.

23. The answer is **E,** page 819.
    Visible jaundice in the first 24 hours of life or a rise in serum bilirubin greater than 0.5 mg/dl/hr should always be considered abnormal and a workup undertaken for hemolytic disease, congenital TORCHS infections (toxoplasmosis, rubella, cytomegalovirus, herpes, and syphilis), and sepsis. Physiologic jaundice is defined as absence of jaundice on day 1 of life with a steady rise to approximately 6 mg/dl on day 3 and a decline by day 10 or 12.

24. The answer is **B,** page 819.
    This infant's bilirubin rose more than 0.5 mg/dl/hr and is abnormal. Exchange transfusion should be considered only in infants with a bilirubin level greater than 20 mg/dl based on their age (see Table 52-9, page 819 in Barkin et al and the answer to question 23.)

25. The answer is **D,** page 820.
    Hypoglycemia and the other choices noted are risk factors for kernicterus. Other risk factors include hypoalbuminemia, hypoxia, hypercarbia, and dehydration. Hyperglycemia is not thought to be a risk factor.

26. The answer is **A,** pages 820 and 821.
    Sickle cell disease or other congenital hemolytic anemias are among the most common causes of unconjugated hyperbilirubinemia in older children. Certain drugs, Gilbert's disease, Crigler-Najjar syndrome, and prolonged fasting are other causes of unconjugated hyperbilirubinemia.

27. The answer is **A,** page 824.
    Gastroesophageal (GE) reflux from a relaxed lower esophageal sphincter is a common cause of vomiting in the well-appearing infant whose only complaint is vomiting. It is more common in the premature infant. Infants with GE reflux are described as "spitting up" beginning soon after birth. Most outgrow GE reflux by 9 months of age. Infants who fail to gain weight and develop aspiration pneumonia or esophagitis require a more extensive workup (barium swallow, esophageal pH monitoring, or radionuclide scans).

28. The answer is **A,** pages 797 and 823 to 825.
    Intussusception is the most common obstructive lesion in infants from age 3 months to 2 years. Other conditions to consider in this age group include volvulus and incarcerated inguinal hernia. (See answer to question 3.)

29. The answer is **B**, pages 813 and 827.

The most common symptom of juvenile polyps is bright red blood on the surface of the stool. Traction on the polyp may cause cramping abdominal pain, and a polyp may be a lead point for colocolic intussusception. The rectum is where 10% of juvenile polyps are found. Although the polyps are nonmalignant, the treatment is polypectomy to be certain the lesions are not premalignant. Although the bleeding is usually minor, the patient may be anemic. (See answer to question 18.) Intussusception is more frequently diagnosed in infants from age 1 month to 1 year. The patient with intussusception may have intermittent abdominal pain, vomiting, and lethargy. The stools can look like currant jelly or be positive for occult blood. The blood is not usually seen as bright red on the surface of the stool. *Salmonella, Shigella, Campylobacter,* and *Yersinia* are bacterial agents commonly associated with bloody diarrhea. Hemorrhoids can cause blood-streaked stools but are uncommon in children, especially young children. Hemorrhoids in children most commonly are external and may be noted on physical examination. Crohn's disease may cause bloody diarrhea or be associated with hemorrhoids if the anus and rectum are involved.

30. The answer is **C**, page 827.

The method of choice for diagnosing suspected rectal juvenile polyps is proctosigmoidoscopy. When a polyp is found, polypectomy should be performed.

31. The answer is **E**, page 827.

The treatment of juvenile polyps is polypectomy after bowel preparation.

32. The answer is **A**, page 827.

Rectal prolapse is an abnormal protrusion of the rectum through the anus. Partial prolapse is most common in children who are younger than 3 years of age. In most cases the cause is unknown. Straining with bowel movements is a provoking factor. Rectal lesions (polyps), cystic fibrosis, sustained cough (pertussis), and *Clostridium difficile* have all been described as precipitating causes of rectal prolapse.

33. The answer is **B**, page 827.

Most rectal prolapses resolve spontaneously. Having a patient avoid straining with defecation and use stool softeners and a child-sized toilet seat is helpful. Manual reduction may be necessary. Prolapses that do not respond to conservative measures may warrant surgical treatment.

34. The answer is **A**, pages 828 and 829.

The patient described here has classic signs and symptoms of acute cholecystitis. The best emergency procedure to support the diagnosis of acute cholecystitis caused by gallstones is ultrasonography. It is rapid, safe, and noninvasive and would be one of the first procedures indicated for this patient in the ED. Cholescintigraphy with 99 mTc-IDA is the procedure of choice for definitively demonstrating cystic duct obstruction. Abdominal radiographs may show calcified gallstones. Patients with acute cholecystitis may have elevated transaminase levels and hyperbilirubinemia.

35. The answer is **E**, pages 828 and 829.

This patient with acute cholecystitis now complains of increasing respiratory difficulty. A chest radiograph is indicated because atelectasis and pneumonia could result from splinting. Other complications include dehydration, electrolyte abnormalities, pancreatitis, necrosis, perforation of the gallbladder, and peritonitis.

36. The answer is **D**, pages 816 and 817.

An ill-appearing febrile infant with hepatosplenomegaly requires a complete sepsis evaluation with lumbar puncture. There is no mention of skin lesions or bruising, the family and medical histories are negative, and no trauma is mentioned, which makes trauma, splenic sequestration, severe liver disease, and bone marrow dysfunction unlikely. The heart is normal without tachycardia, making congestive heart failure less likely and the chest radiograph and ECG less urgent. The lack of adenopathy works against the diagnosis of malignancy, for which an ultrasound would be helpful as a subsequent step. The CBC in the sepsis evaluation would rule out hemolytic anemias.

37. The answer is **D**, page 830.

The majority of GI tract foreign bodies lodge in the esophagus. The three areas of physiologic narrowing in the esophagus are (1) the upper esophageal sphincter (cricopharyngeus), (2) the level of the aortic arch, and (3) the lower esophageal sphincter. Of these, the most common location for a foreign body to lodge is at the level of the upper esophageal sphincter.

38. The answer is **D**, pages 818 to 823.

Hyperbilirubinemia in the nonbreastfeeding infant after the first week of life requires further evaluation. Pyruvate kinase deficiency, spherocytosis, and elliptocytosis may appear as jaundice that persists after the first week of life. Crigler-Najjar syndrome and Gilbert's disease may appear at this time. TORCHS infections, sepsis, urinary tract infection, upper GI obstruction, and congenital hypothyroidism are also in the differential diagnosis of this infant.

39. The answer is **D**, pages 832 and 833.

Most button batteries that reach the stomach pass spontaneously without complications. There is a small risk of leakage associated with exposure to gastric acid. Button batteries lodged in the esophagus need immediate endoscopic removal to prevent mucosal damage and necrosis. Steroids and antibiotics are not indicated. Daily abdominal radiographs will document passage through the pylorus, after which most button batteries pass through the intestinal tract without complications. Endoscopy or surgery is indicated for esophageal location, fixation to GI tract mucosa for a prolonged period of time, and signs of peritonitis. Whole bowel irrigation has not proved beneficial in the management of foreign bodies.

40. The answer is **E**, page 819.

An infant age 49 to 72 hours with a serum bilirubin level of 18 mg/dl or greater should receive phototherapy. Intensive phototherapy should produce a decline of serum bilirubin of 1 to 2 mg/dl within 4 to 6 hours (see Table 52-9, page 819 in Barkin et al).

41. The answer is **E,** pages 833 and 834.

Bloody diarrhea is uncommon in viral gastroenteritis and should alert the physician to the possibility of a bacterial agent as the cause for the diarrhea. Viral diarrhea accounts for 80% of infectious diarrhea in children in the United States. Carbohydrate, lactose, and fat malabsorption may occur. Rotavirus is responsible for 30% to 60% of all severe diarrhea in young children. Norwalk virus and Norwalk-like viruses account for 40% of gastroenteritis outbreaks in older children and adults in schools, camps, institutions, and cruise ships.

42. The answer is **D,** page 829.

Patients with acute cholecystitis should be admitted for observation, pain medications, and IV fluids. Cholecystectomy is best performed after acute inflammation has subsided (48 to 72 hours). Percutaneous lithotripsy to fragment gallstones is a new technology undergoing clinical trials. No data for the pediatric population are available yet. The patient has no evidence of dehydration at this point, so an IV bolus is premature here, although dehydration and electrolyte abnormalities can occur if the vomiting is severe.

43. The answer is **A,** page 834.

Campylobacter is the leading cause of bacterial gastroenteritis in the United States. Newborn puppies and food sources such as chicken and turkeys are reservoirs. *Campylobacter* may be transmitted from person to person or from pet to person, and the incubation period is 2 to 5 days. The patient with *Campylobacter* characteristically has fever, severe abdominal cramps, and watery, mucous, bloody diarrhea, although the patient may be asymptomatic. The illness often resolves spontaneously in a few days. Patients with the dysenteric form of the illness or those in day care should be treated with erythromycin.

44. The answer is **E,** page 834.

With penetration of the lamina propria, patients with *Salmonella* gastroenteritis may develop extraintestinal complications. Reported complications include bacteremia, osteomyelitis, septic arthritis, endocarditis, pneumonia, urinary tract infection, and meningitis.

45. The answer is **A,** page 832.

Esophagoscopy in the operating room with a protected airway is the procedure of choice for removal of a foreign body that is potentially impacted (present for 1 week). Controversy regarding the fluoroscopic Foley catheter technique revolves around safety issues. Risks include lack of control when the object passes through the hypopharynx and potential aspiration if catheterization is performed without airway control. A foreign body lodged in the upper or middle third of the esophagus requires immediate removal because it is unlikely to pass into the stomach and aspiration is a risk.

46. The answer is **B,** pages 834 and 835.

Treatment of *Campylobacter* with erythromycin is indicated in children attending day care centers and children with the dysenteric form of the illness. Antibiotic treatment has been found to have little effect on the diarrhea or abdominal pain. (See answer to question 47.) Patients younger than 3 months of age or toxic patients with suspected *Salmonella* infections should be hospitalized in order to receive IV antibiotics. After infancy antibiotics may prolong the carrier state. *Shigella* is treated with trimethoprim-sulfamethoxazole or ampicillin if susceptible for 5 days. *Yersinia* may be treated with aminoglycosides, cefotaxime, trimethoprim-sulfamethoxazole, or tetracycline to reduce the duration of excretion. Antibiotics may not affect the clinical symptoms. If this child were not in day care, no treatment would be necessary.

47. The answer is **B,** pages 831 and 832.

The most common signs of an esophageal foreign body in a child are refusal to eat, increased salivation, vomiting, and pain or discomfort on swallowing. These symptoms may be followed by a relatively asymptomatic period, especially in the younger child with a diet that is predominantly liquid and soft. All patients with a suspected esophageal foreign body should have PA and lateral neck and chest radiographs, which should rule out radiopaque objects from the hypopharynx to the chest as well as demonstrate mediastinal or subcutaneous air.

48. The answer is **D,** pages 831 and 832.

If lateral and PA neck and chest radiographs are normal, a radiolucent foreign body should be suspected. Further studies are indicated, including fluoroscopic studies with barium examination of the esophagus. Endoscopy is useful for retrieval of the object. CT scan and MRI are beginning to play a role in delineating periesophageal inflammation and abscess formation. Negative imaging procedures do not completely rule out a foreign body.

49. The answer is **E,** page 835.

Single nonfocal seizures occur frequently in *Shigella* infections and may occur before the diarrhea begins. The seizures are associated with a rapidly rising fever.

50. The answer is **A,** pages 835 and 838.

The drug of choice for treatment of *Shigella* is trimethoprim-sulfamethoxazole for 5 days. Ampicillin may be given for susceptible strains.

51. The answer is **C,** page 841.

Susceptible patients who have sexual contact with a person who has a hepatitis B infection should receive hepatitis B immune globulin (HBIG, 5 ml for adults) within 14 days of the last sexual contact or if contact continues. In addition the hepatitis B vaccine series should be started. α-Interferon therapy has been helpful for a few children with hepatitis C.

52. The answer is **B,** page 842.

Signs and symptoms of ulcerative colitis include bloody diarrhea (most common), rectal bleeding, abdominal pain, weakness, weight loss, and fever. Signs of severe colitis include five or more bloody stools in a day, oral temperature greater than 100° F, tachycardia greater than 100 beats per minute, hematocrit value less than 30%, and serum albumin level less than 3 g/dl. The other answers listed can all cause bloody stools, but in uncomplicated cases the patient should not appear as ill as this patient is described.

53. The answer is **C,** pages 842 and 843.

This patient with ulcerative colitis has become sicker with a distended and tender abdomen. The next most appropriate step is abdominal radiographs to look for dilation of the transverse colon and signs of perforation (signs of toxic megacolon). Perforation and hemorrhage are life-threatening complications of toxic megacolon. Any barium study should be undertaken with extreme caution because the barium enema has been implicated in toxic megacolon. The white blood cell count (WBC) would be elevated, and the electrolyte levels may demonstrate dehydration. Sigmoidoscopy and colonoscopy by the gastroenterologist are useful to confirm the diagnosis of inflammatory bowel disease and to help with the ongoing management of these patients. However, they are not useful in this patient with acute abdominal distension. This patient needs parenteral steroids and broad-spectrum antibiotics. Sulfasalazine is useful in the mild attack of inflammatory bowel disease without systemic signs.

54. The answer is **C,** pages 843 to 845.

Abdominal pain with nausea and vomiting is present in 75% of cases of acute pancreatitis. The pain is usually epigastric or periumbilical, sharp, and constant and may radiate to the back or upper quadrants. The abdomen is usually distended and tender. If a mass were palpable, a pseudocyst would be considered. Patients with cholelithiasis (unless accompanied by acute cholecystitis), hepatitis, and renal calculi are less likely to have such severe symptoms. Patients with DKA can have acute abdominal pain and vomiting, but the pain is usually diffuse and does not tend to radiate.

55. The answer is **A,** pages 846 and 847.

This patient with altered mental status, vomiting, and a preceding viral illness must be suspected of having Reye's syndrome. An attempt should be made to elicit a history of toxin or drug exposure, but regardless of history, a toxicology screen should be done. Inborn errors of metabolism may result in vomiting and lethargy but usually do so before an infant is 2, and the patient would have a history of recurrent attacks, delayed growth and development, or a family history of metabolic disorders. An intracranial lesion is unlikely with no evidence of trauma, a nonfocal neurologic examination, and a normal lumbar puncture. A viral syndrome with dehydration may appear this way but would respond rapidly to vigorous hydration. An afebrile child with no evidence of focal infection or skin changes with a normal lumbar puncture is unlikely to have sepsis or meningitis.

56. The answer is **A,** pages 846 and 847.

If lethargy persists after adequate fluid resuscitation, and central nervous system infection and toxic exposure have been ruled out, Reye's syndrome is more likely, and measurements of liver enzymes, serum ammonia, and prothrombin time and partial thromboplastin time (PT/PTT) should be ordered. At this point a urine and serum metabolic screen also should be ordered to rule out inborn errors of metabolism. (See answer to question 55.)

57. The answer is **C,** page 856.

Vomiting is the initial symptom of pyloric stenosis. The vomiting usually begins at approximately 3 weeks of age and becomes progressively worse, becoming projectile. The vomit may be blood streaked if a mucosal tear is present. After vomiting, the infant refeeds hungrily. Constipation may be associated if the infant does not retain enough food. Associated jaundice caused by an immature liver and starvation appears in 1% to 2% of the cases. As the vomiting progresses, a hypokalemic, hypochloremic metabolic alkalosis appears because the infant loses gastric secretions containing large amounts of hydrogen and chloride ions. The kidneys compensate by conserving sodium and wasting potassium and hydrogen. (See answer to question 58.)

58. The answer is **B,** page 856.

If an "olive" (the pyloric mass) can be palpated, further studies are unnecessary and surgical consultation is warranted. In the event an "olive" is not palpable, abdominal ultrasound may demonstrate an increased pyloric diameter, a thickened muscle mass, and an elongated pyloric canal. If sonography is negative, an upper GI series should be performed. It may reveal delayed gastric emptying, indentation of the antrum by the pyloric mass, and an elongated narrowed pyloric channel ("string sign"). Endoscopy is rarely necessary. (See answer to question 57.)

59. The answer is **C,** pages 942 to 945.

The patient has Kawasaki syndrome. Hydrops of the gallbladder, an acute acalculous distension of the gallbladder is a known complication of this disease. A right upper quadrant mass is seen in 75% to 100% of cases. Hydrops of the gallbladder usually begins during the subacute phase, which is marked by the cessation of fever. It is during this period that coronary aneurysms also may occur.

Gynecologic and Obstetric Disorders

Sandra Cunningham

See Barkin et al: Chapter 53.

1. A 4-year-old girl is brought in who has bleeding from the genital area. She states that the area is not painful, although she complains of pain on urination and frequency of urination. She has no vaginal discharge. The child has a seizure disorder, and her mother states that her daughter continues to have four or five seizures each month on her present therapeutic regimen. Physical examination reveals a red-blue mass that obscures the vaginal opening. The mass is symmetric, doughnut shaped, and friable. Which one of the following statements is true?
   A. Recurrence is common after either medical or surgical intervention.
   B. A urine culture will be positive.
   C. The mass represents prolapse of the vagina and subsequent engorgement.
   D. The vast majority of pediatric cases are in African-American girls.
   E. Standard therapy includes hormones administered orally.

2. A mother brings her 15-day-old infant to the ED because she noted breast enlargement with bloody discharge from the infant's nipple. The surrounding skin is not erythematous. The baby is afebrile. Which one of the following statements is true?
   A. The fluid should be expressed to avoid further enlargement of the breast tissue.
   B. This entity occurs in girls only.
   C. Antibiotic coverage for penicillinase-resistant bacteria should be initiated.
   D. The engorgement is generally bilateral.
   E. Breast hyperplasia is associated with an increased risk of fibroadenoma development.

3. A 2-year-old girl is brought to the ED because her mother noted during a bath that the child's labia seemed to be fused. On examination there is a thin bridge of connective tissue across the labia minora. Which one of the following statements is true?
   A. Onset of the condition at this age is pathognomonic for childhood sexual abuse.
   B. The fusion of the labia is always partial.
   C. Treatment will require surgical separation of the labia followed by topical application of an estrogen cream.
   D. The topical use of estrogen cream can result in breast tenderness and vulvar pigmentation.
   E. High estrogen levels are associated with labial adhesions.

4. A 9-year-old girl has a tender mass under one nipple. The mass had been present for approximately 3 weeks before she informed her mother. Appropriate management includes which one of the following?
   A. Warm compresses to the area.
   B. Sonogram of the breast.
   C. No treatment.
   D. Oral antibiotics with coverage for *Staphylococcus aureus* and group A *Streptococcus*.
   E. Needle aspiration of the mass.

5. A 15-year-old girl who is 3 weeks postpartum has a tender, erythematous, palpable mass in one breast. Her temperature is 102.5° F. Which one of the following statements is true?
   A. Lactational mastitis is not associated with an infectious etiology.
   B. Drainage of the abscess is always indicated in lactational mastitis.
   C. Treatment for lactational mastitis differs markedly from that of nonlactational mastitis because of the differing etiologies.
   D. Oral antibiotics are required.
   E. Lactational mastitis occurs only in breastfeeding mothers.

6. The most common sexually transmitted disease in the adolescent population is:
   A. Herpes simplex virus type 2 (HSV-2).
   B. *Neisseria gonorrhoeae.*
   C. *Chlamydia trachomatis.*
   D. *Trichomonas vaginalis.*
   E. Human immunodeficiency virus.

7. Which of the following statements is true concerning *C. trachomatis* infection?
   A. The infection can be asymptomatic in girls but not in boys.
   B. *C. trachomatis* is an obligate intracellular parasite.
   C. The only reliable tool to diagnose it in postpubertal females is a cell culture of endocervical secretions.
   D. Oral azithromycin 1 g daily for 3 days is appropriate treatment for an uncomplicated case.
   E. A complication of the untreated infection is pneumonia.

8. A 14-year-old girl has had multiple vesicles on an erythematous base at the vaginal opening for 3 days. She is sexually active with one partner but denies that he has had similar symptoms. She has no history of lesions in the past. The lesions are painful, and she is having difficulty urinating because of the pain. A test for serum β-human chorionic gonadotropin (HCG) is negative. Appropriate management includes administration of which one of the following?
   A. Oral acyclovir.
   B. Oral azithromycin.
   C. Parenteral acyclovir.
   D. Parenteral ceftriaxone.
   E. No pharmacologic therapy is required.

9. Risk factors for pelvic inflammatory disease (PID) in the sexually active adolescent include which one of the following?
   A. Use of an oral contraceptive.
   B. Pregnancy.
   C. Young age.
   D. Early menarche.
   E. Use of a contraceptive sponge.

10. A 16-year-old girl has lower abdominal pain and cervical motion with uterine adnexal tenderness. She has a purulent vaginal discharge. Gram's stain of the discharge shows gram-negative diplococci. Her temperature is 101.4° F. Her last menstrual period ended 3 days before she came to the ED. A urine test for β-HCG is negative. Appropriate management includes which one of the following?
    A. Laparoscopy.
    B. Inpatient polymicrobial treatment.
    C. Oral azithromycin 1 g × 1 dose plus oral ciprofloxacin 500 mg × 1 dose.
    D. Treatment for gonorrhea alone (with further treatment guided by laboratory analysis of endocervical secretions).
    E. Ultrasonogram.

11. A 5-year-old boy has two painful vesicular lesions on his penis. He has no urethral discharge. He has no other lesions on his body. He attends day care 5 days a week and otherwise is cared for by his mother. Which of the following statements is true?
    A. HSV-1 can be transmitted by hand contact with an infected person.
    B. HSV-2 can be transmitted by hand contact with an infected person.
    C. The lesions are pathognomonic for sexual abuse.
    D. A history of contact can be obtained because the infected source also is symptomatic.
    E. Treatment with oral acyclovir is warranted.

12. A 17-year-old boy has an open, ulcerative lesion on his penis. The lesion is nontender. He admits to having multiple sexual partners and does not use condoms. Which of the following statements is true?
    A. A Venereal Disease Research Laboratory (VDRL) test is always positive during this primary stage.
    B. The patient should be given cefoxitin 2 g every 6 hours intravenously for 48 hours.
    C. Examination of the cerebrospinal fluid (CSF) is indicated.
    D. A maculopapular rash occurs simultaneously with genital lesions.
    E. Treatment is 2.4 million units of benzathine penicillin G administered intramuscularly in 1 dose.

13. A 4-year-old girl has a cauliflower-like mass of nontender lesions at the inner labia minora. Initial appropriate management would include which one of the following?
    A. Referral to a child protection agency.
    B. Inquiry about the presence of cutaneous warts on the child or other family members.
    C. Cauterization of the warts in the ED.
    D. No treatment necessary in the prepubertal child.
    E. Biopsy of a single lesion for definitive laboratory identification.

14. Which of the following statements is true concerning bacterial vaginosis (nonspecific vaginosis) in the postpubertal patient?
    A. The patient's sexual partners should be treated.
    B. The standard treatment of choice is safe for a pregnant patient.
    C. Clue cells may be seen on a wet mount preparation of vaginal discharge.
    D. Vaginal pH will be acidic.
    E. Typical discharge is thick and yellow-green.

15. Which of the following statements is true regarding genital candidiasis?
    A. It is more common in the prepubertal girl because of poor hygiene.
    B. It is more common in girls who use oral contraceptives.
    C. It occurs most commonly in the week before menstruation.
    D. Oral fluconazole 150 mg for 7 days is an appropriate alternative to topical treatment.
    E. Treatment of the patient's sexual partners is advised.

16. A 16-year-old girl has copious, yellow, frothy vaginal discharge. She is sexually active. Microscopic examination of a wet mount of the secretions shows motile trichomonads. Which of the following statements is true?
    A. Clue cells also are present on wet mount.
    B. *Trichomonas vaginalis* is viable away from the body.
    C. Treatment of the patient's sexual partners is unnecessary.
    D. Vaginal discharge has a "fishy" odor.
    E. Standard therapy is safe for pregnant patients.

17. A 14-year-old girl has had painless vaginal bleeding that occurs twice a month and lasts about 7 days for at least 1 year. She does not know the number of sanitary pads she requires per day. Onset of menses was 4 years ago. She reports engaging in sexual activity only two times. She has no history of other bleeding or easy bruising. Which of the following statements is true about her management?
    A. A pelvic examination is not warranted in the hemodynamically stable patient with these symptoms.
    B. All patients with dysfunctional uterine bleeding require hormonal therapy.
    C. Patients with hemoglobin levels greater than 11 g/dl usually do not require treatment.
    D. Hormonal therapy for 1 month is adequate for moderately dysfunctional bleeding.
    E. Estrogen therapy without progesterone is required for the first week of therapy in the patient with moderately dysfunctional bleeding.

18. Which of the following statements is true about spontaneous abortion?
    A. Approximately 15% of pregnancies end in spontaneous miscarriage.
    B. More than 50% of pregnant patients have bleeding in the first half of pregnancy.
    C. A missed abortion refers to partial expulsion of the products of conception.
    D. Missed abortions almost always occur in the first trimester.
    E. Higher doses of anti-D immunoglobulin are required for the Rh-negative patient if she miscarries in the first trimester.

19. Predisposing risk factors for an ectopic pregnancy include which one of the following?
    A. Oral contraceptive use.
    B. Obesity.
    C. Pelvic inflammatory disease.
    D. Middle age.
    E. Congenital uterine abnormalities.

20. A 17-year-old girl has nausea and breast tenderness. She states that her last menstrual period was 4 weeks ago but was lighter than usual and of shorter duration. She is complaining of left lower quadrant abdominal pain. She says she has no vaginal discharge or bleeding. Your differential diagnosis includes ectopic pregnancy. Which one of the following statements is true regarding decisions about her further management?
    A. Ultrasonography with a vaginal probe can first identify an intrauterine pregnancy at β-HCG levels greater than 750 mIU/ml.
    B. Vaginal bleeding or spotting is a constant diagnostic feature of an ectopic pregnancy.
    C. The presence of an intrauterine pregnancy on sonogram definitively rules out an ectopic pregnancy.
    D. Transvaginal ultrasound is no more sensitive than traditional ultrasound in detecting an early ectopic pregnancy.
    E. Culdocentesis is commonly performed to make or confirm the diagnosis of an ectopic pregnancy.

21. A Doppler scan can first detect fetal heart tones at:
    A. 6 weeks.
    B. 8 weeks.
    C. 10 weeks.
    D. 12 weeks.
    E. 14 weeks.

22. A 4-year-old child comes to the ED with allegations of sexual abuse. Which of the following is a correct statement concerning the hymen in a prepubertal girl?
    A. The normal hymen is smooth and semilunar in shape.
    B. A small hymenal opening is inconsistent with penetration.
    C. An approximation of the introital diameter is 1 mm for every year of life.
    D. A fimbriated hymen is consistent with trauma.
    E. Hymenal tears are frequently encountered with a straddle injury.

23. A 6-year-old girl has a palpable, tender mass under her right nipple. Which one of the following is a true statement regarding this patient?
    A. Unilateral breast development in a girl younger than 8 years is abnormal.
    B. Premature genital development can be expected if there is no intervention.
    C. Radiographs of the wrist will reveal an advanced bone age development.
    D. Tenderness of the mass is consistent with early mastitis.
    E. No intervention is necessary in premature thelarche if genitalia development is normal.

24. A 14-day-old infant has erythema, warmth, and induration of one breast. Appropriate management includes which one of the following?
    A. Warm soaks to the area and initiation of oral antibiotics with staphylococcal coverage.
    B. If the infant is afebrile, warm compresses to the area are sufficient with follow-up in 24 hours.
    C. If the results of a full sepsis workup are negative, the child can be discharged with an oral antibiotic regimen.
    D. A full sepsis workup should be performed, and broad-spectrum parenteral antibiotics should be initiated
    E. The condition requires no intervention and will resolve spontaneously.

25. Which of the following statements concerning the uterus during pregnancy is true?
    A. At 6 weeks the uterus can be palpated at the symphysis pubis.
    B. At 12 weeks the uterus is at the level of the umbilicus.
    C. The distance in centimeters from the symphysis pubis to the fundus is equal to the gestational age in weeks.
    D. At 16 weeks the uterus extends beyond the umbilicus.
    E. When the uterus is at the symphysis pubis, fetal movement can be felt by the mother.

26. A 16-year-old girl has had vaginal bleeding and severe lower abdominal cramping for the past 2 to 3 hours. She states that she had a positive pregnancy test 2 weeks ago. Her last menstrual period was approximately 2 months ago. On examination the cervical os is open with tissue at the opening. Initial management would include which one of the following?
    A. Consultation with a gynecologist for a curettage procedure.
    B. No intervention.
    C. Initiation of ergonovine 0.2 mg PO bid.
    D. Performance of pelvic ultrasonography to determine whether evacuation of remaining products of conception is necessary.
    E. Initiation of intravenous (IV) antibiotics.

27. Complications associated with gonococcal cervicitis include which one of the following?
    A. Pyelonephritis.
    B. Pulmonary infection.
    C. Disseminated arthritis.
    D. Chancroid.
    E. Condylomata lata.

28. An 8-year-old girl has burning, itching, and intermittent bleeding of the vulvovaginal and perianal areas. On examination you note excoriation with bleeding, white papular lesions, fine wrinkling and pallor of the vulva with scattered blisters, and no vaginal discharge. Which one of the following is the best diagnosis?
    A. Sexual abuse.
    B. Lichen sclerosus.
    C. Pinworm infection.
    D. Vulvovaginitis.
    E. Candidal infection

29. A 6-year-old girl has pain in the vaginal area, intermittent vaginal bleeding, and a yellow vaginal discharge. On examination you note scant vaginal discharge and vulvar inflammation and excoriation. The child is Tanner stage I. You are considering an infectious, nonsexually transmitted etiology. Which one of the following organisms is associated with vaginal bleeding in the prepubertal girl?
    A. *Haemophilus influenzae* type B.
    B. *Escherichia coli.*
    C. Group B *Streptococcus.*
    D. Group A β-hemolytic *Streptococcus.*
    E. *Salmonella.*

ANSWERS [See Barkin et al: Chapter 53.]

1. The answer is **D,** pages 875 and 876.
   A red-blue mass that is doughnut shaped and friable is characteristic of urethral prolapse. Complaints include bleeding or spotting, frequency of urination, and dysuria. Genital pain is not a usual complaint. The cause is thought to be associated with any condition that causes increased intraabdominal pressure, such as seizures. Approximately 95% of reported cases of pediatric urethral prolapse occur in African-American females. Management is conservative and generally consists of sitz baths and emollient creams applied to the area. Recurrence of a conservatively treated, resolved urethral prolapse is not uncommon. Recurrence after surgical intervention is unlikely.

2. The answer is **D,** pages 873 and 874.
   Maternal hormones can stimulate the neonatal breast, causing engorgement of the breast, accompanied by drops of blood or milk, at 2 to 3 weeks of age. The engorgement generally is bilateral and can occur in either gender. Expressing the milk is contraindicated because this can lead to excoriation and mastitis. Engorgement will resolve spontaneously.

3. The answer is **D,** page 875.

   Labial adhesions are a fusion of the labia minora with a peak incidence at 1 to 6 years of age. Although they have been described in children with a history of sexual abuse, they are not pathognomonic for this. A low estrogen level has been associated with adhesions. The fusion of the labia may be partial or complete. On examination a thin bridge of connective tissue can be seen extending from the posterior fourchette toward the clitoris. Treatment generally requires good hygiene and application of an estrogen cream at bedtime for about 1 month, which will lead to separation of the adhesions. Breast tenderness and vulvar pigmentation is a reversible side effect of the treatment.

4. The answer is **C,** page 874.

   Normal breast development begins after age 8 years. Breast buds, which are usually tender initially, can develop asymmetrically with one breast lagging behind by weeks to months.

5. The answer is **D,** page 874.

   Lactational mastitis occurs because of blockage of milk in the ducts, causing stasis and infection, or from trauma caused by prolonged nursing. Bacterial causes are similar to those for nonlactational mastitis and include group A *Streptococcus, Staphylococcus aureus,* and *E. coli.* Warm compresses and oral antibiotics are generally all that are required. Occasionally drainage of the abscess is necessary.

6. The answer is **C,** pages 876 and 877.

   Adolescent infection rates for *Chlamydia trachomatis* range from 10% to 30%. Because many cases are asymptomatic, the prevalence probably is underestimated.

7. The answer is **B,** pages 876 and 877.

   C. trachomatis is an obligate intracellular parasite. Asymptomatic cases can occur in either boys or girls. Diagnosis in the pubertal patient can be made by cell culture as well as by monoclonal antibodies or enzyme-linked immunosorbent assay. Uncomplicated *C. trachomatis* infection can be treated with azithromycin 1 g for 1 dose or doxycycline 100 mg twice a day (bid) for 7 days (in boys and nonpregnant girls). Pneumonia is a complication of *C. trachomatis* contracted at birth from the genital tract of an infected mother.

8. The answer is **A,** pages 877 and 878.

   The physical examination is consistent with genital herpes. Genital HSV-2 infection is sexually transmitted and is characterized by pain, dysuria, and vulvar pruritus. The incubation period is approximately 1 week. Oral acyclovir 400 mg three times a day (tid) for 7 to 10 days is recommended for primary genital herpes infection in the nonpregnant patient. Azithromycin is the treatment for *C. trachomatis;* ceftriaxone is the treatment for *N. gonorrhoeae.*

9. The answer is **C,** pages 878 to 880.

   A risk factor for pelvic inflammatory disease (PID) is young age; columnar epithelial cells, exposed at the os in the immature cervix, apparently are responsible for this increased risk. Other risk factors include intrauterine devices (IUDs), nonwhite racial background, multiple sexual partners, and a history of PID. The other choices are not known to play any part in the risk of developing PID (see tables on page 879 in Barkin et al).

10. The answer is **B,** pages 878 to 880.

    Because of the significant sequelae associated with nontreatment or treatment failures of PID (e.g., infertility and ectopic pregnancy), early and aggressive treatment is warranted for the adolescent patient, for whom hospitalization and intravenous (IV) antibiotics may be the safest course to ensure compliance with treatment. The Centers for Disease Control and Prevention recommends treatment to provide coverage of *N. gonorrhoeae, C. trachomatis,* and anaerobes.

11. The answer is **A,** pages 877 and 878.

    HSV infection initially appears as erythematous macular lesions that become papular and subsequently progress to vesicular lesions on an erythematous base. The lesions generally are painful. HSV-1 can be transmitted by autoinoculation from a distant site, such as the mouth, or by hand contact with an infected person. HSV-2 is a sexually transmitted disease. Although sexual abuse must be considered on the basis of the physical examination, viral cultures or serologic tests will be helpful in identifying the type of HSV. Contact with another person infected with HSV cannot always be identified, since some carriers are asymptomatic. In the prepubertal child with HSV-1, symptomatic treatment is all that is required. Acyclovir is recommended for the adolescent with primary genital herpes.

12. The answer is **E,** page 880.

    This patient's history and physical examination are consistent with syphilis caused by the spirochete *Treponema pallidum.* Primary syphilis causes an open, ulcerative, nontender lesion of the genitals (chancre). At this stage of the disease, Venereal Disease Research Laboratory (VDRL) and rapid plasma reagin (RPR) tests may be negative. Symptoms of primary syphilis appear 10 to 90 days after exposure, and the lesions heal in approximately 1 week. Secondary syphilis appears 6 to 20 weeks postexposure and consists of a macular papular rash that involves the palms and soles, and may have lymphadenopathy, hepatosplenomegaly, and condylomata lata. Treatment should be initiated in the ED. The treatment of choice for early syphilis is 2.4 million units of benzathine penicillin G administered intramuscularly in 1 dose.

13. The answer is **B,** pages 880 and 881.
    This child's physical examination is consistent with condylomata acuminata caused by human papillomavirus. The lesions are nontender and cauliflower like and remain small in the prepubertal child. Although the virus can be sexually transmitted to the prepubertal child and this issue should be thoroughly investigated, it also can be transmitted by nonintimate contact with an infected person (sharing bath water or bath towels). Inquiry into whether other family members or the child have cutaneous lesions or if the mother had venereal warts during delivery is necessary. The diagnosis is generally based on clinical findings alone. Cryotherapy under general anesthesia is recommended for treatment of venereal warts in prepubertal children (see Fig. 53-12 on page 881 in Barkin et al).

14. The answer is **C,** pages 883 and 884.
    Bacterial vaginosis (formerly referred to as nonspecific vaginitis) is associated with the bacterium *Gardnerella vaginalis.* The normal vaginal flora (lactobacillus) is replaced by anaerobes and *G. vaginalis.* Signs and symptoms include a thin, gray, adherent discharge with a "fishy" odor and may have dysuria, dyspareunia, and pruritus. Vaginal pH will be above normal (greater than 4.5). Clue cells are seen on wet mount. The treatment of choice is metronidazole 500 mg bid for 7 days. It is contraindicated in pregnant patients. Asymptomatic patients and their sexual partners do not require treatment.

15. The answer is **B,** page 884.
    Candidiasis is more common in adolescents than in the prepubertal child because the pH rises after menarche, making the vagina more susceptible to infection with yeast. Additionally estrogen and progesterone can stimulate the growth of yeast, which is why girls who take oral contraceptives are more susceptible. A common time for presentation is in the week after the completion of a menstrual period. Treatment includes topical antifungal creams or vaginal suppositories. Fluconazole 150 mg orally for 1 dose has been shown to be as effective as a 7-day course of topical treatment. Sexual partners generally do not require treatment.

16. The answer is **B,** pages 884 and 885.
    Trichomonas vaginalis is an anaerobic, flagellated protozoan that causes vulvovaginitis. Although it is generally considered a sexually transmitted disease, it is viable away from the body and has been caused by contact with bath towels and swimming pools. Vaginal discharge is copious, yellow-green, and frothy. The odor is described as "musty"; a "fishy" odor is consistent with bacterial vaginosis. A saline wet mount of the discharge will reveal the motile trichomonads. The presence of clue cells is consistent with bacterial vaginosis. Standard treatment is metronidazole in the nonpregnant and nonnursing patient. Sexual partners should be treated to prevent reinfection.

17. The answer is **C,** pages 885 and 886.
    The normal menstrual cycle occurs every 28 days (the range is 21 to 35 days). Dysfunctional uterine bleeding occurs in adolescent girls because of anovulatory cycles. A pelvic examination is warranted in the context of this patient's history and complaints to ascertain the source of the bleeding and to determine the presence of any uterine or adnexal masses. Management is based on the presence of anemia (mild, moderate, or severe). Girls with a hemoglobin (Hgb) level greater than 11 g/dl usually do not require hormonal treatment; however, close follow-up is mandatory. Patients with moderate dysfunctional bleeding (Hgb level 9 to 11 g/dl) require a combination estrogen-progestin oral contraceptive given in a tapering dose over a 21-day period (4 pills per day tapering to 1 pill per day) followed by 1 pill per day for a 4-month period. Iron supplementation is also warranted (see Table 53-1 on page 886 in Barkin et al).

18. The answer is **A,** pages 888 and 889.
    Spontaneous abortion is the natural termination of pregnancy before 20 weeks' gestation. Approximately 15% of pregnancies terminate in spontaneous abortion. About 20% to 25% of pregnant women have some bleeding in the first 20 weeks, and 50% of this group subsequently miscarry. The definition of a missed abortion is an abortion in which the fetus dies but is not expelled. This generally occurs in the second trimester. An Rh-negative patient who aborts in the first trimester requires anti-D immunoglobulin 50 mg, whereas a patient who aborts after the first trimester requires 300 mg.

19. The answer is **C,** page 889.
    A predisposing factor for an ectopic pregnancy is PID. Other factors include the presence of an IUD, previous pelvic surgery, congenitally abnormal fallopian tubes, and previous exposure to diethylstilbestrol (DES).

20. The answer is **A,** pages 889 to 891.
    Although abdominal pain is frequently present with an ectopic pregnancy, it is not a constant feature. The classic triad of pain, bleeding, and a palpable mass is present in only 45% of ectopic pregnancies. Detection of an intrauterine pregnancy on pelvic ultrasound does not definitively rule out an ectopic pregnancy, since the two may be concurrent. A conventional pelvic ultrasound can identify an intrauterine pregnancy at 7 to 8 weeks' gestation, while the transvaginal approach is able to pick up a pregnancy 2½ weeks after conception. β-HCG levels are 750 to 1000 mIU/ml at this point. The transvaginal approach is more sensitive in identifying both early intrauterine and ectopic pregnancies. Culdocentesis is not required for the diagnosis of ectopic pregnancy.

21. The answer is **C,** page 888.
    The Doppler technique can first identify fetal heart tones at 10 weeks' gestation.

22. The answer is **C,** pages 867 and 868.

    The shape of the hymen varies with the individual, the most common being circumferential, fimbriated, and posterior rim shapes. The diameter of the hymenal orifice is not sufficient in most cases to rule out or confirm sexual abuse. However, a rough guideline for introital diameter is 1 mm for each year of life (e.g., a 5-year-old girl will have an introital opening diameter of 5 mm). Hymenal tears are uncommon with a straddle injury and are more consistent with a penetrating injury.

23. The answer is **E,** page 874.

    Although breast development normally occurs after the age of 8 years, premature thelarche is not uncommon. If genitalia development is not advanced, no further intervention is required. Asymmetric breast development and initial tenderness are not unusual. Bone age will not be advanced.

24. The answer is **D,** pages 873 and 874.

    The infant's symptoms are consistent with mastitis. Since mastitis in the neonate is associated with sepsis, a full sepsis workup should be completed, and broad-spectrum antibiotics should be initiated until there is evidence of clinical resolution and culture results of the sepsis workup are negative.

25. The answer is **C,** page 888.

    The uterus is palpable at the symphysis pubis at 12 weeks' gestation and at the umbilicus at 16 to 20 weeks, at which point fetal movement can generally be felt by the mother. A rough estimate of gestational age in weeks is the distance in centimeters from the symphysis pubis to the fundus.

26. The answer is **A,** page 889.

    The history and physical examination are consistent with an incomplete miscarriage, which will require curettage by a gynecologist. If the cervical os had been closed with cessation of bleeding and cramping, it would have indicated a complete miscarriage, in which no intervention is necessary.

27. The answer is **C,** page 877.

    Complications of untreated gonococcal cervicitis include disseminated gonococcal arthritis, PID, tubo-ovarian or Bartholin's gland abscesses, pharyngitis, Fitz-Hugh–Curtis syndrome, and rectal infection.

28. The answer is **B,** page 875.

    Lichen sclerosus is an uncommon, autoimmune phenomenon with a characteristic appearance of the vulva, as in this child's case. Clinical or biopsy confirmation should be sought by a dermatologist. Treatment is conservative and consists of steroid emollients and antifungal treatment for superinfection. Lichen sclerosus is not associated with sexual abuse. Diagnostic workup for other entities includes cultures for β-hemolytic *Streptococcus* and other enteric organisms that cause vulvovaginitis (*Shigella*), cellophane tape test for pinworm, and potassium hydroxide (KOH) for candidiasis.

29. The answer is **D,** pages 867 and 868.

    Organisms most commonly associated with vulvovaginitis and vaginal bleeding in the prepubertal female are group A β-hemolytic *Streptococcus* and *Shigella*. The child may have vulvar irritation, inflammation, and vaginal discharge in addition to vaginal bleeding. Diagnosis can be based on the culture. Local treatment with creams and sitz baths and the administration of oral antibiotics are indicated.

Hematology and Oncology

Robert Lembo

See Barkin et al: Chapter 54.

1. A 6-year-old previously healthy male has a 3-day history of fatigue and dizziness. Physical examination reveals pallor of the nail beds and a palpable spleen tip. The hemoglobin concentration is 8 g/dl and the mean corpuscular volume (MCV) is 80 fL. The most appropriate next step in the evaluation of this patient is to order a (an):
   A. Coombs' test.
   B. Reticulocyte count.
   C. Osmotic fragility test.
   D. Free erythrocyte protoporphyrin test.
   E. Hemoglobin electrophoresis.

2. An 18-month-old boy who recently immigrated to the United States from Southeast Asia with his parents has a temperature of 103.5° F. Examination reveals a well-appearing child with no obvious source of infection. A screening complete blood count (CBC) reveals a hemoglobin concentration of 10.2 g/dl, an MCV of 57 fL, a white cell count of 8300/mm^3, and a platelet count of 189,000/mm^3. Review of the smear confirms microcytosis and hypochromia and shows many target cells. The most likely diagnosis in this patient is:
   A. Iron deficiency.
   B. Bone marrow suppression caused by infection.
   C. Sideroblastic anemia.
   D. Hemoglobin E disease.
   E. Chronic liver disease.

3. A 7-week-old boy born at full term and currently breastfed is brought in for evaluation of nasal congestion. The infant is afebrile, and the examination is unremarkable except for mild, clear rhinorrhea and mild pallor of the nail beds. A CBC reveals a hemoglobin concentration of 10.5 g/dl and an MCV of 95 fL. The most appropriate next step in the management of this infant is:
   A. Oral administration of elemental iron.
   B. Oral administration of pyridoxine.
   C. Oral administration of folic acid.
   D. Injection of vitamin B$_{12}$.
   E. Observation only.

4. A 3-year-old child is irritable and refuses to walk. The parents report intermittent episodes of fever over the preceding 2 months associated with complaints of abdominal pain. Physical examination reveals a thin, irritable boy with mild abdominal distension who refuses to bear weight on the lower extremities. His temperature (T) is 37.9° C and blood pressure (BP) is 120/80 mm Hg. No abdominal mass is noted. The liver is palpable 3 cm below the right costal margin, muscle strength is decreased in the lower extremities bilaterally, and deep tendon reflexes are normal. Both hips have free range of motion, and the spine is nontender. The hemoglobin concentration is 10 g/dl, the total peripheral white count is 8500/mm^3, and the platelet count is 160,000/mm^3. The most likely explanation for the findings in this boy's case is:
   A. Osteogenic sarcoma.
   B. Acute hematogenous osteomyelitis.
   C. Metastatic neuroblastoma.
   D. Nephroblastoma.
   E. Diskitis.

5. A previously healthy 5-year-old boy who is African-American is undergoing an evaluation for acute abdominal pain and nonbilious vomiting. Examination reveals a well-appearing, afebrile child with a mildly tender abdomen, active bowel sounds, and no guarding or rebound tenderness. A CBC reveals a hemoglobin concentration of 11.3 g/dl, an MCV of 65 fL, a red cell count of 5.6 × 10^6/μL, a white count of 8700/mm^3 with 43% polymorphonuclear cells, 2% band forms, 50% lymphocytes, and 5% monocytes, and a platelet count of 187,000/mm^3. Supine and upright films of the abdomen reveal only a nonspecific bowel gas pattern. The most appropriate next step in the management of this patient is to:
   A. Order a sickle cell screening test.
   B. Begin iron replacement therapy.
   C. Measure blood lead levels.
   D. Order an osmotic fragility test.
   E. Continue observation.

6. A 2-year-old boy has mouth sores, swollen neck glands, and low-grade fever. The parents state that he has had six similar episodes over the past 6 months that resolved spontaneously and that he had an episode of pneumonia at age 18 months, which was treated with oral antibiotics. Examination reveals a well-appearing child with T 101° F, shallow ulcers on the buccal mucosa, pharyngeal erythema, and enlarged, mildly tender anterior cervical lymph nodes. A CBC and differential cell count of the child ordered at this time most likely would demonstrate:
   A. Elevated total white count with left shift on differential.
   B. Elevated total white count with right shift on differential.
   C. Normal total white count with lymphopenia.
   D. Normal total white count with neutropenia.
   E. Normal total white count and normal differential.

7. A 3-year-old previously well girl is brought to the ED for evaluation of an abdominal mass noted by the mother while bathing the child. Examination reveals an alert, afebrile, normotensive, well-nourished girl in no distress. The liver edge is at the right costal margin, the spleen tip is not palpated, and a firm, nontender mass is palpable deep in the flank to the left of the midline plane. The right midarm and midthigh circumference is greater than that on the left. A supine roentgenogram of the abdomen reveals displacement of the bowel gas pattern to the right. The most likely explanation for this girl's findings is:
   A. Solitary neuroblastoma.
   B. Wilms' tumor (nephroblastoma).
   C. Polycystic kidney disease.
   D. Renal cell carcinoma.
   E. Beckwith-Wiedemann syndrome.

8. A 3-year-old boy recovering from a 5-day episode of loose stools with intermittent blood streaking has lethargy and decreased urine output. Examination reveals a sleepy, but easily aroused child who is afebrile and has mild skin pallor, moist mucous membranes, and no signs of meningeal irritation. Blood chemistry panel reveals a blood urea nitrogen level (BUN) of 24 mg/dl and a serum creatinine concentration of 1.2 mg/dl. A urinalysis demonstrates a specific gravity of 1.014, 2+ protein, red blood cells, and casts. Of the following choices, the most appropriate next step in the evaluation of this patient is:
   A. Culture of urine and stool.
   B. Examination of peripheral blood smear.
   C. Coombs' test.
   D. Renal biopsy.

9. A 3-year-old girl with a history of a recent mild upper respiratory tract infection has acute, prolonged epistaxis and a 2-day history of bruising. A male cousin is known to have a bleeding disorder. Examination reveals a well-appearing child who is alert and afebrile. Clotted blood is noted in the left anterior naris; scattered red-purple, nonblanching macular lesions of variable sizes are noted over the extremities and trunk; and petechiae are noted on the soft and hard palate. The liver is palpable 1 cm below the right costal margin, and the spleen is not palpated. No cervical, axillary, or inguinal adenopathy is detected. Laboratory assessment of this child is most likely to demonstrate:
   A. Thrombocytopenia, anemia, and leukopenia.
   B. Thrombocytopenia, anemia, and leukocytosis.
   C. Thrombocytopenia, normal hemoglobin concentration, and normal white cell count.
   D. Normal platelet count, prolonged prothrombin time (PT), and normal partial thromboplastin time (PTT).
   E. Normal platelet count and prolonged PT and PTT.

10. A 16-year-old boy is referred for evaluation of poorly characterized pain in his left knee of 3 months' duration. He recalls the onset of pain after he sustained local trauma while playing basketball. Physical examination reveals a well-appearing adolescent who is afebrile and has nontender, nonerythematous swelling over the area of the distal left femur. A roentgenogram of the area of swelling reveals dense sclerosis in the metaphysis along with radial calcification and evidence of a soft tissue mass. Subsequent evaluation of this patient's underlying condition includes each of the following except:
   A. Determination of serum alkaline phosphatase.
   B. Needle aspiration.
   C. Magnetic resonance imaging (MRI) study.
   D. Radionuclide bone scan.
   E. Computed tomography (CT) of the chest.

11. An unaccompanied 14-year-old boy is brought directly to the ED from the airport after a severe headache developed and he began having difficulty speaking en route to the United States from his native country of Ghana. On arrival he is noted to be afebrile, mildly tachycardic, and normotensive with scleral icterus and no hepatosplenomegaly. Neurologic examination shows a blunted level of consciousness and significant weakness of the right arm and leg with intact sensation. The CBC shows a hemoglobin concentration of 7.5 g/dl, an MCV of 86 fL, a total peripheral white cell count of 15,200/mm^3, and a reticulocyte count of 16%. A CT scan of the brain without contrast is unremarkable. The most effective treatment for this patient is:
   A. Simple transfusion of packed red blood cells to raise the hemoglobin level to 14 g/dl.
   B. Intravenous (IV) infusion of heparin.
   C. Exchange transfusion.
   D. IV infusion of streptokinase.
   E. High dose of IV methylprednisolone.

12. A previously well 6-year-old boy has a bulging right eye and complaints of double vision of acute onset. His parents deny recent illness or trauma but acknowledge that the right eye has appeared increasingly larger than the left over the past 2 months. Examination reveals a well-appearing male who is afebrile. There is nontender proptosis of the right eye without accompanying evidence of chemosis, lid edema, or erythema. Limitation of ocular movement is evident, but the pupillary light response and the red reflex are intact. The nasopharynx is unremarkable, and there is no pain to palpation or percussion over the maxillary sinuses. The most likely explanation for this boy's problem is:
    A. Orbital abscess resulting from chronic sinusitis.
    B. Retinoblastoma.
    C. Preseptal (periorbital) cellulitis.
    D. Rhabdomyosarcoma.
    E. Traumatic glaucoma.

13. A 4-day-old full-term girl delivered at home without known perinatal complications has ecchymoses and bleeding per rectum of acute onset. The infant has been breastfed exclusively, and the mother reports that oral intake and activity have been unchanged in the past 24 hours. Physical examination demonstrates an alert, anicteric, afebrile neonate with a heart rate (HR) of 170 beats per minute, BP of 80/60 mm Hg, widespread ecchymoses, and no palpable liver or spleen. There is gross blood per rectum. A CBC reveals a hemoglobin concentration of 16.5 g/dl, a total peripheral white cell count of 12,500/mm³, an MCV of 102 fL, and a platelet count of 176,000/mm³. A coagulation profile indicates an increased PT and PTT and a normal fibrinogen concentration and D-dimer levels. The most likely explanation for this infant's condition is:
    A. Neonatal sepsis.
    B. Hemophilia A.
    C. Vitamin K deficiency.
    D. Neonatal hepatitis.
    E. Von Willebrand's disease.

14. A 3-day-old boy of Southeast Asian ancestry who was delivered uneventfully at term and was discharged as healthy at 18 hours of age is brought to the ED for evaluation of jaundice not present at birth. The infant has been fed formula and has been vigorous over the past 24 hours. Review of the available neonatal screening data indicates that both mother and infant are blood type O+ and that the direct antiglobulin (Coombs') test performed on a sample of cord blood was negative. Examination reveals an alert neonate who is afebrile and deeply jaundiced. There is no hepatosplenomegaly. Neurologic examination is within acceptable limits for the age. The total bilirubin is 24 mg/dl with an indirect reacting fraction of 0.3 mg/dl. A CBC reveals a hemoglobin concentration of 14.8 g/dl, an MCV of 98 fL, a total peripheral white cell count of 11,300/mm³, a platelet count of 155,000/mm³, and a reticulocyte count of 10%. The most helpful test in the evaluation of this infant's jaundice is:
    A. Hepatic transaminase panel.
    B. Kleihauer-Betke test.
    C. Vitamin E level.
    D. Blood culture.
    E. Glucose-6-dehydrogenase assay.

15. A 5-year-old boy is referred for evaluation of intermittent headache and emesis of 2 months' duration. His parents report that over the past 2 days he has been less active than usual, has complained of neck pain, and has had an unsteady gait. Examination reveals an alert, afebrile, mildly pallid boy with resistance to neck flexion and a broad-based, ataxic gait. Limitation of left lateral gaze is noted, and the optic disc margins appear indistinct. Deep tendon reflexes are brisk. At this time the evaluation of this child should include each of the following *except:*
    A. Contrast-enhanced computerized cranial tomography.
    B. Assessment of visual acuity.
    C. Lumbar puncture and cerebrospinal fluid (CSF) analysis.
    D. Complete blood cell count.
    E. Determination of serum electrolytes.

16. A 7-month-old infant who recently arrived with her parents from Jamaica has had 3 days of rhinorrhea, vomiting, and sleepiness of acute onset. Physical examination reveals a pallid, obtunded infant with a temperature of 37.9° C, an HR of 165 beats per minute, a respiratory rate (RR) of 32 breaths per minute, and a BP of 65/48 mm Hg. The anterior fontanelle is soft, the neck is supple, a II/VI systolic murmur is audible over the precordium, the liver is palpable 1 cm below the right costal margin, and the spleen is palpable 4.5 cm below the left costal margin. No motor deficits are noted on neurologic examination. CBC shows a hemoglobin concentration of 4.1 g/dl, an MCV of 84 fL, a total peripheral white blood cell count of 7500/mm^3, a platelet count of 90,000/ mm^3, and a reticulocyte count of 25%. Of the following choices, the most likely explanation for this child's clinical condition is:
    A. Acute cerebral malaria.
    B. Sickle cell splenic sequestration crisis.
    C. Acute meningococcemia.
    D. Hemolytic uremic syndrome (HUS).
    E. Glucose-6-phosphate dehydrogenase (G6PD) deficiency.

17. A 13-year-old boy has intermittent, nonproductive coughing associated with fatigue and decreased appetite. Examination reveals an afebrile male with trace scleral icterus, and a 2 × 3 cm, firm, nontender, nonerythematous mass in the left supraclavicular area. The lung fields are clear to auscultation. No other lymph nodes are palpated, and no edema or hepatosplenomegaly is noted. CBC demonstrates a hemoglobin concentration of 11.2 g/dl; a total peripheral white blood cell count of 8600/mm^3 with 50% polymorphonuclear cells, 40% lymphocytes, and 10% eosinophils; a reticulocyte count of 2.5%; and a sedimentation rate (Wintrobe) of 60 mm/hr. The most likely cause of the findings in this patient is:
    A. Toxoplasmosis.
    B. Atypical mycobacteria infection.
    C. Hodgkin's lymphoma.
    D. Systemic lupus erythematosus.
    E. Visceral larva migrans.

18. An 8-year-old girl is referred for further evaluation of anemia that was detected on a routine office visit. Physical examination is remarkable for pallor, hypoplasia of the thumbnails, atrophy of the thenar eminence, and patchy hyperpigmentation over the neck, chest, and groin. The CBC is remarkable for a hemoglobin concentration of 8 g/dl, an MCV of 80 fL, a total white cell count of 3500/mm^3, and a platelet count of 75,000/mm^3. The most important test to confirm the diagnosis in this patient is:
    A. Reticulocyte count.
    B. Chromosomal analysis.
    C. Bone marrow aspiration and biopsy.
    D. Radiography of the hand.
    E. CT of the head.

19. An 18-month-old is transferred for further evaluation of acute onset of fever to 104° F (40° C) associated with diffuse ecchymoses and peripheral cyanosis. Laboratory assessment of this patient is most likely to reveal:
    A. Prolonged PTT with normal PT and normal thrombin time.
    B. Normal PTT with prolonged PT and normal thrombin time.
    C. Normal PTT, normal PT, and prolonged thrombin time.
    D. Prolonged PTT, prolonged PT, and normal thrombin time.
    E. Prolonged PTT, prolonged PT, and prolonged thrombin time.

20. A 4-month-old boy born after 34 weeks' gestation that was complicated by perinatal group B streptococcal infection has bruising. Examination reveals an afebrile, lethargic infant with stable vital signs and several ecchymoses in varying stages of evolution on the back. Funduscopic examination demonstrates sharp discs and bilateral retinal hemorrhages. The neck is supple, and Kernig's sign is absent. The most likely diagnosis is:
    A. Meningitis.
    B. Child abuse.
    C. Hemophilia A.
    D. Von Willebrand's disease.
    E. Disseminated intravascular coagulation (DIC).

21. A 12-year-old boy with moderately severe hemophilia A is seen in the ED with complaints of forearm pain immediately after a fall from his bicycle. Examination reveals mild swelling of the dorsal and volar aspects of the right forearm with intact sensation and strong radial and ulnar pulses. A roentgenogram reveals no underlying fracture. The most appropriate management of this child is:
    A. Immobilization of the forearm with outpatient follow-up in 24 hours.
    B. Administration of desmopressin (DDAVP) with outpatient follow-up in 24 hours.
    C. Administration of factor VIII concentrate to maintain the level at 30% to 40% with outpatient follow-up in 24 hours.
    D. Administration of factor VIII concentrate to maintain the level at 80% to 100% and admission for observation.
    E. Administration of factor VIII concentrate to maintain level at 80% to 100% and high-dose oral prednisone with admission for observation.

22. A 14-month-old boy with a history of persistent eczema since age 2 months and chronic otitis media has petechiae. Physical examination shows a well-appearing toddler with an extensive eczematous rash, dull tympanic membranes bilaterally, and a spleen tip palpable at the left costal margin. The hemoglobin concentration is 10.5 g/dl, the MCV is 74 fL, the total peripheral white count is 6500/mm^3, and the platelet count is 58,000/mm^3. The most likely diagnosis is:
    A. Infection with human immunodeficiency virus (HIV).
    B. Genital cytomegalovirus (CMV) infection.
    C. Idiopathic thrombocytopenic purpura (ITP).
    D. Diamond-Blackfan syndrome.
    E. Wiskott-Aldrich syndrome.

23. A 12-year-old previously healthy boy has frequent bruising after minor trauma. He has no history of epistaxis or bleeding after circumcision or dental procedures. The family history is negative for bleeding disorders. Examination shows multiple ecchymoses in varying stages of evolution along with areas of thinned, atrophic, and scarred skin. The hemoglobin concentration is 13 g/dl, the MCV is 82 fL, and the platelet count is 156,000/mm^3. A coagulogram reveals a normal PT and PTT. The most likely diagnosis is:
    A. Cutaneous lymphoma.
    B. Henoch-Schönlein purpura.
    C. Ehlers-Danlos syndrome.
    D. Wiskott-Aldrich syndrome.
    E. Von Willebrand's disease.

24. A 3-year-old girl with a 3-day history of upper respiratory infection symptoms is referred for evaluation of fatigue and pallor. Examination shows tachycardia at rest, scattered petechiae on the chest and extremities, and a palpable spleen tip at the right costal margin. The hemoglobin concentration is 7 g/dl, the total peripheral white cell count is 3500/mm^3, and the platelet count is 50,000/mm^3. The peripheral smear shows normochromic red cells and small platelets. The most likely diagnosis in this patient is:
    A. Idiopathic thrombocytopenic purpura.
    B. Transient erythroblastopenia of childhood.
    C. Acute leukemia.
    D. Acquired immunodeficiency syndrome.
    E. Infectious mononucleosis.

25. A 3-year-old child with acute lymphoblastic leukemia who currently receives maintenance chemotherapy is brought to the ED 24 hours after a skin rash consistent with varicella develops in his 7-year-old brother. The 3-year-old is afebrile, and the physical examination is unremarkable. The hemoglobin concentration is 11.5 g/dl and the total peripheral white cell count is 8500/mm^3 with 40% neutrophils and 60% lymphocytes. No blasts are noted on smear. The most appropriate management of this patient is:
    A. Observation in a reverse isolation setting in the hospital.
    B. Administration of IV acyclovir.
    C. Administration of zoster immune globulin (ZIG).
    D. Administration of varicella vaccine.
    E. Continued observation at home.

26. A 3-year-old girl with neuroblastoma on chemotherapy complains of back pain, has a limp, and has not urinated for 12 hours. Physical examination reveals tenderness localized to the spine, increased deep tendon reflex at the right knee, and decreased deep tendon reflex at the right ankle. The most likely diagnosis is:
    A. Tumor metastatic to the distal femur.
    B. Epidural cord compression.
    C. Local tumor invasion involving the iliopsoas muscle.
    D. Chemotherapy-induced peripheral neuropathy.
    E. Tumor metastatic to the motor cortex.

27. A 12-year-old boy with sickle cell disease comes to the ED because of increased fatigue. He is alert and afebrile. Other than mild tachycardia and scleral icterus, the examination is unremarkable. The hemoglobin concentration is 7 g/dl, MCV is 90 fL, total white cell count is 20,000/mm^3, and reticulocyte count is 2%. The most appropriate therapy for this patient is:
    A. Partial exchange transfusion.
    B. Folic acid.
    C. Broad-spectrum antimicrobials.
    D. Digoxin.
    E. Iron.

28. A 22-month-old girl of Mediterranean ancestry is referred to the ED for evaluation of anemia. She is described as a "picky" eater who prefers drinking homogenized cow's milk at meals. Examination reveals a well-appearing child with a spleen tip palpable at the left costal margin and shotty inguinal lymph nodes. The hemoglobin concentration is 11.3 g/dl, the MCV is 64 fL, the red blood cell count is 4.7 x 10^6/µL, the white count is 4500/mm^3 with 40% segmented polymorphonuclear cells and 60% lymphocytes, and the platelet count is 155,000/mm^3. Which of the following is the most appropriate next step in the evaluation of this patient?
    A. Serum ferritin.
    B. Epstein-Barr virus titers.
    C. Quantitative hemoglobin electrophoresis.
    D. Bone marrow biopsy.
    E. Coombs' test.

29. A 5-month-old Caucasian boy has progressive pallor of several months' duration. The infant was born after an uncomplicated full-term pregnancy, labor, and delivery and has been well in all other respects. Examination reveals a pallid infant with tachycardia at rest, no adenopathy or hepatosplenomegaly, and a unilateral triphalangeal thumb on the right hand. CBC shows a hemoglobin concentration of 4 g/dl, an MCV of 108 fL, a reticulocyte count of 0.5%, a total peripheral white blood cell count of 7500/mm³, and a platelet count of 410,000/mm³. Of the following choices, the most likely diagnosis in this child is:
    A. Diamond-Blackfan anemia.
    B. Transient erythroblastopenia of infancy.
    C. Chronic renal disease.
    D. Iron deficiency anemia.
    E. Tumor metastatic to bone marrow.

30. A 10-month-old previously well boy has an acute episode of fever to 101.9° F. Examination reveals a well-appearing infant with mild pharyngeal erythema and injection of the tympanic membranes bilaterally. Screening CBC and differential white count show a hemoglobin concentration of 12.1 g/dl, an MCV of 78 fL, a total white count of 4400/mm³ with 20% polymorphonuclear cells, 2% band forms, 62% lymphocytes, 13% monocytes, and 3% eosinophils, and a platelet count of 151,000/mm³. The most appropriate management of this patient is:
    A. Bone marrow aspiration.
    B. Observation as an outpatient with follow-up in 48 to 72 hours.
    C. Administration of intramuscular ceftriaxone.
    D. Hospitalization for broad-spectrum IV antibiotic therapy.
    E. Administration of G-CSF.

ANSWERS   [See Barkin et al: Chapter 54.]

1. The answer is **B**, page 899.
   The girl in the vignette has normocytic anemia. Such an anemia may be the result of marrow underproduction of erythrocytes, a consequence of increased erythrocyte destruction in the circulation, or loss of blood (e.g., gastrointestinal [GI] bleeding). The reticulocyte count, which reflects the marrow's ability to produce and release erythrocytes, helps differentiate between anemia of underproduction and anemia resulting from increased erythrocyte destruction or blood loss. (See Fig. 46-1.)

2. The answer is **D**, page 899 (Fig. 54-2).
   Target cells reflect an absolute or relative increase in red blood cell surface-to-volume ratio. In conditions in which there is decreased hemoglobin synthesis or abnormal hemoglobin aggregation and as a result decreased red cell volume, a relative increase occurs in the ratio of surface area to volume and target cells are noted on peripheral smear. The child with target cells on peripheral smear described in the vignette also is noted to have a mild anemia and a low mean corpuscular volume (MCV), suggesting a thalassemic hemoglobinopathy.

   One common thalassemic hemoglobinopathy among individuals of Asian ancestry is hemoglobin E disease. The mutation in hemoglobin E disease results in decreased production of a functional β-globin messenger RNA coding for a structural β-globin chain variant. Patients with homozygous hemoglobin E have hemoglobin levels that are in the range of 10 g/dl and mean corpuscular volumes (MCVs) in the range of 50 to 66 fL. Electrophoresis reveals hemoglobin E constituting more than 90% of the total hemoglobin. The major differential diagnostic consideration is iron deficiency. Chronic liver disease may have target cells, but the targeting results from lipid accumulation in the red cells rather than from decreased red cell volume. The sideroblastic anemias are a heterogeneous group of red blood cell disorders characterized by microcytosis, hypochromia, reticulocytopenia, and ineffective erythropoiesis in association with thrombocytopenia and neutropenia. Bone marrow suppression caused by infection is unlikely to be associated with significant microcytosis.

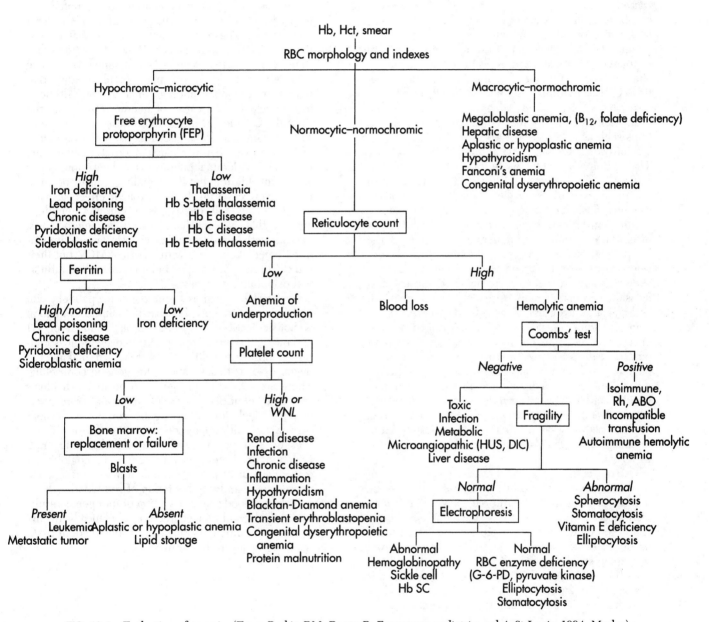

FIG. 46-1   Evaluation of anemia. (From Barkin RM, Rosen P: *Emergency pediatrics*, ed 4, St Louis, 1994, Mosby.)

3. The answer is **E,** page 897.

The infant in this vignette has an appropriate hemoglobin concentration and MCV for his age. A decline in the hemoglobin concentration as well as the MCV is expected in all infants because of rapid increase in blood volume associated with normal growth and the switchover from fetal hemoglobin to adult hemoglobin production. This decline in hemoglobin concentration reaches a nadir at approximately 2 months of age in term infants and has been given the clinical designation of "physiologic anemia of infancy." These infants have adequate iron stores and do not require supplemental hematinics such as folate, pyridoxine, or vitamin B_{12}. The infant with upper respiratory infection (URI) symptoms described in the vignette therefore can be observed as an outpatient with further evaluation reserved for infants with progressive symptoms such as pallor.

4. The answer is **C,** pages 905 and 906, Table 54-3.

The patient described in the vignette is irritable, refuses to bear weight, and has mild anemia suggestive of systemic illness or metastatic disease involving the musculoskeletal system and bone marrow. Neuroblastoma is the most common extracranial solid tumor in children. Originating in neural crest cells of the sympathetic nervous system, neuroblastomas can develop anywhere but most likely originate in the abdomen and extend to surrounding tissue by local invasion. Hematogenous spread to bone marrow, skeleton, and liver, as reflected by the anemia, bone pain, and hepatomegaly noted in the patient described in the vignette, is common. Because the tumor possesses the enzymes for catecholamine synthesis, patients, such as the one described in the vignette, may have hypertension and increased levels of homovanillic acid and vanillylmandelic acid in the urine. Although other malignancies must be considered, nephroblastoma (Wilms' tumor) usually is an asymptomatic mass in the abdomen or flank with or without hypertension.

Osteosarcoma results in localized pain and non-erythematous swelling over long bones, although the flat bones such as the vertebrae, pelvic bones, and mandible may be primary sites affected in very young children. Acute hematogenous osteomyelitis usually produces fever, local warmth, tenderness, and local soft tissue swelling, while diskitis (intervertebral disk space infection) results in back pain and refusal to flex the spine. Hypertension and hepatomegaly would be extremely unusual in these infectious conditions.

5. The answer is **E,** pages 898 and 899.

The child in this vignette has normal white blood cell and platelet counts for his age but a low hemoglobin concentration and an unexpectedly low MCV. α-Thalassemia trait is a syndrome characterized by significant microcytosis and hypochromia of the red blood cells in association with mild anemia and erythrocytosis. The condition occurs with highest frequency among Asian populations but is noted also in African, Mediterranean, and African-American populations. These individuals have normal or low levels of hemoglobin A_2 and F, which distinguishes them from patients with β-thalassemia trait. The diagnosis is made by obtaining family studies that demonstrate similar findings in a parent. Although iron deficiency is a cause of microcytic anemia, the MCV/RBC ratio (Mentzer index) for this patient is 11.6, making iron deficiency less likely than a hemoglobinopathy such as α-thalassemia trait. Lead toxicity may cause abdominal pain associated with microcytic anemia in children, but these findings usually occur in more severe cases in which neurologic effects also are noted. Sickle cell disease is a chronic hemolytic anemia that is not characterized by microcytosis. Patients with hereditary spherocytosis have a compensated hemolytic anemia with a normal MCV, but their red cells lyse more readily in hypotonic saline (abnormal osmotic fragility test).

Because the prognosis is excellent for patients with α-thalassemia trait and because the clinical evaluation is not indicative of specific intraabdominal or GI pathology, the most appropriate management is continued observation. The importance of making the diagnosis of α-thalassemia is for genetic counseling. There are four α-globin genes in normal individuals and four clinical syndromes resulting from their deletion. Deletion of one gene results in a silent carrier state with no hemoglobin abnormalities. Deletion of two genes results in α-thalassemia trait. Deletion of three genes results in hemoglobin H disease characterized by anemia of moderate severity, microcytosis, and fragmentation of red blood cells on peripheral blood smear. Deletion of four genes results in a lethal condition characterized clinically by hydrops fetalis and hematologically by hemoglobin Bart's resulting in severe tissue hypoxia.

6. The answer is **D**, pages 901 and 902.

The recurrent pattern of fever, mouth lesions, and lymphadenopathy in this patient with a history of a serious infection such as pneumonia suggests the rare but well-described clinical entity of cyclic neutropenia. Cyclic neutropenia is characterized by oscillations in the number of peripheral neutrophils from normal to neutropenic levels with a periodicity of approximately 21 days. Other formed elements in blood such as platelets and reticulocytes also may cycle, but the total white count usually remains within the normal range in these patients. Bone marrow aspirates during periods of neutropenia demonstrate either hypoplasia or maturational arrest of the granulocyte series at the myelocyte stage. The etiology of cyclic neutropenia remains uncertain but studies using canine models of the human disease suggest that a regulatory abnormality involving an early hematopoietic stem cell precursor most likely accounts for the condition.

7. The answer is **B**, pages 905 and 906, Table 54-3.

An asymptomatic abdominal mass in a child raises the possibility of benign and malignant disorders, including urinary tract obstructive disease, neuroblastoma, and nephroblastoma (Wilms' tumor). However, the additional finding of hemihypertrophy in this patient strongly suggests the diagnosis of Wilms' tumor. Hemihypertrophy is noted in approximately 2% of cases and may occur ipsilateral or contralateral to the site of the tumor. The cause of hemihypertrophy in patients with Wilms' tumor remains unclear, but the influence of endogenous growth factors is postulated. Neuroblastoma is the most common extracranial solid tumor in children, and the most common site of the primary tumor is the abdomen. Hemihypertrophy, however, is not associated with neuroblastoma. Renal cell carcinoma is typically diagnosed during the sixth and seventh decades and is manifested most frequently with hematuria, but the classic triad of pain, abdominal mass, and hematuria probably occurs in less than 10% of cases. Autosomal recessive polycystic kidney disease usually develops in the newborn period with large kidneys and oliguria and is associated with oligohydramnios during pregnancy. Diagnosis usually is made prenatally with ultrasonography. Autosomal dominant ("adult-type") polycystic kidney disease may present in childhood with flank masses and hypertension, but hemihypertrophy is not a feature of this disorder. Beckwith-Wiedemann syndrome develops in infancy with the classic triad of exomphalos, macroglossia, and symmetric gigantism. The syndrome is closely linked to paternal disomy of chromosome 11 in the domain of the embryonic growth factor IGF-2. Patients with Beckwith-Wiedemann syndrome have an increased risk of neoplasm, including Wilms' tumor.

8. The answer is **B**, page 899, Table 54-2.

The clinical features of a diarrheal prodrome followed by altered mental status, oliguria, and laboratory evidence of azotemia described in this vignette are highly suggestive of hemolytic uremic syndrome (HUS), a disorder that is characterized by microangiopathic, as opposed to a Coombs' positive, hemolytic anemia. A characteristic feature noted on microscopic analysis of a peripheral blood smear in such patients is fragmented erythrocytes, which makes this study the most appropriate next step in the evaluation of the patient. HUS is associated frequently with enteric infection caused by *Escherichia coli* O157:H7, which is known to produce verocytotoxin, a putative agent in the pathogenesis of the syndrome. Routine stool culture techniques, however, will not identify the O157:H7 strain of *E. coli*. Central nervous system involvement has been reported in HUS, and lethargy is a characteristic finding. Renal biopsy at this time would not add significant diagnostic information that could not be obtained in a less invasive manner.

9. The answer is **C**, page 904, Table 54-1, and pages 917 and 918.

The patient has an epidemiologic and clinical picture suggestive of idiopathic thrombocytopenic purpura (ITP). Characteristically these patients have thrombocytopenia that can be profound, normal hemoglobin concentration, and a normal white blood cell count developing after an immunologic challenge or an antecedent nonbacterial infectious disease such as varicella. Because the differential diagnosis includes early aplastic anemia or leukemia and because diagnosis and appropriate therapy for these disorders may be delayed by empirical therapy for ITP with corticosteroids, many hematologists confirm the diagnosis right away with a bone marrow examination. The major risk in patients with ITP is uncontrolled bleeding or bleeding into the central nervous system, neither of which is evident clinically in this patient. However, the risk of central nervous system bleeding increases as the platelet count falls below 20,000/mm^3, and many clinicians would institute therapy at this cut point. Treatment with corticosteroids or γ-globulin has been reported to increase the platelet count in ITP to levels considered protective against spontaneous bleeding. Most clinicians recommend hospitalization until the platelet count stabilizes or increases. This provides a controlled environment to observe the patient receiving therapy who is at risk for central nervous system bleeding or to reduce the risk of traumatic bleeding into the central nervous system. Aspirin or other antiplatelet drugs should not be administered to patients with ITP.

10. The answer is **B,** page 906, Table 54-3.

The patient described in the vignette has clinical and radiographic findings more suggestive of a malignancy than of a local infection of soft tissue or bone. Osteosarcoma (also known as osteogenic sarcoma) and Ewing's sarcoma are the malignancies that account for most primary skeletal cancers in children. Osteosarcoma is more commonly encountered than Ewing's sarcoma, but both occur most frequently in the second decade of life and preponderantly in male patients. Clinically the most common complaint of patients who have osteosarcoma is localized pain and swelling that may be attributed initially to trauma. The tumor most often arises in the metaphysis of the long bones, usually the femur. A palpable mass may be noted on examination. Metastases occur most often to the lungs, lymph nodes, and other locations in the skeleton. Levels of alkaline phosphatase may be elevated if the tumor has significant osteoblastic activity. Plain radiographs may demonstrate sclerosis of bone and periosteal new bone formation. Computed tomography (CT) of the chest and radionuclide bone scanning provide important information regarding the extent of disease beyond the primary lesion. Magnetic resonance imaging (MRI) provides the best assessment of the tumor's extent within the medullary cavity of the affected bone and the adjacent soft tissues.

Acute hematogenous osteomyelitis has local signs of pain and inflammation at the affected site with or without accompanying fever. Findings such as warmth, tenderness, and soft tissue swelling occur in direct proportion to the progression of the inflammatory response through the periosteum and soft tissues. Chronic osteomyelitis has localized signs of inflammation commonly in association with a sinus tract that may drain purulent material. The diagnosis is established through recovery of an organism in blood or more specifically from direct bone aspiration or biopsy. However, direct aspiration is not recommended if a malignant lesion is suspected; biopsy is the preferred method of confirming the diagnosis.

11. The answer is **C,** page 908, Table 54-5, and page 908.

The patient described in this vignette has clinical evidence of a nonhemorrhagic stroke in evolution and both epidemiological and hematological findings consistent with sickle cell disease. Large vessel occlusive disease occurs in sickle cell disease and can produce gross ischemic damage with sequelae. Strokes occur in approximately 7% of patients and are among the more catastrophic acute sequelae of large vessel occlusive disease, frequently resulting in hemiplegia. The initial neurologic signs may resolve completely, improve without resolution, or remain static. However, the mortality rate in untreated patients with cerebrovascular occlusive disease is as high as 20%, and approximately 70% have permanent motor disabilities and deficits in intellectual functioning. A large proportion of untreated patients have a recurrence of cerebrovascular occlusion within 3 years of the initial occlusion.

The treatment of choice for a patient with acute cerebrovascular occlusive disease caused by sickling is exchange transfusion. Exchange transfusion rapidly reduces the circulating level of sickle hemoglobin and limits intracerebrovascular sickling to reduce the progression and extent of vasoocclusive damage. Simple transfusion of packed red cells to reduce the level of circulating hemoglobin S and raise the total hemoglobin level to normal values for age (14 g/dl in this patient) may result in an increase in blood viscosity, which actually could worsen ischemia in the patient with sickle cell disease. The use of corticosteroids, anticoagulants, or thrombolytic therapy remains controversial in therapy for children who have had a stroke, and specific data related to their effectiveness in the treatment of patients with cerebrovascular occlusive complications in sickle cell disease are lacking.

12. The answer is **D,** page 906, Table 54-3.

The patient described in the vignette has findings suggestive of a noninflammatory intraorbital mass lesion. An important cause of intraorbital mass lesions in children is rhabdomyosarcoma, which is the most common soft tissue malignancy in children. The tumors arise from the same embryonic mesenchyme as striated muscle and can occur at virtually any anatomic site. The head and neck region is the most frequent location for rhabdomyosarcoma. Primary lesions arising in the orbit are usually diagnosed early because of the space-occupying effect of the tumor, resulting in proptosis. Other findings may include pain, changes in visual acuity, ptosis, and periorbital edema.

Retinoblastoma develops in the posterior portion of the retina and grows forward over time into the vitreous cavity. Extension of the tumor to the choroid and down the optic nerve can occur and increases the risk of distant metastasis, especially to the central nervous system. Patients usually have leukokoria in the first or second year of life, although decreased visual acuity and strabismus also may be manifestations. The tumor may be bilateral and is usually visualized easily with an ophthalmoscope. Proptosis can occur but usually in the context of advanced disease. Glaucoma usually has the clinical triad of photophobia, epiphora, and blepharospasm resulting from irritation of the cornea. Both corneal and ocular enlargement and decreased visual acuity can occur in glaucoma, but proptosis and gaze limitation are inconsistent with this diagnosis.

Preseptal cellulitis is inflammation of the lids and periorbital tissues caused by trauma, infected wounds, or bacteremia without signs of true orbital involvement. However, inflammatory lesions such as orbital abscess caused by ethmoid sinusitis can produce proptosis, but the normal findings on nasopharyngeal examination and the absence of nasal discharge or facial pain make acute or chronic sinusitis unlikely in the patient described in this vignette.

13. The answer is **C,** page 913, Table 54-8.

The neonate described in this vignette has evidence of a hemorrhagic diathesis in the absence of thrombocytopenia and significant laboratory evidence of fibrinogen consumption. The most common causes of bleeding in a previously well neonate in the context of these findings are vitamin K deficiency and congenital deficiency of coagulation proteins. The classic clinical presentation of vitamin K deficiency is hemorrhagic disease of the newborn characterized by the onset of GI bleeding, ecchymoses, and occasionally intracranial hemorrhage on days 2 to 5 of life. An important risk factor for hemorrhagic disease of the newborn is exclusive breastfeeding because of the low concentration (less than 20 μg/L) of vitamin K in breast milk as compared with proprietary cow's milk formula (~ 800 mg/L). In the absence of intramuscularly administered prophylactic vitamin K administration at birth, the incidence of hemorrhagic disease of the newborn is reported to be as high as one case in 200 infants. The low levels of functional factors II, VII, IX, and X caused by vitamin K deficiency result in a prolongation of both the prothrombin time (PT) and the activated partial thromboplastin time (aPTT) on the coagulogram. Hemophilia A (factor VIII deficiency) and hemophilia B (factor IX deficiency) are the most common congenital disorders producing a hemorrhagic diathesis in newborns. In most infants with hemophilia, hemorrhagic manifestations do not develop until later in the first year of life when the child is more mobile, although approximately 30% of affected boys bleed with circumcision and 1% to 2% develop intracranial hemorrhage. The diagnosis is suggested by a prolonged aPTT and a normal PT on the coagulogram.

Neonatal sepsis can produce disseminated intravascular coagulation (DIC), an acquired hemorrhagic diathesis. Patients with DIC are usually clinically ill and manifest prolongation of both the PT and the aPTT on the coagulogram, decreased concentrations of fibrinogen, and increased levels of D-dimer, indicating degradation of cross-linked fibrin. Evidence of microangiopathy and thrombocytopenia is also found in affected patients. Infants with von Willebrand's disease rarely have hemorrhagic complications in the newborn period. Physiologic levels of von Willebrand factor and the proportion of high–molecular weight multimers are normally elevated at birth and remain high during early infancy, which may account for this observation. The hemorrhagic diathesis caused by liver disease results from the failure of activation of the coagulation and fibrinolytic pathways and abnormally glycosylated proteins. In newborns hepatic dysfunction of sufficient magnitude to produce a hemorrhagic diathesis occurs with hepatitis, hypoxic liver damage, and shock, all of which are unlikely in the patient described in the vignette.

14. The answer is **E,** pages 906 and 907.

The boy of Asian ancestry described in this vignette with neonatal jaundice has significant indirect hyperbilirubinemia associated with a hemoglobin level at the lower limit of normal and an elevated reticulocyte count, suggesting an underlying hemolytic process. The compatible maternal and infant blood types and the negative cord blood direct antiglobulin test make immune-mediated hemolysis an unlikely cause of the hyperbilirubinemia. Nonimmune causes of hemolysis in the newborn include red blood cell enzymopathies such as glucose-6-phosphate dehydrogenase (G6PD) deficiency and membrane abnormalities such as hereditary spherocytosis. The clinical picture of neonatal jaundice caused by G6PD deficiency is characterized by the onset of jaundice out of proportion to anemia usually between days 2 and 3 of life. The severity of neonatal jaundice caused by G6PD deficiency is highly variable, and not all G6PD-deficient infants become icteric in the newborn period. The biologic basis of these observations is not entirely clear. The G6PD gene is located on the X chromosome, and the genetic defect is widely distributed with known concentrations among populations in the Mediterranean littoral, Africa, and the Far East, including China and Southeast Asia. Classic hereditary spherocytosis is an autosomal dominant disorder characterized by osmotically fragile, partially spherical red blood cells caused by abnormalities in the structural protein ankyrin and β-spectrin that are selectively removed by the spleen. An autosomal recessive form of the disease associated with abnormalities in the structural protein α-spectrin is also recognized. Hereditary spherocytosis is the most common hemolytic anemia in northern European populations for whom the incidence is approximately 1 in 5000 individuals. The disorder is infrequent in other racial groups.

Although neonatal sepsis may be associated with hemolysis, patients usually demonstrate signs or symptoms of systemic illness that are not evident in the patient described in the vignette. Patients with neonatal hepatitis have jaundice and an elevation of the direct bilirubin fraction, which is not noted in this patient. The Kleihauer-Betke acid elution test detects the presence of fetal red blood cells in the maternal circulation and is the diagnostic test for confirming fetal-maternal transfusion as the cause of neonatal anemia or hypovolemia.

15. The answer is **C,** page 906, Table 54-3, and pages 921 and 922.

The patient described in this vignette has symptoms and clinical findings suggestive of raised intracranial pressure, probably caused by obstructive hydrocephalus and impending cerebellar herniation. The most likely cause of these findings in a school-aged child is a posterior fossa brain tumor. However, nonneoplastic mass lesions, including those of infectious origin, also should be considered in the differential diagnosis. Brain tumors are the most common solid tumors encountered in children, and they are second only to leukemia as the most common neoplasm in pediatric patients. Approximately two thirds of pediatric brain tumors are infratentorial, and two major histologic cell types predominate—glial cell tumors and primitive neuroectodermal cell tumors. Glial tumors include high- and low-grade astrocytomas and ependymomas. Neuroectodermal tumors include the cerebellar medulloblastoma. Evaluation of the child suspected of having an intracranial mass lesion should include neuroimaging such as contrast-enhanced CT or MRI. Adjunctive testing such as visual field and acuity testing, electrolyte determinations, screening for abnormalities in antidiuretic hormone secretion or cerebral salt-wasting syndrome, and review of the CBC in a search for evidence of a systemic inflammatory response often are indicated. In the presence of raised intracranial pressure and signs consistent with cerebellar tonsillar herniation, however, lumbar puncture is contraindicated.

16. The answer is **B,** page 908, Table 54-5, and page 910. The afebrile infant described in the vignette has a significant normochromic, normocytic anemia, brisk reticulocytosis, mild thrombocytopenia, and marked splenomegaly associated with tachycardia, tachypnea, and hypotension, suggesting hypovolemia caused by acute splenic sequestration. The most likely cause of acute splenic sequestration in a patient from the geographic area described in the vignette is sickle cell disease. Infants with homozygous sickle cell disease whose spleens have not yet undergone infarction and fibrosis may suddenly develop pooling of a significant proportion of their intravascular volume within the spleen. Precipitous declines in the hematocrit level and other formed elements in the blood occur, and hypovolemic shock may ensue, making acute splenic sequestration crisis a life-threatening medical emergency. The usual clinical manifestations of this unpredictable complication include sudden development of weakness, pallor, breathlessness, alteration in mental status, vomiting, and abdominal fullness. Treatment of sequestration crisis is directed at the prompt correction of hypovolemia and restoration of appropriate oxygen-carrying capacity.

Although other causes of hypotension such as septic shock must be considered in this patient, the absence of fever makes meningococcemia less likely. Malaria caused by *Plasmodium falciparum* may result in sequestration of erythrocytes in brain, liver, kidney, and bone marrow. Hemolytic anemia is characteristic of malaria, and profound anemia may be noted in severe infections of *P. falciparum* with some degree of hypersplenism. However, the presence of significant hypersplenism and profound hypovolemia is less likely in malaria than in sickle cell disease. Hemolysis is also characteristic of G6PD deficiency and HUS, but profound hypovolemia is not consistent with these disorders.

17. The answer is **C,** page 906, Table 54-3.
The patient described in this vignette has unexplained unilateral supraclavicular adenopathy, which suggests a pathologic condition within the thorax associated with mild anemia, and reticulocytosis, suggesting hemolysis and an elevated sedimentation rate that may indicate a systemic inflammatory response. These findings taken in the aggregate are consistent with the diagnosis of lymphoma, most likely Hodgkin's disease. Lymphoma is recognized as the third leading cause of cancer among children. Two broad categories are recognized—Hodgkin's disease and non–Hodgkin's lymphoma (NHL). NHL in childhood most frequently is in the abdomen, mediastinum, and head and neck region. Hodgkin's disease usually is painless and results in enlargement of the lymph nodes in the cervical, supraclavicular, or less commonly the axillary or inguinal region. Mediastinal lymph node enlargement is frequent in Hodgkin's disease and may produce coughing or airway compromise. A significant percentage of patients have nonspecific systemic symptoms such as fatigue, anorexia, or pruritus. A smaller percentage have significant systemic symptoms such as fever, night sweats, or weight loss. A variety of immune phenomena are noted in association with Hodgkin's disease, such as autoimmune hemolytic anemia or thrombocytopenia. Cellular immunity is depressed, which places these patients at increased risk for infectious illnesses.

Atypical mycobacterial infections can have unilateral adenopathy, but involvement of a supraclavicular node is unusual. These pathogens affect cervical nodes after they gain access to the lymphatic system through the oral cavity. Acquired toxoplasmosis may have similar systemic symptoms, but the nodes involved usually are those in the posterior cervical chain and hemolysis is not an expected associated finding. Systemic lupus erythematosus may have hemolysis and systemic symptoms, but other clinical features are expected in association, such as rash, fever, photosensitivity, alopecia, and arthralgia.

18. The answer is **B,** page 901.
The patient described in the vignette has a normochromic, normocytic anemia associated with dysmorphic features, hyperpigmentation, and thrombocytopenia. These features are most consistent with Fanconi's anemia, a disorder of unknown etiology associated with chromosome breakage. Both Diamond-Blackfan syndrome and transient erythroblastopenia are characterized by an abnormality only of the red cell line, while the Holt-Oram syndrome is a dysmorphic syndrome involving skeletal and cardiovascular abnormalities not associated with hematopoietic dysfunction.

19. The answer is **E,** page 905, Table 54-2, and pages 912 and 913.

The patient in the vignette has clinical features most suggestive of DIC, an acquired coagulopathy usually associated with systemic infection in young children. Characteristically DIC results in decreases in all coagulation factors as well as platelets and thus manifests abnormalities in the PT, PTT, and thrombin time (TT) on the coagulogram in addition to thrombocytopenia.

20. The answer is **B,** page 903.

The patient in this vignette has clinical features of cutaneous and central nervous system bleeding (retinal hemorrhages) caused by trauma characteristic of child abuse. The absence of fever and meningeal signs does not support acute purulent meningitis, and the patient's sex makes hemophilia A unlikely. In infants DIC usually is associated with systemic infection, which is unlikely in a 6-month-old afebrile infant. Type I von Willebrand's disease tends to produce mucosal bleeding in contrast to deep soft tissue bleeding.

21. The answer is **C,** page 916.

This patient with hemophilia A probably has mild bleeding into the muscle of the forearm. The major risk to this patient is compartment syndrome. The physical examination, however, does not indicate an evolving compartment syndrome. Thus procoagulant therapy and close follow-up are indicated. The recommended level for effective hemostasis in this patient is 30% to 40%. Higher levels are recommended for deep soft tissue injury or central nervous system bleeding, neither of which this patient appears to have. If surgical decompression of the forearm were indicated, a level of 80% to 100% would be indicated (Table 46-1).

22. The answer is **E,** page 903.

The patient with thrombocytopenia has clinical features highly suggestive of Wiskott-Aldrich syndrome. Wiskott-Aldrich syndrome is an X-linked disorder characterized by thrombocytopenia, eczema, and increased susceptibility to pyogenic and opportunistic infection as a result of impairment of both cellular and humoral immunity. The nature of the biochemical and genetic defects in Wiskott-Aldrich syndrome is unclear. Although human immunodeficiency virus (HIV) or cytomegalovirus (CMV) infection can have thrombocytopenia and splenic enlargement, chronic eczema is not a usual accompanying feature. ITP is possible but less commonly encountered in this age group. Diamond-Blackfan syndrome has evidence of impairment in erythrocyte production in contrast to platelets.

TABLE 46-1   Initial Management of Bleeding in Hemophilia*

Degree of hemorrhage	Desired factor level (%)	Factor VIII* (units/kg)	Factor IX* (units/kg)	Typical follow-up
Moderate				
Hemarthrosis	40-50	25	50	Rest, application of ice; telephone follow-up next day
Muscle/soft tissue	30-50			
Laceration requiring sutures	40-50	25	50	Factor correction for 1-10 days depending on severity
Mouth, tongue	40-50 (aminocaproic or tranexamic acid alone if minor)	25	50	Oral aminocaproic or tranexamic acid therapy for several days; close telephone follow-up
Life- or limb-threatening				
Airway	1000	50	100	Hospitalization; maintain normal hemostasis
CNS, spinal cord				
Eye				Surgical intervention as appropriate
Gastrointestinal				
Retroperitoneal				
Compartment syndrome (forearm, calf)	100	50	100	Hospitalization; maintain normal hemostasis Surgical intervention generally not needed
Other				
Head injury—no evidence of CNS hemorrhage	50	25	50	Monitor for head injury; CT scan if delay between injury and factor treatment
Hematuria	0	0	0	Rest and fluids for 48 hr; if no improvement, prednisone 2 mg/kg/day for 4 days

CNS, Central nervous system.
*For patients without inhibitors.

23. The answer is **C**, page 904, Table 54-1.
The patient has clinical features highly suggestive of a vascular cause of purpura and cutaneous findings indicative of type I (gravis) Ehlers-Danlos syndrome. The Ehlers-Danlos syndrome is a heterogeneous group of generalized connective tissue disorders that demonstrate fragility and hyperextensibility of the skin. More than 10 types are recognized. Type I is an autosomal recessive disorder characterized by easy bruising of the skin after trauma, leading to thin, atrophic scars that resemble cigarette paper. The lesions of Henoch-Schönlein purpura, a leukocytoclastic vasculitis, often are raised and can be described clinically as "palpable purpura." Healing of these lesions does not result in scarring. While the normal coagulogram and platelet count do not rule out von Willebrand's disease, the negative history of any mucosal bleeding makes this disorder unlikely. The normal platelet count and the absence of eczema essentially rule out Wiskott-Aldrich syndrome.

24. The answer is **C**, page 903.
The patient has anemia, leukopenia, and thrombocytopenia, the combination of which strongly suggests major bone marrow dysfunction. The normochromic red cells and the small platelets suggest failure of cell production in the marrow. The most likely mechanism of bone marrow failure is either aplasia or replacement with tumor. Thus acute leukemia is high on the differential diagnosis even though the total peripheral white cell count is elevated. Transient erythroblastopenia affects only production of the red cell line. Although HIV and infectious mononucleosis can result in decreases in more than one cell line, it is highly unusual for all three to be depressed. ITP is associated with increased platelet destruction and an intact marrow usually reflected by large platelets on the peripheral smear.

25. The answer is **C**, page 920.
Prevention of infection is a major issue for the clinician managing oncology patients. The patient described here, exposed to an older sibling with active varicella, most likely can benefit from postexposure prophylaxis with zoster immune globulin (ZIG). This is certainly the case if the patient is known to be seronegative. Chemoprophylaxis with acyclovir may be an adjunctive therapy but has not been demonstrated to be superior in efficacy to ZIG. If clinical disease develops in an immunosuppressed patient exposed to varicella, therapy with either parenteral or oral acyclovir is indicated, depending on the severity of the disease.

26. The answer is **B**, page 922.
Asymmetric upper motor neuron findings (hyperreflexia) and urinary retention in this patient are highly suggestive of spinal cord compression. Peripheral neuropathy, which may be caused by the side effects of chemotherapy, is associated with lower motor neuron and sensory abnormalities in the distribution of a peripheral nerve, while motor cortex dysfunction is associated with upper motor neuron findings in the absence of lower motor neuron findings. Localized tumor metastasis to bone or local invasion into muscle does not account for the neurologic findings in this case but may result in a limp.

27. The answer is **B**, page 910.
The patient with sickle cell disease has anemia in the context of an unexpectedly low reticulocyte count (see Table 54-4 on page 907 in Barkin et al). This most likely represents a hypoplastic crisis because sickle cell disease is a chronic hemolytic anemia; the marrow must be hyperactive to maintain hemoglobin levels in the acceptable range. Thus any insult to erythrocyte precursors, such as that produced by parvovirus, can result relatively rapidly in anemia. The therapy for this condition is simple transfusion with packed red cells. Unless the patient is in florid congestive heart failure resulting from hypoplastic crisis, exchange transfusion or inotropic support is not necessary. However, partial exchange transfusion may be indicated in situations such as the acute chest syndrome. An elevated white cell count is expected in patients with sickle cell disease and in the absence of fever does not indicate infection. Iron therapy is not indicated for hypoplastic crisis, and the normocytic red cells do not support iron deficiency as a cause for the low reticulocyte count.

28. The answer is **A**, pages 897 to 899.
The patient of Mediterranean ancestry with a history of poor dietary intake described in the vignette has a mild hypochromic, microcytic anemia and a Mentzer index (MCV/RBC ratio) of 13.6, which is more consistent with iron deficiency anemia than thalassemia. The diagnosis of iron deficiency anemia can be confirmed with a serum ferritin level. Serum ferritin levels less than 10 μg/L at any age indicate depletion of iron stores in the body. The serum ferritin result may be falsely negative, however, in patients with conditions that transiently elevate ferritin levels such as infection, inflammation, or liver disease. The quantitative hemoglobin electrophoresis indicates the presence of β-thalassemia trait by demonstrating increases in hemoglobins A_2 and F. However, coexistent iron deficiency may prevent the expected increases in both of these hemoglobins, leading to a false negative result. Thus in clinical situations in which the differential diagnosis is between iron deficiency and β-thalassemia, the possibility of iron deficiency should be addressed before quantitative hemoglobin electrophoresis is ordered.

29. The answer is **A,** page 901.

The infant with skeletal dysmorphism presented in the vignette has a profound macrocytic anemia and normal white blood cell and platelet counts but an inappropriately low reticulocyte count, suggesting red blood underproduction consistent with Diamond-Blackfan syndrome. Diamond-Blackfan syndrome is a disorder of unknown etiology resulting in a failure of erythropoiesis most likely caused by an as yet uncharacterized defect in the erythroid stem cell. The symptoms are insidious with progressive pallor, irritability, and listlessness usually manifesting within the first 3 months of life. Delayed onset beyond the first year, however, has been reported. Congenital malformations have been reported in approximately a fourth of the affected children. Skeletal dysmorphia of the upper extremity, including triphalangeal thumbs, has been reported most frequently. Patients have no evidence of jaundice, adenopathy, or hepatosplenomegaly, and bone marrow examination demonstrates few or no nucleated erythroid cells and no abnormalities of the granulocyte cell line or the megakaryocytes. Transient erythroblastopenia of childhood (TEC) is an acquired, transient hypoplastic anemia of unknown etiology usually appearing in previously healthy children within the first 3 years of life. The anemia is normochromic, and most children recover spontaneously within 1 to 2 months without recurrence. Parvovirus infection does not appear to be associated with TEC.

Iron deficiency would be an unusual cause of profound anemia within the first 6 months of life in term neonates. Additionally, although the reticulocyte count is depressed in iron deficiency anemia, the red cells are microcytic rather than macrocytic. Tumor replacement of the bone marrow also may produce anemia and a decrease in the reticulocyte count, but other cell lines would also be decreased in numbers in the bone marrow and in peripheral blood. Decreased levels of erythropoietin caused by chronic renal disease result in a hypoplastic anemia, but the red blood cells are normocytic and not macrocytic.

30. The answer is **B,** pages 901 and 902.

The previously healthy, well-appearing, mildly febrile infant described in the vignette has mild leukopenia (total peripheral white blood cell count less than 5000/mm^3), moderate neutropenia (an absolute neutrophil count of 500 to 1000/mm^3), and a compensatory monocytosis without anemia or thrombocytopenia. The most likely cause of transient neutropenia in children outside the immediate newborn period is viral infection. The neutropenia develops during the initial 2 days of illness, usually coincident with viremia, and gradually resolves over approximately 3 to 6 days. Thus continued observation with clinical follow-up of the patient is the most appropriate management strategy.

Neutropenia may occur in the context of a bacterial infection. However, such patients usually appear toxic or have risk factors for or clinical evidence of sepsis. Leukopenia is occasionally the first sign of acute leukemia. The presence of associated cytopenias, adenopathy, or hepatosplenomegaly or the persistence of the leukopenia beyond the duration expected may suggest this diagnosis and necessitate referral for bone marrow examination.

Infectious Disorders

Robert Lembo

See Barkin et al: Chapter 55.

1. A 22-day-old full-term infant who was delivered after an uncomplicated pregnancy and labor is brought in for evaluation of fever. The infant is feeding well although reported to be crying more than usual. There is no history of coughing, vomiting, or diarrhea. The rectal temperature is 38.7° C. The physical examination is unremarkable except for some erythema of the left tympanic membrane. The most appropriate management of this infant is:
   A. Observation only.
   B. Administration of oral amoxicillin with telephone follow-up in 24 hours.
   C. Performance of a complete blood count (CBC) and urinalysis with cultures of blood, cerebrospinal fluid (CSF), and urine; follow-up in 24 hours if screening results are within normal limits.
   D. Performance of a CBC and urinalysis with cultures of blood, CSF, and urine; hospitalization and empiric antimicrobial therapy.
   E. Performance of a CBC and urinalysis with cultures of blood, CSF, and urine; administration of intramuscular (IM) ceftriaxone and follow-up in 24 hours if screening results are within normal limits.

2. A previously well 10-month-old girl has had fever for 2 days. She has no history of coughing, vomiting, or diarrhea. She is reported to have had reduced intake of solids but no change in fluid intake. She is described by her mother as "cranky" for the past day. Examination shows an alert, interactive, and acyanotic infant with a temperature of 40.3° C, stable vital signs, scant clear rhinorrhea without abnormalities in the tympanic membranes, and mild pharyngeal erythema without exudate. The anterior fontanelle is flat, and the neck is supple. The most appropriate management of this infant is:
   A. Screening CBC and blood culture with observation at home if screening CBC is within normal limits
   B. Screening CBC and urinalysis and blood and urine cultures with observation at home if both screening CBC and urinalysis are within normal limits.
   C. Throat culture with observation at home.
   D. Administration of antipyretics to control fever with continued observation at home.
   E. Administration of IM ceftriaxone with follow-up in 12 hours.

3. A 3-year-old previously healthy boy attending day care is brought to the ED after having a 5-minute generalized tonic-clonic seizure. The parents report that he "felt warm" earlier in the day and had a "stomachache" and several loose stools at day care. Examination reveals an alert, well-hydrated boy with a rectal temperature (T) of 102° F, a heart rate (HR) of 110 beats per minute, and a blood pressure (BP) of 96/65 mm Hg. His neck is supple, and no evidence of focal neurologic deficits is present. The abdomen is mildly distended and soft with some poorly localized tenderness to deep palpation but without guarding or rebound tenderness. The bowel sounds are hyperactive. Genitourinary (GU) examination shows the boy has not been circumcised. Of the following choices, the most appropriate test to help establish the cause of this patient's seizure is:

A. Computed tomography (CT) of the head.
B. Lumbar puncture.
C. Urine culture.
D. Stool culture.
E. Urine toxicology screen.

4. A 4-month-old previously well boy returns for reevaluation of unexplained fever to 39.7° C of 3 days' duration. The parents deny exposure to ill contacts or recent immunizations. Examination reveals an alert, mildly irritable, well-perfused infant with a rectal T of 39° C, an HR of 112 beats per minute, and a respiratory rate (RR) of 22 breaths per minute. The anterior fontanelle is flat, the chest is clear, and the abdomen is mildly tender to deep palpation. GU examination reveals the boy is uncircumcised. A CBC obtained at the initial visit demonstrates a hemoglobin concentration of 11.5 g/dl, a total peripheral white cell count of 12,300/mm³ with 56% polymorphonuclear cells and 8% band forms, and a sedimentation rate (Wintrobe) of 30 mm/hr. A catheterized specimen of urine is growing 100,000 colonies of an unidentified organism. Of the following choices the most likely source of this patient's fever is:

A. Occult pneumonia.
B. Early meningitis.
C. Occult gastroenteritis
D. Urinary tract infection.
E. Vasculitis.

5. A 7-month-old infant delivered from a mother known to abuse crack cocaine and heroin has fever and coughing of 6 days' duration. Examination reveals an alert, acyanotic infant with T 38.7° C, RR 60 breaths per minute, intercostal retractions, rales, and intermittent end-expiratory wheezing. Chest radiograph reveals diffuse, bilateral alveolar and interstitial infiltrates with air bronchograms and no hilar adenopathy. Arterial blood gas determination in room air reveals an alveolar/arterial oxygen gradient of 35 torr. The most likely cause of the findings in this infant is:

A. Cytomegalovirus (CMV) infection.
B. *Mycobacterium tuberculosis* infection.
C. *Pneumocystis carinii* pneumonia (PCP).
D. Lymphocytic interstitial pneumonia (LIP).
E. *Mycoplasma pneumoniae* infection.

6. A 3-month-old full-term infant who recently arrived from South America has a history of yellow skin and light-colored stools of 3 days' duration. The birth history includes jaundice in the immediate newborn period resulting from erythroblastosis fetalis, which required double-volume exchange transfusion. Examination reveals an alert, icteric neonate who is afebrile and well perfused. The abdomen is rounded and soft with a liver edge extending 2.5 cm below the right costal margin and no palpable spleen tip. No murmur is audible on chest examination. CBC demonstrates a hemoglobin concentration of 11 g/dl, a total peripheral white cell count of 12,200/mm³, a platelet count of 170,000/mm³, and a reticulocyte count of 0.8%. The total bilirubin is 44 mg/dl with a direct reacting fraction of 2 mg/dl. The alanine aminotransferase (ALT) level is 460 U/L, and the aspartate aminotransferase (AST) level is 320 U/L. The most likely cause of clinical findings in this infant is:

A. Extrahepatic biliary atresia.
B. Epstein-Barr virus infection.
C. Wilson's disease
D. Hepatitis C infection.
E. Early onset congenital syphilis.

7. A 6-year-old boy who recently arrived from Southeast Asia is referred for evaluation of severe pharyngitis, low-grade fever, and weakness of 2 days' duration. Examination shows an ill-appearing boy with T 38.2° C and HR 140 beats per minute. He has cervical adenopathy and a pronounced grayish pharyngeal coating that bleeds when probed with a tongue blade. The oropharynx has a "mousy" odor. He has no stridor, drooling, or trismus. The most likely diagnosis is:

A. Peritonsillar abscess.
B. Infectious mononucleosis.
C. Group A streptococcal pharyngitis.
D. Pharyngeal gonorrhea.
E. Pharyngeal diphtheria.

8. A 4-year-old girl who recently immigrated to the United States is referred for treatment of parasites found in the stool on routine medical examination. The patient has had no fever, abdominal pain, vomiting, or diarrhea. The laboratory report notes the presence of *Blastocystis hominis* and cysts of *Balantidium coli* and *Entamoeba histolytica*. The best treatment for this child is:

A. Observation only.
B. Iodoquinol.
C. Tetracycline.
D. Metronidazole (Flagyl).
E. Praziquantel.

9. A previously well 5-year-old boy has a 2-week history of anorexia, headache, and intermittent fevers to 40° C after a visit to South America. Examination reveals an alert child with a fever of 40.3° C and an HR of 98 beats per minute. He has a palpable spleen tip at the left costal margin. The patient has a "rose spot" rash and watery diarrhea. A CBC is remarkable for a hemoglobin level of 12 g/dl and a total peripheral white cell count of 3800/mm^3 with 15% band forms on differential. The most likely cause of this child's illness is:
   A. Brucellosis.
   B. Leptospirosis.
   C. Typhoid fever.
   D. Malaria.
   E. Amebiasis.

10. A previously well 17-year-old boy visiting the United States from Mexico has fever, coughing, and right upper quadrant pain radiating to the right shoulder of 4 days' duration. Examination reveals an ill-appearing, anicteric boy with an oral T of 39° C, a tender liver edge palpable 2 cm below the right costal margin, and no splenomegaly or adenopathy. Chest roentgenogram reveals an elevated right hemidiaphragm with a small pleural reaction and no evidence of lobar or interstitial infiltrate. The most appropriate therapy for this patient at this time is:
   A. Isoniazid, rifampin, and pyrazinamide.
   B. Cefuroxime.
   C. Surgical removal of the gallbladder.
   D. Metronidazole.
   E. Supportive therapy only.

11. A previously well 16-month-old boy is referred for assessment of a rapidly progressing rash associated with a 1-day history of fever. The child is acyanotic but lethargic with T 39.5° C, HR 165 beats per minute, and BP 85/60 mm Hg. A petechial rash with some areas of confluent ecchymosis covers the face, trunk, and the extremities, including the palms and soles. The most likely diagnosis is:
   A. Group A streptococcal infection.
   B. Measles.
   C. Enteroviral infection.
   D. Meningococcemia.
   E. Rocky Mountain spotted fever.

12. A previously well 3-year-old child has progressive red, itchy skin lesions developing several days after a family vacation trip to a farm in the southeastern United States. Examination reveals an afebrile boy with several erythematous, elevated, serpiginous, "tracklike" lesions on the dorsum of the hands and feet. There is no hepatosplenomegaly. The most appropriate treatment for this child's disorder is:
   A. 1% Hydrocortisone cream.
   B. Amoxicillin.
   C. Thiabendazole.
   D. 5% Permethrin.
   E. Lindane (gamma benzene hexachloride).

13. A 3-month-old boy born at 36 weeks' gestation is brought in for evaluation of increasing lethargy. The parents report that the infant's cry has been "weak" and that his oral intake of a soy-based formula supplemented with honey to increase caloric intake has decreased. The infant has not had a bowel movement in 3 days. Examination shows an alert, anicteric, afebrile infant with stable vital signs, a flat anterior fontanelle, open sutures, poor suck, bilateral ptosis, decreased active and passive tone, decreased deep tendon reflexes, and a hoarse cry. The tongue is of normal size, and no fasciculations are noted. The most likely diagnosis is:
   A. Werdnig-Hoffmann disease.
   B. Hypothyroidism.
   C. Group B streptococcal sepsis.
   D. Guillain-Barré syndrome.
   E. Botulism.

14. A previously well 10-month-old boy is referred for evaluation of fever to 40.2° C persisting for 6 days. He has a T of 39.7° C and an HR of 180 beats per minute. Examination reveals an alert but irritable infant with an erythematous, polymorphic rash over the trunk associated with swelling of the hands and feet. There is scant clear nasal discharge associated with an erythematous oropharynx and conjunctival injection. A soft gallop rhythm is auscultated at the cardiac apex. The most appropriate next step in the evaluation of this child is:
   A. Lumbar puncture.
   B. Throat culture.
   C. Platelet count.
   D. Echocardiogram.
   E. Antinuclear antibody test.

15. A 3-year-old boy who resides with his parents on a farm is brought in for evaluation of lassitude and fever of several days' duration. The mother reports that her son eats soil and has been bitten recently by his puppy. Examination reveals an alert but tired-appearing child who is well perfused and has a temperature of 39° C. The liver extends 3 cm below the right costal margin and is nontender. The spleen is not palpable. Funduscopic examination is unremarkable. A screening CBC reveals a hemoglobin concentration of 10.8 g/dl, a total peripheral white cell count of 14,300/mm^3 with 43% polymorphonuclear cells, 4% band forms, 35% lymphocytes, 3% monocytes, and 15% eosinophils, and a platelet count of 174,000/mm^3. The most appropriate treatment for this patient's underlying disorder is:
   A. Chloroquine.
   B. Metronidazole.
   C. Ivermectin.
   D. Praziquantel.
   E. Thiabendazole.

16. A 4-year-old boy visiting from the Caribbean has a persistent cough. His parents report that he has had complaints of abdominal pain intermittently for the past year. Examination reveals a well-appearing, afebrile child with rales at the right lung base posteriorly. He has no murmur or hepatosplenomegaly. Chest radiograph reveals a patchy infiltrate in the right lower lobe. A CBC reveals a hemoglobin concentration of 11 g/dl, a total peripheral white blood cell count of 8500/mm³ with 45% polymorphonuclear cells, 2% band forms, 35% lymphocytes, 3% monocytes, and 15% eosinophils, a platelet count of 165,000/mm³, and a reticulocyte count of 0.6%. The most appropriate study to perform next in the evaluation of this patient is:
    A. Blood culture.
    B. Sputum culture.
    C. Nasopharyngeal swab for *Chlamydia trachomatis*.
    D. Stool sample for ova and parasites.
    E. Serologic test for *Mycoplasma pneumoniae*.

17. A previously healthy 16-year-old boy has fever, headache, anorexia, and myalgia of 3 days' duration after returning from a summer camping trip 10 days before he comes into the ED. His mother reports that he was exposed to a camper with "the flu" and was bitten by many "bugs" during the trip. Examination reveals an ill-appearing boy with a temperature of 39.7° C, mild tachycardia, and stable blood pressure. No rash or meningeal signs are noted. A CBC demonstrates a hemoglobin concentration of 14 g/dl, a total white blood cell count of 3200/mm³ with 48% polymorphonuclear cells and 4% band forms, and a platelet count of 92,000/mm³. The most likely cause of the clinical findings in this boy is:
    A. Influenza A infection.
    B. *Ehrlichia* infection.
    C. Lyme disease.
    D. Rocky Mountain spotted fever.
    E. System lupus erythematosus.

18. A 13-year-old boy recently discharged from the hospital with extensive partial-thickness burns comes in for evaluation of fever, myalgia, headache, and diarrhea of 2 days' duration. Examination reveals an ill-appearing, disoriented boy with T 39.2° C, HR 128 beats per minute, RR 30 breaths per minute, and BP 86/50 mm Hg. Healing burns on the lower extremities are noted along with diffuse erythema of the skin and mucus membranes and hyperemia of the conjunctivae. The most likely diagnosis in this patient is:
    A. Leptospirosis.
    B. Rocky Mountain spotted fever.
    C. Kawasaki disease (mucocutaneous lymph node syndrome).
    D. *Neisseria meningitidis* sepsis.
    E. Toxic shock syndrome.

19. A previously well 8-month-old girl has persistent fever to 40.2° C and irritability of 4 days' duration. No ill contacts are identified. Examination reveals an alert, interactive infant with a rectal T of 37.6° C, stable vital signs, an open and flat anterior fontanelle, and a supple neck. The patient has mild erythema of the tonsils and pharynx without exudate, mild injection of the tympanic membranes, and palpable suboccipital and posterior auricular lymph nodes. An erythematous, discrete maculopapular rash that is most prominent on the neck and trunk blanches with pressure and was not noted previously. The most likely cause of this infant's illness is:
    A. Group A streptococcal infection.
    B. Transient pneumococcal bacteremia resulting from otitis media.
    C. Rubeola (measles).
    D. Human herpesvirus 6 infection.
    E. Parvovirus infection.

20. An 8-year-old boy has had a progressive rash over the past 3 days. His mother reports that he had an episode of fever, chills, mild headache, and myalgia for 2 days approximately 1 week before she brought him in. He has had no recent exposure to drugs and currently has no complaints. Examination reveals a well-appearing, afebrile boy with a confluent erythematous eruption on the face, involving the cheeks bilaterally but sparing the perioral area, and a new mildly pruritic maculopapular eruption with areas of central clearing on the extremities. He has no adenopathy or hepatosplenomegaly. The most appropriate next step in the evaluation of this patient's rash is:
    A. Perform a rapid group A streptococcal antigen test.
    B. Order Western blot assay for *Borrelia*.
    C. Order immunoglobulin M (IgM) antibody assay for parvovirus B19.
    D. Order liver function tests.
    E. Order antinuclear antibody assay.

21. A 4-year-old girl is referred for evaluation of chronic vaginal discharge that is unresponsive to local hygienic measures and empiric treatment with ceftriaxone. The parents report that there is no suspicion of sexual abuse and no observation of genital manipulation by the child. They are concerned because she awakens at night complaining of an itchy sensation in the perineum. Examination reveals an afebrile, well-appearing girl, an intact hymen with mild inflammation of the vulva and vagina, scant discharge, and multiple excoriations around the perineum and anus without evidence of other skin lesions. Visual inspection of the introitus reveals no foreign body. A vaginal culture obtained a week ago is growing mixed flora of gram-negative organisms, including *Escherichia coli*, but is negative for *Neisseria gonorrhoeae*. The most appropriate test to perform next in the evaluation of this child is:
    A. Pelvic ultrasound.
    B. Culture for *Chlamydia pneumoniae*.
    C. KOH preparation for *Candida albicans*.
    D. Cellophane tape test for *Enterobius vermicularis*.

22. A 1-year-old boy has 4 days of intermittent fever to 40° C, headache, myalgia, vomiting, and a progressive rash shortly after returning from a camping trip. Examination reveals an ill-appearing boy with fever of 39.4° C and a blanching, erythematous, maculopapular rash distributed preponderantly over the palms, wrist, soles, and feet. The total peripheral white blood cell count is 3500/mm^3 with 10% band forms, and the platelet count is 95,000/mm^3. The CSF has 4 white blood cells (WBCs)/mm^3. The treatment of choice for this patient is:
   A. Corticosteroids.
   B. Tetracycline.
   C. Ceftriaxone.
   D. Penicillin.
   E. Amantadine.

23. A previously well 4-year-old boy returning with his parents after a 1-year stay in Southeast Asia has fever for 8 days. The parents report that the child attended day care until 5 days before departure and recall that he was exposed to another child with fever within the preceding 2 weeks. They are particularly concerned that a "brassy" cough, pink eye, and sore throat have developed. Examination reveals an ill-appearing child with a temperature of 39.5° C, mild tachycardia, and stable blood pressure. He has nasal congestion with clear discharge, bilateral conjunctival injection associated with lacrimation, and pharyngeal erythema without exudate. The buccal mucosa opposite the lower molars is noted to have multiple 1-mm white lesions on an erythematous background. The lungs are clear, and no adenopathy is noted. He has no rash on his trunk or extremities. The most appropriate test for ascertaining the cause of this patient's illness is:
   A. Rapid streptococcal antigen detection test.
   B. Serum IgM antibody test to measles virus.
   C. Echocardiography.
   D. Bedside cold agglutinin determination.
   E. Heterophil antibody test.

24. A previously well 16-year-old boy has fatigue and "swollen glands" of 8 days' duration. He reports feeling "achy" and has had a mild sore throat without cough or nasal discharge. Several of his friends with whom he attended a picnic have had similar symptoms within the past week. Examination reveals a well-appearing boy with T 38.1° C and normal HR, RR, and BP. There is diffuse cervical and suboccipital adenopathy without erythema or tenderness. The pharynx is nonerythematous, and the tonsils have no exudate. The abdomen is soft, and no hepatosplenomegaly or rash is noted. A rapid streptococcal antigen test performed on a pharyngeal swab specimen and a heterophil antibody test performed on serum are negative. Of the following choices, the most likely cause of the findings in this patient is:
   A. Epstein-Barr virus.
   B. Rubella.
   C. *Toxoplasma gondii.*
   D. *Mycoplasma pneumoniae.*
   E. Atypical mycobacteria.

25. A 4-year-old child currently in foster care has a 2-week history of persistent nonproductive coughing unaccompanied by fever. Examination is unremarkable except for some palpable right cervical lymph nodes. Chest roentgenogram reveals a right upper lobe infiltrate with a pleural reaction and blunting of the right costophrenic angle. The most appropriate next step in the evaluation of this patient is:
   A. Nasopharyngeal culture for *Bordetella pertussis.*
   B. Nasopharyngeal swab for respiratory syncytial virus (RSV) antigen detection.
   C. Diagnostic thoracentesis.
   D. Mantoux test (PPD).
   E. Acute phase *Mycoplasma pneumoniae* titer.

26. A previously well 7-year-old boy has a facial "droop" of acute onset. His parents deny the boy's having fever, coughing, or recent exposure to ill contacts. He denies facial pain, earache, or hearing loss. Examination reveals an afebrile, well-appearing boy with weakness on the right side of the face in the distribution of the seventh cranial nerve. All other cranial nerves appear intact. The tympanic membrane is normal in appearance and mobility. Cranial computeed tomography is unremarkable. A lumbar puncture reveals 112 total nucleated cells and no red blood cells, a total protein level of 133 mg/dl, and a glucose level of 78 mg/dl. The Gram's stain is negative. The most appropriate test to perform next in the evaluation of this patient is:
   A. Magnetic resonance imaging (MRI) of the brain.
   B. IgG and IgM enzyme-linked immunosorbent assay (ELISA) for antibody to *Borrelia burgdorferi.*
   C. Mantoux intradermal skin test.
   D. Polymerase chain reaction assay of CSF for herpes simplex virus.
   E. Roentgenograms of the paranasal sinuses.

27. A previously well 15-year-old boy has acute testicular pain. He reports having headache, photophobia, and mild abdominal pain for 6 days and the onset of fever on the day before. He denies local trauma, sexual activity, or urethral discharge. Examination reveals a mildly ill-appearing boy with an oral T of 38.6° C who is in considerable pain. The left testicle is in the scrotum and appears swollen and exquisitely tender to palpation. The right testis and the urethral meatus are unremarkable, and a rectal examination reveals no prostate tenderness. The most likely cause of the findings in this boy is:
   A. Acute testicular torsion.
   B. Brucellosis.
   C. Torsion of the appendix testis.
   D. Epididymitis-orchitis caused by *Chlamydia trachomatis.*
   E. Mumps orchitis.

28. A 5-month-old boy has a history of cyanosis and acute cessation of breathing. The parents report that he had had a persistent but intermittent cough for the previous 14 days associated with rhinorrhea and nasal congestion with some lacrimation. Examination reveals an acyanotic, afebrile infant with mild tachypnea and no evidence of respiratory distress. Diffuse moist rales are noted on auscultation of the chest. He has no murmur or wheezing audible. The abdomen is soft, and hepatosplenomegaly is not noted. A chest roentgenogram demonstrates bilateral perihilar infiltrates. A CBC demonstrates a hemoglobin concentration of 11.7 g/dl, a total peripheral white count of 13,600/mm³ with 30% polymorphonuclear cells, 2% band forms, 56% lymphocytes, 10% monocytes, and 2% eosinophils, and a platelet count of 300,000/mm³. The most likely diagnosis in this infant is:

    A. Asthma.
    B. RSV-induced bronchiolitis.
    C. *C. trachomatis* pneumonia.
    D. Pertussis.
    E. Epstein-Barr virus infection.

29. A previously well 18-month-old infant has high fever and refuses to eat. The parents report onset of fever and irritability 2 days ago. No ill contacts are identified. Examination reveals an irritable, poorly consolable toddler with a rectal T of 39.5° C, mild tachycardia, stable blood pressure, and no evidence of dehydration. There are tender anterior cervical nodes bilaterally. The gingiva is erythematous and bleeds when touched with a tongue blade. The tongue has several vesicular lesions, and the anterior and posterior oropharynx is covered with discrete, 1- to 3-mm, shallow gray ulcers on an erythematous base. No lesions appear on the skin of the face, trunk, or extremities. The most likely cause of this child's febrile illness is:

    A. Caustic ingestion with bacterial superinfection.
    B. Primary herpes simplex gingivostomatitis.
    C. Herpangina
    D. Acute necrotizing ulcerative gingivitis (Vincent's infection).
    E. Actinomycosis.

30. A previously well 7-day-old full-term boy is referred for evaluation of lethargy and poor feeding of acute onset. The infant was delivered vaginally without incident to a primigravida mother with a history of primary syphilis treated with penicillin during the second trimester and was discharged at 48 hours. A reactive rapid plasma reagin test was performed on cord blood in a titer of 1:1. The mother complains of persistent vaginal pain, itching, and dysuria beginning just before the onset of labor. Examination reveals a lethargic, moderately icteric neonate with a rectal T of 39.0° C, tachycardia, mild tachypnea, and BP of 75/50 mm Hg. The anterior fontanelle is full with the infant reclining, and both the active and passive muscle tone is decreased. The abdomen is soft, and the liver extends 3.5 cm below the right costal margin. There are no lesions on the skin. The differential diagnosis of this infant includes each of the following *except:*

    A. Group B streptococcal sepsis.
    B. Disseminated herpes simplex infection.
    C. Congenital syphilis.
    D. Galactosemia with *E. coli* sepsis.
    E. Posterior urethral valves with urinary tract infection.

31. A 13-year-old girl has fever and fatigue of 2½ weeks' duration. She also reports decreased appetite, headache, and night sweats. Examination reveals an alert but mildly ill-appearing girl in no respiratory distress with T of 39.1° C and stable vital signs. She has bilateral periorbital edema without ethmoid or frontal sinus tenderness or erythema. Her tonsils are enlarged, erythematous, and covered with exudate, and petechiae are noted on the palate. The posterior cervical nodes are enlarged and nontender. The liver is palpable 2 cm below the right costal margin, and the spleen is palpable 1 cm below the left costal margin. The platelet count is 98,000/mm³. The test most likely to reveal the cause of the findings in this patient is:

    A. Heterophil antibody assay.
    B. Rapid streptococcal antigen test.
    C. Hepatitis B surface antigen test
    D. Antinuclear antibody test.
    E. Bone marrow aspiration.

32. A 7-year-old boy, whose prior health maintenance status is known and whose immunization schedule is up to date, is bitten on the leg by an unidentified fur-bearing animal encountered in a heavily wooded area. The boy states that the attack was unprovoked and that the animal was not recovered. Examination reveals an irregular wound on the medial aspect of the right lower extremity that extends to the dermis without surrounding erythema. The most appropriate management of this child is:

    A. Local wound cleansing and observation for local infection.
    B. Administration of human diploid cell rabies vaccine (HDCV).
    C. Administration of tetanus toxoid and HDCV.
    D. Administration of tetanus toxoid only.
    E. Administration of HDCV and human rabies immunoglobulin (HRIG).

33. A 12-year-old boy with a 2-year history of diabetes mellitus in good control has an acute exacerbation of chronic, recurrent asthma while he is exercising in cold weather during the fall. Examination reveals an afebrile, acyanotic boy with coughing, tachypnea, minimal intercostal retractions, and diffuse end-expiratory wheezing. The peak expiratory flow rate is less than 80% of the predicted value. Urinalysis shows no glucose or ketones. The patient responds to one administration of nebulized albuterol. The peak expiratory flow rate at the completion of therapy is 95% of the predicted value. In addition to an albuterol inhaler, this patient would benefit from:

    A. *Mycoplasma pneumoniae* serologic testing.
    B. Skin testing for inhalant allergens.
    C. Influenza vaccine.
    D. T and B cell quantification.
    E. Pneumococcal vaccine.

34. An 8-year-old girl visiting from Gambia has had intermittent fever for 2 weeks. Her mother reports that she typically has fever to 40° C every 2 days preceded by chills, rapid heart rate, and vomiting, followed by severe headache, nausea, and diaphoresis. Examination reveals an afebrile, alert child with stable vital signs in no distress. Abdominal examination is notable for a liver edge 3 cm below the right costal margin and a spleen tip 1.5 cm below the left costal margin. She has no rash or adenopathy. A CBC demonstrates a hemoglobin concentration of 10 g/dl, an MCV of 80 fL, a total white blood cell count of 3900/mm^3, and a platelet count of 102,000/mm^3. The test most likely to establish a diagnosis in this patient is:

    A. Bone marrow aspiration.
    B. Serial blood cultures.
    C. ELISA assay for HIV antibody.
    D. Thick and thin blood smears.
    E. Epstein-Barr virus IgG and IgM viral capsid antigen titers.

35. A 7-year-old-girl returning with her parents from a 1-week vacation in the Caribbean has fever and headache. The parents are concerned because she had sudden onset of fever to 41° C and complaints of severe retroorbital and muscle pain for 3 days followed by 2 days of improvement before the onset 1 day ago of nausea, vomiting, and abdominal pain. Examination reveals an alert child who is afebrile with stable vital signs. She has generalized maculopapular rash sparing the palms and soles and generalized lymphadenopathy without hepatosplenomegaly. A CBC demonstrates a normal hematocrit and platelet count. The most likely vector for this patient's illness is:

    A. *Aedes aegypti.*
    B. *Ixodes scapularis.*
    C. *Dermacentor variabilis.*
    D. *Loxosceles reclusa.*
    E. *Sarcoptes scabiei.*

ANSWERS   [See Barkin et al: Chapter 55.]

1. The answer is **D,** pages 930 and 931.

Although the management of the young, febrile infant remains controversial, the current consensus continues to favor a highly conservative approach. Thus most clinicians opt to perform a complete clinical and laboratory evaluation to assess risk of major focal (pneumonia, meningitis, and urinary tract infection) or bacteremic infection in the infant less than 1 month of age who has fever. The presence of findings suggestive of otitis media, a frequently encountered minor focus of infection amenable to treatment with oral antimicrobials in an older infant, does not eliminate the possibility of a concurrent major deep soft tissue focus of infection or bacteremia in a young infant. Although ceftriaxone has been used for empiric therapy of older febrile infants who are at low risk for bacterial infection, the drug is not recommended for infants less than 1 month of age.

2. The answer is **B,** page 931.

In the young child with significant elevation of temperature without a defined focus, deep soft tissue major foci of infection (pneumonia, meningitis, and urinary tract infection) and occult bacteremia must be considered in the differential diagnosis. The presence of minor upper respiratory tract symptoms does not argue against either a major deep soft tissue focus or occult bacteremia. Thus an appropriate approach to assessing risk of underlying focal or bacteremic infection in the patient in this vignette is to order a screening CBC and urinalysis along with the appropriate confirmatory tests (i.e., blood and urine cultures). The confirmatory tests, especially the urine culture, should be obtained concurrently with the screening tests because of a significant rate of false negative risk classifications using the results of either the CBC or the urinalysis. Empiric administration of antimicrobials without confirmatory testing is to be discouraged because disease status cannot be ascertained without the results of appropriate cultures. Observation alone is not sufficiently sensitive to assess risk of underlying occult bacteremia, especially in young infants with hyperpyrexia (fever greater than 40° C).

3. The answer is **D,** page 929 (see also page 835).

The patient described in this vignette with a generalized tonic-clonic seizure in association with a fever has gastrointestinal (GI) co-morbidity, suggesting infection with an enteric pathogen such as *Shigella.* Although shigellosis frequently presents with the clinical picture of dysentery, the classic clinical course of infection with *Shigella* organisms starts in the small intestine and progresses subsequently to the large intestine. In the classic case the onset of disease is abrupt and the illness is characterized by fever, toxic appearance, and cramping abdominal pain. Initially the patient has high-volume, watery diarrhea reflecting small bowel involvement followed by low-volume, blood- and mucus-containing stools reflecting large bowel disease. The symptoms of urgency and tenesmus usually herald large bowel involvement. Brief, generalized tonic-clonic seizures are noted in a substantial number of children with *Shigella* infection admitted to the hospital. The incidence of *Shigella*-associated seizures in the community, however, is unclear. Also unclear is the pathogenesis of seizures with *Shigella* infection. Some investigators have implicated Shiga toxin as a factor. Definitive diagnosis of *Shigella* requires isolation of the organism from stool specimens or rectal swabs, using selective growth media. However, even under ideal circumstances, approximately 20% of the infected patients have negative stool cultures. Meningitis or an occult focus of infection must be considered in any patient with fever and seizures. However, the nonfocal neurologic examination and the lack of meningeal signs make intracranial infection unlikely in this case. A first urinary tract infection is a more likely cause of unexplained fever with or without seizures in boys, especially those who are uncircumcised and younger than 6 months old. Toxic ingestions may cause fever and seizure but are often associated with a specific "toxidrome," which assists in clinical recognition.

4. The answer is **D**, pages 929 and 930.

The presence of 10,000 or more organisms in urine obtained by catheterization from symptomatic patients strongly suggests urinary tract infection (UTI). The presence of more than 100,000 organisms in a bagged or clean catch specimen from a girl is presumptive evidence of a UTI. The febrile boy described in this vignette is uncircumcised, which is a recognized risk factor for UTI, and falls in an age range (younger than 6 months) when first UTIs among boys frequently occur. Other serious bacterial infections, such as meningitis and pneumonia, also can occur at this age, and the clinician must be cautious in the approach to the febrile infant. However, the lack of tachypnea or signs of respiratory distress argues against occult ("clinically silent") pneumonia, and the benign clinical appearance, mild degree of irritability, and flat fontanelle argue against both pneumonia and meningitis in this patient. The most common form of vasculitis in young infants is Kawasaki disease (mucocutaneous lymph node syndrome), the clinical features of which are lacking in this baby (Table 47-1).

5. The answer is **C**, pages 931 and 932.

The clinical and laboratory features of the infant in the vignette are highly suggestive of *Pneumocystis carinii* pneumonia (PCP). PCP may be the manifestation of pediatric HIV infection. Specifically, the presence of bilateral mixed alveolar and interstitial infiltrates without hilar adenopathy and the significant room air alveolar-arterial pressure gradient (greater than 20 torr) in the patient described in the vignette suggest PCP rather than *Mycobacterium tuberculosis* or cytomegalovirus. Lymphocytic interstitial pneumonitis usually occurs as a chronic, progressive interstitial lung disorder characterized by a fine reticular or reticulonodular pattern on chest roentgenogram that can impair pulmonary function sufficiently to cause hypoxemia, generally in the second or third year of life. Although pneumonia caused by *Mycoplasma pneumoniae* may be associated with a mixed picture on chest roentgenogram, it is rare in young infants and uncommon in children under 2 years of age.

6. The answer is **D**, page 929 (see also page 841).

The 3-month-old infant described in this vignette has clinical and laboratory evidence of hepatocellular dysfunction and cholestasis consistent with hepatitis rather than hemolysis. An important factor in considering the etiology of hepatitis in this patient is the history of transfusion in the neonatal period. Of the primary hepatotropic viruses that cause hepatitis, hepatitis C, which has an incubation period ranging from 14 to 115 days, can be transmitted via transfusion and, of the choices given, is the most important consideration in this case. Early onset congenital syphilis usually presents with hepatosplenomegaly with or without jaundice as a result of hepatocellular dysfunction at birth. Those infected neonates who are asymptomatic at birth usually become clinically symptomatic within the first 5 weeks of life. Epstein-Barr virus (EBV) infection can cause hepatitis but would be much less common in this age range, although it is well recognized that in socioeconomically underprivileged communities or in developing countries, primary EBV infection occurs early in life. However, most EBV infections early in life are subclinical or at best mildly symptomatic. Extrahepatic biliary atresia (EHBA) is an important cause of cholestasis in early infancy. However, EHBA is a progressive disorder characterized pathologically by obliteration of the extrahepatic biliary system that results in jaundice in otherwise healthy neonates, usually between 21 and 42 days of age. Wilson's disease is an autosomal recessive multisystem disorder that is degenerative and is characterized metabolically by defective mobilization of copper from lysosomes in the liver. It is manifested clinically by variable features such as asymptomatic hepatomegaly, subacute or chronic hepatitis, and portal hypertension after the age of 5 years.

7. The answer is **E**, pages 935 and 936.

Although pharyngeal diphtheria is rare in the United States, it is not uncommon in other areas of the world where rates of childhood immunizations are lower. The patient described in the vignette has findings characteristic of this disorder, including the foul-smelling pharyngeal membrane (composed of fibrin, red cells, inflammatory cells, and epithelial cells) and the striking elevation in heart rate relative to core temperature. Group A streptococcal pharyngitis, gonococcal pharyngitis, and infectious mononucleosis are causes of exudative pharyngitis but are not associated with an adherent pharyngeal membrane. The absence of drooling or trismus makes peritonsillar abscess unlikely in this patient. However, significant underlying tissue edema caused by the necrotic effect of the phage-induced toxin produced by some strains of *Corynebacterium diphtheriae* can produce upper airway obstruction with stridor and must be differentiated from retropharyngeal abscess, bacterial supraglottitis, infectious croup, or bacterial tracheitis.

TABLE 47-1 Criteria for Diagnosis of UTI

Collection method	Probability of infection (based on colony forming units/ml[*])		
	Unlikely	Probable	Likely
Suprapubic	<10³		≥10³
Catheterization	<10³	10³-10⁴	≥10⁴
CCMS			
Male	<10³	10³-10⁴	≥10⁴
Female	<10³	10⁴-10⁵	≥10⁵
Bag	<10³	10⁴-10⁵	≥10⁵

Adapted from Dubin WA: *Pediatr Infect Dis* 3:564, 1984, and from Barkin RM and Rosen P: *Emergency pediatrics,* ed 4, St Louis, Mosby.
UTI, Urinary tract infection; *CCMS,* clean catch midstream.
[*]Pure culture.

8. The answer is **B,** page 937, Table 55-3.

The asymptomatic child described in this vignette has evidence of intraluminal colonic infestation with three protozoan parasites. The importance of *Blastocystis hominis* as a cause of gastroenteropathy is controversial, but both *Entamoeba histolytica* and *Balantidium coli* are well recognized as etiologic agents in human disease. Treatment of asymptomatic cases is important to prevent spread of infection to other individuals by the fecal-oral route and, in the case of *E. histolytica,* to decrease the risk of more serious invasive disease. Both *E. histolytica* and *B. coli* are susceptible to tetracycline, but this drug is not indicated in asymptomatic children under the age of 9 years because the risk of cosmetic deformity caused by dental staining outweighs its antiprotozoal therapeutic benefits. An alternative antiprotozoal agent is the orally administered iodoquinol (diiodohydroxyquin), which is poorly absorbed from the intestinal lumen. Its mechanism of action is unknown, but it is active against *E. histolytica, B. coli,* and *B. hominis.* Thus the therapy of choice for this child would be iodoquinol. Although effective, iodoquinol has clinically important side effects including abdominal cramps, nausea, vomiting, and anorexia at the recommended dosage of 40 mg/kg/day, and more severe side effects such as optic neuritis, optic atrophy, and peripheral neuropathy at higher dosages or with prolonged therapy. Metronidazole (Flagyl) is a bactericidal, amebicidal, and trichomonacidal agent of unknown mechanism of action that has activity against *E. histolytica* in both lumina and tissues. However, it has limited activity against encysted *E. histolytica,* making it more appropriate for the treatment of acute symptomatic intestinal amebiasis and amebic liver abscess. Praziquantel is an antihelmintic drug with a broad spectrum of activity against trematodes, including all pathogenic *Schistosoma* species, and cestodes including *Taenia saginata* (beef tapeworm) and *Taenia solium* (pork tapeworm). Praziquantel is not the drug of choice for treatment of protozoal pathogens.

9. The answer is **C,** page 940.

The patient in this vignette has prolonged hyperpyrexia accompanied by a strikingly low heart rate (temperature-pulse dissociation), reticuloendothelial cell hyperplasia (splenomegaly), and leukopenia, which are clinical features highly suggestive of typhoid fever (*Salmonella typhi*). The history of travel to an endemic area is supportive of this diagnosis. Treatment includes intravenous (IV) fluids and antibiotics such as chloramphenicol, amoxicillin, and trimethoprim-sulfamethoxazole if cultures are positive. If drug resistance is encountered, a third-generation cephalosporin may be used. Invasive amebiasis is encountered in children but usually includes enterocolitis (blood- or mucus-containing stool) or hepatic involvement characterized by right upper quadrant pain and tachypnea. Although malaria is associated with prolonged, intermittent fever, splenomegaly, and leukopenia, there is usually leukocytosis during a febrile paroxysm and anemia. Leptospirosis is an infectious vasculitis that may have either an icteric (approximately 10% of cases) or an anicteric clinical presentation. Anicteric leptospirosis is a biphasic illness characterized initially by fever, headache, myalgia, and abdominal pain, followed by defervescence and then recrudescence of fever associated with uveitis, rash, headache, and meningeal signs. Brucellosis can mimic typhoid fever clinically and epidemiologically. Patients with brucellosis have fever, mild lymphadenopathy, and hepatosplenomegaly. Arthritis and spondylitis also may occur. This diagnosis should be entertained in a patient with an enteric fever–like presentation if a history of exposure to domestic and wild animals is elicited.

10. The answer is **D,** page 937, Table 55-3.

This patient has clinical and radiographic evidence suggestive of a right-sided subdiaphragmatic inflammatory process most consistent epidemiologically with an amebic liver abscess. The drug of choice for treatment of extraintestinal amebiasis is metronidazole (see answer to question 8). The combination of isoniazid (INH), rifampin, and pyrazinamide is appropriate for patients with pulmonary tuberculosis, which is an unlikely diagnosis in this case. Cefuroxime would be an appropriate empiric choice for the initial treatment of community-acquired pneumonia of probable bacterial etiology. However, the clinical and radiographic picture is not consistent with pneumonia in this case. Gallbladder disease, including acute hydrops, cholecystitis, and cholelithiasis, is uncommon in children and adolescents but may have fever and right upper quadrant pain as initial symptoms. However, diaphragmatic and pleural involvement would be highly unusual associated findings.

11. The answer is **D,** page 945.

The patient in the vignette has acute onset of fever and petechial rash that rapidly evolves into a picture consistent with purpura fulminans. The likely cause of purpura fulminans in this patient is meningococcemia. Although Rocky Mountain spotted fever (RMSF) has similar features, the etiologic agent (*Rickettsia rickettsii*) is transmitted by tick bite and the disease usually evolves over several days. The rash in RMSF may be macular or maculopapular initially and then becomes petechial, beginning usually on the distal extremities and moving toward the trunk. Although infection with enteroviruses may include fever and petechial rash, infants and children are usually quite well appearing, unlike the patient in the vignette, and the diagnosis is one of exclusion. Group A streptococcal infection associated with toxin production (scarlet fever) may be associated with erythroderma and petechiae in skin folds (Pastia's lines) but not with purpura. Measles is a potentially serious illness but also evolves over several days with an erythematous, macular rash that becomes confluent beginning on the scalp and neck and descending to the trunk and extremities.

12. The answer is **C,** page 937, Table 55-3 (see also page 701).

The progressive skin eruption described in this child as pruritic and serpiginous is highly suggestive of infection with the larvae of the dog or cat hookworm *Ancylostoma braziliense,* the causative agent of cutaneous larva migrans. Infections with *A. braziliense* are most common among residents of and visitors to warm, humid, and sandy coastal areas, including the states bordering the Gulf of Mexico and the Atlantic Ocean in the United States. Infection is most common in children, and the larvae, which hatch from ova deposited in the feces of infected dogs or cats, penetrate human skin that comes in contact with contaminated sandy areas. The larvae remain in the skin of the accidental host and wander along the epidermal-dermal junction for approximately 4 weeks but can persist for longer periods. The recommended therapy for this nematode infestation is the oral broad-spectrum anthelminthic agent thiabendazole at a dosage of 25 mg/kg/day for 2 to 4 days. However, a significant percentage of patients have side effects such as dizziness, nausea, anorexia, and cramps during oral therapy. Thus some experts recommend topical therapy with 10% thiabendazole suspension at the lead point of the eruption. Hydrocortisone cream has been used as an adjunct to topical thiabendazole but is not the drug of choice for eradication of the parasite. Scabies, caused by the mite *Sarcoptes scabiei,* is recognized by the presence of pruritic papules, vesicles, and linear burrows involving the interdigital web spaces, the axillae, the flexures of the arms and wrists, the beltline, the perigenital area, and the lower buttocks in children and adolescents. Permethrin 5% cream is the topical therapy of choice for scabies in infants and children. Lindane, although effective against *S. scabiei,* is associated with potential toxicity and is not currently recommended as first-line therapy. Amoxicillin has no role in the eradication of either *A. braziliense* or *S. scabiei.*

13. The answer is **E,** pages 934 and 935.

The patient described in the vignette has clinical features of generalized neuromuscular disease. Although Werdnig-Hoffmann disease (spinal muscular atrophy type 1), a degenerative disease of the motor neurons that includes severe hypotonia, generalized weakness, and absence of deep tendon reflexes early in infancy, must be considered in this case, the epidemiologic exposure (honey) and the absence of fasciculations of the tongue are highly suggestive of infantile botulism. The diagnosis of infantile botulism may be indicated by electromyographic (EMG) studies demonstrating brief, small, abundant motor unit potentials (BSAP) and confirmed by identification of the toxin or the organism (*Clostridium botulinum*) in the stool. The absence of fever, the clear sensorium, and the stable vital signs make sepsis unlikely. Landry-Guillain-Barré syndrome (LGB) is a symmetric, ascending polyneuropathy that usually begins suddenly with motor weakness in the lower extremities and may progress to involve the cranial nerves. LGB, however, is much more common in older children than in infants, is usually associated with a prodromal respiratory or GI illness, and is usually accompanied by an increase in CSF protein concentration. The CSF protein concentration is normal in infantile botulism. Congenital hypothyroidism may not appear until 6 to 12 weeks after birth with classic signs such as umbilical hernia, enlarged tongue, prominent posterior fontanelle, coarse facial features, and hoarse cry. Such infants may have a history of neonatal jaundice or transient hypothermia. Because findings may be delayed in onset, thyroid function tests should be part of the initial evaluation of an infant who has feeding problems, hoarse cry, and constipation.

14. The answer is **D,** pages 942 to 944.

The patient in the vignette has clinical features that are highly suggestive of Kawasaki disease (mucocutaneous lymph node syndrome). Myopericarditis can occur early in the course of Kawasaki disease, and a gallop rhythm on auscultation of the heart should suggest its presence. Myopericarditis is usually documented with an echocardiogram (ECG), although the ECG may be useful to indicate its occurrence initially. The platelet count in Kawasaki disease usually does not rise until the subacute phase of the disease and is usually normal when the patient has myocarditis. Although group A streptococcal–associated acute rheumatic fever also is in the differential diagnosis of a patient with fever and carditis, this disease is extremely rare during infancy. The antinuclear antibody test may be positive in patients with systemic lupus erythematosus or pauciarticular juvenile rheumatoid arthritis, but is negative in Kawasaki disease. The patient in the vignette does not have clinical features suggestive of either of those disorders. The lumbar puncture may reveal a low-grade pleocytosis in Kawasaki disease, but this finding has limited diagnostic value.

15. The answer is **E,** page 938, Table 55-3.

The development of a febrile illness in the context of animal exposure should always suggest the possibility of zoonotic infection. The child in this vignette has a history of exposure to dogs (and specifically of a dog bite) and pica, which epidemiologically places him at increased risk for a zoonosis. The clinical features of fever and hepatomegaly suggest a systemic illness, and the presence of significant eosinophilia (more than $500/mm^3$) suggests a host response often noted in the context of tissue invasive parasites. Thus the possibility of visceral larva migrans (VLM) must be strongly considered in this case. VLM is caused by infection with larvae of the roundworm *Toxocara canis* and possibly *Toxocara cati* or *Toxocara leonina*, which are common intestinal parasites of dogs and cats. The eggs are excreted in the animal feces and ingested by humans, usually children between the ages of 1 and 4 years. Following ingestion the larvae penetrate the gut and migrate to the liver, lung, eye, central nervous system, kidney, or heart, where a granulomatous inflammatory host tissue response is usually elicited. The exception seems to be the eye, where the lesions contain eosinophils and mononuclear cells. Because the larvae cannot mature in the accidental human host, they may migrate for months until they are controlled by the host's inflammatory response. Given the potential for significant damage to the retina leading to permanent impairment of vision in this disorder, many experts advise pharmacotherapy with the anthelminthic agent thiabendazole. Ivermectin is a macrocyclic lactone that causes paralysis in nematodes and arthropods by facilitating influx of chloride ions across cell membranes. It is an effective microfilaricidal drug active against *Wuchereria bancrofti* and *Brugia malayi*. It currently is the drug of choice in onchocerciasis. Chloroquine is a synthetic schizonticidal agent active against the asexual erythrocytic forms of most strains of *Plasmodium malariae, Plasmodium ovale, Plasmodium vivax,* and some strains of *Plasmodium falciparum*. It is not effective against *Toxocara* species.

16. The answer is **D,** page 937, Table 55-3.

The presence of patchy pulmonary infiltrates and significant eosinophilia (more than 500/mm^3) in the afebrile but symptomatic patient described in the vignette suggests the diagnostic rubric of Löffler's syndrome. Löffler's syndrome may be an unusual allergic manifestation of the host response to a variety of antigens and not a true clinical entity. Among children Löffler's syndrome is usually the clinical manifestation of helminthic infection, which can be diagnosed by examination of stool for evidence of ova or parasites. Sputum and blood cultures would not be expected to yield pathogens. Common helminthic pathogens include *Toxocara canis, Ascaris lumbricoides,* and *Strongyloides stercoralis.* The differential diagnosis would include vasculitis (polyarteritis or other collagen vascular diseases), asthma, and allergic bronchopulmonary aspergillosis. Although *Chlamydia trachomatis* can cause inclusion conjunctivitis in neonates and afebrile pneumonia with peripheral blood eosinophilia in infants between the ages of 1 and 3 months, it is not well recognized as a cause of Löffler's syndrome in children or adolescents. Although *Mycoplasma pneumoniae* is a recognized pathogen causing interstitial pneumonia or bronchopneumonia among school-aged children, overt illness is less common in preschool-aged children and eosinophilia is not a prominent feature of the disease.

17. The answer is **B,** page 954.

The acute onset of a febrile illness in a patient with antecedent exposure to biting insects suggests a wide range of potential infectious pathogens including protozoa, helminths, and the rickettsiae. An important clinical feature in the patient described in this vignette is the presence of leukopenia and thrombocytopenia, a finding suggestive of human ehrlichial infection. The first recognized case of human ehrlichiosis was reported in Japan and was due to *Ehrlichia sennetsu.* Subsequent reports in the United States implicated the pathogen *Ehrlichia chaffeensis,* which infected mononuclear phagocytes. Granulocytic infection has been recognized recently, and the agent of human granulocytic ehrlichiosis is similar but not identical to *Ehrlichia equi,* which is a pathogen in horses serologically distinct from *E. chaffeensis.* The tick *Ixodes scapularis,* the vector of Lyme disease, supports the growth of *E. equi* and is believed to be the vector for human granulocytic ehrlichiosis. The vector for human monocytic ehrlichiosis is not established. *Ehrlichia* enters the cytoplasm of host cells and multiplies in phagosomes, where multiplication into elementary bodies and maturation into morulae occur. Rupture of the host cell releases the morulae, which reinitiate the infectious cycle. The mechanism of thrombocytopenia is speculative. In animal models, infection with *E. canis* produces antiplatelet antibodies that are associated with thrombocytopenia. The clinical features of human monocytic and granulocytic ehrlichiosis are similar but not identical to those noted with infection with *Rickettsia rickettsii,* the etiologic agent of Rocky Mountain spotted fever. Rash is much less common in the former than in the latter. Infection with *Borrelia burgdorferi,* the cause of Lyme disease, usually presents in its early stage with fever, "flulike" symptoms, and the rash of erythema chronicum migrans. The rash may be absent in 20% to 40% of cases, but the findings of neutropenia and thrombocytopenia are not prominent features of the disease. Systemic lupus erythematosus is associated with both neutropenia and thrombocytopenia, but other features, including malar rash, photosensitivity, alopecia, and joint manifestations, are important features of the disease at presentation. The onset of influenza A infection would be unusual during the summer months in the United States, and although clinical disease can be associated with leukopenia, the presence of concurrent thrombocytopenia would be extremely uncommon.

18. The answer is **E,** pages 951 to 953.

The patient described in the vignette has epidemiologic and clinical features highly suggestive of nonmenstrual toxic shock syndrome (NMTSS). NMTSS has been reported in association with burns, cutaneous and subcutaneous infections, abortions, and respiratory tract infections that include sinusitis, tracheitis, and pneumonia. Although both meningococcemia and Rocky Mountain spotted fever may include fever and hypoperfusion, diffuse erythroderma is not a characteristic feature of these disorders. Kawasaki disease may include erythema of mucous membranes, erythematous polymorphous rash, and fever. The peak age of onset is 18 to 24 months, and the disease is unusual in children older than age 10 years. Leptospirosis is an acute infectious vasculitis that may be associated with icterus (approximately 10% of cases). Virtually all mammals can be infected with the spirochete, which is the etiologic agent, and can transmit it to other mammals. Independent of the vector or the presence of icterus, the disease characteristically follows a biphasic course. The initial phase of disease manifests fever, malaise, headache, and myalgias, followed by lysis of fever. The second phase manifests recrudescence of fever, uveitis, rash, and signs of central nervous system inflammation. The rash may be erythematous, but diffuse erythroderma is not usually characteristic of this disorder.

19. The answer is **D,** page 961.

The patient described in the vignette has a febrile illness associated with the development of a generalized exanthem at the time of defervescence. This clinical picture is diagnostic of roseola infantum, a clinical syndrome often termed exanthem subitum that refers to the sudden and unexpected appearance of the characteristic dermatologic eruption on or about the fourth day of illness. The etiology of the syndrome is now attributed most frequently to infection caused by human herpesvirus-6 (HHV-6), although HHV-6 is not the exclusive agent involved in the pathogenesis of this disorder. Characteristically, infants are affected and manifest the abrupt onset of fever (which may be high-grade) but maintain a benign clinical appearance for 3 to 5 days before defervescence and the appearance of a generalized rash. Associated findings may include nonexudative pharyngotonsillitis, tympanitis, and enlargement of the suboccipital, posterior cervical, and postauricular lymph nodes. Rubeola (measles) is a disorder in which the onset of the exanthem occurs at the height of the febrile illness. These patients appear clinically ill and have cough, coryza, and conjunctivitis. An enanthem (Koplik's spots) involving the buccal mucosa can be noted before onset of the exanthem. Parvovirus infection causes erythema infectiosum, a mild exanthematous illness manifest as low-grade fever, benign clinical appearance, and a biphasic rash beginning on the face as diffuse erythema ("slapped cheek appearance") that spreads to the extremities and trunk as a lacy, reticular erythematous eruption.

20. The answer is **C,** page 961.

The exanthem described in the patient presented in this vignette is the biphasic eruption characteristic of erythema infectiosum, also known as fifth disease. Erythema infectiosum is caused by parvovirus B19. Although the diagnosis most often is based on clinical features alone, laboratory confirmation is sometimes appropriate, especially when there is concern about prenatal infection. Serologic assays demonstrating IgM and IgG specific antibody by enzyme-linked immunosorbent assay (ELISA) technique are widely available. Although usually benign, parvovirus B19 infection is associated with complications such as arthritis (especially in adults) and aplastic crisis in patients with chronic hemolytic anemia. Acquisition of parvovirus B19 during pregnancy has been reported to be associated with fetal loss and nonimmune hydrops fetalis. These appear to be infrequent events, however, and the true risk to the fetus is incompletely understood at this time. Differentiation of erythema infectiosum from stage 1 Lyme disease (erythema chronicum migrans) or systemic lupus erythematosus on clinical grounds is usually not difficult, and adjunctive laboratory testing for these entities is usually not indicated. The confluent rash of scarlet fever is erythematous and raised, giving it a "sandpaper" quality on palpation; it is unlikely to be confused with erythema infectiosum, and a rapid streptococcal antigen test is not likely to provide useful diagnostic information in this patient.

21. The answer is **D**, page 938, Table 55-3 (see also pages 701 and 702).

Persistent vulvovaginitis in the prepubertal child represents a diagnostic challenge for the clinician. The more common etiologies include nonspecific vulvovaginitis and foreign body. Nonspecific vulvovaginitis is a diagnostic rubric and does not imply idiopathic inflammation. Most cases of nonspecific vulvovaginitis are attributable to infection with coliform bacteria resulting from fecal contamination caused by poor perineal hygiene. Other organisms transmitted manually from the nasopharynx such as β-hemolytic streptococci and coagulase-positive *Staphylococcus* also have been associated with nonspecific vulvovaginitis. An often overlooked, but clinically important and treatable, predisposing factor in the development of nonspecific vulvovaginitis is enterobiasis. Pinworms may promote contamination of the perivulvar area with bacteria directly or indirectly caused by the scratching that follows from the pruritus induced by these organisms. Given the symptoms of pruritus and the presence of excoriation on the examination of this child's perineum, a cellophane tape test is clearly indicated. *Candida* vulvovaginitis can also include complaints of severe vulvar pruritus and secondary vulvar dysuria, and findings of discharge and diffuse erythema of the vulva that may extend inferiorly toward the anus. However, in nondiabetic preschool-age children, *Candida* is an uncommon pathogen. One exception to this rule of thumb is the healthy child treated with multiple courses of antibiotics. Bacterial vaginosis is an extremely unlikely cause of vaginitis in the prepubertal girl, and routine examination for clue cells is not recommended. Pelvic ultrasonography may be of limited use in identifying foreign bodies not directly visible but would have limited applicability in the evaluation of vulvovaginitis.

22. The answer is **B**, pages 957 and 958.

The patient described in the vignette has clinical (fever and centripetal rash involving distal extremities initially) and laboratory (leukopenia and thrombocytopenia) findings that are highly suggestive of Rocky Mountain spotted fever (RMSF), an infectious vasculitis caused by *Rickettsia rickettsii* and transmitted to humans through the bite of a tick. Treatment includes supportive care and antimicrobials. Both tetracycline and chloramphenicol are effective against *R. rickettsii*. Tetracycline is usually recommended for patients older than 9 years of age and chloramphenicol for patients younger than 9 years of age. Some infectious disease authorities, however, prefer to treat all seriously ill patients who have RMSF with chloramphenicol. The beneficial role of corticosteroids as adjunctive therapy to specific antibiotic administration has not been established conclusively.

23. The answer is **B**, pages 961 and 962, see Table 55-10, page 962.

The presence of fever and the triad of cough, coryza, and conjunctivitis in the patient described in this vignette is suggestive of measles (rubeola). Koplik's spots, gray-white lesions on a bright red surface located initially on the buccal mucosa opposite the lower molars and subsequently spreading to the labial mucosa are the characteristic enanthem of rubeola. Their identification allows the clinician to make the clinical diagnosis before the onset of the distinctive erythematous rash. The maculopapular exanthem of measles first appears on the forehead at the hairline and behind the ears, and then spreads centrifugally to involve the face, neck, trunk, and extremities. As the rash spreads it becomes confluent, particularly on the face. The patient is usually highly febrile at the time of the exanthem and remains febrile for 3 to 4 days. Measles may require differentiation from Kawasaki syndrome, which can be accomplished serologically by the detection of IgM antibody to measles virus. Echocardiography may demonstrate aneurysmal lesions in 20% of untreated patients with Kawasaki syndrome, but would not be reliable enough for use in differentiating the two diseases. Cold agglutinins can be detected in patients with infection caused by *Mycoplasma pneumoniae* as well as with other viral illnesses. Their presence is thus a nonspecific indicator of disease. The presence of heterophil antibodies, however, is more suggestive of Epstein-Barr virus mononucleosis, but this disorder would be unusual in a 4-year-old patient.

24. The answer is **C**, page 946.

The presence of unexplained adenopathy in an adolescent boy should raise suspicion of infection or malignancy. The acute "flulike" symptoms reported by the patient described in this vignette, which are similar to those reported by other close contacts, suggest an infectious cause. Important ancillary findings are the absence of exudative tonsillitis and hepatosplenomegaly usually seen in patients with Epstein-Barr virus–associated infectious mononucleosis or acute group A streptococcal pharyngitis. An important pathogen to consider in the differential diagnosis therefore is *Toxoplasma gondii*. Acquired toxoplasmosis is usually asymptomatic, but approximately 10% of infected individuals have clinical symptoms and laboratory findings consistent with those described in this patient. Outbreaks of disease have been reported, especially in association with consumption of undercooked meat (such as hamburgers) that are contaminated by oocytes. In most symptomatic cases adenopathy is the primary feature, but in severe infections the liver may be involved and overt evidence of hepatic dysfunction may be noted. Patients with normal immunologic function and mild disease usually do not require treatment. Postnatally acquired rubella is an exanthematous illness that has a prodrome in older individuals consisting of 1 to 5 days of sore throat, headache, adenopathy, and fever before the onset of rash. An interesting but unexplained feature of rubella in its prodromal phase among older patients is severe eye pain. Although rubella is a possibility in this case, the duration of symptoms and the absence of rash make it less likely. Atypical mycobacteria infection is a cause of persistent cervical adenopathy and would also be included in the differential diagnosis. However, the involved nodes are usually in the anterior cervical area or close to the mandible, initially firm to palpation, and then progress to fluctuance. In many cases a characteristic violaceous hue is noted over the involved node.

25. The answer is **D**, pages 959 and 960.

The patient described in the vignette has findings on chest roentgenogram (infiltrate, pleural reaction, and small pleural effusion) that are highly suggestive of primary *Mycobacterium tuberculosis* infection of the lung. Although the differential diagnosis includes infection with other organisms and to a far lesser extent a neoplastic process, the size of the pleural effusion makes diagnostic thoracentesis a difficult procedure in this patient. *Mycoplasma pneumoniae* is relatively uncommon in children under the age of 5 years, and unless the acute phase titer is greater than 1:64, unpaired serology is not helpful clinically for early diagnosis. The clinical and roentgenographic features are not highly suggestive of either respiratory syncytial virus infection or pertussis, which at this age should be more characteristically a triphasic disorder.

26. The answer is **B**, pages 954 to 957.

The patient described in the vignette has clinical features of acute facial nerve (Bell's) palsy and laboratory evidence of central nervous system inflammation consistent with early disseminated (stage II) Lyme disease. In a recent case series only 27% of children with neurologic abnormalities caused by *Borrelia burgdorferi*, the causative agent of Lyme disease, had a history of erythema chronicum migrans, the most common manifestation of primary infection, or arthritis. In such patients seropositivity commonly constituted the primary basis for diagnosis. Thus, despite concern about nonspecificity, seropositivity for *Borrelia burgdorferi* in children with neurologic symptoms usually signifies active neuroborreliosis. The specificity of serologic testing among patients with acute facial palsy and positive immunoassay results may be improved through the use of the IgM immunoblotting technique applied to acute phase sera. Other infectious agents have been associated with isolated Bell's palsy, including herpes zoster (varicella-zoster virus), but herpes simplex would be an unusual pathogen. Infection with *Mycobacterium tuberculosis* can cause meningitis with basilar cranial nerve dysfunction and a negative Gram's stain, but unilateral seventh nerve palsy as the only manifestation would be rare. Paranasal sinusitis may be a cause of an aseptic pleocytosis but would not be likely to cause Bell's palsy.

27. The answer is **E,** pages 947 and 948.

The differential diagnosis of acute onset scrotal pain includes traumatic, infectious and inflammatory, and ischemic disorders. The patient in the vignette has clinical features (prodromal symptoms and fever) strongly suggestive of an infectious and inflammatory disorder. Given the normal position of the testis, acute testicular torsion with ischemia is less likely. Considering the symptoms and clinical course, the most likely infectious agent is the mumps virus. Mumps infection characteristically includes salivary gland swelling, particularly the parotid gland, as well as headache and photophobia, which most likely represent underlying meningitis, and abdominal pain, which most likely represents pancreatitis. The disease also has been associated with orchitis in approximately one third of postpubescent men. The orchitis is usually unilateral and may occur before or in the absence of parotitis. Therapy is supportive, but sequelae such as atrophy and, in cases of bilateral orchitis, sterility have been reported. It is unclear whether corticosteroids can prevent either of these complications. Both epididymitis and urethritis caused by bacterial or chlamydial infection in boys are associated usually with an abnormal urinalysis or urethral discharge. Brucellosis is a zoonosis caused by organisms of the genus *Brucella* that are gram-negative coccobacilli. The distribution is worldwide in both domestic and wild animals. *Brucella* organisms localize in the reticuloendothelial system, leading to characteristic findings of hepatosplenomegaly and adenopathy. The most common localized complication of brucellosis is arthritis, but in men and boys unilateral orchitis or epididymitis is reported to be common. Given the lack of a suggestive exposure by history, it is less likely that the acute orchitis in this patient is indicative of brucellosis.

28. The answer is **D,** pages 948 and 949.

Pertussis characteristically is a triphasic disease comprising relatively distinct stages: catarrhal (1 to 2 weeks), paroxysmal (2 to 4 weeks), and convalescent (1 to 2 weeks). During the catarrhal phase rhinorrhea, lacrimation, conjunctival injection, minimal coughing, and low-grade fever predominate, suggesting a mild upper respiratory tract infection. During the paroxysmal phase the severity and frequency of coughing increase and, characteristically, repetitive paroxysms of multiple, forceful coughs are followed by a single inspiratory effort that produces the characteristic "whoop." Such episodes may be followed by vomiting or prostration. During the convalescent phase the paroxysms of coughing decrease in severity and frequency but may persist for several months. The young infant with pertussis (younger than 6 months), however, may have clinical features including apnea, choking episodes, cyanosis, and coughing paroxysms without the characteristic whoop. Both bronchiolitis caused by respiratory syncytial virus and asthma are disorders that involve lower airways and produce partial or complete obstruction during expiration. The characteristic clinical finding in these patients therefore is wheezing, and chest radiographs usually reveal areas of hyperinflation with or without atelectasis. Pneumonia caused by *Chlamydia trachomatis* usually develops between 1 and 4 months of life. The patients are afebrile, do not manifest evidence of upper respiratory tract findings, and have tachypnea and rales on examination. Chest radiographs may reveal bilateral hyperinflation, diffuse infiltrates that may be interstitial or reticulonodular in appearance, or atelectasis. Peripheral blood eosinophilia (more than 300 cells) is a common laboratory finding.

The diagnosis of pertussis is confirmed by culturing nasopharyngeal secretions obtained with a Dacron or calcium alginate swab on appropriate media (Bordet-Gengou or Regan-Lowe). The culture is most often positive in the catarrhal stage, but false negative results are frequent thereafter. Various rapid diagnostic tests can be performed on nasopharyngeal secretions (direct immunofluorescent test; *Bordetella pertussis* IgA antibody ELISA), but reliability is problematic.

29. The answer is **B,** page 941.

The child described in this vignette has clinical findings consistent with an acute gingivostomatitis. In children the most common etiology of acute gingivostomatitis is infectious, although caustic ingestions must be considered in the differential diagnosis. The most common infectious agents are herpes simplex, coxsackievirus, and *Candida albicans*. Viral infections usually manifest vesicular lesions initially with ulcerations developing subsequently. *C. albicans* produces white plaques that adhere to the mucosa and bleed if mechanical removal is attempted. Given the description of the lesions in this patient and lacking an appropriate exposure history, the most likely etiology of this child's gingivostomatitis is viral. Primary herpes gingivostomatitis is usually differentiated from herpangina caused by coxsackievirus based on the preponderance of vesicles and ulcers in the anterior portion of the oropharynx in the former condition and the preponderance of ulcers in the posterior portion of the oropharynx in the latter condition. Acute necrotizing ulcerative gingivostomatitis (trench mouth) is a periodontal infection caused by fusiform bacilli and spirochetes. Clinically, patients manifest gingival pain and foul breath and taste and have a pseudomembranous necrotic exudate along the gingiva and interdental papillae. Vesicular lesions and discrete ulcers are not characteristic of this disease. Actinomycosis is a suppurative granulomatous disorder caused by *Actinomyces israelii*. The disorder is chronic and often involves the cervicofacial region, where the organism enters the tissues through carious teeth, mucosal trauma, or the tonsils, leading to pain, trismus, swelling, and fistula formation, which are not observed in this patient.

30. The answer is **C,** pages 880 and 940 to 941.

The neonate described in this vignette has evidence of systemic illness suggestive of sepsis or meningitis. In the neonatal period a broad spectrum of pathogens can account for sepsis and meningitis, including group B *Streptococcus (Streptococcus agalactiae)*, *Escherichia coli*, and herpes simplex. Several underlying conditions may predispose to bacterial sepsis in the neonate including galactosemia and urinary tract obstruction caused by posterior urethral valves in the boy. However, the maternal symptoms of vaginal pain, itching, and dysuria commencing before delivery suggest ongoing gynecologic disease consistent with genital infection by herpes simplex. Although serologic evidence suggesting syphilis is noted in the cord blood of this infant at the time of birth, the low titer most likely represents maternally derived antibody and, in the context of appropriate treatment at least 1 month before delivery, is unlikely to reflect neonatal infection. However, congenital syphilis often is asymptomatic at birth, and infected infants may first become symptomatic between 5 weeks and 3 months of age. The presentation may be that of a multisystem disorder involving the central nervous system, lungs, liver, kidneys, skin, and blood, but the acute, more fulminant presentation described for this infant would be quite unusual for a patient with early congenital syphilis.

31. The answer is **A,** pages 945 to 947.

The febrile adolescent girl described in the vignette has exudative pharyngitis, splenomegaly, and mild thrombocytopenia, a clinical picture suggestive of infectious mononucleosis caused by Epstein-Barr virus (EBV). Virtually all patients with classic EBV-associated infectious mononucleosis have a relative lymphocytosis with 20% or more atypical lymphocytes on differential cell count. Approximately 25% to 50% of patients have mild thrombocytopenia. The thrombocytopenia appears to be immune mediated and has been associated with antiplatelet antibodies in some cases. Severe thrombocytopenia with bleeding is rare, however. Although infections caused by group A *Streptococcus* may cause exudative pharyngitis and splenomegaly, thrombocytopenia would be unusual. Systemic lupus erythematosus and leukemia can present with splenomegaly and thrombocytopenia, but exudative pharyngitis would be a highly unusual feature unless there is an intercurrent infection with an upper respiratory pathogen. Neither splenomegaly nor pharyngitis is characteristic of acute infection with hepatitis B virus. Thus the test most likely to reveal the cause of the findings in this patient is the heterophil antibody assay. Heterophil-negative infectious mononucleosis is recognized, and most cases are caused by cytomegalovirus or toxoplasmosis. However, the rapid slide test for heterophil antibody may be falsely negative early in the course of classic EBV infectious mononucleosis. Approximately 60% of these tests will be negative within the first week of illness. However, more specific serologic tests for EBV infection are available and can be used clinically to distinguish acute from remote infection. The most appropriate EBV serologic tests in this situation would be the IgG and IgM anti-EBV viral capsid antigen (VCA) titers. In acute EBV infection both IgM and IgG anti-VCA titers would be elevated, while in remote EBV infection only the IgG anti-VCA titer would be elevated. The anti-Epstein-Barr virus nuclear antigen (EBNA) titer rises much later during the course of infection (weeks to months), and its presence would be useful as a marker of recent or remote infection.

32. The answer is **E,** pages 949 to 951, Tables 55-5 and 55-6, pages 950 and 951.

The patient described in the vignette has sustained an unprovoked bite wound inflicted by an unknown animal vector in a natural geographic setting. Unless it is known with certainty that the natural setting is free of rabies virus or the animal can be recovered, sacrificed, and tested for rabies virus, this wound should be considered at high risk for disease transmission, and postexposure prophylaxis against rabies should begin immediately. The most appropriate approach to management of this patient therefore is local wound care combined with passive and active rabies prophylaxis (if the patient has not been vaccinated previously against rabies). Passive prophylaxis is given as human rabies immune globulin (HRIG) at a dosage of 20 IU/kg injected intramuscularly into the gluteal region. If anatomic considerations allow injection at the wound site, half the dose of HRIG is infiltrated in the soft tissue surrounding the bite, and the remainder is given intramuscularly in the gluteal region. Active prophylaxis is given as a series of human rabies diploid cell rabies vaccine (HDCV) injections in the deltoid muscle immediately and again on days 3, 7, 14, and 28 postexposure. An alternative to HDCV is rabies vaccine adsorbed (RVA), which is administered in the same way as HDCV.

Once initiated, prophylaxis of rabies should *not* be discontinued because of local (soreness, pain, swelling, erythema, itching, induration, burning, or warmth) or mild systemic (nausea, vomiting, abdominal pain, diarrhea, headache, fatigue, low-grade fever, myalgia, arthralgia, and malaise) adverse reactions. Such reactions can be managed successfully in most cases with nonsteroidal antiinflammatory agents. Anaphylaxis is a rare complication of either HDCV or RVA vaccination and may necessitate cessation of active immunization. Local tenderness, soreness, stiffness, urticaria, or angioedema may occur after injection of HRIG. Nephrotic syndrome and anaphylaxis are rare sequelae. Antibodies contained in HRIG may interfere with the immune response to live virus vaccines such as measles-mumps-rubella (MMR). Thus immunobiologic preparations containing live measles virus should not be given to patients receiving HRIG for at least 4 months. Because the health maintenance status of the patient is known and his immunization schedule is current, the patient does not require an additional booster dose of tetanus toxoid.

33. The answer is **C,** page 942.

The patient described in the vignette has two chronic diseases (diabetes mellitus and asthma) that put him at risk for serious complications of acquired infectious disorders such as influenza. Thus this patient would benefit from yearly vaccination with influenza vaccine during "flu" season. The benefit of pneumococcal vaccine in this patient is less compelling. The American Academy of Pediatrics Committee on Infectious Diseases currently recommends the use of pneumococcal vaccine in children 2 years of age or older with chronic disorders associated specifically with increased risk of infection with *Streptococcus pneumoniae* such as sickle cell disease, asplenia, nephrotic syndrome, chronic renal failure, HIV infection, Hodgkin's disease, or other immunosuppressed states and children receiving immunosuppressive therapy. Given the clinical findings in this patient, serologic testing for *Mycoplasma pneumoniae* is unlikely to have diagnostic or therapeutic benefit. Because a recent double-blind, placebo-controlled, and randomized clinical trial found no therapeutic benefit of multiple allergen immunotherapy among allergic patients with perennial asthma treated appropriately with standard medical modalities, it is unlikely that skin testing for inhalant allergens would be useful in this patient. In the absence of findings suggestive of immunodeficiency, T and B cell quantification would offer no benefit diagnostically or therapeutically.

34. The answer is **D,** pages 937 to 939.

The presence of tertian fever (periodicity of 48 hours) in a patient with hepatosplenomegaly, anemia, and an appropriate exposure history is highly suggestive of malaria. Gambia is located in the sub-Saharan area of Africa, where malaria is prevalent. The tertian fever pattern suggests synchronous infection with *Plasmodium vivax*, *Plasmodium ovale*, or *Plasmodium falciparum*. The clinical features described in this case do not reliably differentiate any one of these three species of malaria parasites. During a febrile paroxysm resulting from erythrocytic schizogony the patient usually manifests leukocytosis. However, during the quiescent interval between paroxysms, leukopenia usually is found, and thrombocytopenia is common. The mechanisms underlying these findings are unclear. The diagnosis of malaria is established by examination of thick and thin blood films. The thick film facilitates diagnosis when parasites are present in small numbers, and the thin film is most useful in establishing the species of parasite. Although leukemia would be in the differential diagnosis of a patient with hepatosplenomegaly and pancytopenia, the tertian fever pattern and the epidemiologic history make an infectious etiology more likely, and a bone marrow examination could be deferred until the blood films are examined for parasites and abnormal white cells. Subacute bacterial endocarditis, human immunodeficiency virus infection, and Epstein-Barr virus infection are all less likely possibilities in this patient given the epidemiologic, history, and physical examination findings.

35. The answer is **A,** pages 939 and 940.

The patient described in this vignette has a fever and rash syndrome and a history of travel to an area in which dengue fever is endemic. Dengue fever is an acute febrile illness caused by the dengue subgroup of flaviviruses and transmitted by the mosquito *Aedes aegypti*. After inoculation in the host, the virus disseminates rapidly to regional lymph nodes and then to lymphatic tissue throughout the body including the skin. Virus can be recovered from circulating leukocytes at the end of the viremic period. The illness is characterized by fever that follows a biphasic pattern, myalgia, rash, adenopathy, and leukopenia. *Ixodes scapularis* is the tick vector transmitting *Borrelia burgdorferi*, the etiologic agent causing Lyme disease. Although a flulike illness characterizes many patients with stage I Lyme disease, the rash described in this patient is not consistent with erythema chronicum migrans. *Dermacentor variabilis* is the tick vector transmitting *Rickettsia rickettsii*, the etiologic agent of Rocky Mountain spotted fever (RMSF). Although RMSF is a fever and rash syndrome, the characteristic rash appears first peripherally on the wrists and ankles and moves centrally; it also involves the palms and soles, which is not the case in the patient described in the vignette. *Loxosceles reclusa* is the brown recluse spider whose bite causes necrotic arachnidism. Systemic findings in necrotic arachnidism range from self-limited urticaria to disseminated intravascular coagulation. *Sarcoptes scabiei* is the mite responsible for the papulovesicular pruritic dermatitis referred to clinically as scabies.

Pediatric Neurologic Disorders

Edward E. Conway Jr.

See Barkin et al: Chapter 56.

1. A 4-year-old girl is brought to the ED with a chief complaint of sudden onset of unsteady gait. Vital signs are stable. However, the neurologic examination demonstrates an ataxic gait and symmetric loss of deep tendon reflexes in both legs. Which of the following *best* explains the findings in this patient?
   A. Postinfectious cerebellar ataxia.
   B. Guillain-Barré syndrome.
   C. Acute phenytoin overdose.
   D. Cerebellar tumor.
   E. Lyme disease.

2. Acure cerebellar ataxia is seen *most* commonly following which of the following?
   A. Influenza.
   B. Poliomyelitis.
   C. Herpes simplex.
   D. Mycoplasma.
   E. Varicella.

3. Which of the following statements concerning patients with postinfectious cerebellar ataxia is *incorrect?*
   A. Dysarthria commonly is present.
   B. One half of affected patients have nystagmus.
   C. The head computed tomogram (CT) is normal.
   D. The cerebrospinal fluid (CSF) has a mild pleocytosis.
   E. Residual gait disturbances and abnormal eye movements are seen in 70% of these patients.

4. A 3-year-old boy with a history of posttraumatic epilepsy for which he is taking phenytoin is brought to the ED by his parents, who have noted that "he is walking funny" and complains of headaches. Which of the following is the *best* immediate diagnostic procedure?
   A. Obtain a serum phenytoin level.
   B. Obtain a head CT.
   C. Administer an antihistamine.
   D. Perform a lumbar puncture.
   E. Obtain serum electrolyte measurements.

5. Which of the following *best* describes the findings in a lethargic patient?
   A. Mental blunting with slow responses to stimuli.
   B. Deep sleep requiring vigorous and repeated stimuli for arousal.
   C. Irrational state with disorientation and irritability.
   D. Reduced wakefulness with a defect in attention.
   E. Absence of awareness of self and environment.

6. All of the following are assessed in the Glasgow Coma Scale (GCS) *except:*
   A. Extensor motor response.
   B. Eye opening.
   C. Verbal response.
   D. Deep tendon reflexes.
   E. Response to pain.

7. Coma may be caused by all of the following *except:*
   A. Extensive damage to one cerebral cortex.
   B. Transection of the reticular activating system.
   C. Production of endogenous toxins.
   D. Anoxia.
   E. Hyponatremia.

8. A 5-year-old boy is brought to the ED following a motor vehicle accident. The physical examination demonstrates a decreased level of consciousness, and the patient mumbles something about a headache. The right pupil is 6 mm and nonreactive to light. Which of the following *best* explains these findings?
   A. Herniation of the cingulate gyrus.
   B. Herniation at the foramen magnum.
   C. Medial displacement of the uncus.
   D. Displacement of the thalamus into the posterior fossa.

9. Which of the following is the *most* common cause of nontraumatic coma in pediatric patients?
   A. Intracranial infection.
   B. Anoxic encephalopathy.
   C. Status epilepticus.
   D. Metabolic derangement.
   E. Vascular lesions.

10. A 14-year-old patient has dysconjugate gaze and fixed midposition pupils, has decerebrate posturing, and is noted to be hyperventilating. Where is the *most* likely location of the lesion?
    A. Diencephalon.
    B. Midbrain.
    C. Medulla.
    D. Hypothalamus.

11. Which of the following *best* distinguishes between metabolic and structural causes of coma?
    A. Presence or absence of a pupillary light reflex.
    B. Positive plantar response.
    C. Presence or absence of deep tendon reflexes.
    D. Presence or absence of the oculocephalic reflex.
    E. Presence or absence of the oculovestibular reflex.

12. Damage to the hypothalamus produces which of the following?
    A. Ipsilateral pupillary constriction and anhidrosis.
    B. A unilaterally fixed and dilated pupil.
    C. Midposition, round, fixed, and nonreactive pupils.
    D. Small pupils with preserved light reflexes.
    E. Large, fixed, and nonreactive pupils.

13. A 14-year-old girl is brought to the ED by her friends because they became concerned when she was lethargic and barely able to be aroused after a fight with her boyfriend at a party. She has a known history of an anxiety disorder and takes a benzodiazepine for it. Her mother suffers from depression and is receiving a tricyclic antidepressant. The girl's respiratory rate (RR) is 14 breaths per minute with an oxygen (O_2) saturation of 98%. Her affect is blunted, but she can answer simple questions. Her pupils are 5 mm and reactive bilaterally. Which of the following is the *best* next option for this patient?
    A. Administration of 10% dextrose intravenously (IV).
    B. Administration of naloxone at 10 µg/kg IV.
    C. Administration of naloxone at 100 µg/kg IV.
    D. Administration of flumazenil 10 µg/kg IV.
    E. No pharmacologic intervention is required at this time.

14. All of the following statements concerning the outcome of traumatically induced coma in children are indicators of poor outcome *except* which of the following?
    A. GCS score less than 9.
    B. Age less than 2 years.
    C. Presence of a skull fracture.
    D. Occurrence of a contact seizure.
    E. Bilateral swelling without midline shift.

15. All of the following statements are true regarding pediatric brain death determination *except*:
    A. A 24-hour observation period is required for children less than 1 year of age.
    B. A 48-hour observation period is required for children older than 12 months of age.
    C. Hypothermia must not be present.
    D. Hypotension must be treated aggressively.
    E. The determination of brain death should not be made in the ED.

16. All of the following statements are true concerning headaches in pediatric patients *except*:
    A. Headaches are a common pediatric symptom.
    B. Organic causes are uncommon in children less than 5 years of age.
    C. Large intracranial arteries and veins are sensitive to pain.
    D. Pain originating from supratentorial lesions is referred to the front of the head.
    E. Lesions located in the posterior fossa may refer pain to the neck.

17. All of the following descriptions concerning referred pain in a 3-year-old with sinusitis are paired correctly *except*:
    A. Maxillary sinusitis: facial pain.
    B. Sphenoid sinusitis: occipital pain.
    C. Ethmoid sinusitis: eyeball pain.
    D. Frontal sinusitis: ear pain.

18. A 7-year-old child is brought to the ED complaining of the "worst headache of his life." He describes the pain as both frontal and periorbital on the right side with unilateral nasal stuffiness and tearing of his right eye. Which of the following best represents the type of headache described by this patient?
    A. Classic migraine.
    B. Traction headache.
    C. Tension headache.
    D. Cluster headache.
    E. Vascular headache.

For questions 19 through 26 please match the clinical description listed below with the appropriate movement disorder. Each answer may be used only once.
    A. Chorea.
    B. Athetosis.
    C. Ballismus.
    D. Dystonia.
    E. Torticollis.
    F. Myoclonus.
    G. Tics.
    H. Tremors.

19. _____ Involuntary, rhythmic oscillations that usually affect the hands with onset in adulthood.

20. _____ Quick, stereotyped, and purposeless movements or utterances not associated with an impairment of consciousness.

21. _____ Involuntary, rapid jerks of any body part caused by muscle contractions.

22. _____ Abnormal tilt of the head and neck.

23. _____ Disorder of the basal ganglia characterized by an abnormal posture of the body with or without a facial grimace.

24. _____ Irregular, violent hurling or flailing of one or both limbs.

25. _____ Slow, irregular writhing movement of the extremities usually associated with perinatal injury.

26. _____ A quick, random jerk of any body part with the limbs most commonly affected, occurring months after streptococcal pharyngitis.

27. All of the following statements are true concerning the differentiation between seizures and motor disorders *except:*
    A. Involuntary movements increase during sleep.
    B. Movement disorders do not produce a loss of consciousness.
    C. Movement disorders are more stereotyped than seizures.
    D. An electroencephalogram performed during an abnormal motor movement will be normal.

28. Which of the following findings is present in a patient with a lesion involving the cerebral cortex?
    A. Decreased reflexes.
    B. Increased tone.
    C. Muscle fasciculation.
    D. Significant atrophy of the affected muscle.

29. A 3-year-old child is brought to the ED because he refuses to walk. The child was in good health until 3 days ago, when he was irritable, febrile, and not eating well. A complete sepsis evaluation was performed, including a spinal tap, and the parents tell you that the workup was normal and that they were sent home with no medications. Physical examination reveals a cranky but consolable child who refuses to ambulate. Which of the following is the *most likely* diagnosis for this patient?
    A. Vertebral osteomyelitis.
    B. Epidural abscess.
    C. Transverse myelitis
    D. Guillain-Barré syndrome.
    E. Botulism.

30. A 4-month-old infant who has a history of constipation, vomiting, and abdominal pain is brought into the ED. Physical examination reveals an infant who has generalized muscle flaccidity and a continuous upward gaze. All of the following statements concerning this entity are *true except:*
    A. Antibiotics will not be helpful.
    B. Diagnosis is confirmed by stool assay.
    C. Intubation and mechanical ventilation may be required.
    D. All contacts must receive antibiotic prophylaxis.
    E. It is caused by an endotoxin of *Clostridium botulinum.*

31. A 3-year-old boy is brought to the ED after an acute onset of the inability to move his right side. The infant has a history of congenital heart disease. Which of the following *best* explains the findings in this patient?
    A. Aortic stenosis.
    B. Mitral valve prolapse.
    C. Coarctation of the aorta.
    D. Small ventricular septal defect.
    E. Tetralogy of Fallot.

32. A 13-year-old girl is brought to the ED by her mother, who noted that the patient was feeling warm, was sweating, and complained about feeling lightheaded and having blurred vision. The patient also was limp and unconscious for a brief period on the way to the ED. All of the following statements are correct *except:*
    A. This entity may be precipitated by stress, fear, and anxiety.
    B. Vasodilatation occurs early.
    C. Sympathetic activity decreases.
    D. The heart rate may slow.
    E. Placing the patient in a supine position is contraindicated.

33. A 14-year-old boy comes to the ED with a complaint of cough, fever, and malaise for 10 days. He is currently taking terfenadine as an antihistamine. You decide to treat the patient's clinical pneumonia. Which *one* of the following antibiotics may cause QT prolongation when taken concomitantly with terfenadine?
    A. Amoxicillin.
    B. Clavulanic acid.
    C. Tetracycline.
    D. Erythromycin.
    E. Ciprofloxacin.

34. A 14-year-old is brought in to the ED by her friends after she fainted at a party. They are unsure if she ingested anything, but she did not have any alcohol. Her heart rate (HR) is 80 beats per minute, respiration rate (RR) 14 breaths per minute, and blood pressure (BP) 110/60 mm Hg supine. Which of the following *best* demonstrates orthostatic changes in this patient?
    A. HR of 110 beats per minute when the patient sits up.
    B. Systolic blood pressure of 130 mm Hg when the patient sits up.
    C. Feeling of dizziness when going from a sitting to supine position.
    D. RR of 16 breaths per minute when sitting.
    E. Systolic blood pressure of 140 mm Hg sitting, decreasing to 110 mm Hg while supine.

35. Which of the following is the *most* common cause of vertigo in pediatric patients?
    A. Antihistamine overdose.
    B. Otitis media.
    C. Brainstem tumor.
    D. Basilar skull fracture.
    E. Cerebellar tumor.

36. A mother brings her 3-year-old son into the ED because, as they were out toy shopping and the child wanted a costly toy that he wasn't allowed to have, he suddenly became limp and blue and had several "jerky movements." The mother has a history of seizures as a child. In the ED the child is alert and awake. All of the following statements are true concerning this patient's condition *except:*
    A. The child had a petit mal seizure.
    B. Ocular compression may reproduce the symptoms.
    C. Bradycardia or asystole may occur in these children.
    D. Treatment usually involves only reassurance.
    E. The event is related to increased vagal discharge or sensitivity.

37. Which of the following statements concerning bacterial meningitis in pediatric patients is *incorrect?*
    A. It occurs most commonly between 3 and 8 months of age.
    B. Nearly 90% of cases occur before the age of 5 years.
    C. Hematogenous transmission of organisms is uncommon.
    D. The upper respiratory tract is the major reservoir of pathogens.
    E. One third of children have a distant focus of infection.

38. Which of the following organisms is the *most* likely cause of meningitis in a 9-month-old infant?
    A. *Streptococcus pneumoniae.*
    B. *Staphylococcus epidermidis.*
    C. *Escherichia coli.*
    D. *Staphylococcus aureus.*
    E. *Neisseria meningitidis.*

39. Which of the following organisms is the *most* common cause ventriculoperitoneal CSF shunt infections?
    A. *S. aureus.*
    B. *Listeria monocytogenes.*
    C. *Staphylococcus epidermidis.*
    D. *E. coli.*
    E. *S. pneumoniae.*

40. When a ventriculoperitoneal shunt is being assessed, which of the following statements is *most correct?*
    A. Distal obstruction occurs more frequently.
    B. If the reservoir cannot be depressed, a distal block is present.
    C. If the reservoir pumps but does not refill, a distal block is present.
    D. The distal catheter usually resides in the peritoneum.

41. A 4-month-old infant is brought into the ED by paramedics who had been called by the baby-sitter. The infant fed well an hour earlier and was noted to be blue and not breathing by the baby-sitter. Physical examination reveals a pale, lethargic infant who is not responsive to touch. Capillary refill time is 5 seconds, and the right pupil is fixed and not reactive. Vital signs show an HR of 170 beats per minute and BP of 140/96 mm Hg. Which of the following is the best initial management for this patient?
    A. Administration of 0.5 g/kg IV mannitol.
    B. Administration of 1 mg/kg IV furosemide
    C. Administration of 20 ml/kg of 0.9% NaCl.
    D. Intubation of the patient's trachea.
    E. Performance of an immediate subdural tap via the anterior fontanelle.

42. A 6-month-old infant is being evaluated for possible meningitis, and the CSF reveals 400 white blood cells (differential pending), glucose 35 mg/dl, and protein 120 mg/dl. The CSF/glucose ratio is 0.3. Which one of the following is the *most* likely cause of this patient's illness?
    A. *S. pneumoniae.*
    B. Enterovirus.
    C. *Mycoplasma pneumoniae.*
    D. Herpes simplex.
    E. *Toxoplasma gondii.*

43. Which one of the following is the most common etiology of aseptic meningitis?
    A. Herpes simplex.
    B. *Candida albicans.*
    C. Enterovirus.
    D. Arbovirus.
    E. Varicella-zoster.

44. A 7-month-old infant is found to have meningitis caused by *N. meningitidis.* She is immediately intubated in the ED. It was a difficult intubation, requiring the physician to have prolonged contact with the patient's oropharyngeal secretions. The infant lives at home with her parents and three siblings and attends day care for 48 hours per week. All of the following people should receive chemoprophylaxis *except:*
    A. The patient's 34-year-old mother.
    B. The patient's 4-year-old sibling.
    C. The physician who intubated the infant.
    D. The other children in the day care center.
    E. All of the above should receive chemoprophylaxis.

45. Which one of the following statements concerning migraines is *incorrect?*
    A. Migraines are more common in adolescent girls.
    B. Half of the patients who have migraines have their first attack before age 20.
    C. The patient often has an associated history of motion sickness.
    D. Migraineurs have a higher incidence of epilepsy than the general population.
    E. A prodrome occurs in more than 95% of the patients.

46. A 19-year-old woman has a severe headache and diplopia. A computed tomogram both with and without contrast of the head is normal. A spinal tap reveals clear fluid with an opening pressure of 250 cm H$_2$O. Which of the following *best* explains the findings in this patient?
    A. Pseudotumor cerebri.
    B. Supratentorial tumor.
    C. Infratentorial tumor.
    D. Subarachnoid hemorrhage.
    E. Arteriovenous malformation.
47. Which of the following entities is the *most* common cause of seizures in pediatric patients?
    A. Hypoxia.
    B. Fever.
    C. Hypoglycemia.
    D. Hyponatremia.
    E. Ischemia.

48. Which one of the following is the *most* common cause of seizures in the newborn period?
    A. Hypoxic-ischemic encephalopathy.
    B. Hypoglycemia.
    C. Central nervous system hemorrhage.
    D. Drug withdrawal.
    E. Inborn errors of metabolism.
49. Which of the following *best* predicts the risk of a future afebrile, nonprovoked seizure?
    A. Family history of epilepsy.
    B. Duration of the seizure.
    C. Age at first seizure.
    D. Status epilepticus.
50. Which of the following is *most* frequently associated with febrile seizures?
    A. Upper respiratory tract infections.
    B. Otitis media.
    C. Acute gastroenteritis.
    D. *Roseola infantum.*
    E. Urinary tract infection.

ANSWERS   [See Barkin et al: Chapter 56.]

1. The answer is **B,** pages 972 to 974.
   The conditions that most commonly cause ataxia include drug intoxication, postinfectious acute cerebellar ataxia, and posterior fossa tumors. Weakness may be mistaken for ataxia, and thus patients with Guillain-Barré syndrome, transverse myelitis, tick paralysis, or myasthenia gravis may all have an ataxic gait. Of the choices listed, only Guillain-Barré syndrome produces an ataxic gait and symmetric loss of deep tendon reflexes.
2. The answer is **E,** pages 972 to 974.
   Acute cerebellar ataxia occurs after an antecedent nonspecific viral illness. It occurs after influenza, poliomyelitis, coxsackievirus B, echovirus type 6, herpes simplex virus, mononucleosis, *Mycoplasma* infection, and most commonly varicella.
3. The answer is **E,** pages 972 to 974.
   Patients with acute postinfectious cerebellar ataxia have severe ataxia, and most have dysarthria; half have nystagmus. The head CT is normal, and the CSF usually has a mild pleocytosis. The course of illness usually is benign with the ataxia resolving within a few weeks to months. Residual symptoms, such as persistent gait disturbances, truncal tremor, abnormal eye movements, and impaired speech may persist for up to 6 years after the initial episode in about one third of the patients.
4. The answer is **A,** pages 972 to 974.
   Drug ingestion is one of the most common causes of acute ataxia. Patients taking anticonvulsants, especially phenytoin, may have toxic levels and thus ataxia. Other drugs and toxins that may produce ataxia include alcohol, tricyclic antidepressants, hypnotics, sedatives, benzodiazepines, heavy metals (lead), insecticides, and drugs commonly abused such as phencyclidine hydrochloride (PCP).

5. The answer is **D,** page 974.
   Coma is the absence of awareness of self and environment. Lethargy is a term describing a reduced wakefulness in which the primary defect is one of attention. A confused patient misrepresents incoming stimuli, particularly visual ones. Delirium is a more floridly abnormal state characterized by disorientation, fear, irritability, misrepresentation of sensory stimuli, and visual hallucinations. Obtundation is mental blunting manifested by slow responses to stimuli and an increase in sleep time. Stupor is a deep sleep from which the patient can be aroused only by vigorous and repeated stimuli.
6. The answer is **D,** page 974.
   The Glasgow Coma Scale (GCS) is a practical, user friendly, rapid assessment of neurologic dysfunction. It allows the assessment of motor and verbal responses and eye opening, and patients with scores less than 8 are considered comatose. Assessment of deep tendon reflexes is not part of the GCS score.
7. The answer is **A,** pages 974 to 980.
   Coma is the absence of awareness of self and environment. It is caused by damage either to both cerebral cortices or to the reticular activating system. Nontraumatic causes involve the inadequate delivery of substrates, inadequate removal of a toxin, or production of an endogenous toxin. Other causes include anoxia and hormonal or electrolyte abnormalities.

8. The answer is **C,** pages 974 and 975.

Both traumatic and nontraumatic causes of coma can cause herniation-displacement or compression of the brain tissue against the dural folds that support it. There are three major foci for herniation. If supratentorial structures are shifted laterally, herniation of the cingulate gyrus may occur under the falx cerebri. Clinical signs may include the loss of leg function from compression of one or both of the anterior cerebral arteries. In transtentorial herniation the diencephalon (thalamus and hypothalamus) is displaced through the foramen magnum into the posterior fossa with compression and ischemia to the brainstem. This usually occurs as the result of elevated intracranial pressure affecting both hemispheres equally. The third and *most* frequent location for herniation is at the tentorial edge from the supratentorial to the infratentorial compartment. This is referred to as uncal herniation and usually results from an expanding mass lesion that occupies the middle cranial fossa or parenchyma of the temporal lobe. Clinical signs include headache, decreased level of consciousness, and ipsilateral pupillary dilatation caused by compression of the oculomotor nerve by the medially displaced uncus of the temporal lobe. (See Table 56-1 on page 975 in Barkin et al.)

9. The answer is **A,** page 975.

Reviews of etiologies of pediatric coma patients have shown that intracranial infection is the most common cause of nontraumatic coma, followed by anoxic encephalopathy, status epilepticus, metabolic derangement, and vascular lesions (Box 48-1).

10. The answer is **B,** page 976.

Central neurogenic hyperventilation is a serious condition found in patients with lesions of the midbrain. Midbrain lesions also cause clear-cut pupillary findings resulting in midposition round regular pupils that are light fixed but may fluctuate in size spontaneously.

11. The answer is **A,** page 977.

The pupillary pathways are relatively resistant to metabolic insults, and the presence or absence of a light reflex is the single most important physical finding that distinguishes structural from metabolic causes. Most metabolic conditions that affect the central nervous system lead to pupils that are constricted but that remain sensitive to light. A magnifying glass may be required to appreciate this finding in patients with constricted pupils. (See Fig. 56-1 on page 977 in Barkin et al.)

Box 48-1
Coma Mnemonic
"TIPS from the Vowels (AEIOU)"

Trauma/tumor	**A**lcohol/Abuse
Insulin and hypoglycemia	**E**pilepsy/Encephalopathy
Intussusception	**I**nfection/Inborn errors
Poisoning/psychogenic	**O**piates
Shock	**U**remia

---

12. The answer is **A,** page 977.

Hypothalamic damage usually produces ipsilateral pupillary constriction associated with ptosis and anhidrosis (Horner's syndrome). Pupillary function usually is preserved.

13. The answer is **E,** page 979.

Patients with suspected metabolic causes of coma can have a trial of naloxone or glucose (1 g/kg of 50% dextrose) while en route to the hospital if a narcotic ingestion or hypoglycemia is suspected. Flumazenil is a benzodiazepine antagonist that can be administered in "pure" benzodiazepine overdose situations. It must be used with caution for patients with known seizure disorders and for patients who may have ingested proseizure drugs, since the flumazenil may antagonize the protective effect of the benzodiazepine in a mixed ingestion. The patient described here had access to both tricyclics and benzodiazepines, but the physical examination demonstrates normal reactive pupils and respiratory status. Since the patient is clinically stable, no immediate intervention is required.

14. The answer is **D,** page 980.

The prognosis in cases of traumatic pediatric coma is better than in the adult counterparts. Age appears to be a major factor affecting both morbidity and mortality. Predictors of poor outcome include a GCS score less than 9, age less than 2 years, presence of a skull fracture, presence of a mass lesion, and bilateral swelling with or without midline shift.

15. The answer is **B,** pages 980 and 981.

The guidelines for pediatric brain death determination of the American Academy of Pediatrics (AAP) involve an observation period of a minimum of 24 hours for children younger than 1 year and 12 hours for children older than 1. The emergency physician must identify and correct any reversible condition, especially the detection of toxic and metabolic disorders.

16. The answer is **B,** pages 981 to 984.

Headache is defined as pain involving the scalp, skull, or intracranial contents. Because children less than 5 years of age rarely complain of headaches, an organic cause is likely in these patients. All of the other statements concerning headache are correct.

17. The answer is **D,** page 981.

Fever is a common cause of headache pain that tends to be frontal or bitemporal and have a vascular throbbing quality. Maxillary sinusitis causes facial pain rather than headache whereas sphenoid sinusitis produces occipital pain, and ethmoid sinusitis results in eyeball pain. In the absence of pain and prolonged upper respiratory symptoms, frontal headache in young children whose frontal sinuses have not pneumatized should not be attributed to sinusitis.

18. The answer is **D,** page 982.

Cluster headaches, although rare in pediatric patients, are paroxysmal and unilateral. They tend to be retroorbital, periorbital, or frontal. Unilateral autonomic symptoms may develop and include nasal stuffiness, lacrimation, and Horner's syndrome. They are not usually associated with an aura.

19. The answer is **H,** page 984.
Tremors are involuntary, rhythmic oscillations that usually affect the hands. Essential (familial) tremor is inherited as an autosomal dominant trait. Its onset is usually in adulthood.

20. The answer is **G,** page 984.
Tics or habit spasms are stereotyped, quick, and purposeless movements or utterances not associated with an impairment of consciousness. Face, neck, and shoulders are commonly involved. Tics increase in frequency when the patient is under stress or excited.

21. The answer is **F,** page 984.
Myoclonus involves involuntary, rapid jerks of any body part caused by muscle contractions. The jerks can be symmetric or asymmetric, rhythmic, focal, or generalized. They can be activated by visual or tactile stimuli (reflex myoclonus) or by purposeful movements (action myoclonus).

22. The answer is **E,** page 984.
Torticollis is an abnormal tilt of the head and neck.

23. The answer is **D,** page 984.
Dystonia is a disorder of the basal ganglia characterized by an abnormal posture of the body with or without a facial grimace resulting from simultaneous contraction of agonist and antagonist muscles. Dystonia can affect the limbs, trunk, or face. Acquired dystonias can be acquired from trauma, infections, intoxication (carbon monoxide), hypoxic-ischemic encephalopathy, tumors, and hydrocephalus.

24. The answer is **C,** page 984.
Ballismus is an irregular, violent hurling or flailing of one or more limbs and is associated with infectious causes including viral encephalitis or a stroke involving the subthalamic nucleus.

25. The answer is **B,** page 984.
Athetosis is a slow, irregular writhing movement of the extremities. It is associated with perinatal injury, including hypoxia, ischemia, and kernicterus.

26. The answer is **A,** page 984.
Chorea is a quick, random jerk of a part of the body. Any body part can be included, but the limbs are most commonly affected. Sydenham's chorea, which may occur months after streptococcal pharyngitis, is one of the major Jones criteria for the diagnosis of rheumatic fever.

27. The answer is **A,** page 985.
It may be difficult to differentiate between a motor disorder and a focal seizure. Helpful clues include the following: (a) involuntary movements usually disappear during sleep, but seizures do not; (b) movement disorders do not produce a loss of consciousness; (c) movement disorders are more stereotyped than seizures; and (d) an electroencephalogram (EEG) performed during an abnormal movement will be normal.

28. The answer is **B,** page 986.
Acute paraplegia or quadriplegia is a neurologic emergency. It is important to localize the lesion either to the upper motor neuron, which arises in the cerebral cortex and traverses the brainstem and spinal cord, or to the lower motor neuron unit, which includes the anterior horn cell, the neuromuscular junction, and the muscle. Lesions of the upper motor neuronal unit usually affect whole muscle groups, produce increased tone and deep tendon reflexes, and do not demonstrate fasciculations or atrophy. (See Table 56-5, Page 986 in Barkin et al.)

29. The answer is **B,** pages 986 and 987.
Refusal to walk or stand is often the first symptom of a subacute process and is often interpreted by the child or parent as leg weakness or pain. This patient has a history of trauma (spinal tap). An infectious cause of paraplegia is epidural abscess, and the initial symptoms may be similar to diskitis and osteomyelitis. Most epidural abscesses are due to hematogenous spread of bacteria, especially *Staphylococcus aureus,* rather than extension from osteomyelitis; therefore it is important to elicit a history of preceding infection or trauma to the back. Vertebral osteomyelitis also is due to hematogenous spread of bacteria, but the patients usually have more systemic signs such as fever, anorexia, and back pain. Diskitis usually includes walking difficulties in children under 3 years of age.

30. The answer is **D,** pages 836, 934, and 987.
Botulism is a toxin-mediated neuromuscular disease. The toxin produced by *Clostridium botulinum* binds irreversibly to the neuromuscular junction, preventing the release of acetylcholine, and causes paralysis. Weakness proceeds in a symmetric, descending fashion beginning with the cranial nerves. Definitive diagnosis requires identification of the toxin in the stool. A trivalent antitoxin is available but is not helpful in the infantile form of botulism because not much toxin is circulating. Antibiotics play no role in this disease.

31. The answer is **E,** pages 988 and 989.
The acute onset of hemiplegia implies a vascular disorder or epilepsy. Predisposing illnesses associated with cerebrovascular disease include sickle cell disease, congenital heart disease (cyanotic), and vasculopathies such as systemic lupus erythematosus. Cyanotic heart disease may cause acute hemiplegia as the result of venous thrombosis associated with dehydration and polycythemia or by atrial embolization of a thrombus or vegetation. Of the choices listed only tetralogy of Fallot allows a cerebral emboli via right-to-left shunting.

32. The answer is **E,** pages 989 to 993.

Syncope is a sudden, transient loss of consciousness caused by inadequate blood, oxygen, or substrate to the brain. It is usually brief and precipitated by intercurrent illness, hypovolemia, anemia, vasodilation, drug use, prolonged bed rest, or inactivity. Warning signs are common and include nausea, a feeling of warmth, perspiration, lightheadedness, dizziness, blurred vision, and pallor. The period of unconsciousness usually is brief. Placing the patient in a supine position with the head down usually results in a return of consciousness.

33. The answer is **D,** page 991.

QT prolongation, ventricular dysrhythmias, and torsades de pointes have resulted from overdoses of antidysrhythmic drugs such as procainamide and quinidine as well as from normal use of tricyclic antidepressants, phenothiazines, and nonsedating antihistamines such as terfenadine and astemizole, especially if administered with erythromycin or ketoconazole.

34. The answer is **A,** page 992.

The patient's vital signs, including orthostatic vital signs, should be measured (i.e., pulse and blood pressure measurement in the supine and sitting [legs dependent] or standing position). A positive test would be the increase in HR by 20 beats per minute, the development of bradycardia, a decrease in systolic blood pressure by 20 mm Hg when erect, or the feelings of dizziness when going from supine to any other position.

35. The answer is **B,** page 993.

The most common cause of vertigo in pediatric patients is otitis media.

36. The answer is **A,** pages 995 and 996.

Cyanotic breath-holding spells result from cerebral hypoxia. They are more common than the pallid breath-holding spell in which the child begins to cry because of anger, frustration, or fear and stops breathing with cyanosis ensuing rapidly followed by limpness and loss of consciousness. The child may resume normal behavior or continue crying after awakening. Posturing and tonic-clonic movements may occur, and the child may remain sleepy for a period after the attack. All of the remaining statements are true concerning breath-holding spells.

37. The answer is **C,** pages 996 to 1008.

Meningitis is an inflammatory process of the meninges surrounding the brain. It occurs most commonly between 3 and 8 months of age with 90% of all cases occurring before the age of 5 years. The upper respiratory tract is the major reservoir of pathogens, and hematogenous transmission is common with bacteremia often preceding the onset of meningitis. Up to one third of children have a distant focus of infection.

38. The answer is **A,** page 997.

S. pneumoniae is the most common, followed by *Haemophilus influenzae* type B and *N. meningitidis.* They cause meningitis in 90% to 95% of the cases involving children over 2 months of age. (See Table 56-6, Page 997 in Barkin et al.)

39. The answer is **C,** page 998.

S. epidermidis is the most common pathogen responsible for ventriculoperitoneal shunt infections, followed by *S. aureus* and gram-negative organisms.

40. The answer is **B,** page 998.

To assess shunt function, the reservoir is pumped, and if it cannot be depressed, a distal block is present; if it pumps but does not refill, it is blocked proximally at the ventricular end. Proximal obstructions occur more commonly than distal obstructions.

41. The answer is **D,** page 999.

The infant described in this scenario appears to have increased intracranial pressure, possibly from shaken baby syndrome. The most important approach is the standard ABCs (airway, breathing, and circulation), and therefore the infant's trachea should be intubated. Hyperventilation to obtain a $Paco_2$ of approximately 35 mm Hg should help to decrease the cerebral blood volume.

42. The answer is **A,** page 1000.

The CSF glucose level is usually low in patients who have bacterial meningitis. The normal CSF/serum glucose ratio is approximately 0.6, and there is a greater specificity for bacterial meningitis with a ratio of 0.3. (See Table 56-8 on Page 1001 in Barkin et al.)

43. The answer is **C,** page 1002.

Children with aseptic meningitis or meningocephalitis usually manifest fewer symptoms than children with a low-grade fever. Enterovirus accounts for approximately 85% of all cases of aseptic meningitis.

44. The answer is **E,** page 1003.

Chemoprophylaxis is recommended for all household contacts regardless of age in households with at least one contact younger than 48 months. Day care facilities with children under 2 years of age with 25 or more hours of contact per week usually should initiate prophylaxis.

45. The answer is **E,** pages 1004 to 1008.

Migraine is an episodic headache that is unilateral or bilateral, pulsating, of moderate to severe intensity, and exacerbated by physical activity. Migraines are more common in adolescent girls, and half of the patients who have migraines have the first one before the age of 20 years. Migraineurs have an incidence of epilepsy of 2% to 8%, which is higher than the general population. A prodrome of psychologic, neurologic, and constitutional symptoms occurs in approximately 60% of the patients.

46. The answer is **A,** pages 1008 and 1009.

Pseudotumor cerebri (idiopathic intracranial hypertension) is a syndrome characterized by the clinical manifestations of increased intracranial pressure with normal CSF constituents and a normal brain shown by head CT. Common predisposing conditions include otitis media, corticosteroid use, obesity, and mild head trauma. Papilledema is present in virtually all cases.

47. The answer is **B,** pages 1009 to 1011.

A seizure is a sudden, paroxysmal, excessive electrical discharge of neurons within the cerebral cortex. The most common cause of seizures in pediatric patients is fever.

48. The answer is **A,** page 1011.
    The most common cause of perinatal seizures within the first 48 to 72 hours of life is perinatal anoxia or hypoxia, often intrauterine hypoxia. In full-term and premature infants 50% to 65% of seizures are due to hypoxic-ischemic encephalopathy.
49. The answer is **A,** page 1012.
    After a first nonfebrile, unprovoked seizure, the risk of recurrence depends on several factors and ranges from 27% to 61%. Definite risk factors include an abnormal EEG and an underlying neurologic abnormality. Other risk factors include the type of seizure (partial), family history of epilepsy, and a history of prior febrile seizures.

50. The answer is **A,** page 1017.
    Viral infections are associated with 80% of febrile seizures for which a cause has been determined. Upper respiratory infections represent 38% to 40% of cases, otitis media 15% to 23%, pneumonia 15%, acute gastroenteritis 8%, roseola 5%, and influenza 1.4%.

49

Orthopedic Disorders

Dennis Heon • Adriana Manikian

See Barkin et al: Chapter 57.

1. A 7-year-old boy comes to the ED with a limp and temperature (T) up to 39° C for 2 days. Your physical examination reveals erythema, swelling, and decreased active range of motion of the left knee. Laboratory data include white blood cells (WBCs) 17,000 cells/mm^3, erythrocyte sedimentation rate (ESR) 80 mm/hr, and C-reactive protein (CRP) 25 mg/L. You decide to perform arthrocentesis. Which of the following is most consistent with septic arthritis?

Appearance	Leukocytes (cells/mm^3)	Percentage of neutrophils	Percentage of glucose synovial/ blood	Mucin clot
A. Clear	90	25	60	Good
B. Turbid	40,000	50	60	Poor
C. Turbid	80,000	25	20	Poor
D. Bloody	4,000	30	60	Good

2. An 8-year-old girl complains of back pain. Probable causes include all of the following *except:*
   A. Psychogenic cause.
   B. Spondylolisthesis.
   C. Pyelonephritis.
   D. Leukemia.
   E. Intervertebral diskitis.

3. A 6-year-old girl has had bilateral leg pain for 2 months. She describes the pain as being in her thighs and behind the knees. She states that the pain is worse in the evenings and is gone by morning. The physical examination is unremarkable. The complete blood count (CBC) with differential count, ESR, and CRP are within the normal limits. Plain knee radiographs are normal. Which is the most appropriate next step in the management of this child's condition?
   A. Order a radionuclide bone scan.
   B. Obtain Lyme disease titers.
   C. Order magnetic resonance imaging (MRI) of the knee.
   D. Refer the patient for physical therapy.
   E. Reassure the parents that the condition will resolve spontaneously.

4. A 5-year-old boy has had an antalgic limp for 2 months, and it is slowly getting worse. He has stiffness of the right hip as well as decreased abduction and medial rotation. A radiograph is obtained and shown in Fig. 49-1. Which of the following statements about the condition described above is true?
   A. The condition is more common in adolescents.
   B. Bone age of affected individual is normal for age.
   C. ESR is elevated.
   D. Bone scan is positive.
   E. Arthrocentesis is diagnostic.

5. An 8-year-old boy with sickle cell disease has osteomyelitis. The most likely recovered pathogen is which of the following?
   A. *Haemophilus influenzae.*
   B. *Staphylococcus aureus.*
   C. *Salmonella.*
   D. *Pseudomonas aeruginosa.*
   E. *Streptococcus.*

6. A 4-year-old girl has had low back pain for 7 days. She is febrile to 38.2° C. The pain is worse with flexion of the spine, walking, or straight leg raising. Lumbar spine radiographs show narrowing of the L1-L2 intervertebral disk space. Which of the following is true about the above condition?
   A. It affects children from all age groups.
   B. ESR is normal.
   C. Blood cultures are likely to be positive in most cases.
   D. Aspiration and biopsy of the disk space are necessary for diagnosis.
   E. Bed rest and immobilization of the spine are necessary, and antibiotics should be administered.

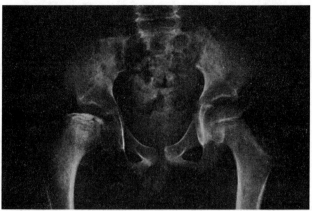

FIG. 49-1

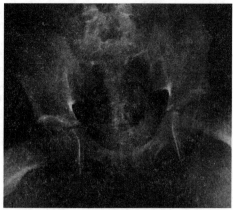

FIG. 49-2

7. A 3-year-old boy has had a limp and temperature up to 39° C for 1 day. He has redness, swelling, and warmth over the right knee. The patient does not voluntarily move the affected joint and keeps his knee in 35 degrees of flexion. Which of the following is a true statement about the diagnosis in this patient?
    A. Widening of the joint space on plain radiograph is the first finding.
    B. WBC count greater than 15,000/mm^3 is found in more than 90% of the cases.
    C. The most common mechanism of infection is direct inoculation.
    D. The most common organism found is *S. aureus*.
    E. Delay in diagnosis by 1 day is associated with increased morbidity.

8. A 16-year-old boy twisted his ankle while playing basketball and is now limping. Physical examination reveals moderate swelling around the lateral malleolus, a positive anterior drawer test, and a negative talar tilt test. The patient has no point tenderness. An x-ray film of the ankle shows only soft tissue swelling. What is the most likely injury in this patient?
    A. Posterior talofibular ligament injury.
    B. Anterior talofibular ligament injury.
    C. Anterior talofibular ligament and calcaneofibular ligament injury.
    D. Salter-Harris type I fracture of the distal tibia.
    E. Salter-Harris type I fracture of the distal fibula.

9. A 14-year-old boy has a 2-month history of anterolateral thigh and knee pain. The pain is intermittent and dull and increases with exercise. Physical examination reveals decreased internal rotation of the left hip. A radiograph of the hips is shown in Fig. 49-2. Which one of the following is true about the underlying condition?
    A. It is a nondisplaced Salter-Harris type I fracture.
    B. Body habitus is noncontributory.
    C. The condition is usually bilateral.
    D. Plain radiograph is diagnostic.
    E. Management is nonoperative.

10. A 5-year-old boy has a limp favoring the right leg. The patient has full range of motion in the knee and a mild decrease in abduction and medial rotation of the hip. He is afebrile. He had upper respiratory infection (URI) symptoms 1 to 2 weeks ago. Laboratory tests and radiographs of the hip and knee are normal. The most likely diagnosis is which of the following?
    A. Toxic synovitis.
    B. Slipped capital femoral epiphysis (SCFE).
    C. Legg-Calvé-Perthes (LCP) disease.
    D. Septic arthritis.
    E. Trauma.

11. A 14-year-old boy has knee pain after he exercises. Physical examination localizes the pain to the anterior tibial tuberosity. The most appropriate treatment for this condition is which of the following?
    A. Decreased level of physical activity for 3 months.
    B. Ice packs for 3 days followed by hot packs for 1 week.
    C. Prednisone 1 mg/kg for 1 week.
    D. Long leg splint for 2 weeks.
    E. Immediate orthopedic referral.

12. A 15-year-old girl has a 1-month history of left knee pain that is worse at night. She remembers falling on her knee several months ago. She reports that the pain is worsening and that there is a lump over the medial surface of her right knee that is enlarging. Which of the following is the most appropriate first step in the evaluation of this adolescent?
    A. CBC with differential count and ESR.
    B. Biopsy of the mass.
    C. MRI of the knee.
    D. Radiograph of the knee.
    E. Radionuclide bone scan.

13. A 7-year-old girl has had pain in her right leg and fever for 2 weeks. Physical examination reveals pain along the femur, as well as warmth and erythema. Laboratory studies demonstrate WBCs 14,000 cells/mm³, ESR 70 mm/hr, and CRP 65 mg/L. A radiograph of the femur shows periosteal elevation and a small amount of lytic destruction. What is the best antibiotic regimen for this patient?
    A. Nafcillin intravenously (IV) for 6 weeks.
    B. Nafcillin IV for 2 weeks, then oral dicloxacillin for 4 weeks.
    C. Nafcillin and cefotaxime IV for 4 weeks.
    D. Ticarcillin-clavulanate IV for 4 weeks.
    E. Oral cephalexin for 6 weeks

14. A 15-month-old girl has had a limp for 4 hours. Physical examination is unremarkable. The patient is afebrile. Medical history is noncontributory. The most likely diagnosis is which of the following?
    A. Growing pains.
    B. Toxic synovitis.
    C. Early bacterial infection of a bone or joint.
    D. Slipped capital femoral epiphysis.
    E. Traumatic injury that was not witnessed.

15. A 16-month-old boy is unable to bear weight on his right leg. The parent states that he jumped off the couch onto the floor, cried, and would not walk. Physical examination reveals point tenderness over the distal tibia. A radiograph is obtained and is shown in Fig. 49-3. What is the most appropriate course of action?
    A. Obtain a skeletal survey and notify the child protection team.
    B. Prescribe rest, ice, and elevation, and wrap the leg in an Ace bandage.
    C. Place the leg in a cast for 3 to 6 weeks.
    D. Make an emergency orthopedic referral.
    E. Begin workup for a pathologic fracture.

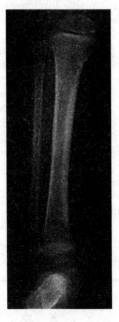

FIG. 49-3

16. A 4-year-old girl has a 2-week history of intermittent fever up to 40° C, malaise, anorexia, pain, and swelling in both wrists and ankles. The physical examination shows an ill-appearing febrile child with a salmon-red morbilliform rash mainly on the trunk. She has a pericardial rub, marked hepatosplenomegaly, and tender, edematous ankles and wrists. Which of the following sets of laboratory data best describes this child's condition (*WBC*, white blood cell; *ESR*, erythrocyte sedimentation rate; *ASLO*, antistreptolysin O; *ANA*, antinuclear antibodies; and *RF*, rheumatoid factors)?

	WBCs (per mm³)	Diff. (w/left shift)	ESR (mm/hr)	ASLO	ANA	RF
A.	14,000	None	5	1:200	Neg	Neg
B.	35,200	Marked	113	1:200	Neg	Neg
C.	7,500	None	95	1:200	Pos	Neg
D.	15,000	Minimal	80	1:1000	Neg	Neg
E.	8,000	None	11	1:200	Neg	Neg

17. A 3-month-old boy is brought to the ED by social services staff because abuse is suspected. Radiographic studies reveal an epiphyseal fracture (bucket-handle or corner fracture) of the tibia. Which of the following is a true statement about this condition?
    A. It is caused by accidental trauma.
    B. It is common in older children.
    C. It is commonly confused with an ossification center.
    D. It is easily seen on plain radiographs.
    E. It is associated with shaken baby syndrome.

18. A 13-year-old boy has had right elbow pain for 1 month, and it is becoming progressively worse. He plays tennis regularly and denies any trauma to the elbow. Physical examination reveals tenderness over the lateral epicondyle and pain on forced flexion of the extended wrist. Radiographs of the elbow are normal. What is the most appropriate next step in the management of this child's condition?
    A. Administer aspirin 100 mg/kg/day.
    B. Administer nonsteroidal antiinflammatory drugs (NSAIDs).
    C. Tell the patient to rest until symptoms resolve.
    D. Refer the patient for physical therapy.
    E. Administer oral corticosteroids.

19. Avascular necrosis of the femoral head can be caused by all of the following except:
    A. Legg-Calvé-Perthes (LCP) disease.
    B. Sickle cell disease.
    C. Gaucher's disease.
    D. Chronic steroid use.
    E. Hemophilia.

20. A 6-year-old boy has had bilateral knee and ankle pain and swelling for 3 days. Today the mother noticed a raised purpuric rash over his buttocks and lower extremities. The boy also is complaining of intermittent abdominal pain. CBC, coagulation studies, and serum electrolyte levels are normal, and urinalysis shows trace protein and 50 to 100 red blood cells (RBCs)/high-power field (HPF). Which of the following is a true statement regarding this child's arthritis?
    A. Arthritis is transient and has an excellent prognosis.
    B. Arthritis rarely occurs in this disorder.
    C. Arthritis is severe with residual deformities.
    D. Arthritis requires treatment with corticosteroids.
    E. Effusions, if present, are hemorrhagic.

21. A 16-year-old gymnast has had right knee pain for 1 month. She states that the pain is worse after exercise and after prolonged periods of sitting. Physical examination reveals crepitation on passive motion of the patella and mild quadriceps wasting. Which of the following is the most likely diagnosis?
    A. Patellar dislocation.
    B. Chondromalacia patellae.
    C. Osgood-Schlatter disease.
    D. Prepatellar bursitis.
    E. Anterior cruciate ligament injury.

22. A 14-year-old girl has idiopathic thoracolumbar scoliosis. Which of the following statements best describes her condition?
    A. It is frequently associated with significant back pain.
    B. It is most common in children in the first years of school.
    C. It is frequently confused with Scheuermann's disease.
    D. It is best treated surgically in children.
    E. There is a relationship between the restrictive lung disease and the magnitude of the curve.

ANSWERS [See Barkin et al: Chapter 57.]

1. The answer is **C,** pages 1039 to 1040.
   Normal values for a joint aspirate are listed in choice A. A high glucose level is more consistent with an inflammatory process like juvenile rheumatoid arthritis (JRA) or rheumatic fever than with septic arthritis. It also can be seen in viral arthritis. A bloody tap is most consistent with a traumatic injury.

2. The answer is **A,** pages 1028 to 1031.
   Although back pain is a common adult complaint, it is rare in children (2% referrals to orthopedists). Significant illness or injury must be ruled out before labeling a complaint psychosomatic.

3. The answer is **E,** pages 1026 and 1027.
   Growing pains typically occur in children who are between 2 and 8 years old and affect boys more than girls. Growing pains have no specific joint or extraarticular manifestations and are associated with normal laboratory values (CBC with differential, ESR, and rheumatologic studies). Radiographs of the hips, knees, and ankles are normal. Treatment is not necessary, and the condition resolves spontaneously.

4. The answer is **D,** pages 1027 and 1033 to 1034.
   The patient has Legg-Calvé-Perthes disease (LCP). It affects children who are between 4 and 10 years old. Bone age usually is delayed. The ESR is normal. The bone scan is positive early in the course of the disease. Arthrocentesis is indicated if there is a concern about septic arthritis, but would not be diagnostic in this case.

5. The answer is **C,** page 1036.
   Salmonella is the most commonly recovered pathogen of osteomyelitis in patients with sickle cell disease. *Haemophilus influenzae* was formerly the second most common pathogen of osteomyelitis in normal children, but with widespread immunization, the incidence is decreasing. *Staphylococcus aureus* is the most common cause of osteomyelitis in normal children and the second most common cause of osteomyelitis in sickle cell disease. *Pseudomonas* is found in penetrating injuries to the foot and in drug abusers. *Streptococcus* is a less common cause of osteomyelitis in normal children under the age of 2 years.

6. The answer is **E,** page 1029.
   This child's symptoms and radiographic findings are consistent with intervertebral diskitis. It affects children younger than 10 years old, but the majority of cases occur by age 5. The patients have back pain that worsens with movement of the spine and splinting of the paravertebral muscles. Nonverbal children can have a paradoxic cry when picked up or during diaper changes. The ESR is elevated, WBC count is usually normal or mildly elevated, and blood cultures are negative in most cases. Diagnosis is made by spine radiograph, which shows narrowing of the lumbar intervertebral disk space and end plate irregularities of the adjacent vertebral bodies. Bone scan may be helpful in the early stages of the process when the radiographic changes are not present. Aspiration and biopsy of the disk space are reserved for children who do not respond to treatment. Only 25% of the aspirates have positive cultures, and in most cases *S. aureus* is the pathogen. Treatment consists of bed rest, immobilization (bracing) of the lumbar spine, and administration of antistaphylococcal antibiotics.

7. The answer is **D,** pages 1038 and 1039.

The patient has septic arthritis. *S. aureus* is the pathogen in more than 50% of the cases with a known pathogen. Displacement of the normal fat lines is the earliest finding on plain radiographs. Widening of the joint space and bony destruction are late findings. A WBC count greater than 15,000/mm^3 is seen in only half of the cases. The most common mode of infection is hematogenous spread. A delay in diagnosis of more than 4 days has been associated with increased morbidity and complications.

8. The answer is **B,** page 1032.

The anterior talofibular ligament is the weakest of the three major lateral ankle ligaments. A positive anterior drawer test is indicative of this injury. The posterior talofibular ligament is the strongest of the three, and injury to this ligament is rarely an isolated event. The anterior talofibular ligament and the calcaneofibular ligament must be torn completely to cause gross lateral ankle instability (positive talar tilt test). Fractures are more common than sprains in young children because the ligaments are stronger than the physis of the bones. A Salter-Harris type I fracture is through the physis, and thus no fracture is visible on the x-ray. Point tenderness is common with this type of injury.

9. The answer is **D,** pages 1027 and 1032 to 1033.

The patient has a slipped capital femoral epiphysis (SCFE). It is a displaced Salter-Harris type I fracture. Of patients with this condition, 88% are obese, and 10% of the fractures are bilateral. Anteroposterior (AP) and frog leg views on plain hip film are diagnostic. The treatment is surgical pinning.

10. The answer is **A,** pages 1025 and 1032.

The patient has toxic synovitis, a nonspecific inflammation and hypertrophy of the synovial membrane. It occurs in young children (1 to 7 years old) and is more common in boys. Often the patient has a history of upper respiratory infection. Laboratory and radiologic tests are normal. SCFE and LCP disease would have abnormal radiographs. If the diagnosis of septic arthritis cannot be ruled out, arthrocentesis is indicated but would be normal in the above patient. A 5-year-old should be able to describe a traumatic injury even if it was not witnessed by others.

11. The answer is **A,** pages 1027 and 1032 to 1033.

The patient has Osgood-Schlatter disease. It is a traction apophysitis of the tibial tubercle from repeated episodes of microtrauma. It is common in physically active boys during adolescence. The condition results from overuse. Recommended treatment is to decrease the level of physical activity for several months and allow the tibial tubercle to fuse to the diaphysis of the tibia.

12. The answer is **D,** pages 1027 and 1032.

Any rapidly growing bony mass in an adolescent is considered malignant until proven otherwise. Given the location of this patient's mass, distal femur or proximal tibia, the most likely diagnosis is osteogenic sarcoma. Plain radiographs are the first step in the evaluation of the mass and usually show a lytic or sclerotic lesion in the metaphysis of the involved bone, cortical disruption, and marked periosteal reaction with new bone formation ("sun-burst pattern"). MRI of the primary lesion, radionuclide bone scan, and chest CT often are obtained for staging purposes. Biopsy of the lesion gives the definitive diagnosis. CBC and ESR are normal in the early stages of the disease.

13. The answer is **B,** pages 1037 and 1038.

The patient has osteomyelitis. The most common pathogen is *S. aureus.* All patients with osteomyelitis require admission and intravenous (IV) antibiotics. The therapy currently recommended is 1 to 2 weeks of parenteral antibiotics followed by 3 to 6 weeks of oral antibiotics. The addition of cefotaxime is indicated for osteomyelitis in newborns (less than 1 month old) or in patients with sickle cell disease. An antipseudomonal penicillin is indicated for penetrating wounds of the foot and for drug abusers. Oral therapy alone is inadequate.

14. The answer is **E,** pages 1025 and 1031.

The most common cause of limp in this age group is trauma that was not witnessed. Sometimes focal physical examination findings exist, but often the patient just has a limp. SCFE occurs in adolescents. All of the other choices occur in this age group but are statistically less likely.

15. The answer is **C,** pages 1031 to 1034.

The patient has a toddler's fracture, which occurs in infants and young children because of seemingly trivial traumatic events. The fracture is a spiral fracture of the diaphysis of the tibia caused by torsional forces applied from a fall or by twisting against resistance. The fibula is intact. This type of fracture is common because the bone is still a woven matrix and has not ossified fully yet. A spiral fracture of the femur and humerus without a story consistent with a twisting mechanism raises suspicion of child abuse. The location of this patient's injury and the intact fibula make child abuse less likely. The patient has a nondisplaced fracture and requires immobilization for 3 to 6 weeks. The patient does not need emergency orthopedic referral because circulation to the limb is intact; however, nonemergency orthopedic follow-up is advised. Open reduction with internal fixation is not indicated. The injury is not consistent with a pathologic fracture.

16. The answer is **B,** pages 1025 to 1028.

This child has classic symptoms for systemic onset JRA. A markedly elevated WBC count with a leukemoid reaction, high ESR, anemia, and negative ANA and RF are all consistent with this diagnosis. Pauciarticular JRA type I is the most common type of JRA and is ANA positive in 90% of the cases. The WBC count and differential are usually normal, ESR is elevated, and RF is usually negative. Common laboratory findings in rheumatic fever are leukocytosis with a left shift, elevated ESR, and positive ASLO titers.

17. The answer is **E,** page 1025.

A bucket-handle or corner fracture is a metaphyseal-epiphyseal fracture, usually of the proximal tibia or distal femur. It is pathognomonic for child abuse and is associated with shaken baby syndrome. The injury is caused by either a rapid acceleration-deceleration force or torsion. Bucket-handle fractures do not produce a significant periosteal reaction because of the intact periosteum in most cases. The incidence of these fractures is underestimated because they are overlooked easily.

18. The answer is **C,** page 1025.

This patient has "tennis elbow," an inflammation of the aponeurosis of the extensor carpi radialis brevis and extensor communis aponeurosis. Radiographs of the elbow are normal. Treatment consists of rest until resolution of the symptoms followed by a gradual increase in activity to strengthen the forearm muscle. NSAIDs, although not contributory to the resolution of the condition, may be used for pain relief.

19. The answer is **E,** pages 1031 to 1034.

Hemophilia is associated with hemarthrosis. The most commonly involved joints are the knees and the elbows. Avascular necrosis is a complication of all the other answer choices.

20. The answer is **A,** pages 798 to 799 and 1026 to 1027.

This child has Henoch-Schönlein purpura (HSP). Patients typically have nonthrombocytopenic palpable purpura that is usually on the buttocks and lower extremities, arthritis, abdominal pain, and nephritis. Arthritis is present in two thirds of the patients with HSP. It is transient and has an excellent prognosis. The most commonly involved joints are the knees and ankles. Effusions seldom occur and are serous, not hemorrhagic. Corticosteroid therapy is reserved for severe nephritis. NSAIDs or aspirin may be indicated for symptomatic relief in patients with arthritis.

21. The answer is **B,** pages 1032 and 1033.

The patient has chondromalacia patellae, a common degenerative disorder caused by trauma, overuse, or disturbances in patellar function. It is most common in adolescent girls. There is crepitation on passive motion of the patella and quadriceps muscle wasting (usually vastus medialis). Treatment consists of non–weight-bearing exercises, ice application, and NSAIDs or aspirin. In cases of treatment failure, arthroscopic debridement and patellar realignment are indicated.

Osgood-Schlatter disease is a traction apophysitis of the tibial tuberosity. The pain is worse on exertion, especially with flexion of the knee, and improves with rest.

Patellar dislocation is a traumatic tear of the medial patellar retinaculum. Attempts to extend the knee cause severe pain. Treatment consists of relocation of the patella by extending the knee after adequate pain control.

Prepatellar bursitis occurs in people who kneel for long periods of time. Painful swelling on the anterior aspect of the patella without an associated effusion is typical. NSAIDs, knee pads, and restriction of the precipitating activity resolve the condition.

Anterior cruciate ligament injury is caused by hyperextension of an already extended knee. In most cases the patient hears a "pop." The injury is followed by restricted range of motion in the knee and, in 90% of the cases, by acute hemarthrosis. In mild cases conservative treatment (physical therapy and bracing) is sufficient. Operative repair is indicated for an unstable knee.

22. The answer is **E,** pages 1029 to 1030.

Idiopathic scoliosis is lateral deviation of the spine in the coronal plane. It occurs most commonly in adolescence and in girls more than boys but sometimes is seen in infancy and early childhood. It rarely causes back pain, unless there is significant impingement of nerve roots. The mainstay of therapy is early recognition, close follow-up, and bracing. Surgical treatment is indicated for curvature greater than 40 degrees and in rapidly progressing disease. A linear relationship exists between the magnitude of the curve and the severity of the restrictive lung disease. Scheuermann's kyphosis is excessive curvature (more than 45 degrees) in the thoracic spine. It has an autosomal-dominant inheritance and is more common in males.

CHAPTER

50

Psychiatric and Behavioral Disorders

Theodore M. Barnett

See Barkin et al: Chapter 58.

1. An 8-year-old boy has nocturnal enuresis. He never has been continent at night but has no daytime wetting. Physical examination and a urinalysis are normal. Your recommendation to the parents is:
   A. Administration of imipramine.
   B. Administration of desmopressin (DDAVP).
   C. A behavioral pediatrics appointment.
   D. An appointment with the child's pediatrician.
   E. A urologic consultation.

2. A 6-year-old girl has a 2-week history of nocturnal enuresis. She has been toilet trained since she was 18 months old and had not previously wet the bed for a year. Physical examination and urinalysis are normal. Your next step is:
   A. Urodynamic studies.
   B. Measurement of serum electrolyte levels, blood urea nitrogen, creatinine, and glucose.
   C. Trial of phenazopyridine.
   D. Renal ultrasound.
   E. Obtainment of additional family and social history.

3. A 5-year-old boy has a 6-week history of soiling his underwear. He has a history of painful, difficult bowel movements since early infancy. He has a normal physical examination except for a distended abdomen with palpable feces. Of the following, the most useful evaluation is:
   A. Barium enema.
   B. Psychometric testing.
   C. Social services evaluation of the family.
   D. Magnetic resonance imaging (MRI) of the lumbosacral spine.
   E. Abdominal ultrasound.

4. Childhood sleep problems usually are brought to the ED because of:
   A. The child's anxiety about not sleeping.
   B. The child's falling asleep at school.
   C. Disturbance of parental sleep.
   D. Side effects of medication.
   E. The child's refusal to sleep.

5. The parents of a 3-year-old complain that she has been waking up in pain the last two nights. She wakes up agitated and screaming within an hour or two of going to bed and cannot be consoled. After about 15 minutes, she seems to become more comfortable and goes back to sleep. The child denies having any problem. After examining the child and finding no abnormalities, you conclude that she is suffering from:
   A. Nightmares.
   B. Sleep terrors.
   C. Normal night awakenings.
   D. Colic.
   E. Childhood schizophrenia.

6. You are seeing a 9-month-old who has listlessness. Her mother appears exhausted and reports her husband is overseas in the military. She is concerned that the baby has seemed to be less interested in playing for the past 3 weeks. As you consider the differential diagnosis in this patient, which of the following statements is true?
   A. Evidence of neglect on physical examination precludes a diagnosis of depression.
   B. Weight gain is not related to depression in infants.
   C. Depression in infants is a result of endogenous factors and is rarely a product of environment
   D. Depression should not be considered in patients less than 1 year old.
   E. Developmental delay can be a result of depression.

7. An adolescent has been referred for medical screening before admission to a psychiatric facility. Your evaluation shows a sad, tearful young man who is otherwise normal physically. A urine drug screening test is pending. As you await the results, the patient discloses he has been using marijuana daily for the past month since his mother was diagnosed with a manic episode. Which of the following statements regarding the patient described above is true?
   A. Drug abuse excludes the diagnosis of depression.
   B. Admission is not needed unless a patient has a major depressive disorder.
   C. A major depressive episode may last up to a week.
   D. A family history of bipolar disorder increases the incidence of depression.
   E. Suicidal ideation does not occur before 8 years of age.

8. A teenager is in the ED for "problems with hyperactivity." He was diagnosed with attention-deficit hyperactivity disorder (ADHD) 2 weeks ago and started taking methylphenidate. His parents are concerned because "he's just getting worse." For the past month he has been irritable, talking constantly in school, and sleeping very little and has experimented with cocaine. He has not gotten a passing grade in 3 weeks. You suspect the patient is suffering from:
   A. A side effect of methylphenidate.
   B. Bipolar disorder.
   C. ADHD with inadequate control.
   D. Secondary effects of polydrug abuse.
   E. Cyclothymic disorder.

9. A 6-year-old girl has abdominal pain. Her mother reports ten visits to her family doctor for the same symptoms. The patient has no associated fever, vomiting, change in stools or diet, or weight loss. The pain occurs only on school mornings and resolves by 10 AM if the child is allowed to stay home. Examination is entirely normal, and the patient is pain free at present. The child's physician reports that an extensive workup, including urine, blood, and upper gastrointestinal (UGI) studies and an abdominal ultrasound, was negative. The two of you agree the patient is best treated by:
   A. Admission to the hospital for further studies.
   B. Surgical consultation.
   C. Oral diazepam each morning to control anxiety.
   D. Daily enemas until pain resolves.
   E. Reassurance, close follow-up, and firm insistence on school attendance.

10. A 9-year-old is brought to the ED because she is unable to move her right foot. Although the child does not seem to be bothered by this, the mother is quite distressed and begins to tell you about their recent house fire and subsequent relocation. Complete physical examination and plain radiographs are normal. While considering the possibility of conversion disorder, you remember that:
   A. Conversion disorder is an involuntary act.
   B. Prepubertal boys and girls are equally likely to be affected.
   C. Children of higher socioeconomic status have a higher incidence.
   D. Most conversion reactions in children have bizarre or unusual manifestations and are easily recognized.
   E. Normal vital signs differentiate conversion reaction from organic disease states.

11. A 7-year-old boy with attention-deficit-hyperactivity disorder (ADHD) is brought to the ED because "he needs more Ritalin." His mother has an appointment with his pediatrician in a week but has enough medication for only 3 days. Vital signs and physical examination are normal, but the child fidgets when sitting. Appropriate ED management includes:
   A. Measurement of methylphenidate (Ritalin) level.
   B. Prescription for a week's supply of methylphenidate (Ritalin) at the patient's present dosage.
   C. Consultation with the patient's pediatrician.
   D. Reduction of the dosage so that the medication will last a week.
   E. Change in the medication to pemoline.

12. Which of the following statements regarding medications used to treat ADHD is true?
   A. The primary agents used are antidepressants.
   B. Increased appetite is a common side effect of these medications.
   C. All children with ADHD will benefit from medication.
   D. A side effect of many of these agents is tics.
   E. Decreasing dosage can lead to manic episodes.

13. A 10-year-old is brought in by police for abrasions on his hands. He was caught breaking store windows and is well known to the police for truancy and vandalism. His mother reports that he "lies all the time" and cannot be controlled at home or in school. Which of the following is true?
   A. Conduct disorder can be fully assessed in the ED.
   B. Physical threats and assault may be part of conduct disorder.
   C. Conduct disorder rarely interferes with school activities.
   D. Conduct disorder is normal in toddlers.
   E. Oppositional defiant disorder is more severe than conduct disorder.

14. Medical disorders that can trigger pica in young children include:
   A. Iron-deficiency anemia.
   B. Pneumonia.
   C. Hepatitis A.
   D. Chronic parotitis.
   E. Peptic ulcer disease.

15. A 15-year-old girl is brought to the ED by her mother, who is concerned about her daughter's eating habits. Examination reveals an emaciated adolescent. Which of the following characteristics distinguishes anorexia nervosa from bulimia?
    A. Disturbed eating behavior.
    B. Use of laxatives or purgatives.
    C. Normal serum electrolyte levels.
    D. Body weight less than 85% that predicted by age and height.
    E. Concern about body shape.

16. The 15-year-old in question 15 has lost 10 pounds in the last 2 weeks but has normal serum electrolyte levels. The patient has no regular physician, and the mother reports that they just moved to this area while she looks for a job. Indications for admission of adolescents with eating disorders include:
    A. Serum potassium level less than 4 mEq/dl.
    B. Weight loss of over 2 pounds per week for more than 2 weeks.
    C. History of using stimulant medications for weight loss.
    D. Blood urea nitrogen (BUN) level less than 12 mg/dl.
    E. Uncertain outpatient follow-up.

17. A 10-year-old boy has a 2-week history of intermittent jerking movements (flexion) of his left arm. Which of the following is consistent with a diagnosis of transient tic disorder?
    A. The movement never occurs when the patient is asleep.
    B. The movement increases when the patient is distracted or studying.
    C. The movement is accompanied by altered mental status.
    D. The movement is slow and writhing.
    E. The movement stops when the patient is instructed to stop it.

18. Tourette's syndrome is manifested by which of the following?
    A. Multiple motor and vocal tics associated with loss of consciousness.
    B. Vocal tics only for any length of time.
    C. Multiple motor and vocal tics persisting for more than a year.
    D. Multiple motor and vocal tics persisting for no more than 2 months.
    E. Vocal tics only persisting for more than a year.

19. A 6-year-old boy comes to the ED with a history of "hallucinations" for the past 6 hours. The child insists that there are "three dogs in the room talking" to him. He just returned from visiting a friend's house. His mother reports that he has never experienced anything like this before. A true statement about psychotic symptoms in childhood is:
    A. Most cases have a functional cause.
    B. Most cases have an organic cause.
    C. Toxicologic causes of psychosis are rare.
    D. Most cases are a result of traumatic head injury.
    E. Most cases are a result of inherited psychiatric illness.

20. A 5-year-old boy who previously was found to have autism is pulling at his ears. He fights your examination violently. Autistic disorder may be distinguished from childhood schizophrenia by which of the following characteristics?
    A. Unusual movements.
    B. Social isolation.
    C. Onset before 36 months.
    D. Disinterest in normal activities.
    E. Self-stimulating behavior.

21. A 14-year-old girl is brought to the ED by ambulance after she reportedly ingested ten 25-mm diphenhydramine capsules. A friend found the patient at home alone, difficult to arouse, and called the ambulance. The patient reports that she "wants to see her mother" who died a year ago and that "I knew if I went to sleep I wouldn't wake up." Which of the following factors is the best predictor for future suicide attempts?
    A. Substance ingested.
    B. Arrival by ambulance instead of car.
    C. Age of the patient.
    D. Sex of the patient.
    E. Intent of the patient.

22. Boys outnumber girls in completed suicides because:
    A. They attempt suicide more frequently.
    B. Boys have a higher incidence of substance abuse.
    C. Boys choose more lethal methods.
    D. Boys have a higher incidence of mood disorders.
    E. Boys are less likely to leave suicide notes.

ANSWERS [See Barkin et al: Chapter 58.]

1. The answer is **D**, pages 1042 and 1043.
   About 7% of 8-year-olds have primary nocturnal enuresis. Although several therapeutic modalities for treating primary enuresis exist, longitudinal care and positive support and encouragement are essential. Pharmacologic agents rarely are necessary.

2. The answer is **E**, pages 1042 and 1043.
   This school-age girl with a normal examination and urinalysis is unlikely to have a urinary tract infection (UTI) or structural abnormality. The enuresis in this example may be a result of psychosocial problems such as stress or maltreatment, and possible causes should be addressed with the patient and family. A normal examination does not exclude child abuse.

3. The answer is **A,** pages 850, 1043-1044.

Although functional bowel problems such as stool retention during toilet training are the most common cause of encopresis, Hirschsprung's disease must be considered in any child who has had encopresis and a history of bowel movement problems since infancy. Diagnosis is important, since this is a surgically correctable problem that has life-threatening complications if left untreated.

4. The answer is **C,** pages 1044 and 1045.

Children rarely if ever complain about their own sleep problems. Parental sleep frequently is disrupted by childhood sleep difficulties (for whatever cause), and this is usually the trigger for an ED visit.

5. The answer is **B,** pages 1044 and 1045.

Onset early in the sleep cycle and amnesia for the event are classic signs that this child is having night terrors. Children with nightmares may be difficult, but not impossible, to console and usually remember the episode. This child is too old to have colic, and normal night awakenings should not have inconsolability. Childhood schizophrenia should not cause solely nocturnal symptoms.

6. The answer is **E,** pages 1047 and 1048.

Depression in infancy often results in poor weight gain and developmental delay. Lack of a nurturing environment, such as child neglect, is thought to be the primary etiology.

7. The answer is **D,** pages 1047 and 1048.

A family history of any mood disorder increases the likelihood of an occurrence in other family members. Drug abuse may cause altered mood but does not exclude a diagnosis of mood disorder. The decision to admit must be based on patient status and not on the diagnosis. Major depressive episodes are defined as lasting for at least 2 weeks. Suicidal ideation may be seen in very young children.

8. The answer is **B,** pages 1047 to 1049.

Bipolar disorders are underdiagnosed in adolescents because of confusion with ADHD and conduct disorders. Primary drug abuse must be considered as a cause, but the patient's irritability, constant talking, sleep disturbance, and drug use, combined with failing grades for 3 weeks, meet the criteria for a manic episode. His symptoms predate the methylphenidate. Symptoms of overdose with methylphenidate include decreased appetite, somatic complaints, insomnia, or tic disorders.

9. The answer is **E,** page 1048.

This child has complaints of abdominal pain only on school days with no associated signs, a normal examination, and a normal (and extensive) ancillary evaluation. Negative reinforcement (such as enemas) or medication is not indicated for school phobia. Reassurance, follow-up with a primary care physician, and firm insistence on school attendance are the hallmarks of care in this disorder.

10. The answer is **A,** pages 1048 and 1049.

Conversion disorder is an involuntary act, which distinguishes it from malingering. Girls are affected about twice as often as boys. More sophisticated children may have quite believable symptoms, and normal vital signs do not exclude an organic cause.

11. The answer is **C,** page 1049.

Methylphenidate is a controlled substance with abuse potential. Medication and dosage changes for patients with ADHD should be made only in consultation with the child's physician, who will be providing follow-up. Methylphenidate levels rarely are clinically useful.

12. The answer is **D,** page 1049.

Pharmacologic management of ADHD is usually stimulant medication. Side effects include decreased appetite, growth and sleep disturbance, and tic disorders. Children with ADHD almost always benefit from a structured environment with fewer distractions, but not all will benefit from medication.

13. The answer is **B,** page 1050.

Conduct disorder is evidenced by functional impairment in an academic or social setting accompanied by intimidation, threats or assaults, theft, lying, and serious rule or law violations. Oppositional defiant disorder is less severe. Oppositional behavior is normal in toddlers. Longitudinal follow-up is essential in the management of this disorder.

14. The answer is **A,** pages 1050 and 1051.

Iron deficiency is the most common nutritional deficiency to trigger pica. Other conditions associated with pica include mental retardation, autism, and schizophrenia. The condition also can occur without apparent organic or psychiatric cause.

15. The answer is **D,** pages 1050 and 1051.

Anorexia nervosa is characterized by the inability to maintain a body weight more than 15% below the weight predicted by height and age. Anorexic patients may use laxatives or purgatives. Bulimia nervosa is characterized by binge eating followed by purging without the emaciation seen in anorexia.

16. The answer is **E,** pages 1050 and 1051.

Longitudinal follow-up is mandatory for patients with eating disorders. Malnutrition and electrolyte disturbances can lead to death if not treated. The decision to admit should be made based on the patient's clinical examination, adequacy of follow-up, hydration status, and serum electrolyte levels.

17. The answer is **A,** page 1051.

Transient tic disorder is defined by the presence of single or multiple tics for at least 2 weeks. The tics may include blinking, nodding, grunting, twitching, or more complex behaviors. Slow, writhing movements suggest athetosis. Tics usually disappear or lessen during sleep or with distraction. Stress or focusing on the tic may make it worse.

18. The answer is **C,** page 1051.

Tourette's syndrome is characterized by multiple motor and vocal tics persisting for more than a year. If only motor or vocal tics occur, the patient has chronic motor or chronic vocal tic disorder respectively. Alteration of mental status is not a characteristic of Tourette's syndrome.

19. The answer is **B,** pages 1051 and 1052.
    Functional psychotic disorders are uncommon in children. A diligent search for an organic etiology should be made. Prescription drugs and drugs of abuse frequently are the cause of psychotic episodes in younger patients.

20. The answer is **C,** pages 1051 and 1052.
    Childhood schizophrenia probably does not exist before age 5, whereas autism is defined as having an onset before 36 months. Both disorders may have unusual movements, social isolation, disinterest in normal activity, and self-stimulatory behavior.

21. The answer is **E,** page 1053.
    Patient intent is the key to the risk of further suicide attempts. Although the method chosen in this case was not particularly lethal, the girl apparently believed the method would be effective, and she was only discovered by chance. These factors suggest she had a strong intent to commit suicide.

22. The answer is **C,** pages 1053 and 1054.
    Girls are more likely to attempt suicide, but boys are more likely to be successful in their attempts. The latter results from boys' using more lethal methods such as firearms and hanging.

Respiratory Disorders

Jackie Grupp-Phelan

See Barkin et al: Chapter 59.

1. A 2-week-old full-term infant arrives in the ED after experiencing an episode of apnea at home. Which of the following initial diagnostic evaluations is most appropriate?
   A. Computed tomogram (CT) of the head.
   B. Determination of serum electrolyte levels.
   C. Barium swallow.
   D. Head ultrasound.
   E. Electroencephalogram.

2. A 1-month-old infant with a 5-day history of a severe cough has a temperature (T) of 100.4° F (38° C). Which of the following statements is most correct regarding this patient?
   A. A congenital airway anomaly should be suspected.
   B. Cough equivalent asthma is common in this age group.
   C. A trial of dextromethorphan should be considered in this infant.
   D. *Bordetella pertussis* is unlikely in this infant.

For Questions 3 to 6, indicate which answer is associated with the characteristics described. Each answer may be used once, more than once, or not at all.
   A. Aspiration of a foreign body.
   B. Allergy or infection.
   C. Croup.
   D. Psychogenic cough

3. Cough that worsens at night or during sleep. _____

4. Dry hacking cough; not present at night. _____

5. Cough that worsens with exercise. _____

6. Dry barking cough during sleep. _____

7. Which of the following statements regarding cyanosis is *most* correct?
   A. Cutaneous pigment and thickness of the skin has little influence on the detection of cyanosis.
   B. Cyanosis is determined by the absolute amount of reduced hemoglobin in the blood.
   C. The rate of blood flow through the capillaries has little effect on the detection of cyanosis.
   D. The most common cause of cyanosis in children is carboxyhemoglobinemia.

8. An ill-appearing 2-year-old boy is brought to the ED with a viral illness that has progressed to stridor, copious amounts of purulent sputum, and fever of 104.5° F. Of the following, which is the most likely cause of his stridor?
   A. Bacterial tracheitis.
   B. Peritonsillar abscess.
   C. Croup.
   D. Retropharyngeal abscess.

9. An 11-year-old child has a 7-day history of temperature to 101.4° F and cough. The mother started giving the child amoxicillin 1 day after the symptoms began. On examination the respiratory rate (RR) is 35 breaths per minute, heart rate (HR) is 88 beats per minute, blood pressure (BP) is 95/68 mm Hg, and pulse oximetry reading is 95%. Physical examination shows a minimally ill-appearing child with bilateral rales. Which of the following is the appropriate management for this child?
   A. Discontinue the amoxicillin and administer intramuscular (IM) penicillin.
   B. Discontinue all antibiotics and observe the child.
   C. Administer oral (PO) erythromycin rather than the amoxicillin.
   D. Admit the child to the hospital for intravenous (IV) antibiotics.
   E. Discontinue the amoxicillin and administer ciprofloxacin.

10. All of the following criteria support the diagnosis of acute life-threatening event (ALTE) *except:*
    A. The duration of apnea is greater than 10 seconds.
    B. The apnea occurs while the patient is asleep or awake.
    C. The apnea is associated with pallor or cyanosis.
    D. There is a short interval between feeding and an apneic episode.

11. A 20-month-old has temperature of 104° F (40° C) and the sudden onset of severe inspiratory stridor. The child is irritable, looks ill, and is not speaking. Which of the following is most appropriate in the management of this child?
    A. Airway visualization in the operating room.
    B. Racemic epinephrine nebulizer treatment.
    C. Administration of humidified oxygen via nonrebreathing mask.
    D. Examination of the hypopharynx in the ED.
    E. Lateral neck radiograph.

12. A 12-year-old girl with a history of asthma is in moderate respiratory distress with periods of agitation. Her vital signs are T 100° F (37.8 ° C), HR 120 beats per minute, and RR 28 breaths per minute. A blood gas study reveals pH 7.30, Paco$_2$ 35 mm Hg, and Pao$_2$ 75 mm Hg. She has minimal wheezing and poor air entry bilaterally. The patient has not responded to albuterol, subcutaneous epinephrine, IV theophylline, ipratropium, and steroids. The next appropriate intervention is:
    A. Administer lorazepam 0.5 mg for anxiety.
    B. Intubate the patient's trachea and institute mechanical ventilation.
    C. Administer continuous high-dose inhalation of albuterol.
    D. Administer IV theophylline.

13. All of the following statements regarding childhood asthma are correct *except:*
    A. The single most important risk factor for morbidity is the failure to diagnose asthma in children who have a history of recurrent wheezing.
    B. Adolescents are at highest risk of death from this disease.
    C. Most deaths occur after the patient is admitted to the hospital.
    D. β$_2$-Agonists themselves do not directly cause death when used appropriately.

14. A 10-month-old boy has moderate respiratory distress, wheezing, and rhinorrhea. His vital signs are T 102.2° F (39° C), RR 60 breaths per minute, and HR 120 beats per minute with a pulse oximetry reading of 91% on room air. After two albuterol treatments by inhalation the patient has improved aeration, RR 40 breaths per minute, and pulse oximetry of 95% on room air. Which of the following is the next appropriate step in the management of this child?
    A. Observe for 1 hour in the ED, then discharge the child home with no medications.
    B. Arrange home nebulizer or spacer treatment with β-agonist inhalation therapy.
    C. Administer ipratropium by inhalation.
    D. Prescribe a 5-day course of oral prednisone.

15. A 6-month-old has fever of 102.2° F (39° C), cough, tachypnea, and lethargy. Which of the following organisms is *least likely* to play a role in this child's illness?
    A. *Streptococcus pneumoniae.*
    B. *Staphylococcus aureus.*
    C. *B. pertussis.*
    D. Group B streptococci.
    E. *Haemophilus influenzae.*

16. An 8-year-old child with a history of asthma is seen in the ED with moderate respiratory distress. The child is not taking asthma medication at home. The best initial therapy is:
    A. Epinephrine 0.01 ml/kg subcutaneously.
    B. Albuterol 0.01 to 0.03 ml/kg by nebulizer.
    C. Methylprednisolone (Solu-Medrol) 2 mg/kg intravenously.
    D. Albuterol 0.15 mg/kg/dose orally.
    E. Prednisone 2 mg/kg orally.

17. A 3-year-old child is seen in the ED with the acute onset of stridor, barking cough, and fever. The child appears alert and playful but has marked inspiratory stridor. Which of the following is the most appropriate management of this child?
    A. Have the child sit in the mother's lap, start a cool mist, and observe for 2 hours before discharge.
    B. Administer nebulized racemic epinephrine and then discharge the patient.
    C. Obtain a lateral neck radiograph.
    D. Administer intramuscular dexamethasone (Decadron), observe for 2 hours, and discharge to home.

18. A 6-year-old child with congenital heart disease and asthma who is maintained on digoxin, furosemide, and albuterol has a history of dyspnea and tachypnea. On physical examination the child is afebrile and has RR 65 breaths per minute, HR 110 beats per minute, and BP 92/70 mm Hg. The patient has decreased breath sounds bilaterally, and rales are auscultated in the bases. All of the following interventions would be helpful in this patient *except:*
    A. Administer a 20 ml/kg IV fluid bolus.
    B. Administer 100% O$_2$ by face mask.
    C. Maintain the patient in an upright position.
    D. Administer furosemide.

19. A 12-year-old girl has dyspnea at rest, nonproductive cough, and chest pain. A radiograph shows bilateral pleural effusions. Which of the following is the most likely pathogen in this patient?
    A. *S. aureus.*
    B. *S. pneumoniae.*
    C. *Pneumocystis carinii.*
    D. Epstein-Barr virus.

20. All of the following interventions should be considered in the management of the patient with bacterial tracheitis *except:*
    A. Emergency intubation of the trachea.
    B. IV cefuroxime.
    C. IV nafcillin.
    D. Endoscopy in the operating room.
    E. IV methylprednisolone (Solu-Medrol).

21. All of the following statements regarding radiographs in children with pneumonia are correct *except:*
    A. Chest radiographs should be obtained for all children seen in an ED in significant respiratory distress.
    B. A lateral decubitus radiograph can help to define an associated pleural effusion.
    C. Classic radiographic findings consistent with a viral process include distinct consolidation localized to one or two lobes.
    D. If a foreign body of the airway is suspected, inspiratory and expiratory or bilateral decubitus radiographs should be obtained.

22. A 1-week-old infant with an unremarkable birth history is brought to the ED after experiencing many brief pauses in breathing occurring up to five times a minute. The infant is otherwise well appearing with good tone and is feeding vigorously. The mother is concerned that the infant will stop breathing. Which of the following is most appropriate in the management of this patient?
    A. Reassure the mother that this is normal periodic breathing of the newborn.
    B. Admit the patient for observation overnight and discharge if no further apneic events occur.
    C. Send the child home with an apnea monitor and arrange follow-up for the next morning.
    D. Obtain specimens for blood, urine, and cerebrospinal fluid (CSF) cultures.

23. A 9-year-old child has an 8-day history of intermittent fever to 102.2° F (39° C), purulent nasal discharge, headache, and cough that is worse at night. Which of the following is most appropriate in the management of this patient?
    A. Trial of a β_2-adrenergic agent.
    B. Sinus radiographs.
    C. Chest radiographs.
    D. A 7-day course of oral penicillin.

24. An afebrile 2-month-old child with a history of persistent cough is seen in the ED. What is the most likely diagnosis in this child?
    A. Cystic fibrosis.
    B. Food allergy.
    C. Pneumonia caused by *Chlamydia trachomatis.*
    D. Pneumonia resulting from *B. pertussis.*

25. Which of the following entities is the *most* common cause of pleural effusion in pediatric patients?
    A. Extensive burns.
    B. Juvenile rheumatoid arthritis.
    C. Infectious causes.
    D. Systemic lupus erythematosus.
    E. Leukemia.

26. A 2-week-old with fever and a localized infiltrate on a chest radiograph is seen in the ED. Which of the following is the most likely cause of the infiltrate?
    A. Group A streptococci.
    B. Group B streptococci.
    C. *S. aureus.*
    D. *B. pertussis.*

27. All of the following statements regarding intubation in patients with severe status asthmaticus are true *except:*
    A. Intubation is indicated in patients with persistent hypoxia and hypercarbia despite maximal therapy.
    B. Intubation is indicated in patients fatiguing or failing to respond to aggressive bronchodilation therapy.
    C. Magnesium sulfate may be effective for asthmatic patients refractory to other treatment measures.
    D. Ketamine is contraindicated in children requiring ventilation.

28. All of the following statements regarding corticosteroids are true *except:*
    A. Steroids increase the number and affinity of β-adrenergic receptors.
    B. Steroids have a direct bronchodilator effect with an onset of action within 1 hour.
    C. Orally administered corticosteroids are not as effective as those administered intravenously.
    D. Steroids should be administered as soon as possible after arrival to the ED.

ANSWERS [See Barkin et al.: Chapter 59.]

1. The answer is **B,** page 1056.
   The evaluation and workup for a child with apnea focus on identification of the underlying cause of apnea. A complete history and physical examination should be performed. Laboratory and radiologic evaluation should be tailored to the specific suspected diagnosis. Routine screening tests may include a complete blood count (CBC) and measurements of serum glucose, calcium, and magnesium. An electrocardiogram (ECG) also may be obtained.

2. The answer is **A,** page 1061.
   Infants with severe cough should be carefully examined for airway anomalies. In infants with a fixed congenital airway problem the cough may be present only during intercurrent viral illness. Asthma is the most common cause of cough in preschool and school-aged children but is an unlikely cause of cough in infants. Infants less than 1 year of age constitute 50% to 70% of all cases of *Bordetella pertussis* infection, which therefore should be considered in this infant.

Questions 3 to 6 are based on material found on pages 1061 to 1063 of Barkin et al.

3. **B**
4. **D**
5. **B**
6. **C**
7. The answer is **B**, pages 1063 to 1064.

   Cyanosis is determined by the amount of reduced hemoglobin in the blood; the amount of oxygenated hemoglobin has little influence. Cyanosis is clinically evident when at least 5 g of reduced hemoglobin is in 100 ml of capillary blood. The detection of cyanosis is influenced by different factors, including the cutaneous pigment and thickness of the skin and the rate of blood flow through the capillaries. Carboxyhemoglobinemia does not cause cyanosis but may produce a cherry-red flush of the skin, retina, or mucous membranes in extreme intoxications.

8. The answer is **A**, page 1067.

   Bacterial tracheitis has features of both croup and epiglottitis. It is often a secondary infection caused by *Staphylococcus aureus* or *Haemophilus influenzae*. Since it is a subglottic lesion, it can mimic croup. It also shares specific features with epiglottitis such as bacterial etiology, high fever, and toxic appearance. A frequently reported feature of bacterial tracheitis is copious amounts of purulent sputum.

9. The answer is **C**, page 1061.

   Mycoplasma pneumoniae is a common cause of pneumonia in this age group. The children look surprisingly well. Treatment with oral erythromycin is reasonable in a child who shows few symptoms.

10. The answer is **D**, page 1056.

    An acute life-threatening event (ALTE) is defined as cessation of breathing for 20 seconds or longer and a shorter respiratory pause associated with bradycardia, cyanosis, or pallor. It may occur when the patient is asleep or awake. A short interval between feeding and apnea is more likely related to reflux and is not usually associated with ALTE.

11. The answer is **A**, pages 1094 to 1097.

    The clinical scenario presented in this case is suggestive of epiglottitis. The next step in management should be to mobilize an interdisciplinary team (including but not limited to an anesthesiologist, otolaryngologist, and pediatric critical care physician) and proceed to the operating room for examination of the airway under anesthesia. Lateral neck x-ray films may delay treatment and are not indicated.

12. The answer is **C**, pages 1087 and 1088.

    Agitation and diminished level of consciousness may signify arterial hypoxemia and hypercapnia. This patient is ill and must be treated in a rapid manner. A trial of high-dose continuous albuterol by inhalation may be preferable to intubation and its potential complications (pneumomediastinum, pneumothorax) in patients with asthma. Theophylline has not been shown to improve pulmonary function when added to β-agonist therapy in the patient with severe asthma.

13. The answer is **C**, pages 1079 and 1088.

    Asthma is associated with considerable morbidity. The single most important risk factor for morbidity is the failure to diagnose asthma in children with a history of recurrent wheezing. Adolescents are at the highest risk of death as a result of overreliance on bronchodilators, which is associated with a delay in seeking medical care. Deaths caused by asthma within the hospital are rare.

14. The answer is **B**, pages 1088 to 1091.

    The patient described in this question has responded well to two doses of albuterol by inhalation. After a period of observation the stable patient (nontoxic appearance, pulse oximeter reading greater than 94%, RR less than 40 breaths per minute, and able to feed) may be sent home with a nebulizer to administer albuterol every 4 hours. Ipratropium and prednisone have not been shown to change the outcome in infants with bronchiolitis. Close follow-up of these patients is essential.

15. The answer is **D**, page 1104.

    All of the organisms listed except group B streptococci are common pathogens in infants older than 3 months and young children. Group B streptococci usually occur in infants under the age of 1 month.

16. The answer is **B**, page 1087.

    The child described in the clinical scenario is in moderate distress and should be treated with albuterol by nebulization or metered-dose inhaler. Subcutaneous epinephrine may be considered if there is no response to albuterol. Steroids are indicated yet may take several hours to show an effect.

17. The answer is **D**, pages 1093 and 1094.

    The patient in this scenario has marked stridor and should benefit by the early administration of steroids and racemic epinephrine via nebulization. Following this treatment the patient should be observed for at least 2 hours and discharged if stridor at rest is not present.

18. The answer is **A**, pages 1110 to 1112.

    The child described in this question has dyspnea and possible congestive heart failure. The differential diagnosis includes asthma and pneumonia. Appropriate interventions include oxygen, bronchodilator, and diuretic therapy. Administering 20 ml/kg IV normal saline in a euvolemic patient in respiratory distress may increase the risk for pulmonary edema.

19. The answer is **A**, page 1099.

    S. aureus is the most frequently isolated pathogen in patients like the one described in this question. *S. pneumoniae* and Epstein-Barr virus also can cause exudative pleural effusions. *Pneumocystis carinii* is a common cause of pleural effusion in immunocompromised patients.

20. The answer is **E,** page 1098.
The approach to the child with tracheitis is similar to that for the child with epiglottitis. Emergency intubation usually is required. Endoscopy may be beneficial, not only for early diagnosis and cultures, but also for the removal of the copious obstructive secretions. Antibiotics should be initiated as soon as the airway is controlled. Antibiotic coverage should use agents that cover staphylococcal and streptococcal species. The administration of steroids has no role in the treatment of patients with bacterial tracheitis.

21. The answer is **C,** page 1106.
Classic radiographic findings consistent with a viral infection of the lower respiratory tract are perihilar or peribronchial infiltrates.

22. The answer is **A,** page 1116.
Normal newborns may demonstrate periodic breathing, which is a regular recurrence of respiratory pauses of 3 seconds or more followed by a breathing period of 20 seconds or less that is repeated at least three times. Unlike a patient in an apparent life-threatening event, the infant described in this scenario exhibits no change in color, loss of muscle tone, or gagging.

23. The answer is **B,** pages 1062 and 1063.
The clinical picture in this patient is consistent with sinusitis. Children with a history of protracted cough and nasal symptoms should be evaluated for sinusitis. Sinus films have variable reliability. Films in children older than 6 years of age are easier to interpret. For small children in whom maxillary sinusitis is suspected, a single Waters' view is appropriate.

24. The answer is **C,** pages 1103 to 1106.
Chlamydia trachomatis is recognized as one of the most common types of pneumonia during the first 3 months of life. Fever is usually present in children with pneumonia but may not be present in infants infected with *C. trachomatis*. Documentation of nasopharyngeal carriage of *C. trachomatis*, along with its detection in conjunctival scrapings by direct immunofluorescent antigen or culture, can confirm the diagnosis of *Chlamydia* pneumonia. Treatment is with oral erythromycin.

25. The answer is **C,** page 1099.
All of the diagnoses in this question may cause an exudative pleural effusion. Pleural fluid exudates primarily result from diseases on the pleural surface. Infectious agents are the *most common cause* of pleural inflammation in the pediatric age group.

26. The answer is **B,** page 1104.
Group B streptococci is the most likely choice for this age group. See Table 59-4 on page 1104 in Barkin et al for other etiologic agents listed by age group.

27. The answer is **D,** page 1087.
Patients with severe asthma, in respiratory failure, having persistent hypoxemia and hypercarbia on maximal therapy, and fatiguing or failing to respond to aggressive bronchodilation management may require intubation. Ketamine, a sedative and bronchodilator, may be a useful agent in children with asthma who require ventilation.

28. The answer is **C,** pages 1085 and 1086.
Corticosteroids may increase the number and affinity of β-adrenergic receptors. Steroids appear to produce a direct bronchodilator effect that is supported by a more rapid onset of action. Orally administered corticosteroids are as effective as IV therapy.

Urinary and Renal Disorders

Larry B. Mellick • Laura C. Carlson

See Barkin et al: Chapter 60.

1. A 15-year-old boy has a low-grade fever, mild facial swelling, and malaise. On examination he is found to have pain in the left testicle, tenderness, and swelling. The most common etiologic agent of this illness is:
   A. Adenovirus.
   B. Enterovirus.
   C. Arbovirus.
   D. Myxovirus.
   E. Paramyxovirus.
2. Which of the following statements is correct concerning the diagnosis in the patient described in question 1?
   A. Urethral discharge, dysuria, and a tender prostate are common findings.
   B. Half of the patients affected have subsequent testicular atrophy.
   C. Serologic testing for the viral agent should be performed routinely.
   D. Steroid is the drug of choice.
   E. Infertility is a common complication.
3. Drugs that have been found to cause red urine in children include all of the following except:
   A. Quinine.
   B. Doxorubicin (Adriamycin).
   C. Salicylates.
   D. Phenobarbital.
   E. Phenazopyridine (Pyridium).
4. A 12-year-old boy has a bicycle accident. He is brought to the ED with a straddle injury and a large scrotal hematoma. The most appropriate management of this patient is:
   A. A urinalysis to screen for hematuria.
   B. Reassurance and a discharge to home.
   C. Immediate surgical consultation.
   D. Observation in the ED for 6 hours.
   E. A warm compress for comfort.
5. The most common complication of circumcision in infants is:
   A. Infection.
   B. Hemorrhage.
   C. Adhesion.
   D. Obstruction.
   E. Necrosis.

6. A normal 1-year-old toddler has an expected mean plasma creatinine level of:
   A. 0.32 mg/dl.
   B. 0.48 mg/dl.
   C. 0.60 mg/dl.
   D. 0.77 mg/dl.
   E. 0.97 mg/dl.
7. An 8-year-old boy has sudden onset of scrotal erythema and edema but no pain. He has no fever, and urinalysis shows no proteinuria. The most appropriate management of the patient is:
   A. Urine collection for 24 hours.
   B. Testicular ultrasound.
   C. Intravenous (IV) pyelogram.
   D. Reassurance and discharge.
   E. Surgical consultation.
8. Measures to prevent dysuria in the adolescent girl include all of the following *except:*
   A. Wiping the anus from front to back after bowel movement.
   B. Urinating before intercourse.
   C. Avoiding the use of bubble baths.
   D. Using warm water instead of soap to clean the genital area.
   E. Wearing cotton undergarments.
9. A 4-year-old black boy has had a painful sustained erection for 3 hours. His medical history is most likely positive for what other illness?
   A. Diabetes mellitus.
   B. Hyperstimulation syndrome.
   C. Sickle cell disease.
   D. Idiopathy.
   E. Leukemia.
10. Appropriate management of the patient described in question 9 may include all of the following except:
    A. Discharge to home.
    B. Administration of analgesics.
    C. Transfusion.
    D. Surgical intervention.
    E. Hydration.

11. Which of the following statements concerning phimosis in the pediatric population is correct?
    A. Phimosis is a common problem in children.
    B. Surgical consultation is necessary in most cases.
    C. The ability to retract the foreskin in children is age related.
    D. It is characterized by the inability to retract the foreskin over the glans.
    E. Urinary outlet obstruction is a common complication.

Use the following clinical scenario to answer questions 12 and 13.
A 3-year-old girl has fever, cramping abdominal pain, and bloody diarrhea. On examination she is irritable and hypertensive, and has a petechial rash. Her urine is scant and grossly bloody.

12. Organisms implicated in the development of this illness include all of the following except:
    A. *Salmonella.*
    B. *Shigella.*
    C. *Pseudomonas.*
    D. *Escherichia coli.*
    E. *Streptococcus pneumoniae.*

13. The most efficient early intervention for this illness is:
    A. An immunosuppressive agent.
    B. Heparin infusion.
    C. An antiplatelet agent.
    D. Vitamin E.
    E. Peritoneal dialysis.

14. Which of the following statements concerning testicular tumors in the pediatric population is correct?
    A. They constitute approximately 10% of pediatric tumors.
    B. They occur most commonly at age 2.
    C. They are painful, firm, asymmetric scrotal masses.
    D. Treatment includes immediate surgical consultation.
    E. Computed tomographic (CT) scan is the study of choice.

15. Which of the following is the most common cause of acute tubular necrosis in children?
    A. Heavy metal poisoning.
    B. Myoglobinuria.
    C. Hemoglobinuria.
    D. Renal ischemia.
    E. Nonsteroidal antiinflammatory drugs.

16. A 13-year-old boy is seen in the ED after waking up 2 hours earlier with acute pain in the left testicle. The cremasteric reflex is absent, and a twist of the cord is palpable. Manual reduction is unsuccessful. The most appropriate management of the patient is:
    A. Magnetic resonance imaging (MRI) scan.
    B. CT scan.
    C. Scintigraphy.
    D. Surgical consultation.
    E. Ultrasound.

17. Which of the following statements concerning testicular torsion is correct?
    A. Peak incidence is at age 10.
    B. Leukocytosis is present 90% of the time.
    C. Painless swelling is present 10% of the time.
    D. Testicular rescue is successful 50% of the time.
    E. It is typically associated with a urethral discharge.

18. A 12-year-old girl has fever, abdominal pain, malaise, edema, and scant production of dark-colored urine. Which of the following laboratory data is *inconsistent* with the most likely diagnosis?
    A. Elevated blood urea nitrogen (BUN) level.
    B. Elevated antistreptolysin (ASO) level.
    C. Elevated total serum complement.
    D. Red cell casts in the urine.
    E. Reduced fractional excretion of sodium.

19. In the patient described in question 18, progression to anuria and renal failure is expected what percent of the time?
    A. 2%.
    B. 5%.
    C. 10%.
    D. 25%.
    E. 50%.

20. Pathognomonic findings for testicular torsion include all of the following *except:*
    A. Abnormal testicular axis in the contralateral side.
    B. Absence of cremasteric reflex.
    C. Elevated testicle on the ipsilateral side.
    D. Scrotal edema.
    E. Palpable twist of the cord.

21. A 10-year-old white girl has cough and congestion. Except for a low-grade fever, her vital signs are normal. Urinalysis shows 2+ protein. She has normal serum blood urea nitrogen and creatinine levels. Which one of the following is the next appropriate step in the management of this patient?
    A. Arrange for an IV pyelogram.
    B. Schedule a follow-up urinalysis.
    C. Obtain a nephrology consult in the ED.
    D. Obtain a 24-hour urine collection for protein and creatinine clearance.
    E. Admit the patient with a diagnosis of nephrotic syndrome.

22. Which of the following statements about hydroceles is correct?
    A. Reduction of a hydrocele is possible with ice, analgesia, and gentle pressure.
    B. Hydroceles more commonly are located on the left side.
    C. Fluid accumulation within the tunica vaginalis of the scrotum results in a hydrocele.
    D. Aspiration of a scrotal swelling is the treatment of choice.
    E. Hydroceles most frequently occur in the pubertal male.

23. Which of the following findings is common in nephrotic syndrome?
    A. Edema.
    B. Hypoproteinemia.
    C. Acute renal failure.
    D. Proteinuria.
    E. Hyperlipidemia.
24. A 2-month-old girl has hypertension, a heart murmur, and diminished femoral pulses. What is the most likely diagnosis?
    A. Pheochromocytoma.
    B. Williams syndrome.
    C. Renal artery thrombosis.
    D. Coarctation of the aorta.
    E. Neuroblastoma.
25. A 7-year-old boy has an erythematous, maculopapular, blanching rash that began on the legs and buttocks. He also complains of cramping abdominal pain. Physical examination demonstrates a migratory arthritis with swelling of the hands and feet. Which is the most likely diagnosis?
    A. Henoch-Schönlein purpura (HSP).
    B. Meningococcemia.
    C. Rocky Mountain spotted fever.
    D. Thrombocytopenic purpura.
    E. Lyme disease.
26. Which of the following statements is *incorrect* regarding hypercalciuria as the cause of hematuria in children?
    A. It is a familial autosomal dominant condition.
    B. It may be present in 3% to 6% of asymptomatic children.
    C. Enuresis and rickets may occur in severe cases.
    D. Dietary calcium and sodium should be limited to 500 to 600 mg/day.
    E. It is more common in black children.

27. In patients with Henoch-Schönlein purpura (HSP) who have severe renal involvement, which of the following treatments is recommended?
    A. Oral broad-spectrum antibiotics.
    B. IV immune globulin and steroids.
    C. Renal transplant.
    D. Acetaminophen.
    E. Plasmapheresis.
28. A 14-year-old boy is seen in the ED with vomiting, flank pain radiating to the groin, and gross hematuria. His pain has not been relieved by multiple doses of a narcotic. The next appropriate step in the management of this patient is:
    A. Testicular ultrasound.
    B. CT scan of the abdomen and pelvis.
    C. Hospital admission for continued observation.
    D. IV pyelogram.
    E. Scintigraphy.
29. Organisms implicated in the development of acute prostatitis include all of the following except:
    A. *Pseudomonas.*
    B. *Streptococcus.*
    C. *Chlamydia.*
    D. *E. coli.*
    E. *Enterobacter.*
30. A 6-year-old child has acute renal failure. Her blood pressure is 150/100 mm Hg. She has normal mental status. Which of the following is the most appropriate initial treatment?
    A. Furosemide 1 mg/kg IV.
    B. Diazoxide IV bolus.
    C. Nitroprusside infusion.
    D. Fluid restriction.
    E. Nifedipine 0.25 mg/kg sublingually.

ANSWERS   [See Barkin et al: Chapter 60.]

1. The answer is **E,** page 1151.
Mumps (paramyxovirus) is the most common viral agent in primary orchitis. All of the other viruses listed have also been implicated but much less frequently. Other viral agents reported to be associated with orchitis include Epstein-Barr virus (EBV), dengue (arbovirus), and arenavirus (agent of lymphocytic choriomeningitis).
2. The answer is **B,** page 1151.
Fifty percent of patients with orchitis (mumps) subsequently have testicular atrophy. Urethral discharge, dysuria, and a tender prostate are uncommon findings and imply a concurrent epididymal infection. Steroid therapy is not indicated in the treatment of orchitis. Fertility usually is maintained because the testicular infection typically is unilateral.

3. The answer is **D,** page 1130.
The anticonvulsant phenobarbital has not been shown to cause red urine, but the color change has been reported with phenytoin. All of the other drugs have been implicated. Refer to the table on page 1130 of Barkin et al for a complete list of conditions that cause urine to be red.
4. The answer is **C,** page 1141.
A large hematoma may represent a significant testicular injury and requires surgical consultation. The presence of red blood cells (RBCs) in the urine is an expected finding with trauma. A period of observation would only delay appropriate interventions. A warm compress might increase swelling and is not recommended.
5. The answer is **B,** page 1142.
Hemorrhage is the most common complication of circumcision both during and after the procedure. Bleeding typically is minor and usually can be controlled by the application of pressure. Infection and adhesions are not common complications of the circumcision procedure. Although obstruction and necrosis also are recognized complications, they are rare.

6. The answer is **A,** page 1128, Table 60-1.

A 1-year-old has a mean plasma creatinine level of 0.32 mg/dl. The mean plasma creatinine level for an 8-year-old is 0.48 mg/dl, for a 12-year-old is 0.59 mg/dl, for the average adult woman is 0.77 mg/dl, and for the average adult man is 0.97 mg/dl. A normal adult plasma creatinine level would represent a significant change in glomerular filtration rate (GFR) for a 1-year-old child.

7. The answer is **D,** page 1141.

Idiopathic scrotal edema (ISE) is seen in prepubertal boys with 77% of the cases occurring before 10 years of age. This condition is characterized by a sudden onset of edema and erythema without pain. The swelling may extend to the phallus, and fever is rare. Because of its characteristic findings and symptoms, an allergic etiology has been postulated. ISE typically resolves spontaneously within 1 to 4 days.

8. The answer is **B,** page 1129.

Urinating after intercourse, not before, may help prevent urethritis, urinary tract infections, and dysuria. Wiping the anus from front to back improves perineal hygiene and decreases contamination of the female genitourinary tract and incidence of infection (vulvovaginitis). Chemical irritation from bubble bath and soap can cause dysuria. Avoidance of these and other products such as shampoo and feminine hygiene products is both preventive and curative. Wearing cotton undergarments decreases moisture and may prevent conditions conducive to dysuria.

9. The answer is **C,** pages 1153 and 1154.

Sickle cell disease is the most common cause of priapism in the pediatric population. Sludging of sickle cells in the sinusoids impairs normal venous drainage. The local acidosis and hypoxia that follow sets up a cycle for more sludging and obstruction of venous outflow. Priapism does occur with diabetes, with hyperstimulation, with leukemia, and idiopathically, although much less commonly.

10. The answer is **A,** pages 1153 and 1154.

These patients should be hospitalized for pain control and monitoring for urinary retention, which may complicate the disease. Other coexisting conditions such as a painful crisis or infection should be investigated. Narcotic analgesics and hydration are the mainstay of supportive care. Some patients do require red blood cell transfusion or exchange to decrease the sickle cell load. Surgical intervention is indicated when priapism does not resolve with aggressive medical therapy.

11. The answer is **C,** pages 1152 and 1153.

Phimosis is characterized by the constriction of the distal prepuce, preventing easy passage over the glans. The ability to retract the foreskin in children is clearly age related. At 6 months of age the foreskin will retract in only 25% of boys. True phimosis is relatively rare and is characterized by the presence of decreased urinary stream, hematuria, and pain in the area of the prepuce. Reassurance and education constitute appropriate management of age-related inability to retract the prepuce, and parents should be cautioned against forceful foreskin retraction.

12. The answer is **C,** pages 1145 and 1146.

Pseudomonas organisms have not been implicated in hemolytic uremic syndrome (HUS). The organism found most frequently in association with typical cases of HUS is a cytotoxin producing *E. coli* (serotype O157:H7). In underdeveloped countries *Shigella* and *Salmonella* have been associated with HUS, which also has been associated with neuraminidase-producing *S. pneumoniae*.

13. The answer is **E,** pages 1146 and 1147.

Peritoneal dialysis has been the most efficient therapy in improving the outcome of patients with HUS. Dialysis is performed most frequently when severely affected HUS patients have had at least 24 hours of anuria or simultaneous seizures, hypertension, and oliguria. Heparin, immunosuppressants, antiplatelet agents, and vitamin E have not been consistently beneficial.

14. The answer is **B,** page 1141.

Testicular tumors occur most commonly in 2-year-old boys, with another peak in the prepubertal years. Less than 2% of all solid tumors in children occur in the testicle and have an incidence in prepubertal boys under 15 years of age of 0.5 per 100,000. A testicular tumor usually is a painless, heavy, firm, asymmetric scrotal mass. Hemorrhage or necrosis in the tumor is the only condition that may cause pain. Testicular tumors can be referred to a surgeon on a nonemergency basis. Ultrasound is the preferred diagnostic study for confirmation.

15. The answer is **D,** pages 1155 and 1156.

The most common cause of acute tubular necrosis (ATN) in both children and adults is renal ischemia. Hypovolemia usually is responsible for the renal ischemia. Myoglobinuria, hemoglobinuria, heavy metal poisoning, and nonsteroidal antiinflammatory drugs can cause ATN but do so much less frequently.

16. The answer is **D,** pages 1162 to 1164.

Imaging studies never should delay the surgeon's evaluation or impede the patient's transition to the operating room. Surgical exploration is the treatment of choice for patients with pain less than 12 hours in duration and a history suggestive of torsion. Imaging is reserved for those patients further along in the course of their disease or in whom the likelihood of torsion is small.

17. The answer is **C,** page 1162.

Surprisingly, about 10% of patients with testicular torsion have painless swelling. The peak incidence of this condition occurs at around 13 years of age. About 50% of the patients with testicular torsion have leukocytosis, and a left shift is seen in approximately two thirds of the cases. Testicular salvage rates are 96% and 93% when surgical intervention occurs at less than 4 hours and between 4 and 8 hours, respectively. The presence of a urethral discharge is more suggestive of epidymitis.

18. The answer is **C**, pages 1144 and 1145.
In poststreptococcal glomerular nephritis the total serum complement, and specifically C3, is depressed in 90% to 100% of patients in the first 2 weeks of the illness. After 3 to 4 weeks these values return to normal. All other laboratory data are expected to be abnormal as described.

19. The answer is **A**, page 1144.
Anuria and renal failure occur in 2% of the patients who have poststreptococcal glomerular nephritis. The spectrum of physical findings associated with acute glomerulonephritis (AGN) depends on the length of the illness and ranges from mild facial swelling, extremity edema, and minimal blood pressure elevation to pulmonary edema, malignant hypertension, and cardiac dysrhythmias.

20. The answer is **D**, page 1162.
Pathognomonic findings for torsion include an elevated testicle with a palpable twist of the cord, an abnormal axis of the testicle, an abnormal position of the epididymis in the scrotum, the absence of a cremasteric reflex, and an abnormal testicular axis in the contralateral testis. Scrotal edema is not pathognomonic for torsion.

21. The answer is **B**, pages 1138 to 1140.
Trace to 2+ proteinuria is not uncommon in the acute care setting of stressed, febrile, or dehydrated patients. Consequently, children with less than 3+ proteinuria should be referred for a follow-up urinalysis. For a patient with 3+ or 4+ proteinuria, referral for an urgent renal evaluation is appropriate if blood pressure, serum proteins, and renal function are normal.

22. The answer is **C**, page 1141.
A hydrocele results from fluid accumulation within the tunica vaginalis of the scrotum. Ice, analgesia, and gentle pressure usually reduce inguinal hernias but not hydroceles. Hydroceles more commonly are located on the right side, not the left. Hydroceles never should be aspirated. Hydroceles typically are present at birth, whereas varicoceles may be found in the pubertal boy.

23. The answer is **A**, pages 1143 and 1144.
The presence of edema is the usual sign in a child with nephrotic syndrome (NS). The edema is noted first around the eyes but is frequently attributed to a cold or allergies. With progression and more widespread distribution of the edema the parents may assume that the child simply is gaining weight. On occasion the disease is diagnosed early in its course with the discovery of asymptomatic proteinuria. Acute renal failure is uncommon in NS and if present is attributed to severe intravascular volume depletion, bilateral renal vein thrombosis, or severe hypertension.

24. The answer is **D**, page 1138, Table 60-5.
A murmur, hypertension, and decreased femoral pulses are some of the physical findings associated with coarctation of the aorta. Pheochromocytoma in older patients includes flushing, palpitations, diarrhea, and tachycardia. Williams syndrome has a characteristic elfin facies. Renal artery thrombosis occurs in premature infants with a history of umbilical catheterization. Children with hypertension and a neuroblastoma may have an abdominal mass.

25. The answer is **A**, pages 1147 and 1148.
This clinical scenario is typical of Henoch-Schönlein purpura (HSP), a vasculitis that usually has a rash most concentrated on the lower body, hematuria, abdominal pain, and often arthritis. In addition to other features distinctive of these febrile diseases, the rashes of meningococcemia and Rocky Mountain spotted fever may begin on, but generally are not concentrated on, the lower extremities and buttock. Thrombocytopenic purpura typically has a low platelet count. The rash of Lyme disease, erythema chronicum migrans, is distinctive and begins as a small macule with a rapidly expanding annular border.

26. The answer is **E**, page 1131.
Hypercalciuria and its associated hematuria are more common in white children than in black children. Hypercalciuria is an autosomal dominant condition that occurs in 3% to 6% of asymptomatic children. Enuresis and rickets may occur in severe cases. A large daily fluid intake is recommended in addition to calcium and sodium dietary restrictions.

27. The answer is **B**, pages 1147 and 1148.
IV immune globulin is the treatment of choice for patients with severe renal involvement. High-dose, pulsed steroids may be beneficial for the associated glomerulonephritis, joint swelling, and gastrointestinal symptoms. Antibiotics, plasmapheresis, acetaminophen, and renal transplant are not beneficial.

28. The answer is **D**, pages 1168 and 1169.
This clinical scenario describes classic renal colic. An IV pyelogram is indicated for this patient to rule out complete obstruction of the affected side. Testicular torsion may have groin pain. However, the absence of other physical findings does not support the need for a testicular ultrasound. If the patient's pain is relieved and no evidence of an infected stone is found, a discharge to home with urology follow-up is appropriate. Scintigraphy is not indicated.

29. The answer is **B,** pages 1154 and 1155.
Streptococcus is not known to cause prostatitis. The most common urinary pathogens, *E. coli, Klebsiella, Enterobacter, Proteus, Pseudomonas,* and *Staphylococcus* species, also are the organisms routinely implicated. In postpubertal patients *Neisseria gonorrhoeae* and *Chlamydia trachomatis* are most frequently associated. Prostatitis is exceedingly rare in prepubertal patients.

30. The answer is **A,** pages 1155 to 1159.
In acute renal failure euvolemic patients without evidence of obstruction respond well to furosemide initially. The correct dosage is 1 mg/kg with its maximum effect expected in 30 minutes. Furosemide can be administered up to a total of 6 mg/kg. If an encephalopathy results from the hypertension, administration of diazoxide, nitroprusside, or nifedipine is appropriate. A normal intravascular volume must be maintained, and fluid restriction would not be recommended unless the patient was overloaded with fluid.

Important Mnemonics, Facts, and Formulas

Stuart M. Caplen • *Edward E. Conway, Jr.* • *David H. Rubin* • *Martin G. Hellman*

TOXICOLOGY

Anion Gap

$Na - (Cl + HCO_3)$
Normal anion gap = 12 to 14 mEq/L

Causes of Anion Gap Acidosis (MUDPILES)

Methanol
Uremia
Diabetes
Phenformin, **P**araldehyde
Iron, **I**soniazid, **I**nhalants (cyanide, carbon monoxide, hydrogen sulfide)
Lactic acidosis
Ethanol, **E**thylene glycol
Salicylates

Osmolar Gap

Osmolar gap is defined by a difference between the calculated and measured osmolarity of greater than 10 mOsm.

$$\text{Serum Osmolarity} = 2\,(Na) + \frac{\text{Glucose}}{18} + \frac{\text{BUN}}{2.8}$$

Causes of Osmolar Gap (IGAME)

Isopropanol
Glycerol
Acetone
Methanol, **M**annitol
Ethylene glycol, **E**thanol

Hydrocarbons Requiring GI Decontamination (CHAMP)

Camphor
Halogenated hydrocarbons (carbon tetrachloride)
Aromatic hydrocarbons (benzene)
Metals
Pesticides

Organophosphate Overdose (SLUDGE OR DUMBELS)

(Cholinergic symptoms)
Salivation
Lacrimation
Urination
Diarrhea
Gastrointestinal
Emesis
OR
Diarrhea
Urination
Miosis
Bronchorrhea, **B**ronchospasm, **B**radycardia
Excitation (anxiety, seizures, muscle fasciculations)
Lacrimation
Salivation

Anticholinergic Overdose

Hot as Hades
Blind as a Bat
Dry as a Bone
Red as a Beet
Mad as a Hatter

Radiopaque Substances (CHIPS)

Cocaine packets, **C**arbon tetrachloride, **C**hloroform
Heavy metals (arsenic, lead, iron), **H**ealth foods (vitamins, bone meal)
Iodine, **I**ron
Psychotropics (TCA's), **P**henothiazines
Sustained-release or enteric-coated potassium or salicylates

Drugs That Cause Miosis (COPS)[1]

Cholinergics, **C**lonidine
Opiates, **O**rganophosphates
Phenothiazines, **P**ilocarpine
Sedative-hypnotics

Drugs That Cause Mydriasis (AAAS)[1]

Antihistamines
Antidepressants
Atropine
Sympathomimetics, **S**copolamine

Drugs That Cause Seizures[1] (OTIS CAMPBELL)

Organophosphates
Tricyclics
Isoniazid, Insulin
Sympathomimetics
Camphor, Cocaine
Amphetamines
Methylxanthines
Phencyclidine (PCP)
Benzodiazepine withdrawal, Botanicals (water hemlock)
Ethanol withdrawal
Lithium, Lidocaine
Lead, Lindane

Drugs That Cause Pneumonitis Or Pulmonary Edema (MOPS)[1]

Meprobamate, Methadone
Opiates
Phenobarbital, Propoxyphene
Salicylates

Differential Diagnosis of Coma

1. AEIOUTHIPS
   Alcohol
   Encephalitis, Electrolytes
   Infection, Insulin
   Opiates
   Uremia
   Trauma
   Hypertension or Hypotension, Hyperthermia or Hypothermia
   Intussusception
   Psychiatric (catatonia)
   Seizures, Syncope
2. I SPOUT A VEIN
   Insulin
   Shock
   Psychogenic
   Opiates
   Uremia (other metabolic)
   Trauma
   Alcohol
   Vasculitis
   Encephalitis
   Infection, Insulin
   Neoplasm

Drugs That Can Be Hemodialyzed (ISTUMBLE)

Isopropanol
Salicylates
Theophylline
Uremia
Methanol
Barbiturates
Lithium
Ethylene glycol

Drugs That Cause Hypothermia (COOLS)[1]

Carbon monoxide
Opiates
Oral hypoglycemics, insulin
Liquor
Sedative-hypnotics

Causes of Hyperthermia (NASA)[1]

Neuroleptic malignant syndrome, Nicotine
Antihistamines
Salicylates, Sympathomimetics
Anticholinergics, Antidepressants

Symptoms of Lead Poisoning (ABCDEFG)

Anemia
Basophilic stippling
Colic
Dementia
Encephalopathy
Foot drop
Gingival pigmentation

Symptoms of Narcotic Withdrawal (WITHDRAWAL)

Wakefulness
Irritability
Tremulousness, Temperature instability
Hyperactivity, High-pitched cry, Hyperreflexia
Diarrhea, Diaphoresis
Rhinorrhea, Respiratory distress
Apnea, Autonomic dysfunction
Weight loss
Alkalosis
Lacrimation

Carbon Monoxide Half-Life

4 to 5 hours—room air
90 minutes—100% oxygen
20 minutes—hyperbaric chamber

Local Anesthetics

1% lidocaine has 10 mg/ml
Toxic dose of lidocaine 4.5 mg/kg
Toxic use of lidocaine with epinephrine 7 mg/kg

Amides

All have two i's. There is no cross reactivity between esters and amides.
Lidocaine
Bupivacaine
Dibucaine
Mepivacaine

Esters

Procaine
Cocaine
Benzocaine
Tetracaine

ELECTROLYTES, FLUIDS, RENAL

Causes of Hypokalemia (ILL ADD POTASIUM)

Insulin
Leukemia
Liddle's disease (renal tubular defect)

Alkalosis
Diuretics
Diarrhea

Periodic paralysis
Oral loss (vomiting)
Tubular acidosis (RTA)
Adrenocorticoid excess
Starvation
Ileostomy
Ureterosigmoidostomy
Milk of magnesia (laxative abuse)

Causes of Hyponatremia (PISS)

Psychogenic water intoxication, Pseudohyponatremia (hyperglycemia)
Iatrogenic water administration (D_5W IV)
SIADH (syndrome of inappropriate secretion of antidiuretic hormone)
Sodium content normal with water excess (CHF, nephrotic syndrome)

Effect of Glucose on Sodium

Each 100 mg/dl increase in plasma glucose level decreases serum sodium level by 1.6 mEq/L.

Indications for Calcium

Calcium channel blocker overdose
Hypermagnesemia
Hyperkalemia
Hypocalcemia

Cystic Fibrosis

CAN CAUSE: Hyponatremia, hypochloremia, metabolic alkalosis

Pyloric Stenosis

CAN CAUSE: Hypokalemia, hypochloremia, metabolic alkalosis

Maintenance Fluid Requirements for Children

100 ml/kg/24 hr for first 10 kg of body weight
50 ml/kg/24 hr for next 10 kg up to 20 kg of body weight
20 ml/kg/24 hr for each kg of body weight over 20 kg
For example, in a 22-kg child:

$10 \times 100 = 1000$ ml
$10 \times 50 \ \ = \ \ 500$ ml
$2 \times 20 \ \ \ = \ \ \ \underline{40}$ ml
1540 ml (maintenance fluids for 24 hours)

Rule of Nines for Burns

Can be used for determining percentage of total body surface area in burns *in older children* (not infants).
9% each—head, each arm
18% each—chest, back, each leg
1%—perineum

Parkland Burn Formula

4 ml/kg per % total body surface area per 24 hours
50% given in first 8 hours, 50% over next 16 hours

Evaluation of Renal Failure:

	Prerenal	Intrarenal	Postrenal
Ultrasound	Normal	Increased density/ swelling	Dilated bladder or kidney
Serum BUN/Cr	>15:1		
Urine Na	<15 mEq/L	>20 mEq/L	Index not helpful
Urine Osm	>500 mOsm/ kg H_2O	<350 mOsm/ kg H_2O	
Creatinine urine/ plasma	>40:1	<20:1	
Fractional excretion of sodium	<1 (<2.5 in neonates)	>2 (>2.5 in neonates)	

Differentiation of Diabetes Insipidus and SIADH

	Diabetes Insipidus	Syndrome of Inappropriate Secretion of Antidiuretic Hormone (SIADH)
Urine Osm	Decreased (<150 mOsm/L)	Increased
Serum Osm	Increased (>290 mOsm/L)	Decreased

FACTS AND FORMULAS

Circulation

For age greater than 1 year,

The lowest acceptable systolic blood pressure = $(2 \times Age) + 70$

Circulating Blood Volume

Blood volume in a child is approximately 80 ml/kg.

Respiratory

$$\text{Endotracheal tube size} = \frac{\text{Patient age in years}}{4} + 4$$

Children under age 7 or tube size under 5.5 mm usually requires an uncuffed endotracheal tube.

Drugs That May Be Delivered Via Endotracheal Tube (LEAN)

Lidocaine
Epinephrine
Atropine
Narcan

Respiratory Difficulty in the Intubated Patient (DOPE)

Dislodgment
Obstruction
Pneumothorax
Equipment failure

A-a Gradient

Normal = 10 to 15 mm Hg

Short formula: $P(A-a)o_2 = (145 - Pao_2) - 1.2(Paco_2)$ at sea level
Standard formula: $P(A-a)o_2 =$
  (Barometric Pressure – PH_2O) $(FiO_2) - (1.2)Paco_2 - Pao_2$
$PH_2O = 47$ at sea level

Oxygen Content

$$Cao_2 = (Hemoglobin)(1.34)(Sao_2/100) + (Pao_2)(0.003)$$

Respiratory Rate

A respiratory rate greater than 60 breaths per minute is considered abnormal in all age groups.

Children's Weight

As an approximation, Weight in kilograms = $(2 \times Age) + 8$.
Weight rule of 4-40-40: A 4-year-old weighs 40 pounds and is 40 inches tall.
Weight rule of 7-11: An infant usually gains 7 kg in the first 11 months.
An infant doubles its birth weight at 4 to 5 months and triples its weight by 1 year.
Normal weight gain in the neonate is ½ to 1 ounce (15 to 30 g) per day.
Newborns lose 7% to 10% of birth weight in the first few days before they start to regain it.

Blood Gas

A pH of 0.01 unit is a result of a base change of 0.67 mEq/L.
An acute change in $PaCO_2$ of 10 mm Hg is associated with an increase or decrease of 0.08 unit.

"Mosts"

- The most common cause of rectal bleeding in the first year of life is anal fissure.
- The most common type of growth plate fracture is Salter-Harris type II.
- The most common cause of cyanotic congenital heart disease is tetralogy of Fallot.
- Anterior oral vesicles most commonly denote herpes simplex; posterior oral vesicles denote coxsackie A herpangina.
- The purpuric rash of Henoch-Schönlein is most often seen below the waist.
- Physiologic jaundice most commonly peaks on the third or fourth day in full-term infants, second or third day in premature infants.
- Inverted T waves as a normal variant on electrocardiogram (ECG) are most commonly seen until adolescence.
- The most common cause of chest pain in preadolescents and adolescents is costochondritis.
- On lateral elbow films the posterior fat pads are always abnormal and indicate effusion in the joint.
- Most teeth erupt at 1 per month after 6 months. It's a "poor man's bone age."
- Most PrEEmies Extend while Full terms Flex

Jones Criteria for Acute Rheumatic Fever (CANCER)

Carditis
Arthritis
Nodules
Chorea
Erythema marginatum
Rheumatic fever

Reference

1. Erickson TB: Dealing with the unknown overdose, *Emergency Medicine* June, 1996.

Index